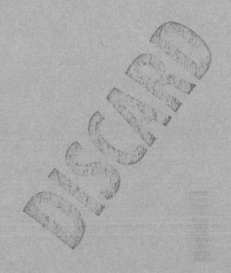

CELL PATHOLOGY

CELL PATHOLOGY

NORMAN F. CHEVILLE, D.V.M., Ph.D.

THE IOWA STATE UNIVERSITY PRESS / AMES

1 9 7 6

NORMAN F. CHEVILLE is head, Pathology Research Laboratories of the National Animal Disease Center, Ames, and holds an appointment also as professor of Veterinary Pathology, Iowa State University. His research interests have centered on the pathology of viral diseases, including especially Newcastle disease and hog cholera. He holds the M.S. and Ph.D. degrees from the University of Wisconsin and the D.V.M. degree from Iowa State University. In 1968 he did postdoctoral research at the National Institute of Medical Research, London. Besides this book he is author of *Cytopathology in Viral Disease* (1975) and more than fifty articles dealing mostly with the ultrastructure of viral diseases.

ⓒ 1976 The Iowa State University Press
Ames, Iowa 50010. All rights reserved

Composed and printed by
The Iowa State University Press

First edition, 1976

Library of Congress Cataloging in Publication Data

Cheville, Norman F. 1934–
     Cell pathology.

        Includes bibliographies and index.
        1. Pathology, Cellular. I. Title. [DNLM:
1. Pathology. 2. Veterinary medicine. SF769 C543c]
RB25.C43   636.089′1′0181   75–20441

ISBN 0–8138–0310–1

C O N T E N T S

Cell Pathology was written for the professional person who must deal medically with sick animals. While this encompasses zoologists caring for wild species and physicians interested in comparative medicine, the text was developed to conform with the discipline of pathology as it exists within the field of veterinary medicine.

The book was begun to provide an introduction to the ultrastructural aspects of anatomical pathology. The goal was to bridge the gap between what is seen in the electron microscope by the experimental pathologist and what the prosector encounters in the postmortem room. During the initial assembly of candidate micrographs, it became obvious that an atlas could not provide the intended message. Thereupon, the manuscript evolved into an interpretation of general pathology as it applied to the vertebrate species with emphasis on the pathologic changes in cell ultrastructure. Diseases such as uremia, diabetes, leukemia, influenza, tuberculosis, and others that involve fundamental abnormalities have been used repeatedly to explain disease processes.

The subject matter of *Cell Pathology* represents lesions of *nonhuman* vertebrate animals. The animal kingdom is divided into the *lower animals* (up to the phylum chordata) and the *higher animals* which include the cyclostomes, bony and cartilaginous fishes, amphibians, reptiles, birds, and mammals. This latter category is the realm and the responsibility of the veterinary pathologist. The need to constantly compare the biology of one species with another imparts a distinguishing character to veterinarians and zoologists and that character is an underlying principle of this book.

In the text, I have tried to avoid becoming an urbane purveyor of scientific data, and to get down on paper the substance of what I believe to be true. In dealing with controversial evidence, I have tried to avoid experiments that do not satisfy the traditional canons of scientific research and have resisted using in vitro studies when in vivo experiments or naturally occurring diseases were available. Human models of animal disease are occasionally used in clarification of certain mechanisms. Medical eponyms have been avoided. These silly and often outlandish designations are generally not used in the veterinary and zoological literature and should not be transferred to animal diseases from what appears to be their human counterpart. I have not avoided the use of such words as "normal," "identical," "injection," etc., whose meaning in relation to disease is usually relative to many variants. For those readers who develop aggressive and nervous tendencies over such words, I recommend that good judgment be applied.

It is hoped that the book will find use in undergraduate studies. There will be students (and I fear some academicians) who insist that a knowledge of ultrastructure is not necessary to the practicing biomedical professional person. Possibly. Against that logic can be cited the difference between the scientific and the technical faces of biomedicine. Acceptance of the title "doctor" is acceptance of the responsibility for understanding disease, not merely knowing how to deal with it technically. One cannot condone those planners of curricula who, while insisting on rigorous preprofessional courses in mathematics and physics, willingly constrict the courses that provide the very foundation of medical knowledge.

To those who will use this text in reference to the analysis of postmortem material, it must be emphasized that appropriate sampling is the important facet preceding the examination of tissue. The application of careless tissue sampling and unscientific examination results in useless, and sometimes harmful, information. Biologists who utilize microscopy in that fashion are the very ones who criticize the static nature of histology as not being "scientific" and who often thereupon proceed to draw lines between points of equally dubious physiologic samplings. The anatomical pathologist should not be cornered into intellectual paranoia by such nonsense. Those experimentalists who, by being conditioned from their familiarity with biochemical reactions, bypass entirely the fundamental changes in cell structure should be appropriately reprimanded. A quotation from Huxley is pertinent: "All progress in . . . biology involves straight description, comparative observation and analysis, and experiment, with a constant interplay between them all."

ACKNOWLEDGMENTS

To the many colleagues who have contributed to the inception and development of this book, I am deeply grateful. Dr. Harley Moon has written valuable textual material on intestinal pathology. Dr. Arlis Boothe has contributed several micrographs and reliably maintained the microscopy laboratory at the National Animal Disease Center so that those concerned with ultrastructural pathology could proceed with their research relatively untroubled by technical failure. Mr. Joe Gallagher contributed scanning electron micrographs.

I am also grateful to the following microscopists who have generously contributed micrographs: M. Aikawa, Western Reserve University; C. C. Capen and J. C. Geer, Ohio State University; G. L. Kelley, University of Kansas; I. M. Reid, Institute for Research on Animal Disease, Compton (England); K. Rhoades, R. Cutlip, and J. Proctor, National Animal Disease Center; C. Simpson, University of Florida; A. Takeuchi, Walter Reed Army Institute of Research; J. Venable, Oklahoma State University; and W. Wegmann, University of Zurich.

Acknowledgment is given to the following journals for permission to publish micrographs: *American Journal of Medicine*, Fig. 10.8; *American Journal of Pathology*, Figs. 2.6, 2.7, 4.4, 4.21, 5.9, 5.20, 9.6, 11.4, 11.6; *American Journal of Veterinary Research*, Fig. 3.24; *Journal of Cell Biology*, Fig. 3.24; *Journal of Pathology*, Fig. 2.22; *Journal of Parasitology*, Fig. 9.8; *Laboratory Investigation*, Figs. 3.21, 5.4, 5.5, 5.7, 5.9, 5.13, 5.14, 5.19; *Veterinary Pathology*, Figs. 2.17, 3.4, 4.6, 4.13, 4.14, 5.3, 5.23, 5.26, 6.10, 11.12; *Zentralblatt für Veterinärmedicin*, Fig. 7.1.

The former director and director of research of the National Animal Disease Center, Drs. C. A. Manthei and W. S. Monlux, have allowed the facilities and time required for the accumulation of the necessary material. I must also acknowledge the untiring help of my secretary, Mrs. Leah Oppedal, who patiently transformed my writing into typescript. Mr. Gene Hedberg provided excellent drawings. I must acknowledge indebtedness to those friends and graduate students who have used portions of the rough manuscript and have contributed to its completion. Drs. R. C. Cutlip and C. C. Capen have reviewed portions and I am appreciative of their comments. I am grateful to the staff of the Iowa State University Press, particularly Mrs. Rowena James and Mrs. Nancy Lewis, who have done a patient and thorough job of editing the manuscript.

I have come to realize that it is through the forbearance, over long periods of ill-temper, of those closest to one that books are written. In final words, therefore, I offer thanks to my wife, Beth, who made this writing endurable, to my parents who made it possible, and to my children who make it all worthwhile.

CELL PATHOLOGY

CHAPTER ONE

Introduction to Cell Pathology

Pathology, in the broadest sense, is abnormal biology. As a biological science, it encompasses all abnormalities of structure and function. It involves the study of pathologic cells, tissues, and organs and is the link between the basic sciences and clinical studies in the biomedical curriculum. In practice, animal pathology is partitioned into three distinct disciplines: *invertebrate pathology,* concerned with the lower animals; *medical pathology,* concerned with diseases of humans; and *veterinary* (or comparative) *pathology,* concerned with the disease processes of the vertebrate species of animal life.

Pathology is essentially the search for and the study of *lesions:* those abnormal structural and functional changes which have developed. Their detection requires the techniques used in the study of anatomy and physiology. Pathologists tend to divide their approach to pathology along these lines; that is, they become specialized in either anatomical or clinical pathology. This text is biased toward the former, and particularly toward changes in cell ultrastructure. The reader is cautioned, therefore, that the separation between pathologic structure and function is an artificial one. Some lesions are detectable only by microscopy and others only by biochemical methods. For every chemical change in a cell, however, there is a corresponding structural change. The challenge to the anatomical pathologist lies in finding it.

PATHOGENESIS

The study of lesions necessitates a consideration of the multiple factors involved in their *pathogenesis:* the development of a disease process. Causal agents such as microorganisms, chemicals, or physical forces may vary in their capacities to injure cells. On the other hand, tissues of different species (or even of different individuals) may not respond in the same way or as intensely to the same agent. The pathologic processes of inflammation, immunoreactivity, and blood coagulation do not always progress uniformly or sequentially.

Students not adept at dealing with normal biologic variance will find pathology exceedingly confusing. Disease produces great exaggerations in the spectrum of structural and functional cell responses which are considered normal. As animals age, the limits of normality become increasingly vague. Vascular lesions are usually present in aged animals and although they are pathologic, by some they may be considered part of the "normal" aging process. The regression of the thymus in young adults is a "normal" process, yet it involves degeneration and death of cells.

The time involved for the development of lesions is important in their structural appearance. Acute (sudden) processes may differ greatly from their chronic (slow, occurring over a long time) counterparts. For example, the cellular responses are markedly different in acute and chronic inflammation. Inflammatory lesions may therefore be especially confusing when acute processes are superimposed upon chronic ones.

Similar pathologic processes in different organs may cause differences in clinical manifestations. Foci of acute and chronic inflammation confined within subcutis are often painful but, as space-occupying lesions, do not endanger the life of the animal. The same type of lesion in the brain is life-threatening, for the brain tissue cannot expand beyond the confining limits of the cranium.

One of the most misleading apects of the examination of pathologic tissues involves multiplicity of causation. Two or more agents may be involved in tissue injury. Tumors ulcerate through epithelium and become infected. The superimposition of severe inflammation may mask the more serious primary lesion. Viruses may induce a respiratory disease of little importance, yet in so doing predispose the lung to severe secondary bacterial infection. When two or more processes such as these are combined, they must be differentiated and the dominant causal factor of the lesion determined. The isolation of a microorganism from tissue does not necessarily mean that it has caused the lesion in question!

PHYLOGENY

Phylogeny, the evolution of a group of animals, is a basic concern of the student of veterinary or comparative pathology. It is impossible to develop a practical approach to pathobiology without an awareness of the differences (and similarities) among species. There is an intriguing tendency for closely related species to suffer similar metabolic, neoplastic, and infectious diseases. Specific pathogenic microorganisms generally will also infect animals which are close, in the phylogenic scheme, to the original host.

Animals have evolved fascinating and complex mechanisms for sustaining life in the face of severe conditions of the environment. The kangaroo rat can go an entire lifetime without taking a single drink. The pupfish, which lives in hot desert springs, can tolerate water much saltier than the sea. Tadpole shrimp eggs can survive broiling heat and freezing cold, for years if necessary, until fresh rains hatch them. The study of these mechanisms, while significant in its own right, often provides valuable insight into the ways in which cells respond in the injured animal.

In this text we deal with diseases of vertebrate species. These are considered the "higher animals" in contrast to the lower, nonvertebrate species. Occasionally disease processes in the latter will be considered where they provide useful models

for a basic disease process. The spontaneous diseases which occur in these species are not mirrors of their counterparts in vertebrates. The biological processes, however, are similar and at the level of the cell may even be identical. One of the most exciting eras of pathology was begun by observations of the inflammatory response of the water flea.

CELL RESPONSE

The cellular protoplasm is divided by the nuclear membrane into nucleoplasm (karyoplasm) and cytoplasm (Fig. 1.1). Control of function and development resides chiefly in the nucleus; metabolic and synthetic processes occur in the cytoplasm. The cytoplasmic matrix (cytosol), which is the gel substance in the cytoplasm, contains various organelles and inclusions. On the basis of tradition (now somewhat outdated) organelles are considered the internal functioning organs of the cells. Inclusions are lifeless accumulations of metabolites (lipid globules, glycogen, protein crystals, and pigments) that are not required to maintain cell life.

The cell may respond in one of two broad pathways in its interaction with factors which injure or stimulate: (1) cell growth which includes enlargement, reduplication of organelles, and cell proliferation, or (2) cell regression with degeneration, shrinkage, and death. Within tissue these processes are not mutually exclusive. They can occur simultaneously and, in many pathologic tissues, one pattern is followed by the other.

A century of microscopic examination has given us traditional categories of pathologic cell growth and degeneration. The German pathologist Virchow (1821–1902) laid the foundation for modern anatomical pathology. His lectures on cellular pathology introduced the classic terminology for cell growth disturbances and degeneration which we follow. The introduction of the electron microscope in the 1960s radically altered some of these fundamental concepts of cytopathology. Ultrastructural research provided immediate answers to many problems of cell structure that pathologists had struggled with, in obliquely designed experiments, for decades.

The observation of abnormal cells in

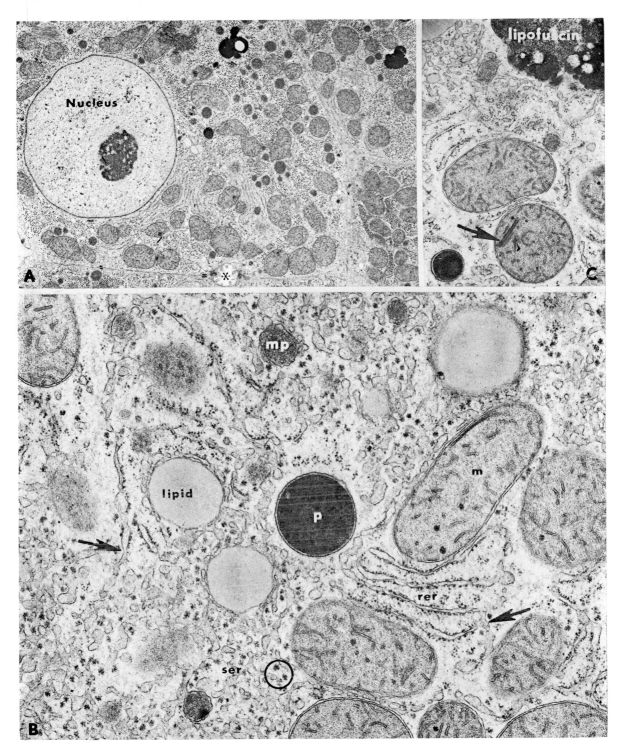

Fig. 1.1. Ultrastructure of an hepatocyte, aged dog. A. Typical
distribution of organelles. Note bile canaliculus (asterisk) between
apposed plasma membranes. B. Enlargement of cytoplasmic organelles.
Note relationship of rough (rer) and smooth (ser) endoplasmic
reticula that communicate at arrows. Large lipid globules,
mitochondria (m), microperoxisomes (mp), and peroxisomes (p).
Glycogen granules are encircled. C. Reduplication of mitochondrial
cristae (arrow) and lipofuscin.

vivo or in their living state following biopsy is tedious and time-consuming, and the results are not sufficiently reproducible for application to routine pathologic examination of sick animals. Limited use is made of cell cultures derived from pathologic tissues (particularly from tumors and from viral infection), but the processes in vitro do not mimic cytopathology in vivo. The evaluation of pathologic material therefore has been largely restricted to cells fixed by formaldehyde, glutaraldehyde, and other special solutions. Fixation of cells followed by staining to accentuate special structures allows the pathologist to evaluate degenerative changes on the basis of established and reproducible disease processes. It is essential in examining pathologic tissue to be aware of all abnormal conditions existing in the animal. Without this information, making a direct analogy between cellular change and its cause is likely to result in error.

In the ultrastructural examination of pathologic tissues, the status of individual cell responses can be determined when sampling and fixation are properly done. Appropriate sampling is the important facet in the analysis of biopsy and postmortem material. Fixation, staining, and microtomy are but techniques to be mastered. Sampling, in contrast, differs in each postmortem examination and demands a thorough knowledge of anatomy and cellular structure. Careless tissue sampling and unscientific examination result in useless, and sometimes harmful, information.

For good ultrastructural examination, fixation must be immediate. If standard osmium and glutaraldehyde fixative is not available, formalin may be used for diagnostic purposes. In rapidly metabolizing tissues, such as adrenal cortex and liver, it is best to fix in cold solutions and to trim the tissue pieces immediately over ice.

CELL GROWTH

HYPERTROPHY

The word *hypertrophy* is classically applied to tissues and organs that have increased in size without an increase in the number of their cells. Although hypertrophy may be seen in any tissue, it occurs in pure form only in those composed of cells that do not reproduce themselves readily. Muscle (both skeletal and cardiac) hypertrophies in response to an increased work load. There is an increase in the length and diameter of the cells but not in their number. When one kidney is removed, the other enlarges. No new nephrons have formed and the increase in size of the remaining kidney is due to enlargement of the existing tubule cells.

In cytopathology, hypertrophy is used to indicate cell enlargement, as distinct from cell swelling. Cellular organelles are larger than normal and their size is increased in proportion to their increased functional capacity. The hypertrophic muscle cell is larger than normal, contains larger mitochondria, and its myofilaments are increased both in length and number.

Some of the most striking examples of hypertrophy occur in secreting glands when they are stimulated by the appropriate endocrine hormone. In females, the acinar cells of the mammary gland undergo marked hypertrophy in late gestation under the influence of the hormone prolactin. In intact males, the prostate gland becomes hypertrophic with advancing age. The hypertrophy that is common in aged dogs is causally related to testicular function. Canine prostatic epithelium has a remarkable affinity for testosterone, which it converts to dihydrotestosterone (Gittinger and Lasnitzki 1972; Gloyna et al. 1970). Individual prostatic epithelial cells become

Fig. 1.2. Hypertrophy (left) and atrophy (right) of the prostate. A. Hypertrophic gland (from an aged intact dog) encircles the urethra and constricts flow of urine from bladder (b). B. Histology. Prostatic epithelial cells are enlarged. C. Ultrastructure. Cytoplasm is filled with dense secretory granules. D. Atrophy of the prostate in an aged castrated male dog. E. Histology. Epithelial cells are small and surrounded by bands of collagen. F. Ultrastructure. Nuclei are relatively structureless, cytoplasmic organelles are vacuolated, and autophagosomes (a) are present.

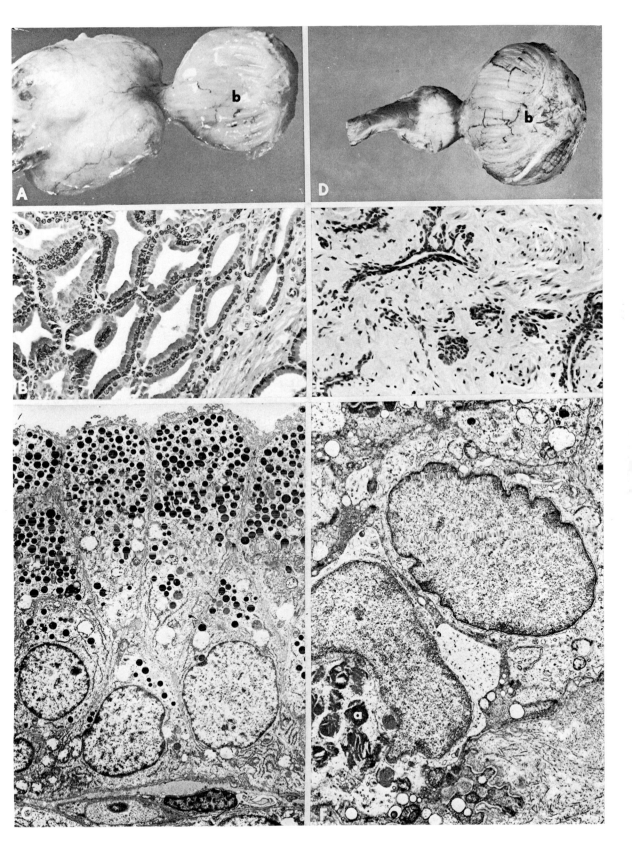

markedly enlarged, their cytoplasm is filled with secretory granules, and there is reduplication of the organelles involved in protein synthesis (Fig. 1.2). Castration, which removes the source of testosterone, produces prostatic cell atrophy—the opposite effect of cell enlargement.

HYPERPLASIA

Hyperplasia is a quantitative increase in the number of cells in a tissue. As in hypertropy, the hyperplastic cell and its organelles are not qualitatively abnormal. They are simply present in greater numbers. One of the most common causes of hyperplasia is chronic irritation. Parasite infestation of the skin, gut, respiratory tract, or urogenital system is noted for inducing epithelial hyperplasia. A callus in the skin is due to hyperplasia of keratinocytes within the epidermis. Papilloma viruses produce warts by inducing extensive epidermal hyperplasia. In both of these cases the epidermis is thickened by large increases in the number of cells. Some hyperplasia may occur in the endocrine-stimulated mammary gland and prostate lesions just described, although the processes in the main are hypertrophic.

METAPLASIA

Metaplasia is the occurrence of a cell type in a tissue where it is not normally present. It represents the replacement of vulnerable cells by cells more resistant to the inciting stress. The transformation is orderly and there is faithful reproduction of the new cell type (Kroes and Teppema 1972; Triche and Harkin 1971). Vitamin A deficiency results in widespread changes of simple types of epithelium to stratified squamous epithelium (Hayes et al. 1970). Foci of hyperplastic basal cells develop in the respiratory epithelium and expand, causing it to desquamate. As the basal cells enlarge, they gradually convert to keratin production (Wong and Buck 1971). Cellular metaplasia entails dedifferentiation followed by redifferentiation along a different pathway.

DYSPLASIA

Dysplasia means abnormality of development. It is most commonly used in reference to developmental defects in the skin, brain, and skeletal system. By definition, dysplasia applies to cells which are malformed during maturation. For example, spermatozoa are dysplastic when the head and tailpiece are structurally abnormal or improperly aligned. Classically, although somewhat erroneously, dysplasia is also applied to disorganized tissues which have peculiar cell forms but which are not clearly neoplastic. *Fibrous dysplasia* in bone indicates that fibrous connective tissue has replaced normal bone, but its growth will not progress in the manner of a tumor.

NEOPLASIA

Neoplasia is the uncontrollable growth of cells. The factors which control cell proliferation no longer limit mitotic activity. Cells develop into large masses visible as tumors in the host. In most neoplasms, the pattern of growth clearly differentiates the tissue from hyperplasia and characterizes it as benign or malignant. In some, however, the borderline between hyperplasia and neoplasia is ill defined, and proper classification becomes lost in vague and imprecise definitions of the word neoplasm. The *differentiation* of neoplastic cells refers to the extent to which these cells resemble their normal forebears. Tumors with poorly differentiated cells are apt to be highly malignant. *Anaplasia* means lack of cell differentiation and anaplastic tumors contain cells with marked pleomorphism, that is, variations in size and shape.

CELL REGRESSION

ATROPHY

Atrophy is the decrease in size of cells that have gained full development. The muscle wasted away in disuse, the mammary gland shrunken in old age, and the diminished size of genitalia after castration —all are examples of atrophy. Atrophy represents an adaption to a changed environment for the cell. Cells shrink when their level of work is diminished or when their source of nutrition or stimulation is removed. Obviously, when large numbers of parenchymal cells shrink, the organ involved will decrease in size commensurably.

Some examples in which cells are decreased in size after once functioning in full capacity follow. The prefaces used indicate the various causes associated with the process but do not reflect the complex interplay which often exists between them. *Disuse atrophy* may result from inactivity or a limitation in movement. It is particularly important in muscle when limbs are restrained by casts or other mechanisms. *Neurogenic atrophy* is loss of innervation due to peripheral nerve injury or loss of central control due to brain or spinal cord injury. *Endocrine atrophy* results from lack of pituitary trophic hormones and decreased metabolism. *Vascular atrophy* is a consequence of loss of blood supply. *Pressure atrophy* comes from direct pressure on the cell; most instances involve pressure on the blood supply or blockade of a duct (Donath et al. 1973).

"Senile atrophy" is sometimes applied to changes which involve the slowly progressive loss of parenchymal cells with advancing age. The reproductive organs atrophy first followed by muscles, bone, and later the nervous system. "Physiologic atrophy" is applied by some to the programed disappearance of embryonic tissues which degenerate as part of their normal life cycle, a process we shall refer to as necrobiosis.

Atrophic cells are smaller than normal and, except for lysosomes, their organelles are fewer in number and size. The liver of starved animals is smaller than normal. Hepatocyte volume is reduced up to 50% and both smooth and endoplasmic reticulum are reduced in mass. The number of mitochondria may remain unchanged, but individual mitochondria are increased in size by excessive matrix material (Riede et al. 1973).

Autophagy (autophagocytosis) is the phenomenon by which cell atrophy occurs (Cole et al. 1971). Autophagic vacuoles (cytosegresomes), which develop from the Golgi complex, engulf degenerate cellular organelles. When prostatic epithelial cells are deprived of androgens by castration, they cannot produce secretion-granules. The rough endoplasmic reticulum is strikingly diminished in volume and the Golgi complexes are absent or diminished. The autophagic vacuoles that develop degrade these organelles with lysosomes and they persist in atrophic cells as membrane-bound

bodies of dense debris (Fig. 1.2). Portions of the cytoplasm bleb from the cell surface, are released, and are phagocytized by adjacent cells which process the fragments by lysosomal digestion—a process called *apoptosis* (Helminen and Ericsson 1972; Kerr and Searle 1973; Paris et al. 1972).

HYPOPLASIA AND APLASIA

Hypoplasia is the failure of organs, tissues, or cells to obtain full size. The cause of these conditions may relate to faulty blood supply, pathologic innervation, absence of specific nutritive elements, or congenital defectiveness. A striking example of the latter is the panleukopenia virus-induced hypoplasia of the cerebellum responsible for ataxia of kittens. Panleukopenia virus traverses the placenta, infects the fetal brain, and replicates in and destroys primordial cells in the cerebellum. These cells thereupon fail to develop and the cerebellar folia are stunted and fail to function properly.

Aplasia is complete failure of an organ to develop. The organ may be totally absent (agenesis) or may be represented by a rudimentary structure composed of connective tissues.

CELL DEGENERATION AND DEATH

Degenerative reactions in cells are separated into two phases: cell degeneration and cell death. *Necrosis* is death of tissue in the living animal. It may be used to indicate dead tissue or the process of dying. Cellular degeneration becomes cellular necrosis when the point of irreversibility is reached in the degenerative process. Like the exact moment of death in the animal itself, however, that point is not precisely discernible.

Dying is the most complex process the pathologist must consider. When it is short, as in the action of cyanide on the cell enzyme cytochrome oxidase, the cellular lesions produced are subtle and beyond the scope of routine ultrastructural methods. When dying extends over long periods of time, the lesions are often so extensive, multiple, and interrelated that they are difficult to interpret. The excitement of discovering, studying, and integrating these pieces of evidence toward an acceptable thesis on the causes of death, however, is

Table 1.1. Mechanisms of anoxia in cellular injury

Mechanism	Example
Mitochondrial lesion	Cyanide poisoning
Plasmalemmal defect in O_2 acceptance	Oubain poisoning
Arterial blockade	Infarction
Circulatory failure	Cardiac (heart) failure
Erythrocyte deficiency (in numbers)	Anemia
(in quality)	Pyruvate kinase deficiency
Alveolar wall destruction (degeneration)	Senile emphysema
(inflammation)	Pneumonitis
Blockade of the alveolus (by fluid)	Pulmonary edema
(by cells)	Pneumonia
Blockade of the upper respiratory tract	Foreign body obstruction
Oxygen deficiency of inspired air	Asphyxiation

the reward of the thorough pathologic examination.

FACTORS THAT COMPLICATE CELL RESPONSES

Systemic disease, whatever the cause, produces alterations in the vital constituents of plasma and other body fluids. Many of these changes are important secondary contributors to cell degeneration and death. When superimposed upon some exogenous form of injury, they are often responsible for the death of the animal due to their effect on vital organ systems.

ANOXIA

Oxygen deficiency in the cell is the most common cause of degeneration. When combined with increased body temperature, it becomes a potent cause of cell death. Oxygen deficiency may be brought about by one cause or a combination of mechanisms that prevent oxygen from reaching its ultimate goal, the mitochondrion (Table 1.1). The mechanisms involved may be generalized or precisely directed to specific cell organelles or enzyme systems. For example, cyanide quickly causes death of the animal by the precise and rapid inhibition of cytochrome oxidase in the mitochondria of brain cells. Cell anoxia develops because there is interference with the utilization of oxygen, and this results in damage to neurons and white matter (Hirano et al. 1967). On the other hand, in death due to oxygen deficit from asphyxiation (suffocation), anoxia develops more slowly and tissue injury is much more widespread.

Cytopathology resulting from systemic anoxia varies according to the severity and duration of the oxygen deficiency. The consequences are greater in visceral organs such as brain, heart, liver, and kidney whose parenchymal cells are metabolizing to a high degree. These organs have elaborate vascular systems with shunts, anastomoses, and double blood supplies which protect them from lesser degrees of injury. They are vulnerable, however, when several mechanisms which produce anoxia are operable. Within the brain, susceptible neurons shrink and become electron dense. Their mitochondria become swollen and vacuolated. The adjacent astrocytes usually are "watery" and show evidence of dissolution of chromatin and cytoplasmic ribosomes (Shay and Gonatus 1973).

In those diseases in which cell degeneration is clearly due to exogenous agents, anoxia may still play an important secondary role in the production of cell degeneration and necrosis (Bakay and Lee 1968; Glinsmann and Ericsson 1966; Sulkin and Sulkin 1965). Anoxia is particularly important in embryos and fetuses that develop vascular damage of the embryonic membranes. Abortion and defective embryogenesis may be the serious consequences.

DEFICIT OF INORGANIC IONS

The classic studies of Ringer utilizing the perfusion of isolated frog hearts clearly demonstrated the importance of sodium (Na^+), potassium (K^+), and calcium (Ca^{++}) ions for normal function of the heart. Deficiencies of these cations can cause death due to myocardial failure. Early signs of ionic deficiency in the cardiovascular system include an irregular heartbeat, an abnormal electrocardiogram, and a drop in blood pressure. *Tetany,* a syndrome of convulsive seizures associated with twitching and spasms of skeletal muscle, occurs when there is a deficit of Ca^{++}, K^+, or Mg^{++} in the circulating blood. The deficiency or imbalance of these ions leads to irritability of the neuromuscular junction. In addition to their being required for muscle contractility, the inorganic cations also participate in maintenance of proper osmolarity of body fluids and proper acid-base balance.

Sodium is the paramount cation in the extracellular fluid, a heritage from primitive unicellular organisms which evolved in sea water. Deficiencies occur as direct loss in severe vomiting and in diarrhea, which is most serious in newborn animals whose kidneys are less able to reabsorb Na^+. Renal disease in adults may be accompanied by failure of Na^+ reabsorbtion. In Na^+ deficiency there may be an excess of intracellular water since water passes into the cell by osmotic attraction.

Potassium is the chief cation of the animal cell. Deficits affect the myocardium. Excesses which occur in renal disease may affect the cardiac conduction system. The kidney is designed to retain Na^+ (by tubular reabsorption) and to excrete K^+, contrasting mechanisms which are governed in part by aldosterone of the adrenal.

ACID-BASE IMBALANCE

In plasma and interstitial fluid, it is extremely important that the hydrogen ion (H$^+$) concentration be maintained within narrow limits. The normal pH of body fluids in mammals is 7.4 (7.36–7.44). Death certainly results below pH 7.0 (acidosis) and above pH 7.8 (alkalosis). The H^+ constant of extracellular fluids is a result of a balance between acids and bases. Carbonic acid (H_2CO_3), formed from $CO_2 + H_2O$, is the most important acid in plasma. It is expired via the respiratory system as it is formed during the metabolism of organic compounds. Bicarbonate (HCO_3^-) is the principal base. To combat disturbances of acid-base balance, the body uses three fundamental mechanisms: (1) chemical buffering, the major system being $HCO_3^- \rightleftharpoons H_2CO_3$; (2) release of blood CO_2 through the lungs; and (3) excretion of H^+ by the kidneys.

Cells are relatively tolerant to changes in pH. In terms of H^+, pH 7.8 represents 40% and pH 7.0 represents 250% of the H^+ at pH 7.4. How the increase and decrease of H^+ is manifested as cytopathology is not precisely known, but these changes have obvious effects on electrolyte balance and on water intake and egress of the cell.

DEHYDRATION

Decrease of body water may occur due to deficient intake or excessive loss. If dehydration is progressive, intracellular dehydration leads to enzyme defects that are reflected in mitochondrial degeneration (Bartok et al. 1973). This is particularly important in infectious diseases. The febrile animal requires greater amounts of water, yet if incapacitated is unable to drink. Some amphibians may lose water by evaporation equivalent to 50% of body weight and survive if rehydrated. Mammals in contrast may die after losing 12% (especially if plasma sodium rises accordingly).

HYPOGLYCEMIA AND STARVATION

Any severe fall in the concentration of glucose in plasma rapidly affects the central nervous system and results in progressive disorientation and prostration. Surprisingly, this is rarely a major contributing factor in death. Glucose levels are maintained within relatively normal ranges even in fasting and the early stages of starvation. Hypoglycemia may accompany the parasitemic phases of protozoal infections because of the excessive glucose utilization within infected erythrocytes. Although precipitous drops in blood glucose occur in animals that die, this appears to play only a minor role in the process of death (Love and McEwen 1972).

The mammalian nervous system consumes about two-thirds of the circulating glucose and most of the remainder goes to skeletal muscles and erythrocytes. Liver stores of glycogen can supply the brain's needs for only a few hours of fasting and, in the interval between night and morning feedings, amino acids from skeletal muscle protein breakdown provide material for hepatic glucose production. Free fatty acids derived from adipocyte triglyceride breakdown supply energy to tissues other than those of the nervous system.

In early starvation, the loss of muscle protein and Ca^{++}, K^+, and Mg^{++} causes substantial loss of water associated with these substances and this is responsible for weight loss. Of the amino acids appearing in plasma, alanine is the principal substrate for hepatic glucose production and alanine given by injection can increase synthesis of glucose in the liver. An alanine cycle, the conversion of alanine to glucose and reconversion to alanine, recycles a fixed supply of glucose and is an efficient means of transporting nitrogen to the liver from amino acids liberated by muscle breakdown.

As starvation progresses, the greater weight losses are accounted for by consumption of body fat, a much richer source of energy than protein. Circulating fatty acids are oxidized in the liver to acetoacetic acid and other ketones and ketosis signals a response to depletion of body glucose. The brain of a starved animal uses ketones as a substitute source of energy.

TEMPERATURE VARIATION

In all the warm-blooded (homeothermic) vertebrates, body temperature is virtually independent of environmental temperature. The selective advantage of having a body temperature determined by the energy of metabolism and controllable by cellular mechanisms is shown by the fact that this pattern of body temperature has evolved phylogenetically several times. Homeothermy is not without its price, for even under the least demanding circumstances birds and mammals devote 90% or more of their total energy metabolism to the maintenance and regulation of body temperature.

The energy cost of homeothermy increases markedly as the environmental temperature decreases. Animals such as hummingbirds, bats, ground squirrels, and hedgehogs have daily or seasonal dormant periods to avoid excessive expenditure of energy. The importance of environmental temperature to poikilothermic (cold-blooded) animals is obvious considering that their body temperatures vary directly with the environmental temperature. The rates of most chemical reactions double with each increase of 10° C. This is a particularly valuable influence on defense mechanisms such as phagocytosis. In most vertebrates the complex reactions of in-

flammation are plainly enhanced by the increases in body temperature known as fever.

In fish, heat loss is not due to surface heat lost in a cold water medium but to the process of respiration. The low oxygen content (2.5% of that in air) and high capacity for heat absorption of water render homeothermy extremely difficult in aquatic animals. The low oxygen in blood allows for little accumulation of metabolic heat and this small accumulation is lost immediately in passage though the gills. Large, rapidly swimming fish (and all aquatic mammals) require the adaptive advantage of elevated body temperature to enhance muscle power. In these animals, the rete mirabile, a network of arteries and veins below the backbone, provides a counter-current thermal barrier against heat loss. It short-circuits heat flow from muscle to gill and shunts accumulated heat back to the dark swimming muscles.

AGING

Increasing age is inevitably accompanied by degenerative disease even though individual cells may remain viable longer than the life span of the animal itself. Many aging changes are secondary to diminished function of supportive structures. Bone, joints, and connective tissues become increasingly rigid. Interstitial spaces are expanded by deposition of collagen and ground substance. The cardiovascular system has a diminished capacity to respond and brain, muscle, and viscera suffer from the decreased perfusion by circulating blood. Neurons, myocytes, and other cells slowly accumulate metabolic products that remain in the cell. The progressing cycles of diminished function and structural change inevitably reach a point where the tissue is more susceptible to injury. This in turn hastens the progression of tissue senescence.

In some specific diseases, the capacity of groups of cells to remain functional is related to factors of blood supply, innervation, endocrine stimulation, and combinations thereof. Loss of nerve supply is a direct cause of cell death locally. If thyroid and adrenal hormones are diminished, so is the viability of the cells which are stimulated by these hormones.

Starvation is a common cause of death in aged animals. In some insects with short life spans there is a genetically programed loss of key enzymes in the digestive tract. In others, crucial mouthparts drop off during metamorphosis and the insect dies after fat reserves are exhausted. These same mechanisms affect vertebrates, though less dramatically. Aged mammals, for example, may die from malnutrition brought about by loss of teeth.

In viewing aging in the biologic sense, it is necessary to distinguish primary causal mechanisms from secondary expressions of cell damage. Cells becoming aged accumulate a multiplicity of abnormal gene products that can represent molecular mischief. The relations within and between cells begin to break down, destroying the feedback mechanisms that orchestrate cell functions in the efficient multicellular organism. Within cells, key enzymes and the mechanisms for their production appear to become increasingly sluggish. The repair mechanisms for the major macromolecules, DNA, RNA, and protein become less efficient and the breaks that occur in the molecules are repaired with some defectiveness. Aging is also associated with abnormal antigens on the cell surface which predispose to autoallergic disease and malignancy.

Immunologic theories implicate the lymphoid system in aging. Death is allegedly hastened due to the progressive loss of the capacity to rid the animal of unwanted protein antigens (Aoki and Teller 1966). The disappearance of the thymus and its hormone (thymosin) is implicated in this loss of immunologic surveillance.

Dwarfs regularly appear in litters of the Snell-Bagg mouse line due to a defective recessive gene. Life span of the dwarf mice is about 5 months, one-quarter that of normal littermates. Growth is impaired, animals never reach normal size, and in a few months cataracts develop, the skin thins, the hair grays, and the mouse dies. This happens because the pituitary is not producing hormones that activate thyroid and adrenal glands which initiate and stimulate growth. If dwarfs are injected with pituitary hormones at weaning, life span is doubled and it appears that this effect is mediated in part through the development of the lymphoid system, particularly the thymus. If dwarfs are injected with lymphocytes from normal littermates the life span is similarly doubled (Fabris et al. 1972).

Senescence also occurs in cells grown in vitro and longevity is inversely correlated with age of the donor (Martin et al. 1970). This type of senescence is characterized by the progressive shrinkage of both cytoplasm and nucleus. Organelles involved in synthesis of proteins, carbohydrates, and lipids decrease in size while those concerned with intracellular digestion increase (see autophagy, Chapter 2). Free radical mediated pathology contributes to the aging process, and life spans of cells in culture can be extended with vitamin E which inhibits the activity of free radicals in the cytoplasm.

In some of the lower vertebrates, excess adrenal cortical activity is associated with senescence. Pacific salmon undergo an intriguingly rapid pattern of aging and death after their migration from the sea to freshwater rivers to spawn. After eggs are ejected and fertilized, the adults become increasingly sluggish and die within a few days. Adrenal cortical toxicosis is allegedly the cause of the rapid aging process. The changes that occur are associated with the onset of sexual maturity and include atrophy of the digestive tract, muscles, and viscera. Castration suppresses adrenal activity and allows an increased life span (Robertson and Wexler 1962).

REFERENCES

Aoki, T. and Teller, M. N. Aging and cancerigenesis. III. Effect of age on isoantibody formation. *Cancer Res.* 26:1648, 1966.

Bakay, L. and Lee, J. C. The effect of acute hypoxia and hypercapnia on the ultrastructure of the central nervous system. *Brain* 91:697, 1968.

Barták, I., Virágh, Sz. and Menyhárt, J. Prompt divisions and peculiar transformation of cristae in liver mitochondria of rats rehydrated after prolonged water deprivation. *J. Ult. Res.* 44:49, 1973.

Cole, S., Matter, A. and Karnovsky, M. J. Autophagic vacuoles in experimental atrophy. *Exp. Mol. Path.* 14:158, 1971.

Donath, K., Hirsch-Hoffmann, H.-U. and Seifert, G. Zur Pathogenese der Parotisatrophie nach experimentelle Gangunterbindung. Ultrastructurelle Befunde am Drüsenparenchym der Rattenparotis. *Virch. Arch. A* 359:31, 1973.

Fabris, W. et al. Lymphocytes, hormones and aging. *Nature* 240:557, 1972.

Gittinger, J. W. and Lasnitzki, I. The effect of testosterone metabolites on the fine structure of the rat prostate gland in organ culture. *J. Endocrin.* 52:459, 1972.

Glinsmann, W. H. and Ericsson, J. L. Observations on the subcellular organization of hepatic cells. *Lab. Invest.* 15:762, 1966.

Gloyna, R. E., Siiteri, P. K. and Wilson, J. D. Dihydrotestosterone in prostatic hypertrophy. *J. Clin. Invest.* 49:1746, 1970.

Hammerling, V. et al. New visual markers of antibody for electron microscopy. *Nature* 223:1158, 1969.

Harder, F. H. and McKhann, C. F. Demonstration of cellular antigens on sarcoma cells by an indirect ^{125}I-labeled antibody technique. *J. Nat. Cancer Inst.* 40:231, 1968.

Hayes, K. C., McCombs, H. L. and Faherty, T. P. The fine structure of vitamin A deficiency. I. Parotid duct metaplasia. *Lab. Invest.* 22:81, 1970.

Helminen, H. J. and Ericsson, J. L. E. Ultrastructural studies on prostate involution in the rat. *J. Ult. Res.* 40:152, 1972.

Hess, F. A., Weibel, E. R. and Preisig, R. Morphometry of dog liver: Normal base-line data. *Virch. Arch. B* 12:303, 1973.

Hirano, A., Levine, S. and Zimmerman, H. M. Experimental cyanide encephalopathy. *J. Neuropath. Exp. Neurol.* 26:200, 1967.

Howe, C., Morgan, C. and Hsu, K. C. Recent virologic applications of ferritin conjugates. *Progr. Med. Virol.* 11:307, 1969.

Kerr, J. F. R. and Searle, J. Deletion of cells by apoptosis during castration-induced involution of the rat prostate. *Virch. Arch. B* 13:87, 1973.

Kroes, R. and Teppema, J. S. Development and restitution of squamous metaplasia in the calf prostate after a single estrogen treatment. *Exp. Mol. Path.* 16:286, 1972.

Love, J. N. and McEwen, E. G. Hypoglycemia associated with Haemobartonella-like infection in splenectomized calves. *Am. J. Vet. Res.* 33:2087, 1972.

Martin, G. M., Sprague, C. A. and Epstein, C. J. Replicative life-span of cultivated human cells. *Lab. Invest.* 23:86, 1970.

Nakane, P. K. and Pierce, G. B. Enzyme-labeled antibodies. *J. Histochem. Cytochem.* 14:929, 1966.

Paris, J. E. et al. Effect of castration on histochemistry and biochemistry of acid hydrolases in rat prostate gland. *J. Nat. Cancer Inst.* 49:1685, 1972.

Riede, U. N. et al. Einfluss des Hungers auf die quantitativ Cytoarchitektur der Rattenbeberzelle. *Beitr. Path. Bd.* 150:246, 1973.

Robertson, O. H. and Wexler, B. C. Histologic changes in the organs and tissues of senile castrated kokanee salmon *(Oncorhynchus nerka kennerlyi)*. *Gen. Comp. Endocrin.* 2:458, 1962.

Shay, J. and Gonatus, N. K. Electron microscopy of cat spinal cord subject to circulatory arrest and deep local hypothermia (15 C). *Am. J. Path.* 72:369, 1973.

Sulkin, N. M. and Sulkin, D. F. An electron microscopic study of the effects of chronic hypoxia on cardiac muscle, hepatic and autonomic ganglion cells. *Lab. Invest.* 14:1523, 1965.

Triche, T. J. and Harkin, J. C. An ultrastructural study of hormonally induced squamous metaplasia in the coagulating gland of the mouse prostate. *Lab. Invest.* 24:596, 1971.

Weibel, E. R., Kistler, G. S. and Scherle, W. F. Practical stereological methods for morphometric cytology. *J. Cell Biol.* 30:23, 1966.

Wong, Y.-C. and Buck, R. C. An electron microscope study of metaplasia of the rat tracheal epithelium in vitamin A deficiency. *Lab. Invest.* 24:55, 1971.

C H A P T E R   T W O

Cell Death and Degeneration

CELL DEATH

NECROSIS (DEATH OF CELLS IN THE LIVING ANIMAL)

Necrosis includes those changes in the cell beyond the point at which degeneration is reversible. Necrotic cells are shrunken and their intercellular attachments are broken. Their structural appearance depends not only upon the type of degeneration but also upon the time elapsing between injury and fixation for microscopic study. Sufficient time must elapse for pathologic changes to occur.

In histologic preparations, necrotic cells appear distorted, smudged, and homogeneous. Nuclei are contracted and their state may be described as: *pyknotic* (shrunken and dense with irregularities in the nuclear membrane); *karyorrhectic* (rupture of the nuclear membrane with fragmentation and release of nuclear contents); or *karyolytic* (complete dissolution of the nucleus with loss of chromatin material). If necrosis is recent, cells may stain deeply with eosin; but if autolysis (dissolution by their own enzymes) has occurred, the cells take up little stain.

Ultrastructurally, the architecture of the necrotic cell is effaced (Fig. 2.1). Protein and lipid debris are strewn through the cytoplasm (Vogt and Farber 1968). Debris-filled autophagosomes are usually present and are evidence of *autophagy*, the process whereby degenerate organelles are removed from the cell (Shelbourne et al. 1973). During some types of cell death, ribosomes and protein crystal lattices develop (Mottet and Hammer 1972). Nuclear changes include progressive clumping of chromatin and dissolution of the nuclear membrane.

PATTERNS OF NECROSIS

Foci of necrosis in tissue often have characteristics which lead the pathologist in certain directions regarding etiology. Some of the patterns that can be recognized and which vary according to the nature of the destructive agent are listed below.

In *coagulation necrosis*, the cell is homogeneous and opaque due to coagulation of protein. The coagulated cell persists after cell detail has disappeared. Interruptions in the arterial supply, bacterial toxins, or severe febrile illnesses may be responsible. The affected area of necrotic tissue is sharply delimited from the surrounding normal tissue.

Rapid enzymatic dissolution of the cell which results in complete destruction is called *liquefactive necrosis*. It is seen in bacterial infection leading to pus formation, in which proteolytic enzymes are released from leukocytes. The brain responds to anoxic injury with rapid enzymic digestion and foci of dissolution.

Caseation necrosis occurs when dead cells are converted into a granular friable mass resembling cottage cheese. It is present in diseases such as tuberculosis and tularemia. The presence of special lipids and the chronicity of the cellular reaction prevent liquefaction.

In *enzymic necrosis of fat*, lipases split the neutral fat in adipose cells, releasing the lipid and imparting a granular eosinophilic appearance to the fat cell (Davis and Gorham 1954). This type of necrosis is seen in trauma of adipose tissue and com-

15

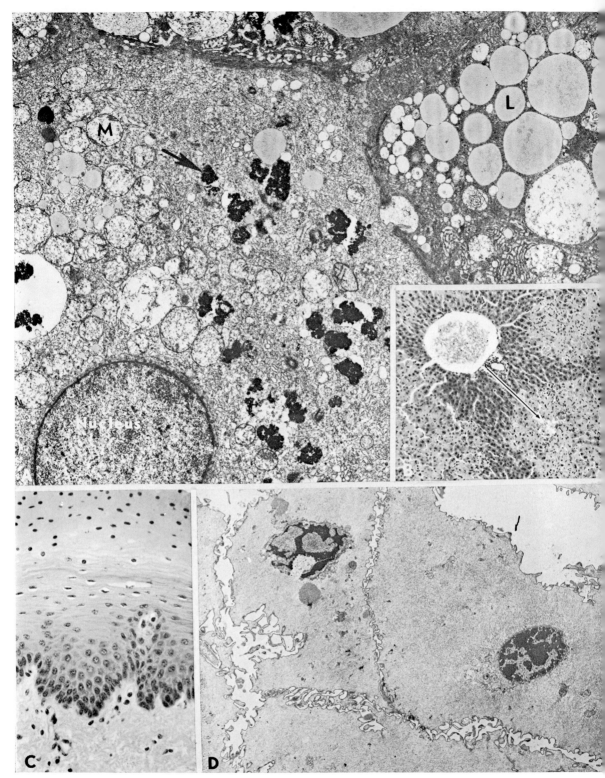

Fig. 2.1. Necrosis and necrobiosis. A. Necrosis of hepatocyte in
CCl_4 poisoning, rat. Note mitochondria (M), lipid globules (L), and
bile pigment (arrow). B. Histology. Centrolobular necrosis. Arrow
traverses blood flow from portal triad to central vein. C.
Necrobiosis in stratified squamous cells of normal esophagus. D.
Ultrastructure. Squamous cell nuclei are degenerate, cell junctions
are separated, and cytoplasm is homogeneous and lacks organelles.

monly accompanies pancreatic injury. Unidentified enzymes released from damaged pancreatic acinar cells free lipases in adipose cells, which cause autodigestion of triglycerides (Panabok'ke 1958). Fat, free in connective tissues, incites inflammation and phagocytosis which separate enzymic necrosis from autolysis. Cholesterol clefts, giant cells, and calcium are often present.

The superimposition of the growth of saprophytic bacteria upon necrosis results in a histologic pattern which is a mixture of coagulation and liquefactive necrosis. This *gangrenous necrosis* may occur due to bacterial invasion of an infarct or as a result of restriction of blood supply in an established bacterial infection by collection of fluid and intravascular clotting.

Gangrene is also applied to necrosis of tissues in an extremity wherein vascular occlusion has resulted in coagulation necrosis. When bacterial infection does not occur the tissue mummifies and the condition is referred to as *dry gangrene*. Affected tissue is cool, dry, and discolored. There is a sharp demarcation of inflammatory tissue preventing systemic infection. When organisms invade, the combination of ischemia and infection produce putrefactive, foul-smelling tissues, a lesion called *moist gangrene*.

NECROSIS DUE TO VASCULAR BLOCKAGE

Ischemia, the local loss of blood from a tissue, is commonly responsible for coagulative necrosis. When the blood supply to tissue is shut off the cells quickly degenerate and die. In cardiac failure stasis of blood in the hepatic veins causes progressive cell death backwards from central vein to portal triad (Fig. 2.2).

An *infarct* is a local area of necrosis caused by ischemia due to obstruction in the arterial tree. Infarction may result from the local development of a clot or thrombus or by embolism.

Infarcts are classified on the basis of bacterial contamination (septic or bland) and color (anemic or white and hemorrhagic or red). Red infarcts are filled with blood. The amount which escapes into the deprived area is determined by the age of the infarct, the type of injury, and the type of tissue. Infarcts of the kidney are generally white; those of the lung red. Most infarcts

are transiently hemorrhagic, becoming pale in a very short period. The capillaries at the border of the infarct undergo dissolution and blood may seep into the area of necrosis.

Rarely, infarction occurs due to emboli in veins. Venous infarcts are intensely hemorrhagic. Generally, peripheral venous drainage develops and prevents necrosis.

Embolism is the sudden blocking of an artery or vein by an obstruction which has arrived in the bloodstream. Emboli can be thrombi, neoplastic cells, lipid globules, air bubbles, or foreign particles. Thromboemboli break away from some distant focus of thrombosis and are especially common causes of infarction and necrosis. Septic thromboemboli not only cause infarction but disseminate infection throughout the body of the animal. Emboli of neoplastic cells may dislodge from a primary tumor, circulate, and take up residence in the lung or other viscera to initiate secondary tumor growth. In the dog, emboli of degenerate intervertebral disc ground substance break away and become impacted in vertebral veins and arterioles where they produce necrosis of the central gray matter of the spinal cord.

NECROBIOSIS (CELL DEATH DUE TO NORMAL CYTOLOGIC PROCESSES)

In *necrobiosis*, cell death is programed and the cytopathic changes evolve in orderly and reproducible sequences. Necrobiosis occurs in adult animals as a part of normal cell turnover. An example is the loss of cornified squamous cells of skin. Keratinocytes become filled with keratin, nuclei degenerate, and plasma membranes no longer adhere. As desmosomes disintegrate, cells desquamate from the skin surface (Fig. 2.1). Necrobiosis is also seen in erythrocytes which die when their hemoglobin molecules begin to precipitate and new hemoglobin cannot be resynthesized. In erythrocytes the process actually begins immediately after maturation when nuclei degenerate. Their genome is no longer required for protein synthesis and, in mammals, they are shed from the cell. Cell death occurs without sequelae because cell function has been fulfilled and the cells have been replaced with new erythrocytes.

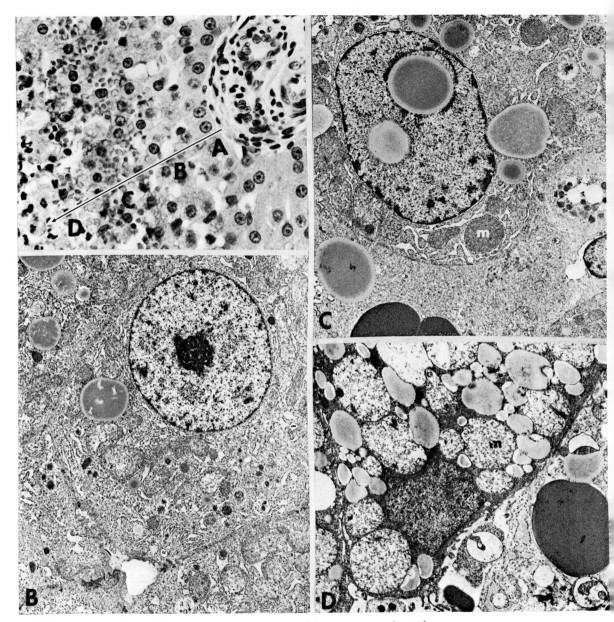

Fig. 2.2. Centrolobular liver necrosis, cat with severe anemia and heart failure. *Upper left:* Stasis of blood in hepatic vein causes degeneration to be progressively worse along the pathway of blood flow from portal triad (top right) to central vein (arrow). Zones of effect labeled A (normal hepatocyte), B (early change), C (severe degeneration), and D (necrosis) correspond to micrographs labeled B, C, and D. Note the progressive accumulation of lipids in the cytoplasm.

Necrobiosis is a prominent feature of embryonic development and histogenesis (O'Connor and Wyttenbach 1974). An intriguing model for study has been the tail breakdown in tadpole amphibians during metamorphosis. The tail regresses because of a thyroxin-dependent autolysis initiated in the myocyte. Early cytoplasmic changes include folding of myofibrils and loss of striation; these develop before gross signs of tail atrophy occur. Degeneration of mitochondria is also an early change and is followed by disorganization and disintegration of sarcoplasmic reticulum and the development of lysosomes. Macrophages replace and destroy the myocytes. (An earlier erroneous interpretation stated that rupture of lysosomes with liberation of hydrolizing enzymes was the initiating reaction in destruction of tail tissue. It has been demonstrated, however, that lysosomes appear in response to autolysis of the myocytes. While they may release hydrolytic enzymes within the cell, lysosomes do not initiate the necrobiotic process) (Fox 1973; Weber 1964).

POSTMORTEM DEGENERATION (CELL DEATH ACCOMPANYING DEATH OF THE ANIMAL)

The interpretation of lesions is often clouded by changes which have taken place between the time of death and the necropsy. Postmortem changes vary in the rapidity with which they occur according to environmental temperature and humidity (Table 2.1). The condition of the animal also influences the rapidity of change. The layers of fat, hair, or feathers act as insulators against heat loss after death.

Postmortem degeneration is due to total diffuse anoxia. Autolytic changes mimic early ischemic change and in fact have a hypoxic basis. Organelles degenerate according to the oxygen requirements and the differences in postmortem change are reflected in these requirements. In ultrastructural examination of cells, timing and preservation techniques are critical. Postmortem autolysis is characterized by relatively uniform destruction of the cell. Protein disintegrates into small granules which are distributed throughout the cell. Cells with rapid metabolic activity (liver and adrenal) are best fixed in cold solutions which immediately retard degenerative phenomena.

Rigor mortis, or stiffening of the muscles, occurs 6–12 hrs after death. Immediately after the circulation of blood ceases there is a progressive decrease in the pH of muscle. Oxygen, ATP, and creatine phosphate are also decreased. Muscle fibers shorten as they pass into rigor. This movement resembles contraction in vivo in several ways. It is initiated by an efflux of calcium from the sarcoplasmic reticulum, it uses ATP as an energy source, and the ultrastructural changes resemble those of contraction (Henderson et al. 1970; Stromer et al. 1967).

Rigor begins earliest in cardiac muscle and expresses the blood from the left ventricle. Failure indicates antemortem degeneration. Of the skeletal muscles, the head and neck are first affected, with progression to the extremities. Rigor disappears as putrefaction begins: a matter of 1–2 days depending upon external factors. Rigor

Table 2.1. Postmortem changes

Algor mortis (cooling)—aids in estimating time of death

Rigor mortis (rigidity) —begins 6–12 hrs after death

Postmortem clotting (thrombi are antemortem)

Postmortem imbibition (hemolytic staining)

Hypostatic congestion (dependent lividity)—due to gravity

Pseudomelanosis—$Fe + S = FeS$ giving shades of green and black

Autolysis—invokes no inflammatory response

Putrefaction—may cause rupture and displacement of organs

Emphysema (due to gas-producing bacteria)—may cause rupture of organs

Biliary imbibition

mortis is enhanced by high metabolic activity and temperature before death and in diseases such as strychnine poisoning. It is delayed by starvation, cachexia, and cold.

CELL DEGENERATION

The injured cell exhibits changes in cell movement, size, and density. During early stages of degeneration, cell motion and metabolism are often increased and manifested as reduplication of organelles, intake of water, deformation of the plasma membrane, and accumulation of cellular products such as glycogen, lipid, and protein. Severe degeneration is characterized by lessened activity and cellular shrinkage. When degeneration becomes irreversible, necrosis begins.

CELL SWELLING

Cell swelling is the fundamental expression of injury. It is manifested by increase in cell size and regressive changes in organelles. It includes a spectrum of morphologic and physiologic changes which begin with increased uptake of water and extend to the diffuse disintegration of intracellular proteins. Cell swelling must be distinguished from cell enlargement (hypertrophy), which is due to increased size with concomitant increase in normal cell organelles.

Cell swelling is often a subtle change and is best seen in the rapidly metabolizing parenchymal cells of the liver, kidney, and heart (Bassi and Bernelli-Zazzera 1964; Majno et al. 1960). It commonly occurs in diseases associated with fever, toxemia, and cachexia. Although cell swelling is reversible in these situations, the changes may be a prelude to more severe alterations.

GROSS APPEARANCE OF TISSUES

Tissues and organs whose component cells are severely affected by cell swelling are themselves swollen. They are larger and heavier than normal and tend to be of paler coloration. Organs such as kidney and liver bulge beneath their capsules and organ contours are more rounded. A quick assessment of cell swelling can be made at the postmortem examination by comparing the specific gravity of normal and affected tissues. This can be done in a crude manner in a graded series of copper sulfate solutions that vary from 1.010 to 1.110 (at 5 unit intervals) specific gravity. A small slice of the two tissues is placed in each solution and the specific gravity noted by sinking or floating of the tissue. Cell swelling causes the specific gravity of tissue to decrease.

MICROSCOPIC APPEARANCE

The early changes in cell swelling are due to excess water uptake which dilutes the cytoplasmic matrix and gives the cell a pale, lucid, ground-glass appearance. Histologically, tissue architecture is maintained but the cells are larger and paler than normal. Component parts are disorganized and intercellular junctions are compressed. Well-defined structures are blurred and vacuoles are often prominent in the cytoplasm. In skeletal muscle, myofilaments are smudged and less obvious. Renal tubular epithelial cells project into the tubule lumen and have irregular luminal borders. Endothelial cells, which are one of the most overlooked sites of cell swelling, intrude upon and often obliterate the vascular lumen.

CELL SURFACE CHANGES

The swollen cell, as viewed by scanning electron microscopy, bulges from its normal limits. It infringes upon its neighbors and, if present on a tissue surface, extends outwards into the surrounding cavity or lumen. The cell surface is irregular and bulbous and is apt to be lacking surface structures characteristic of the particular cell type involved.

Two consistent patterns of structural change occur in the plasma membrane during cell swelling. First, there is destruction of specialized surface structures such as cilia, microvilli, and junctional complexes. The microfilaments which function in these structures are broken and fragmented. If fluids accumulate extracellularly, cells may remain attached only at specialized attachment devices such as desmosomes (Fig. 2.3). These structures persist

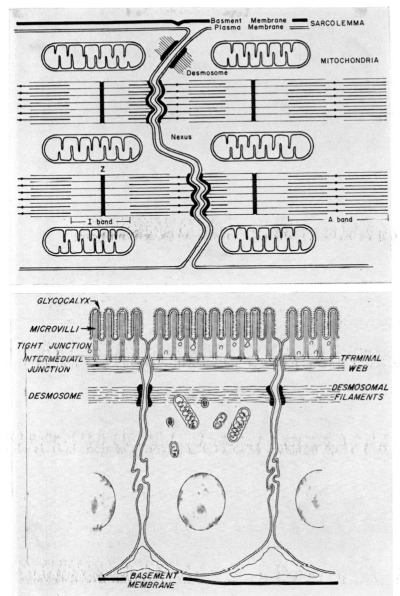

Fig. 2.3. Cell attachment devices on myocardial cells (top) and intestinal epithelial cells (bottom).

in cell swelling and are remarkably resistant to most types of injury. In the absence of calcium, however, desmosomes and hemidesmosomes loosen and cleave (Hays et al. 1965; Scaletta and MacCallum 1972).

The second consistent change in the plasma membrane of swollen cells is the formation of blebs of cytoplasm at the cell surface. If the plasma membranes at the stalk of the bleb fuse, portions of the cytoplasm may be lost into the intercellular spaces: a process referred to as *cytoplasmic ecdysis.*

CYTOPLASMIC CHANGES

Electron microscopic examination of thin sections of properly fixed tissues reveals the true nature of cell swelling. In general, the cytoplasmic matrix is markedly expanded without a concomitant increase in ribosomes or other organelles. The cytocavitary network is invariably involved; the endoplasmic reticulum and Golgi complexes are usually dilated and their cisternae filled with tiny precipitates. The cytocavitary network is fragmented into myriads of small vesicles (Figs. 2.4 and 2.5). Plasma membranes, which are compressed, usually exhibit degenerate surface structures and are thrown into folds or uropods which project from the cell surfaces.

As cell swelling progresses, proteins precipitate in the cytoplasmic matrix and within organelles (Fig. 2.6). Traditional histopathologists called this change cloudy swelling (or albuminous degeneration) due to the cloudiness and granularity of the cytoplasm. The cloudy appearance seen in light microscopy is due to diffuse deposition of protein in the cytoplasmic matrix and the granularity to dense, swollen mitochondria (Ericcson and Glinsman 1965). Cell proteins may aggregate, redistribute, disintegrate, and disappear. There is segmental loss of endoplasmic reticulum. In most tissues collected at necropsy, postmortem degeneration so complicates the picture that many experimental pathologists doubt the validity and existence of "cloudy swelling."

VARIATIONS IN CELL SWELLING

Red blood cells that degenerate usually lose the integrity of their plasma membranes and take in excessive amounts of water. The expanding mammalian erythrocyte loses its discoid shape and becomes round; its hemoglobin is dispersed. These cells, which are called *spherocytes,* lack the normal deformability which is necessary for circulation. Spherocytosis is most common in older erythrocytes for, as erythrocytes age, the enzyme components which maintain energy production gradually wane. There is concomitant decrease in ATP, plasma membrane function is affected, and the normal biconcave shape becomes spheroidal (see Fig. 3.20).

Histologically, the hallmark of *hydropic degeneration of epithelia* is the presence of translucent vacuoles within the cytoplasm which do not stain for fat or glycogen. When examined by electron microscopy, the vacuoles are seen to represent markedly swollen mitochondria, Golgi complexes, or endoplasmic reticulum. Water

has selectively accumulated within these injured organelles. Hydropic degeneration is characteristic of degenerative processes in epithelium, endothelium, pulmonary alveolar walls, and renal tubular epithelium (particularly in electrolyte imbalance).

Cytoplasmic proteolysis is the term used to identify expanding foci of clearing of cytoplasmic structures and is characteristic of several viral diseases. Lysis of proteins begins in the perinuclear zones and extends outward to involve entire cells. Proteolytic foci may contain delicate microfibrillar material. The poxviruses induce *ballooning degeneration* caused by the accumulation of water and stretching of the plasma membrane. Keratin fibrils are lysed and cellular organelles are dissolved, leaving a massive fluid-filled, turgid cell (Fig. 2.7).

Swelling of neurons accompanied by lysis of cytoplasmic rough endoplasmic reticulum (Nissl substance) is referred to as *chromatolysis* (not to be confused with chromotolysis relating to disintegration of nuclear chromatin). The neuron is expanded by excessive water accumulation and the basophilic Nissl substance, which is the large dense area of rough endoplasmic reticulum, is removed from the cytoplasm (Fig. 2.6). Neuronal chromatolysis is characteristic of traumatic injuries wherein the axon of the nerve is sectioned. It is also seen in many viral infections.

MECHANISMS OF CELL SWELLING

Cell swelling may be caused by any agent that alters the ionic content and water balance of the cell. Injury to the plasma membrane, either directly or secondary to cessation of metabolic activities in organelles or cytoplasmic matrix, is ultimately responsible for excessive water uptake. How and where water accumulates in the cell depends upon the type of injury and the site at which pathologic change is initiated.

Normally, water traverses the cell passively, that is, by diffusion equilibrium. Intracellular water is regulated by modification of electrolyte composition which thereby controls cell volume (Trump and Ginn 1969). The unequal distribution of sodium (Na^+) and potassium (K^+) across the plasma membrane is due to active trans-

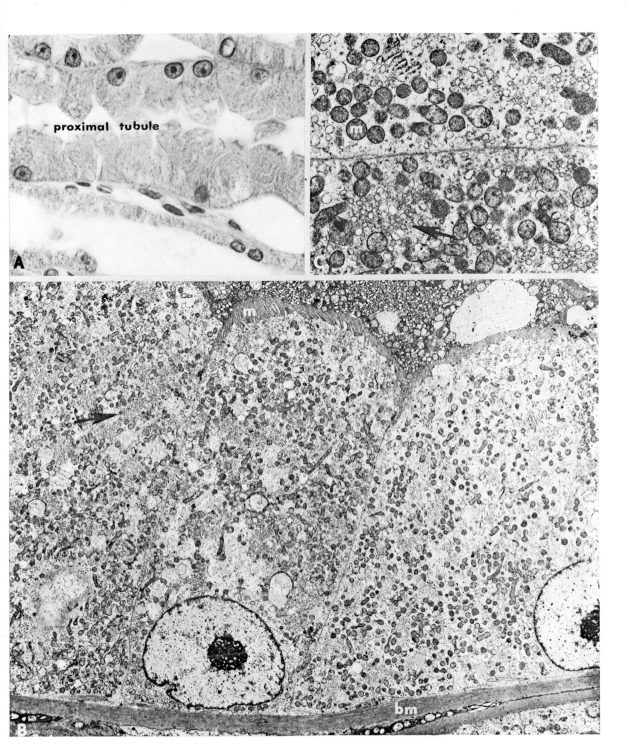

Fig. 2.4. Cell swelling of renal proximal convoluted tubule, dog.
B. Ultrastructure. Cells are enlarged and cytoplasmic matrix is
rarified. Endoplasmic reticulum has fragmented into vesicles (arrow).
Note distortion and smudging of microvilli (m) and thickened
basement membrane (bm). C. Enlargement of vesicle (arrow) and
dense shrunken mitochondria (m).

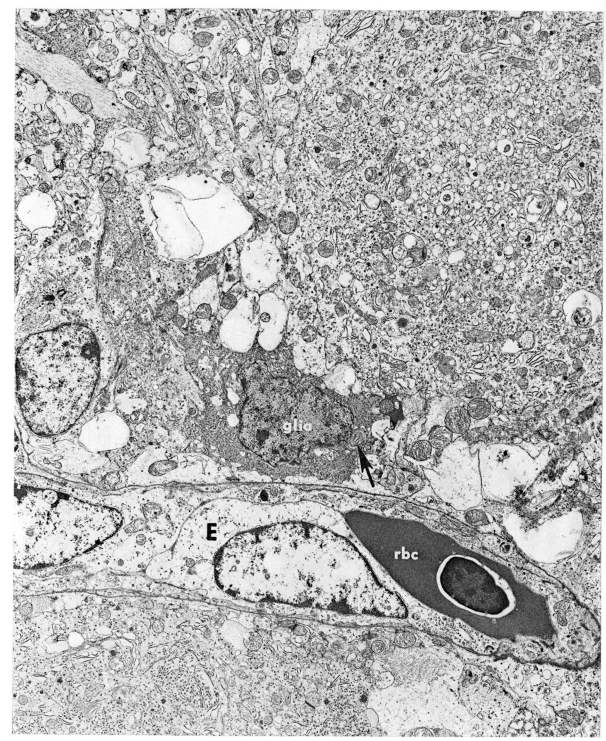

Fig. 2.5. Cell swelling Purkinje cell layer, cerebellum, chicken, avian (viral) encephalomyelitis. Endothelial cells (E) are transparent and obliterate capillary lumen. Degenerate neurons are swollen and vacuolated and endoplasmic reticulum is fragmented. Glial cells are necrotic and contain myelin figures (arrow).

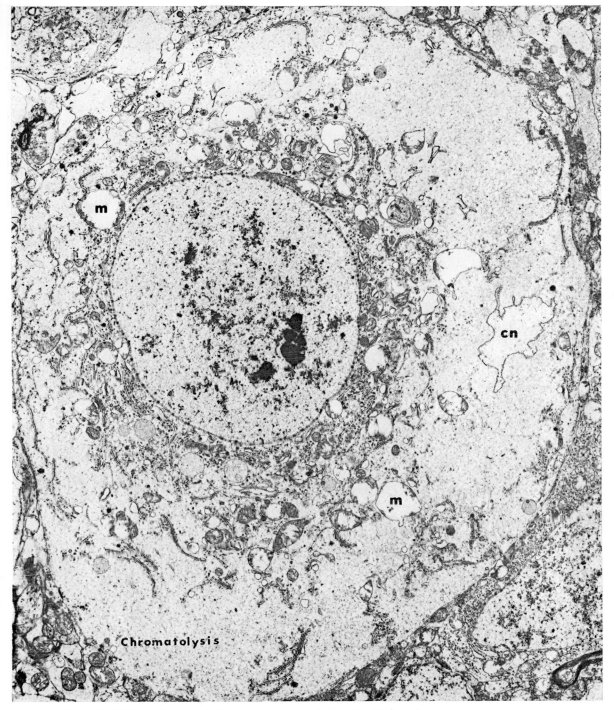

Fig. 2.6. Cell swelling and chromatolysis, cerebellar Purkinje cell, pig with porcine (picornaviral) encephalomyelitis. Note expansion of cell volume with dilatation of mitochondria (m) and cytocavitary network (cn). Destruction of the rough endoplasmic reticulum is responsible for the term chromatolysis. Precipitates of protein are present in the cytoplasmic matrix and nucleoplasm.

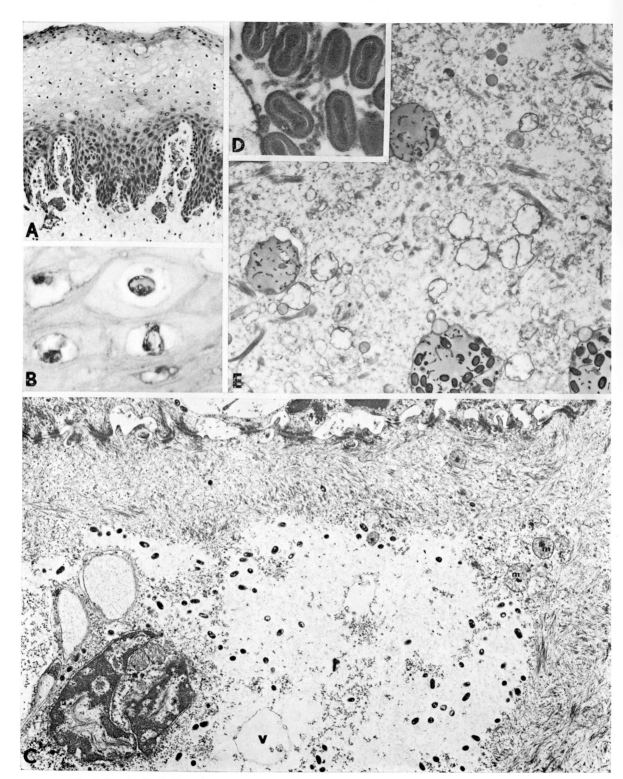

Fig. 2.7. A.–C. Ballooning degeneration, bovine papular stomatitis.
A. Lesion in esophagus. Note subepithelial hyperemia. B. Degenerate epithelial cells with keratinolysis, nuclear swelling, and
tiny cytoplasmic inclusions. C. Ultrastructure. Central, perinuclear
lysis leaving spaces containing delicate filaments and a peripheral
zone of keratin filaments. Note pox virions, degenerate mitochondria
(m), and vacuoles (v). D. Fowlpox virions. E. Early lipid-containing
fowlpox inclusion bodies.

port which drives the Na⁺ out and the K⁺ in. If these transport mechanisms are interfered with, cells take up fluid and both cell volume and intracellular hydrostatic pressure are increased. When overhydration becomes severe, the plasma membrane may rupture, producing lysis of the cell (Crocker et al. 1970).

The active movement of ions across membranes from low to higher concentration utilizes ATP to move against thermodynamic gradients. The plasma membrane hydrolyzes ATP at the inner surface and uses the energy released to pump Na^+ out. For the cell to maintain a low intracellular Na^+ concentration, it must extrude Na^+ against the higher concentration on the outside. It must also do this against an electrochemical barrier, for the plasma membrane is negative on the inside and positive on the outer surface. This *sodium pump* utilizes a Na^+-K^+-activated ATPase and underlies such important functions as renal electrolyte regulation, nerve excitability, and muscle function (Table 2.2). Injury to the pump results in the net entry of Na^+ and Cl^- together with water into the cell, causing it to swell.

EXPERIMENTAL CELL SWELLING

Direct injury to the plasma membrane can be produced by chemical poisons, ultraviolet light, antigen-antibody-complement complexes, or mechanical injury. Under experimental conditions, the plasma membrane becomes "leaky," Na^+ enters the cell, K^+ leaves, and water enters the cell passively. One of the more precise plasma membrane poisons is *ouabain*, a plant glycoside used by primitive Africans who painted it on arrows used for hunting. It is a current therapeutic agent for heart failure. Ouabain depresses Na^+-K^+-activated ATP-ase and thereby prevents the extrusion of sodium from the cell. Na^+ and water move into the mitochondria and endoplasmic reticulum causing cell swelling and degeneration.

Drugs that interfere with sulfhydryl groups (SH) of the membrane can disrupt transport mechanisms and result in increased permeability (Sahaphong and Trump 1971). When organic mercury is used to experimentally block sulfhydryl groups on the plasma membrane, water and Na^+ enter the cell and move to the cisternae of the endoplasmic reticulum and nuclear envelope which become markedly dilated. The stretching of membranes causes secondary damage, and calcium leaks into the cell where it concentrates in the swollen mitochondria.

Most causes of cell swelling are indirect in regard to the plasma membrane and can be reproduced experimentally by interrupting cellular respiration and glycolysis. Iodoacetate and antimycin A have been used to suppress ATP synthesis in cytoplasmic membranes. They produce injury that mimics acute ischemic injury such as occurs in infarction. The plasma membrane is affected secondarily and is responsible for entrance of water into the cell.

Active transport of soluble substances by the plasma membrane has been illustrated experimentally in models utilizing isolated, intact preparations of renal tubules, toad bladder, and frog skin. For example, if tubule cells are isolated and immersed in a solution containing phenol red, this vital dye soon passes through the cells and becomes concentrated in the tubule lumen. The greater concentration in the lumen than in the surrounding medium demonstrates that the renal tubule cells are secreting the dye against a concentration gradient. After induction of selective injury to the plasma membrane, disturbed transport of dye occurs and swelling of the cell by expansion of the cytoplasmic matrix can be seen structurally.

SEVERE CELL SWELLING

In severe cell swelling, there is entrance of larger molecules such as plasma proteins into the cell, in addition to water and electrolytes. If cardiac myocytes are killed by

Table 2.2. **Ionic concentration (in mEq) in mammalian intra- and extracellular fluids**

	Interstitial Fluid	Intracellular Fluid (Cytosol)
Cations		
Na+	145	12
K⁺	4	155
Anions		
Cl⁻	120	4
HCO₃⁻	27	8
Organic anions	7	155

anoxia due to experimental ligation of the blood supply to the heart muscle, they can be demonstrated to contain large amounts of albumin, globulin, and fibrinogen (Kent 1969).

The rate of entry of proteins into injured cells can be studied experimentally by the intravenous infusion of small tracers such as lanthanum (which penetrates spaces as small as 2nm) into normal and injured animals. Upon ultrastructural examination of normal muscle, the infused lanthanum is found only within the vascular system and interstitium. In injured muscle, however, it is also present within the damaged cell and among the muscle fibrils (Fahimi and Cotran 1971).

Intracellular substances escape into the interstitial spaces when the cell is severely injured. Soluble enzymes and other proteins in the cytoplasmic matrix leave the cell. In some cases of myocardial and liver damage, the plasma levels of these released enzymes are sufficiently high to be useful clinically in predicting the severity of cell injury. During the extensive degeneration that develops in bovine blackleg, remarkable increases in glutamic oxaloacetic transaminase and other enzymes can be demonstrated in plasma.

SPECIFIC CHANGES IN CELL ORGANELLES AND INCLUSIONS

PLASMA MEMBRANE

Maintenance of the permeability characteristics of the plasma membrane is an important function of living cells. The lipid nature, electrical surface charge, glycocalyx, and pores of the membrane are influences on the extent and rate of passive permeation into and out of the cytoplasmic matrix. All of these have an important bearing on the control of cell swelling (Loewenstein 1966).

The plasma membrane consists of a blanket of phospholipid molecules whose water-soluble heads are exposed to the outer surfaces of the membrane. The molecular tails are hydrophobic and are buried, back-to-back, in the interior of the membrane. The phospholipids anchor the protein molecules that are embedded in the membrane and project from its surface (Fig. 2.8).

The cell surface consists of a highly reactive microenvironment of acidic mucopolysaccharides, sialic (neuraminic) acid, and substances such as globulin which may adsorb to the cell periphery. Studies with

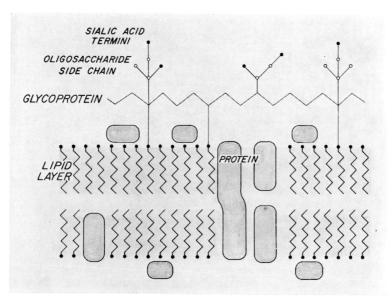

Fig. 2.8. Model of plasma membrane. Polar lipid layers are interrupted by protein molecules and surface glycoproteins with reactive termini. Surface-absorbed substances such as globulin are not shown.

erythrocyte membranes reveal that glycoproteins are oriented so that their carbohydrate segments are exposed. Specific enzymatic hydrolysis of components of the glycocalyx is important in several injuries to cells. The glycocalyx is especially important in the epithelial cells of the intestinal mucosa and pulmonary alveolar wall (Weiss 1969).

Many cellular functions depend upon the arrangement of plasma membrane components. The biologic behavior of normal and pathologic cells can be altered as a result of changes in distribution of surface proteins and glycoproteins, some of which act as receptors for antibodies, hormones, and microorganisms. Some of the protein molecules that are distributed randomly over the cell surface are capable of moving over the surface to assume a nonrandom distribution. Substances that bind to cell surface components (ligands) and induce migration of ligand-receptor molecule complexes include antibody molecules; bacteria; and lectins, plant proteins (such as concanavalin A) that bind to specific plasma membrane carbohydrates. The aggregation of ligand-receptor molecules is referred to as capping.

The cell attachment devices associated with the cell surface are vital to the cell's integrity. The gap of the desmosome contains a central dense lamella composed of neuraminidase-resistant glycoprotein. At high power it is seen as a zigzag structure with lateral extensions to the outer surface of the plasma membrane. In epitheliotropic viral infections the desmosome is often attacked, leading to separation of cells and dehiscence of the epithelium. In vesicular stomatitis the desmosome appears to be specifically affected; this is responsible for the widespread separation of keratinocytes. Familial acantholysis of angus calves, a disease characterized by shedding of epidermis, is due to an anomalous development of desmosome-tonofilament complexes that allows detachment of intercellular junctions (Jolly et al. 1973).

MECHANICAL DAMAGE

Severe mechanical injuries to the plasma membrane are usually lethal to the cell. In rupture wounds where the cytoplasmic constituents are not lost, however, the plasma membrane can heal by reduplication and regrowth. This has been demonstrated experimentally in single cells such as ova. Artificially induced tear wounds caused loss of cytoplasm but healed by undulation and reduplication of the margins of the torn plasma membrane (Bluemink 1972). Small holes and other defects in the plasma membrane are associated with loss of selective permeability and can be demonstrated in some systems by vital dye staining or by determination of changes in electrical surface charges.

PLASMA MEMBRANE AND VIRAL INFECTION

The structures of the plasma membrane act as receptors for viral infection. Fusion of virions with the plasma membrane is especially mechanistic with those viruses whose outer envelopes resemble the cellular plasma membrane. In the influenza virus, two polypeptides (identified as hemagglutinin and neuraminidase) are contained in surface projections of the virion. Attachment of the virion to the host cell plasma membrane (on respiratory tract cilia) occurs by the complexing of hemagglutinin projections to cell surface mucoproteins: more precisely, to acetylated sugars of the oligosaccharide chain (Fig. 2.9).

After intracellular replication is complete, influenza virus is released from the cell by an induced local change in the plasma membrane. When the viral nucleocapsid touches the plasma membrane, projections of neuraminidase and hemagglutinin are formed. This focus is then used as a final coat for the virion as it buds from the cell (Fig. 2.10). The mechanism of release involves the removal of plasma membrane sialic acid termini by viral neuraminidase which permits separation of virions from the cell.

PLASMA MEMBRANE–HORMONE INTERACTION

Most hormonal instructions given to the cell are translated by the plasma membrane to a biological activator, cyclic-3′5′-adenosine monophosphate (cyclic AMP or cAMP) which in turn initiates appropriate action in the cytoplasm. For example, hor-

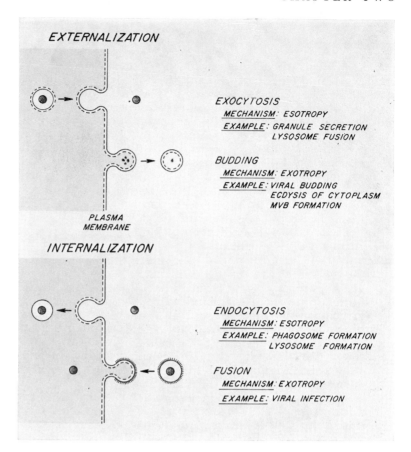

EXTERNALIZATION

EXOCYTOSIS
   MECHANISM: ESOTROPY
   EXAMPLE: GRANULE SECRETION
           LYSOSOME FUSION

BUDDING
   MECHANISM: EXOTROPY
   EXAMPLE: VIRAL BUDDING
           ECDYSIS OF CYTOPLASM
           MVB FORMATION

PLASMA
MEMBRANE

INTERNALIZATION

ENDOCYTOSIS
   MECHANISM: ESOTROPY
   EXAMPLE: PHAGOSOME FORMATION
           LYSOSOME FORMATION

FUSION
   MECHANISM: EXOTROPY
   EXAMPLE: VIRAL INFECTION

Fig. 2.9. Models of externalization and internalization of cells. Exotropy is protusion of a membrane into a space; esotropy is invagination into the cytoplasmic matrix.

mones such as epinephrine attach to the plasma membrane and activate adenyl cyclase. Adenyl cyclase transforms ATP (located in the inner plasma membrane) into cAMP which then diffuses into the cell, translating information of the hormone into biochemical activity. Destruction of this mechanism in hepatocytes is particularly important in glucose metabolism.

PLASMA MEMBRANE AND IMMUNOREACTIVITY

Plasma membrane structural proteins and lipoproteins are important in changes involving immunoreactivity where membrane proteins participate as antigens (Aoki et al. 1969). The reaction of antibodies with antigens in the plasma membrane induces striking configurational changes. The attachment of antibody to plasma membrane viral antigens induces movement of antigen-antibody complexes to clusters and this "capping" is followed

by ecdysis and endocytosis. Plasma membranes of adjacent cells may be induced to fuse to form syncytia (giant cells). Fusion involves coalescence of two double-tiered membranes to form a single triple-layered membrane and necessitates a rearrangement of proteins and phospholipids to globular form (the close adhesiveness of two plasma membranes is not fusion). In other types of immunoreactivity on the cell surface, small (10 nm) holes may be produced in the plasma membrane by the action of complement; this leads to cell lysis.

NUCLEUS

The nucleus is not markedly affected during the early phases of cell swelling. The *nuclear envelope,* the two membranes enclosing the perinuclear space, is a barrier to ions (Wiener et al. 1965). It is continuous with and considered an integral part of the cytocavitary network. Nuclear pores

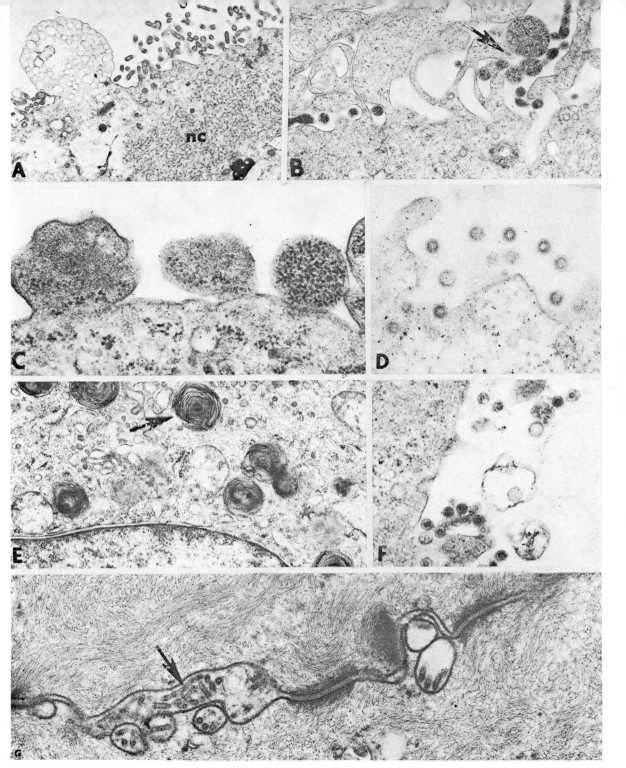

Fig. 2.10. A. Cell surface changes, measles virus infection. Herniation of cytoplasm due to viral-induced defect in plasma membrane
(also may be seen as fixation artifact). Aggregates of nucleocapsids
(nc). B. Measles virions (arrow). C. Parainfluenza virions budded
from cell surface. D. Coronavirus at cell surface. E. Dense myelin
figures (arrow). F. Arenavirus virions. G. Lysis and disorganization
of desmosomes and intercellular junctions of keratinocytes.
Vesicular stomatitis, cow. Virions (arrow).

(or annuli), which are considered potential avenues for exchange of water and ions between the cytoplasm and nucleus, are traversed by a delicate septum or diaphragm which appears to selectively control movement of water unless specifically injured.

The nucleus of hyperplastic cells is often much changed. Accumulations of fibrils, tubules, and other proteins may develop. Large inclusion bodies develop in a variety of situations where the transcription of genetic information is altered (Fig. 2.11). In intranuclear viral infections, lattices of viral-induced proteins crystallize in the nucleus. In other cases, lysis of proteins in the nucleus leaves a background of delicate fibrils.

The nuclear membrane may exhibit reduplication and the formation of extensive undulations. This is common in malignant neoplasms. The nuclear membrane of thymic and malignant lymphocytes characteristically folds inward upon itself, forming false nucleoplasmic inclusions (Miller 1969; Weber et al. 1969). Similar changes occur in neutrophils in specific genetic diseases (Lutzner and Hecht 1966). Changes in the nucleus are often striking in rapidly metabolizing cells which have been selectively poisoned (Allen et al. 1970; Karasaki 1970). Massive enlargement is accompanied by unorthodox configurations in most nuclear structures. The toxicities involving heavy metals such as lead are characterized by the formation of intranuclear protein matrices upon which the metallic ions are deposited (Goyer et al. 1970).

The significance of selective injury to the nucleus depends upon the stage of the cell cycle when it occurs. In general, cells are most susceptible during the G phases of the cycle. It is clear, however, that some postmitotic cells can function in the absence of a nucleus as evidenced by the mammalian erythrocyte or the removal of cell nuclei by experimental cell surgery.

In lethal injury, the components of the nucleus disintegrate as the cell degenerates. The nuclear membrane breaks apart and elements of the karyoplasm mix with the cytosol. *Chromatin,* which is the structural form of the DNA-histone complexes, dissociates and disappears. Chromatin is present in the normal cell in two interchangeable states. *Euchromatin* is dispersed and stains poorly. It becomes concentrated into deeply staining chromosomes during mitosis, i.e., the M phase of cell cycle. *Heterochromatin* is the condensed region of the chromosome which persists during interphase (because of its inactivity in RNA synthesis). It remains in the dying cell as dense, shrunken masses of granules.

NUCLEAR CONTROL OF PROTEIN SYNTHESIS

The central dogma of genetics is that its information is encoded in the sequences of subunits that constitute the genes. A gene is simply a specific sequence of base-pairs in DNA. The genetic message is transmitted by first the copying of the base-pair sequence of DNA onto mRNA molecules (transcription) and the mRNA then directing amino acid assembly into protein (translation). From the gene code, or primary template, the living cell is able to replicate thousands of different proteins, each with several hundred amino acids arranged in a highly specific sequence.

Transfer of information from the gene DNA involves transcription of DNA into three types of RNA: (1) messenger RNA (mRNA) which serves as a template on which amino acid subunits are assembled; (2) ribosomal RNA (rRNA) which originates in nucleoli and forms the ribosomes where translation is accomplished; and (3) transfer RNA (tRNA) which carries the amino acid subunits of protein to their proper site along the mRNA template (Fig. 2.12).

Ribonucleotides in the nucleus are polymerized during transcription through action of RNA polymerase to form RNA molecules patterned directly from DNA strands. Remarkable electron micrographs of protein synthesis in bacteria have depicted these changes (Miller and Hamkalo 1972). The secondary template, messenger RNA, carries the information required for synthesis of a specific protein. Messenger RNA leaves the nucleus and becomes incorporated into ribosomes of the cytoplasm where it directs protein synthesis.

The DNA in the different cells of an individual contains the same genetic information but only a limited amount is expressed. The cells' genetic program not only can be switched on and off (as in mitosis) but also can be selectively expressed. Thus the neuron and the keratinocyte have very

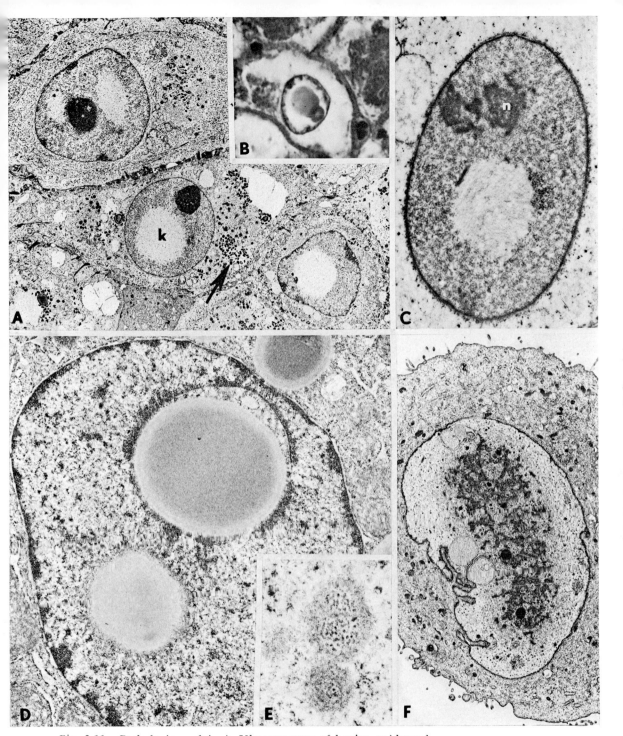

Fig. 2.11. Pathologic nuclei. A. Ultrastructure of benign epidermal monkeypox. Foci of karyolysis in nuclei (k). Virions are present in cytoplasm (arrow) but not nucleus. B. Histology of A. C. Microfilaments remain in karyolytic zones of the nucleus (swinepox). Note nucleolar disaggregation (n). D. Neutral lipid globules in nuclei of an hepatocyte. Left globule is within cytoplasmic indentation and only appears to be in the nucleus. Right globule is free in nucleoplasm. E. Nuclear bodies. F. Intranuclear inclusion in an adenovirus-infected cell. Virions are embedded in the dense protein matrix.

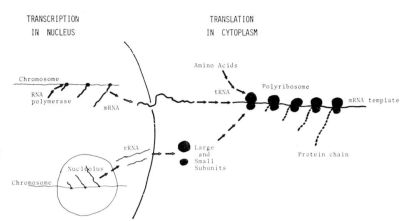

Fig. 2.12. Pathways of
DNA transcription and
translation.

different functions even though their DNA contains the same basic information. In mammalian cells, the chromosomal proteins regulate genetic expression. Histones keep genes turned off; nonhistone proteins selectively turn them on. Histones function as nonspecific repressors of RNA synthesis and are involved in the maintenance of chromatin structure. They block transcription by binding to DNA and by stabilizing the DNA helix. The chromosomal nonhistone proteins include a variety of enzymes and other proteins that recognize defined gene loci and thereupon regulate the transcription of specific genetic information.

DNA BREAKAGE AND REPAIR

The DNA molecules are not permanently fixed in their structural configuration but slowly undergo decay. This necessitates mechanisms of repair that, after toxic or irradiation injury to DNA, are of extreme significance in maintaining the normal cellular genome. These elaborate procedures to protect the DNA molecule against mutagenic agents include two major pathways. First, the altered portion of the molecule may be repaired in situ (with or without enzymes). Second, removal of the damaged segment and replacement with newly synthesized DNA units may occur by complex enzymic processes. The excision or "cut-and-patch" repair of this second category, when dissected into individual phases, includes: (1) incision of the damaged segment by an endonuclease, (2) its

excision by an exonuclease with subsequent degradation, (3) repair DNA-replication initiated by a polymerase, and (4) rejoining of the new segment into the DNA molecule by activity of a ligase. The repair-synthesis of new DNA segments is referred to as "unscheduled synthesis" since it occurs outside of the S-phase or normal DNA replication in the cell growth cycle.

The analysis of abnormalities in the functional integrity of the DNA repair mechanism has been applied to the genetic disease xeroderma pigmentosum of man. This disease is characterized by extreme sensitivity to ultraviolet rays in sunlight that cause epidermal cell injury. The cellular defect involved is a lack of ultraviolet endonuclease. This suppresses the normal repair of DNA molecules after ultraviolet irradiation injury and is responsible for mutiple carcinomas (Regan et al. 1971).

The concept of DNA repair has enormous consequences in terms of cancer-causing viruses, the genomes of which are passed from one cell generation to the next by becoming integrated into the host cell genome. DNA breakage facilitates the integration into the host cell DNA and the opportunity for insertion is greatly extended when there are delays or failures in DNA repair.

NUCLEOLUS

The normal interphase nucleolus consists of spongelike aggregates of dense granules (RNA, 10–15 nm diameter), fibrils (loose fibrillar reticulum, 5 nm diameter), and intranucleolar chromatin (DNA), all embedded in an amorphous protein matrix. Pathologic change in the nucleolus may be described under the headings of enlargement, segregation, disintegration, or shrinkage.

Nucleolar segregation is the rearrangement of granular and fibrillar components into two or more distinct zones. If the mechanism involved precisely affects the nucleolus, segregation leads to disintegration. Cytochemical studies with uridine-H^3 (to measure normal uptake in nucleolar RNA) indicate that disintegration progresses in the order: nucleolus-associated chromatin, fibrillar reticulum, and dense granules (Geuskens and Bernhard 1966). Dispersion is followed by disappearance of the nucleolar material or clumping in large abnormal protein aggregates (Fig. 2.13).

Specific injury to the nucleolus is caused by many toxins, antimetabolites, and carcinogens (Reddy and Svoboda 1968). Most of these act as inhibitors of RNA polymerase and in preventing its formation of mRNA. Poisoning with the antibiotic actinomycin, with aflatoxin, and with Amanita toadstool toxin will be examined as models of nucleolar injury.

Actinomycin, an antibiotic produced by the bacterium Streptomyces, interferes with transcription. It depresses mRNA formation by binding tightly to DNA and thereby inhibiting the RNA polymerase from building mRNA chains. A few minutes after a single injection of actinomycin into a rat, nucleolar damage can be detected in hepatocyte nucleoli. Chromatin is cleaved away and nucleolar macromolecules are segregated and redistributed into distinct zones. Later, they are dispersed and only disoriented fibrils remain (Smuckler and Benditt 1965; Stenram 1965).

Ingestion of the destroying angel toadstool *(Amanita phalloides)* causes liver necrosis that is initiated in the nucleolus. In contrast to most other poisonous mushrooms (which produce extremely rapid disease by acting upon the gastrointestinal tract), action is delayed and death is lingering. In hepatocytes, the nucleolar fragmentation and subsequent cytopathic action of the Amanita toxins are a consequence of toxin binding to RNA polymerase which depresses the activity of that enzyme (Marinozzi and Fiume 1971). The fungal metabolite aflatoxin, which also causes liver ne-

crosis, impairs the emergence of ribosomal subunits. It destroys RNA polymerase and this leads to the suppression of RNA and protein synthesis within the endoplasmic reticulum and the fragmentation and disintegration of this system (Moulé 1973).

Degenerative changes in the nucleolus have been reported during infection by many viruses (Jacob 1968; Weiss and Meyer 1972) and some mycoplasmas (Jezequel et al. 1967). The message for transcription and translation in the viral genome is activated with ensuing destruction of nucleolar structure and function. The DNA-containing adenoviruses and papovaviruses are known to replicate within the nucleolar amorphous matrix (Fig. 2.13). Disintegration follows shutdown of cell function by viral-induced enzymes.

Injury to other parts of the cell is often reflected in secondary damage to the nucleolus. Unfortunately it is rarely possible to distinguish between these nonspecific effects and specific damage described above. Cells of starved animals usually have small nucleoli; this is best seen in liver and pancreatic acini. Feeding of a high protein diet is followed by return to normal size.

Enlargement of nucleoli accompanies general cell enlargement. It is also frequent in neoplastic cells and some cytotoxic reactions. Remarkable increases in size occur in experimental thioacetamide-induced liver cirrhosis in rats (Salomon et al. 1962). Increased RNA and protein synthesis with blockade of transport of these nucleolar products to the cytoplasm are responsible.

NUCLEAR BODY

The nuclear body is a small body of variable size and structure associated with highly active cells. It is usually composed of a core of dense particulate or tubular material and a peripheral fibrillar zone (Dumont and Robert 1971; Weber and Fromme 1963). Differences in the central area have given rise to the application of adjectives such as "simple," "granular," and "beaded" to the nuclear body. Sequential study of nuclei has indicated that nuclear bodies originate by the segregation of ribonucleoprotein fibrils and granules from nucleoli (Dupuy Coin and Bouteille 1972). Their function in the cell remains a mystery. Glycogen has been seen in the central area (Caramia et al. 1967). Nuclear

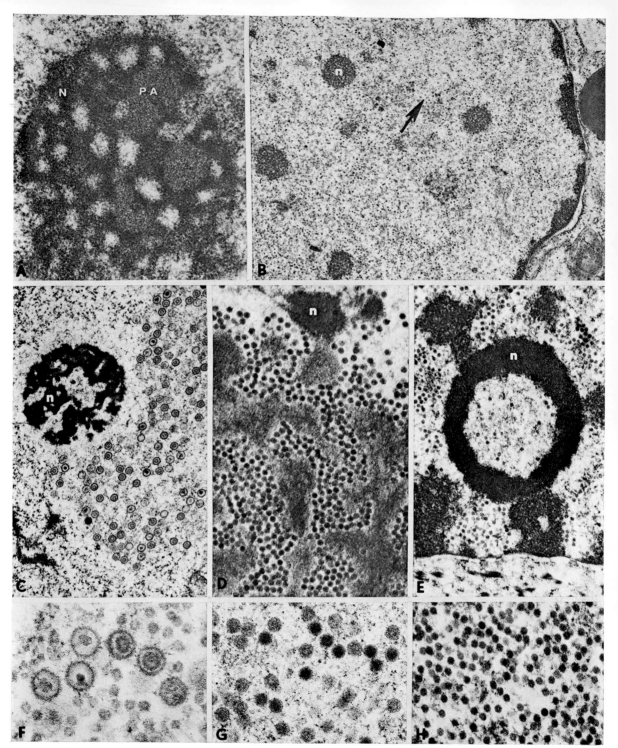

Fig. 2.13.   Nucleolar pathology. A. Nucleolar enlargement in tumor
cell. Nucleonema (N), pars amorpha (PA). B. parvoviruses (arrow)
in early intranuclear inclusion body. Disaggregation of nucleolus
(n). Virions are distributed throughout the nucleus but cannot
be distinguished at this power (micrograph, A. D. Boothe). C.
Nucleolar shrinkage (n), herpesvirus-infected hepatocyte. D. Nucleolar
disintegration (n), adenovirus-infected macrophage. Viral proteins
and virions make up the nuclear inclusion body. E. Ring-shaped
nucleolar aggregation (n), equine papillomavirus–infected keratinocyte. F. Herpes virions. G. Adeno-virions. H. Papilloma virions.

bodies are rarely present in degenerate cells but are common in cells of malignant tumors (Brooks and Siegel 1967; Krishan et al. 1967). Changes in structure develop in different phases of cellular activity (Reid 1973b; Reid and Isenor 1972).

RIBOSOMES

The ribonucleoprotein granules identified as ribosomes are formed by the interaction of ribosomal RNA and complex types of protein. They function in the cell for the assembly of amino acids into protein. Ribosomes occur in the cytoplasm in two forms: attached and free. Proteins synthesized by those ribosomes attached to the membranes of the endoplasmic reticulum are inserted into the cisternae. Polyribosomes are clusters of ribosomes held together by a tiny filament of mRNA that is formed in the nucleus (associated with DNA) and carries the appropriate code for the amino acid sequence.

RIBOSOMES IN PROTEIN SYNTHESIS

Free amino acids in the cytoplasmic matrix are enzymatically coupled to ATP yielding activated amino acids. These attach to small molecules of tRNA dissolved in the cytoplasmic matrix which transfer the amino acids to a specific location on the strand of mRNA attached to the ribosome. A different tRNA exists for each amino acid. When all the amino acids are aligned on the mRNA in specific sequence, they are linked together by the enzymatic formation of peptide bonds and released from the matrix of ribosomal RNA.

PATHOLOGIC CHANGES IN RIBOSOMES

Disruption of the RNA molecules or their enzymatic machinery in any phase of protein synthesis may be responsible for ribosomal destruction. Ribosomes detach from membranes of the rough endoplasmic reticulum and polyribosomes disaggregate (Reid et al. 1970). Their disappearance is manifest histologically as loss of cytoplasmic basophilia. This is the usual accompaniment to cell swelling.

In most instances of pathologic protein metabolism there occur defects in the rough endoplasmic reticulum. Early degeneration involves loss of normal architecture initiated by the removal of ribosomes from the membranes (Fig. 2.14). Where a specific block in enzymatic machinery occurs, protein substrate may accumulate in the cytoplasm. Proteins with abnormal structure may be produced which cannot be catabolized and they accumulate in the cell. Crystal-shaped lattices of ribosomes and protein are frequently encountered in degenerating cells. It has been hypothesized that hypothermia and cooling of the cell cause the formation of ribosomal tetramers that develop into lattices of ribosomes (Simoni et al. 1973).

Disruption of ribosomes may result from toxicity or from deficiencies in specific nutrients. Deletion of amino acids, sources of energy, or hormones (insulin, growth hormone, thyroxin, etc.) can have serious consequences. Many of the pathologic alterations in cytoplasmic ribonucleoprotein synthesis result from primary defects in the nucleus. We have seen how aflatoxin, Amanita toxin, and actinomycin influence cytoplasmic ribosomes secondarily by inhibiting nucleolar RNA polymerase. A direct toxic model of ribosomal destruction in liver cells can be induced with ethionine. Ethionine, an analogue of methionine, causes rapid depletion of hepatocyte ATP and disaggregation of polyribosomes. Ethionine impairs protein synthesis by reducing the rate of its initiation. This results in failure of certain proteins to reassociate with ribosomes and a reduction in the rate of peptide chain initiation. Ribosomal monomers accumulate and are not incorporated into polyribosomes (Kisilevsky et al. 1973).

In several viral infections large masses of viral ribosomes appear in the cytoplasm of infected cells. The protein-synthesizing machinery of the cell is usurped and directed to produce protein utilized in the assembly of virions. Excess protein accumulates in the form of inclusion bodies of ribosomes, protein fibers, or virion-protein aggregates. In most instances the virions are sufficiently distinct to be identified. Only the tiny parvoviruses and picornaviruses are so like ribosomes that they cannot be distinguished.

The neurotropic picornaviruses (such as the enteroviruses that cause avian encephalitis, porcine polioencephalomyelitis, and

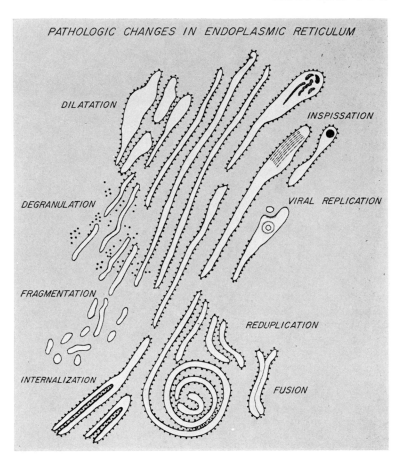

Fig. 2.14. Pathologic changes in endoplasmic reticulum.

human poliomyelitis) replicate in the cyto-plasmic matrix of neurons. The single-stranded RNA of the viral genome serves as a direct template for the formation of new strands of viral RNA (there is no inter-mediate step of transcription). As this proc-ess develops, normal ribosomal function is shut down and the rough endoplasmic reticulum, which dominates the normal neuron, fragments and disintegrates. This progressive lysis of the Nissl substance (rough endoplasmic reticulum) constitutes chromatolysis (Fig. 2.6).

The genome of influenza virus is a single-stranded RNA molecule which acts by in-ducing a new messenger RNA that is com-plementary in base sequence. Synthesis of new virions is initiated by an RNA-de-pendent RNA polymerase contained in the influenza virion which causes transfer of in-formation by base-pairing from the genomic (+) RNA to its complementary (−) RNA. New (+) strands are then syn-thesized from the (−).

Vaccinia virus (a poxvirus) replicates through the information transmitted in a more complex double-stranded DNA genome. After the virion attaches to and enters the cell, it is uncoated. This process releases the genome which contains enough DNA to code for several hundred polypep-tides. Information is transferred not only for synthesis of new viral DNA and pro-tein but for proteins that regulate virion uncoating and cell shutdown. Within 2–3 hrs after infection in vitro, foci of lysis of cytoplasmic ribosomes and endoplasmic reticulum can be seen and in their place develop regions of dense granular viro-plasm.

CYTOCAVITARY NETWORK

The endoplasmic reticulum, Golgi com-plex, nuclear membrane, and cytoplasmic vesicles are components of a membranous system; they are related structurally and functionally (Fig. 2.15). This *cytocavitary*

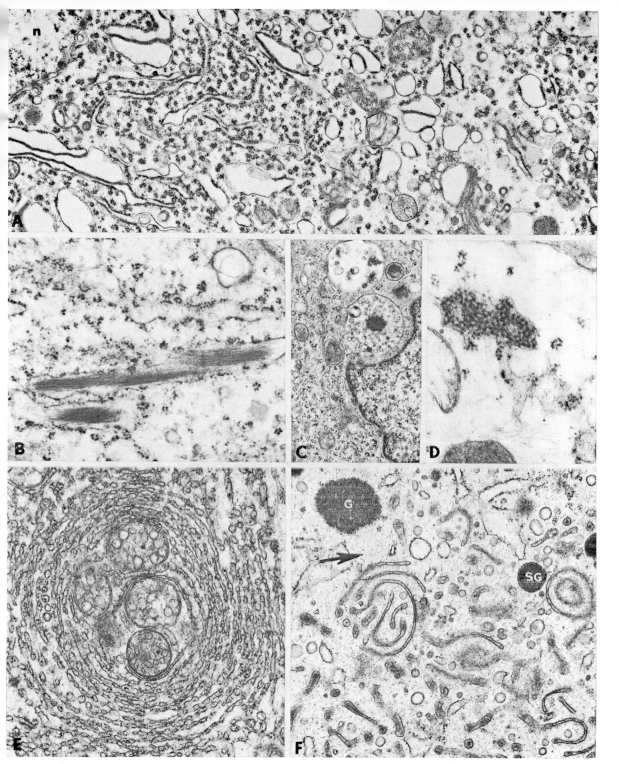

Fig. 2.15. Pathologic change, cytocavitary network. A. Dilatation
and vesiculation of ER in neuron (chromatolysis). Nucleus (n)
is at left, severe fragmentation at right. B. Intracisternal fibrils. C.
Multivesicular bodies. D. Accumulation of rodlets in the ER
cisternae. E. Reduplication of smooth ER with whorling around
mitochondria (m), adrenal cortex, dog. F. Fusion and fragmentation
of ER in a tumor cell. Microfilaments (arrow), dense granular
material (G), secretory granule (SG).

network includes all membrane-bound cavities other than mitochondria. It is extensively involved in cell swelling. Where overhydration is severe, water accumulates in the cisternae of these organelles causing dilatation (hydropic degeneration), loss of ribosomes, and fragmentation.

ENDOPLASMIC RETICULUM

The rough endoplasmic reticulum (ER) is active in synthesis of export proteins such as collagen, serum proteins, lipoproteins, and many protein secretion granules (Claude 1970). It is not usually involved in synthesis of proteins such as hemoglobin that are designed for intracellular use. Protein molecules which are discharged from the ribosomes penetrate the cavity of the ER and are stored and segregated for transport outside the cell.

Alterations in lipoprotein synthesis lead to accumulation and inspissation of lipoprotein droplets (liposomes) within the ER cisternae. Chemical interference with any of these metabolic processes is reflected in structural changes of the ER. Rough ER degenerates to smooth dilated vesicles when the membranes are segmented and ribosomes detach. For example, the ER of liver cells is destroyed during carbon tetrachloride poisoning when enzymes in the membrane transform the drug into highly toxic metabolites. Tolbutamide, a drug that alters pancreatic islet β-cell structure and function, induces severe dilatation, ribosome loss, and vesiculation (Williamson et al. 1961).

Smooth endoplasmic reticulum is involved in detoxification. Reduplication of smooth ER is seen in the early stages of poisoning by drugs such as phenobarbital, alcohol, and dilantin. Chronic carbon tetrachloride intoxication is characterized by massive development of smooth ER (Meldolesi et al. 1968; Stenger 1966). This is seen by light microscopy as large dense eosinophilic inclusion bodies in the cytoplasm. The induction of drug-metabolizing enzymes associated with smooth endoplasmic reticulum is allegedly the mechanism involved in the pathologic changes.

The catabolism of phenobarbital in the liver is a widely studied model of detoxification. After intravenous injection of this drug there are parallel increases in smooth ER and drug-metabolizing enzymes (Burger and Herdson 1966; Orrenius et al. 1965). Hepatocytes enlarge; greater cell volume is due to increased surface area and volume of the smooth ER. Mitochondria and peroxisomes show little change. Cell recovery occurs after withdrawal of the drug and the smooth ER returns to normal within 15 days (Bolender and Weibel 1973).

Reduplication of smooth endoplasmic reticulum is not restricted to toxic injury; it is commonly seen in cells of the liver and adrenal. In hepatocytes it has also been associated with high carbohydrate diets (Ruebner et al. 1972).

Peculiar distortions of the endoplasmic reticulum are often encountered in the examination of pathologic tissue. For most of these there is no established mechanism of formation (Pham et al. 1972). Fusion, fragmentation, reduplication, and vesiculation all occur as nonspecific changes that accompany cell degeneration (Fig. 2.15). Peculiar large dense tubules within the cisternae of the endoplasmic reticulum are commonly found in abnormal cells, particularly in neoplastic cells (Schaff et al. 1973; Thake et al. 1971).

GOLGI COMPLEX

The flattened sacs of the *Golgi complex* act as condensation membranes for the concentration into granules of products such as enzymes, hormones, bile, and yolk which are elaborated at other sites. Carbohydrates are conjugated to proteins. Experimentally, radioactively labeled sugar (H^3-glucose) becomes incorporated into glycoproteins in the Golgi complexes of goblet cells (Haddad et al. 1971; Neutra and Leblond 1966). The membranes of the Golgi complex also contain the enzymes required for the transfer of inorganic materials such as sulfate to acceptor molecules (Young 1973).

The Golgi complex is enlarged in hypertrophic cells, particularly those which are involved in the formation of secretory granules. The dictyosomes, or stacks of Golgi lamellae, are large and contain granular material. Electron-lucent Golgi vesicles form from the ends of the flattened Golgi lamellae. Other transport vesicles appear to originate in the Golgi complex, particularly the "coated" transport vesicles or acanthosomes.

In exhausted and atrophic cells the Golgi complex is apt to be small. The dictysomes degenerate by segregation of lamellar sacs into small, irregular vesicles (vesiculation). They become empty spaces lined by smooth membranes. Golgi vesicles progressively disappear. Degenerative changes in the Golgi complex are commonly seen in toxic damage to cells (Arstila and Trump 1972; Estes and Lombardi 1969).

ANNULATE LAMELLAE

Annulate lamellae are stacks of cytoplasmic membranes with pore structures similar to nuclear pores. They allegedly arise by evagination of the nuclear membrane (Kessel 1968; Wischnitzer, 1970). They are associated with rapidly proliferating cells and are frequently observed in embryonic and neoplastic cells. Annulate lamellae have been reported in the nuclei of cells in culture.

TUBULORETICULAR STRUCTURES

Tubuloreticular structures are complex formations of interconnected dense tubules, 20–30 nm in diameter, which develop within the cisternae of the endoplasmic reticulum (Fig. 2.15) They are seen in abnormal lymphoreticular cells, particularly endothelial cells and lymphocytes, in disease conditions of differing independent pathogenesis. They have been reported in neoplasms, autoimmune diseases, and viral infections. Their biologic significance is unresolved but cytochemical studies indicate that they consist of phospholipids and acidic glycoprotein (Schaff 1973).

PHAGOSOMES

Phagosomes are formed by the fusion of the advancing edges of pseudopodia during the process of phagocytosis (Fig. 2.16). Phagocytosis is a two-phase process. The initial phase represents attachment, either by nonspecific chemicoabsorption to the cell surface or by fusion with a specific surface receptor site. The second phase is endocytosis, which arises from plasma membrane movement initiated by contraction of the actomyosin myofilament system associated with the membrane. Cytochalasian B, by virtue of its inhibitory effects on microfilaments, is used experimentally to suppress phagosome formation.

Phagosomes contain the particulate substances that had previously attached to the cell surface. The internal surface of the limiting membrane represents the exterior face of the cellular plasma membrane. The internal milieu is relatively inert and devoid of enzymatic reactions. In general, phagosomes are concerned with intracellular transport. By fusion with enzyme-laden lysosomes, they become phagolysosomes which function in intracellular digestion.

PINOCYTOTIC VESICLES

Pinocytosis is considered a variant of phagocytosis whereby soluble materials are taken up in endocytic invaginations of the plasma membrane. The phagosomes involved in pinocytosis are smaller and are referred to as *pinocytotic vesicles*. These smooth-surfaced structures are easily differentiated from the transport vesicles which have an outer fringe of projections.

AUTOPHAGOSOMES

Autophagy (autophagocytosis) is sometimes referred to as "intracellular phagocytosis." During autophagy, portions of the cytoplasmic matrix and its organelles are incorporated into membrane-bound autophagosomes which subsequently fuse with lysosomes. Autophagy is a common reaction in sublethally altered cells, and is the mechanism whereby damaged organelles are removed from the cell (Arstila 1971).

MULTIVESICULAR BODIES

Multivesicular bodies are large phagosomes filled with tiny vesicles. The vesicles have budded from the surface of the phagosomal membrane by the extrusion of bits of cytoplasmix matrix (Fig. 2.15). Multivesicular bodies are transformed into autolysosomes by fusion with acid-hydrolase containing primary lysosomes and function in autodigestion.

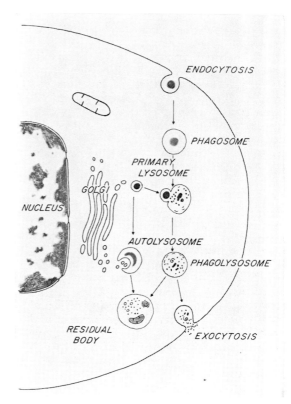

Fig. 2.16. Phagosome-lysosome pathways. Primary lysosomes discharge enzymes to the exterior or fuse with phagosomes to form secondary lysosomes (phagolysosomes). They also incorporate damaged organelles as autolysosomes (autophagic vacuoles) and persist as residual bodies.

LYSOSOMES

Lysosomes are membrane-bound granules filled with hydrolytic enzymes, proteins, and mucopolysaccharides (Table 2.3). Because of their potent hydrolytic enzymes, they are essential for the processes of intracellular digestion. Lysosomal proteins are synthesized in ribosomes, transported into the endoplasmic reticulum, and put in proper order and packaged within the Golgi complex.

The *primary lysosome* is a small dense granule released by the Golgi complex with its enzymes in an inactive state by some association with acidic mucopolysaccharides. During intracellular digestion, primary lysosomes unite with phagosomes to form secondary (active) lysosomes, also termed *phagolysosomes.* Phagolysosomes are digestive vacuoles within which enzymatic degradation of ingested material takes place. They either remain in the cell as residual bodies or provide a mechanism for excretion of debris from the cell by exocytosis (Fig. 2.18).

The induction of lysosome formation occurs in many types of cell injury and parallel increases in hydrolytic enzymes can be demonstrated histochemically (Axline and Cohn 1970; Morrison and Panner 1964)

Fig. 2.17. Pathologic change, cytocavitary network. A. Intracisternal rods (arrow), thyroid carcinoma cell. B. Annulate lamellae, cross section (arrow) and longitudinal section (left), interstitial cell tumor, testis, dog. C. Atrophy with vesiculation of lamellae of Golgi complex (arrow), intensely secreting exhausted cell, adrenal medulla, dog with uremia. Nucleus (N), mitochondria (M), lipid globule (L). D. Phagocytosis, entrance of bacterium *(Salmonella choleraesuis)* into phagosome. E. Various organelles concerned with phagocytosis. Phagosome formation at cell surface, phagosome containing bacterium (top center), lysosome (L), and fusion of phagosome and lysosome (arrow).

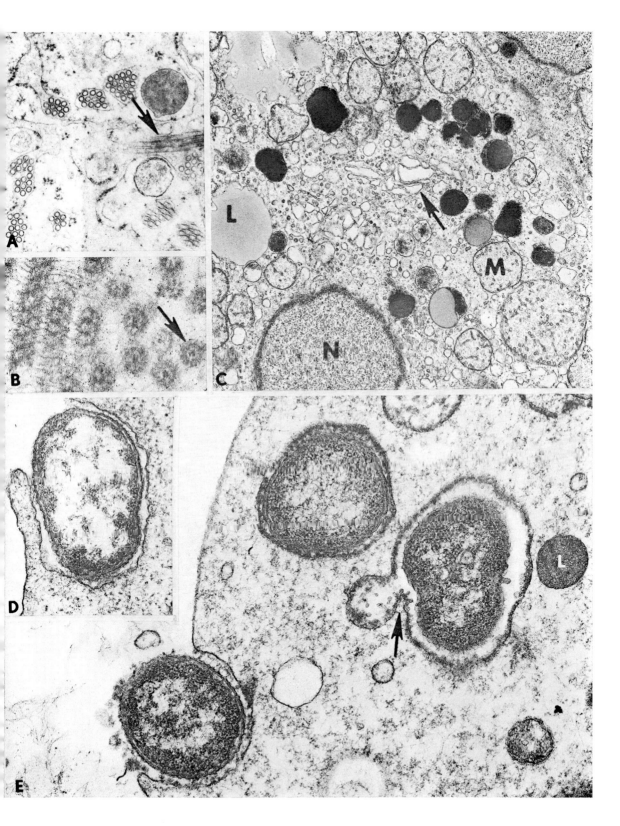

Table 2.3. **Biologically active substances identified in lysosomes**

Substance	Histochemical Identification	Function
Acid hydrolases	Acid phosphatase	Intracellular digestion.
Arginine-rich proteins	Acridine orange	Implicated in histamine release. Also as pyrogen, fibrinolytic agent, and coagulation inhibitor.
Acidic mucopolysaccharides	Alcian blue	Stabilize and repress other enzymes until utilization.

During autophagy, lysosomes produce limited focal areas of autolysis in cells which recover (Arstila 1971). It is also proposed that rupture of lysosomes with release of hydrolytic enzymes within injured cells is a mechanism of cell death (Allison et al. 1966; Brandes et al. 1969). When the stability of the lysosomal membrane is altered, lysosomes act as "suicide bodies" by causing lysis of the cell from within.

RESIDUAL BODIES

Residual bodies are large, secondary lysosomes filled with necrotic debris and damaged cellular components. Lipoproteins and other lipids make up most of the debris and their accumulation reflects the lack of sufficient quantities of lipase in most phagolysosomes. Lipoprotein membranes may accumulate in residual bodies in concentric lamellar formations called myelin figures or myeloid bodies. Myeloid bodies are characteristic of degenerative processes in brain, myelinated nerves, and other cells with large amounts of lipoprotein membranes (Hruban et al. 1972). Some intracellular lipids become oxidized to pigmented autofluorescent lipofuscin (aging pigment). Lipofuscin can be discharged from the cell or, as in the case of neurons and cardiac myocytes, remain within the residual body.

LYSOSOMAL STABILIZATION

Pharmacologically, some drugs stabilize lysosomal membranes, making them inoperable. Cortisone (Weissman and Thomas 1962) and chloroquine (Read and Bay 1971) are potent lysosomal stabilizers. In animals treated with large doses of cortisone, there is failure of lysosomes to fuse with each other, with phagosomes, and with the plasma membranes, and the process of intracellular digestion is retarded. It has been suggested that cortisone restricts the movement of phospholipid acyl chains in membranes. In contrast, vitamin A, carbon tetrachloride, and bacterial endotoxin are lysosomal labilizers; that is, they promote the lysis of the lysosomal membranes and release of acid hydrolases into the cytosol.

LYSOSOMAL DISEASES

Many hereditary diseases have been discovered which are caused by specific absence or abnormality of lysosomal enzymes (Malmqvist et al. 1971; Prieur et al. 1972; Resibois et al. 1970). The lysosomal diseases are usually manifested in one of two ways: (1) by the absence of a hydrolytic enzyme that causes the substrate of that enzyme to accumulate, or (2) by defective enzymatic hydrolysis wherein substrates are hydrolyzed to nondegradable products which accumulate in the cell. Many of the lysosomal diseases are genetic defects known as lipid storage diseases which involve the brain or reticuloendothelial system. Affected cells are engorged with abnormal lipid complexes. The Chediak-Higashi syndrome is a different lysosomal disease that afflicts many species. Structurally, there is a distinct abnormality in smooth endoplasmic reticulum associated with packaging termini of the Golgi (Essner and Oliver 1974). The lysosomes that form in these areas cannot migrate to phagosomes and fuse properly. The delay in intracellular digestion causes a peculiar susceptibility to some infectious diseases.

PEROXISOMES

Peroxisomes are small membrane-bound dense granules that represent a primitive form of organelle containing enzymes. Like lysosomes, they originate from the endoplasmic reticulum (Essner 1967; Reddy and Svoboda 1973a). In vertebrates, peroxi-

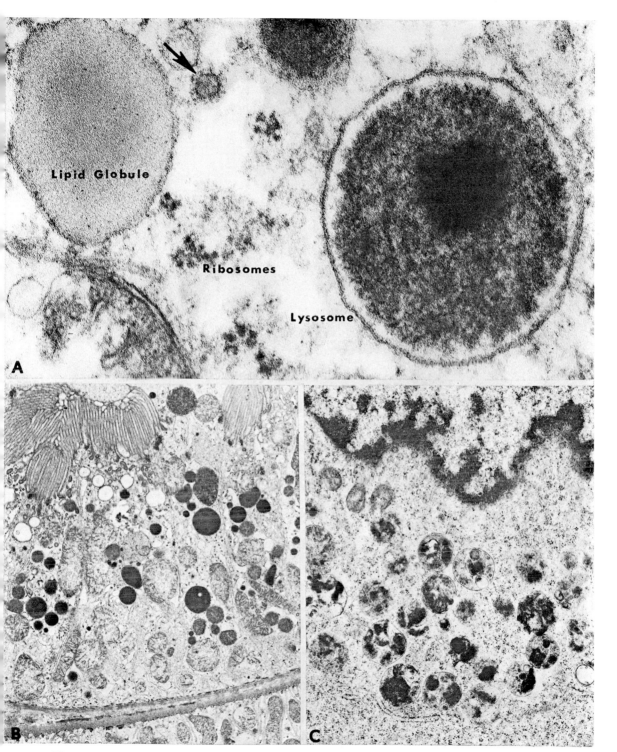

Lipid Globule

Ribosomes

Lysosome

A

B

C

Fig. 2.18. Lysosomes. A. Large primary lysosome, activated macrophage of tuberculosis. Transport vesicle (arrow). B. Accumulation of lysosomes and adsorption granules in proximal convoluted tubule during protein loss of nephritis in a dog. C. Accumulation of residual bodies and phagolysosomes, macrophage.

somes are most prominent in hepatocytes, renal tubular cells, and steroid-synthesizing cells but can be found in most cells.

In the liver, peroxisomes were first identified as microbodies. The function of their enzymes (catalase, urate oxidase) is largely peroxidative, hence the designation as peroxisomes (De Duve and Baudhuin 1966). They are detected by a diaminobenzidine staining procedure (Novikoff and Novikoff 1973). Hepatic microbodies contain an internal "nucleoid" which has been related to uricase content. Dalmatian dogs, which have an hereditary uricase deficiency, allegedly have smaller internal nucleoids than do other dogs (Afzelius 1965). Two congenital peroxisomal diseases have been reported in animals: acatalasemia in mice and an enzymatic defect in human infants called the cerebrohepatorenal syndrome of Zellweger (Goldfischer et al. 1973).

Peroxisomes are markedly enlarged in toxic injury to renal tubule cells (Lavin and Koss 1971). They are known to be especially altered by drugs such as salicylates and lithocholic acid. Peculiar tubules either singly or in crystalline arrangements have been reported in degenerate peroxisomes (Gorius and Houssay 1973; Hruban et al. 1974; Reddy and Svoboda 1973b).

De Duve, the discoverer of peroxisomes, proposed that catalase in these bodies existed to oxidize hydrogen peroxide that formed in cell injury and thereby represented a protective mechanism. An association between catalase-producing peroxisomes and serum lipids exists. Experimentally, agents that inactivate catalase or block its synthesis produce hyperlipemia. Catalase administered intravenously has a hypercholesteremic effect. Congenitally acatalasemic mice tend to have lower serum levels of triglycerides. Antilipidemic drugs have been shown to act by increasing the number of microbodies and the synthesis of liver catalase (Svoboda and Reddy 1972). A mechanistic role in atherosclerosis has therefore been hypothesized.

The progenitors of peroxisomes are small $(0.15–0.25\mu)$ circular bodies whose delimiting membrane is continuous with the smooth ER (Fig. 2.19). Called *microperoxisomes*, they contain catalase but lack the nucleoid of larger peroxisomes (Novikoff and Novikoff 1973) (see Fig. 1.1).

MICROTUBULES AND MICROFILAMENTS

Microtubules function in the movement of cilia, the tails of spermatozoa, and the spindle apparatus of dividing cells (Behnke and Forer 1967; Goldman and Follett 1970). They are also important in the exocytotic extrusion of secretion granules from the cell and appear to be related to other forms of intracellular movement. The analogy has been made that microtubules and microfilaments act as bone and muscle respectively in producing movement of the cell.

Microtubules disappear in several types of cell injury but their roles in producing or in responding to injury are vague. They are known to be altered by changes in intracellular ions, particularly calcium (Schlaepfer 1971). Halothane inhibits protein synthesis and microtubule formation and this has been suggested as a mechanism in anesthesia (Allison and Nunn 1968).

Colchicine, vincristine, and other antimitotic drugs damage microtubules and induce excessive microfilament formation. When injected into the subarachnoid space of rats, they induce a degenerative pattern that mimics the neuronal degeneration which accompanies aging. There is proliferation of microfilaments with loss of microtubules (neurotubules), allegedly due to blocking of microfilament coiling in the process of forming neurotubules (Schochet et al. 1968; Wisniewski and Terry 1967).

MITOCHONDRIA

Enzymes which catalyze oxidative phosphorylation, the mechanism for energy production, are embedded in the complex inner membrane of the mitochondrion. Acetyl coenzyme A which is formed in the cytosol from the degradation of glucose penetrates the mitochondrion and the acetate group enters the Krebs cycle. Pairs of electrons are removed by dehydrogenases and enter the respiratory chain. The only fuels required for the mitochondrion are phosphate and ADP; the final products are ATP plus CO_2 and H_2O.

Mitochondria are exquisitely sensitive to changes in water and electrolyte balance, oxygen tension, pH, and temperature (Fig. 2.20). When these changes occur, as in cell swelling, they directly affect the mitochon-

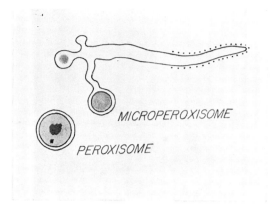

Fig. 2.19. Development of microperoxisome and peroxisome.

drion. Oxygen is required for oxidative phosphorylation, and structural changes in mitochondria are reliable indicators of anoxic injury to the cell. In addition to these nonspecific factors, many substances, such as cyanide, selectively affect the terminal respiratory chains in the mitochondrion and produce irreversible injury in a few seconds.

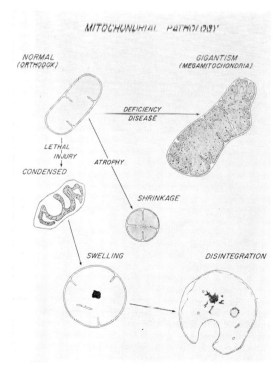

Fig. 2.20. Pathologic changes in mitochondria.

MITOCHONDRIAL DEGENERATION

Mitochondria behave as osmometers and the swelling that develops after injury reflects entry of solutes and water. In lethal injury, mitochondria pass through a reproducible sequence of changes that involves altered volume control, redistribution of components, and the appearance of new substances in the matrix. The progression, as shown experimentally by treating cells in culture with specific poisons, involves: (1) rapid condensation which is associated with loss of ions and water from the inner compartment due to depression of active pumping systems, (2) reinflation with transitory resemblance to the normal conformation, (3) swelling, associated with loss of capacity to synthesize ATP at the inner membrane (swelling exhibits an inverse correlation with ATP concentration), (4) flocculation of matrical proteins (an absolute sign of irreversible injury), and (5) deposition of calcium (Fig. 2.21)

Toxic injury to mitochondria is, in most cases, mediated via action of the biochemical system located in the mitochondrial matrix and inner membrane. The ultrastructural changes in many toxicities have been documented (Table 2.4). Fluoroacetate is a classic example of a mitochondrial metabolic inhibitor. It causes a competitive inhibition of aconitrate hydrolase that leads to unbalanced citrate turnover and accumulation. Structural changes that occur in the mitochondrial matrix reflect the presence of this enzyme at this site (Pucci 1964). Hormones appear to alter mitochondria by interfering with protein synthesis (Finegold and Green 1970; Gustafsson and Tata 1963; Volk and Scarpelli 1966). For example, thyroxin is known to stimulate the incorporation of amino acids into mitochondrial protein. Well-defined mitochondrial changes have also been reported in neoplastic conditions (Tandler et al. 1970).

In mitochondrial gigantism, enormous mitochondria called megamitochondria (or chondriospheres) form by progressive deposition of protein in the matrix. Early enlargement cannot be separated from simple hypertrophy but the degenerative phase is characterized by *cristolysis:* the disorganization and loss of cristae. The matrix areas of these enlarging mitochondria become increasingly dense.

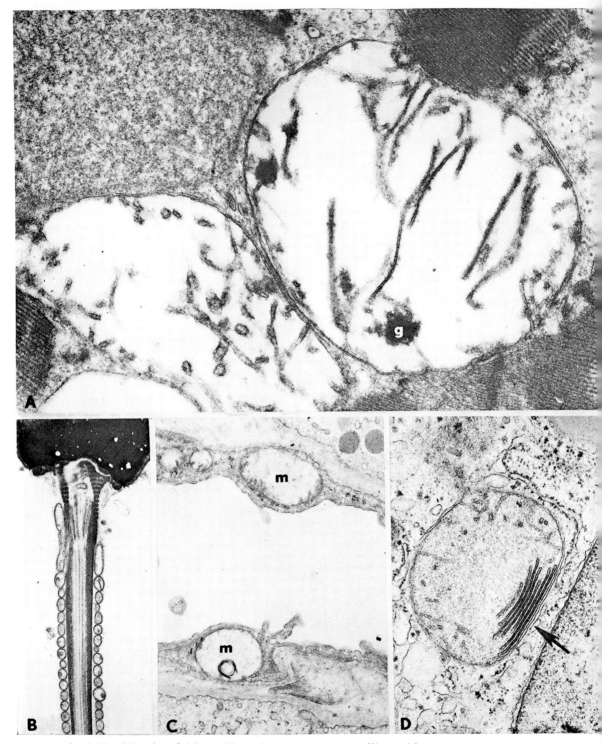

Fig. 2.21. Mitochondrial swelling. A. Acute severe swelling with disintegration of cristae, development of dense matrix granules (g). Matrix areas are cleared. Skeletal muscle, malignant edema, lamb. B. Degenerate mitochondria surrounding neckpiece of spermatozoa, bull semen ejaculated 12 hrs previously. C. Chronic swelling of mitochondria (m) with formation of myeloid bodies. Membranous pneumocytes, lung of dog, severe cardiac failure and hypoxia. D. Reduplication of cristae (arrow), dog hepatocyte.

Table 2.4. Lesions of the mitochondrion demonstrable in vivo

Toxicity	Tissue (Reference)
Acriflavin	Rat myocardium (Laguens, *J. Molec. Cell. Cardiol.* 4:185, 1972)
Aminoglutethimide	Rat adrenal (Racella, *Lab. Invest.* 21:52, 1969)
Chloramphenicol	Human bone marrow (Smith, *J. Cell Sci.* 7:501, 1970)
Clofibrate	Pig liver (Lee, *Exp. Mol. Path.* 20:387, 1974)
Clostridial toxin	Muscle (Grossman, *Am. J. Path.* 50:77, 1967)
Digoxin	Rat myocardium (Arcasoy, *Lab. Invest.* 20:190, 1969)
E. coli toxin	(White, *Ann. Surg.* 174:983, 1971)
Ethanol	Rat liver (Rubin, *Lab. Invest.* 23:620, 1970)
Emetine	Dog myocardium (Pearce, *Arch. Path.* 91:8, 1971)
Hypoglycin	Rat liver (Brooks, *Am. J. Path.* 62:309, 1971)
Oxygen	Rat lung (Yamamoto, *Am. J. Path.* 59:409, 1970)
Reserpine	Dog myocardium (Wilcken, *Science* 157:1332, 1967)
Rotenone	Cow myocardium (Harris, *Science* 165:700, 1969)
Tetanus toxin	Mouse muscle (Zacks, *J. Neuropath. Exp. Neurol.* 23:306, 1964)
Uranium	Kidney (Carafoli, *Lab. Invest.* 25:516, 1971)
Choline	Mouse liver (Wilson, *J. Cell Biol.* 16:281, 1963)
Fatty acids	Myocardium (Vitali-Massi, *Virch. Arch.* 342:38, 1968)
Iron	Rat erythroblast (Dallman, *Blood* 35:496, 1970; *J. Cell Biol.* 48:79, 1971)
Manganese	Mouse liver (Bell, *Lab. Invest.* 29:723, 1973)
Oxygen	Mouse liver (Sulkin, *Lab. Invest.* 14:1523, 1965)
Protein	Rat pancreas (Svoboda, *Lab. Invest.* 15:731, 1966)
Riboflavin	Mouse liver (Tandler, *J. Cell Biol.* 41:477, 1969)
Thiamin	Rat myocardium (Wu, *Virch. Arch.* 9:97, 1971)
Vitamin E	Rat liver (Lantos, *Exp. Mol. Path.* 18:68, 1973)

Mitochondrial gigantism is seen in deficiencies of vitamins, particularly vitamin E and riboflavin. Mice placed on a riboflavin-free diet for 6 wks develop extensive enlargement of mitochondria: some organelles become larger than the nuclei. Except for size, they are not distinctly abnormal; that is, they are not distorted, disorganized, or filled with debris even though they are "rich in matrix and poor in cristae." As cells degenerate, however, mitochondria begin to degenerate also. If riboflavin is given intraperitoneally, mitochondria return to normal, allegedly by the development of dividing membranes and division (Tandler et al. 1969).

Mitochondrial swelling involves overt swelling with loss of cristae and matrix. The matrix areas become less dense than normal and the cristae are shorter and disoriented. In severe reactions, excess water uptake transforms mitochondria into large, structureless vacuoles that give the cell the typical appearance of hydropic or vacuolar degeneration. Swelling is the reaction to deficiencies of oxygen and is the most common mitochondrial lesion seen in pathologic material. Vacuolar mitochondria are widespread in cells during disease accompanied by fluid imbalance, edema, prolonged high fevers, metabolic disease, and most specific mitochondrial poisons. In advanced lesions, debris fills the mitochondrial matrices, reduplication of membranes produces lamellar structures in the matrix, and lipids and protein lattices are usually present.

Dense matrix granules are associated with binding of calcium and other divalent cations that occur in cell swelling. Calcium (Ca^{++}) is bound organically to the granules and the number of Ca^{++} ions which accumulate during respiration-supported uptake bears a precise relationship to the number of energy-conserving sites traversed by electrons flowing down the respiratory chain (Greenwalt et al. 1964). Excessive calcium intake such as occurs in potassium deficiency (Heggtveit et al. 1964) may be manifested as an increased number and size of dense matrix granules. In extensive injuries, large deposits of mineral develop within the mitochondrion (D'Agostino 1964).

Shrinkage of mitochondria with fragmentation, dispersion, and lysis is seen in atrophy, hypoplasia, and some other disturbances in growth. In rapid, severe injury in which metabolic processes have not had sufficient time to alter structural elements, mitochondria may appear in this small "atrophic" form.

Several factors complicate the ultrastructural interpretation of pathologic mitochondria. (1) Mitochondria are extremely labile and, even with careful fixation techniques, artifacts are common. Often there is artifactual change which is accentuated because of pathologic swelling of the mitochondrion. (2) Mitochondrial structure is highly variable in normal cells. Mitochondria in liver cells have few cristae and abundant matrix; those in muscle have numerous cristae and little matrix. (There is a correlation between number of cristae and rate of respiration.) Mitochondria in actively secreting adrenal cortical cells are tubular or pear-shaped. (3) Mitochondria can vacillate between two basic conformational states depending upon the metabolic state. Orthodox configuration is the common form observed in intact cells. Granular matrix material fills the mitochondrion. It is alleged that energy transformation changes the membrane structure to the condensed configuration, characterized by contraction of the inner membrane accompanied by fluid in the intermembranous space. The matrix is homogeneous and markedly diminished in volume. The condensed state is rarely observed in situ, for it requires special fixation techniques. The correlation between mitochondrial structure and different energy states is amply demonstrated in vitro but is rarely seen in cells fixed in situ.

Structural changes in the inner membrane result from the reaction of isolated mitochondria in vitro and specific mitochondrial poisons. Bordetella endotoxin, for example, induces the transformation from the condensed to the orthodox configuration (Harris et al. 1968). These changes have not been demonstrated in vivo.

DNA filaments also occur in some mitochondria (Nass et al. 1965), but their significance in pathologic cells has not been demonstrated. It is alleged that mitochondria are self-replicating and, to some extent, independent of nuclear control. Mitochondrial DNA codes for the RNA component of the mitochondrial protein synthesizing system and its unique ribosomal strands.

CELLULAR GLYCOGEN AND BLOOD GLUCOSE

Glycogen is the storage form of glucose and exists free in the cytoplasmic matrix of the cell. It is a normal component of many cells; major deposits occur in liver, muscle, and kidney. Glycogen is best detected histologically with the periodic acid-Schiff stain (PAS). Control slides digested with diastase (ordinary saliva will do) must be used to rule out glycoproteins which also accept this stain. Diastase digests out the glycogen but not the more complex glycoproteins.

Ultrastructurally, three types of glycogen particles can be demonstrated. Alpha particles, or glycogen rosettes, are the visible morulae of 150 (50–200) nm. Beta particles are ovoid, 15–30 nm in diameter, and are called monoparticulate glycogen. When β-particles are broken down they are seen to be composed of elongate particles (3–20 nm in length) termed γ-particles (de Bruijn 1973; Drochmans 1962) (Fig. 2.22).

GLUCOSE-GLYCOGEN CONVERSIONS

The levels of blood glucose are maintained in the normal animal by dietary sources and by conversion of hepatocytic glycogen to glucose. In the liver, glucose is either converted to glycogen or glycogen is broken down to glucose for return to the bloodstream. Blood glucose is lowered by insulin and is raised by epinephrine, glucocorticoids, and glucagon.

INSULIN

Insulin, the secretion product of the pancreatic islet β-cell, depresses the critical

Fig. 2.22. Glycogen infiltration, liver. A. Histology. B. Glycogen-filled nucleus with "glycogen body" (arrow), hepatocyte, cow (Micrograph, I.M. Reid). C. Low-power micrograph of glycogen removal in prolonged glutaraldehyde fixation. D. High power of glycogen. Small aggregates of β-particles (arrow) form the α-rosettes. E. Glycogen (arrow) in hepatocyte of dog fixed in cold OsO_4. Note intrahepatic canaliculus (c) and mitochondria (m).

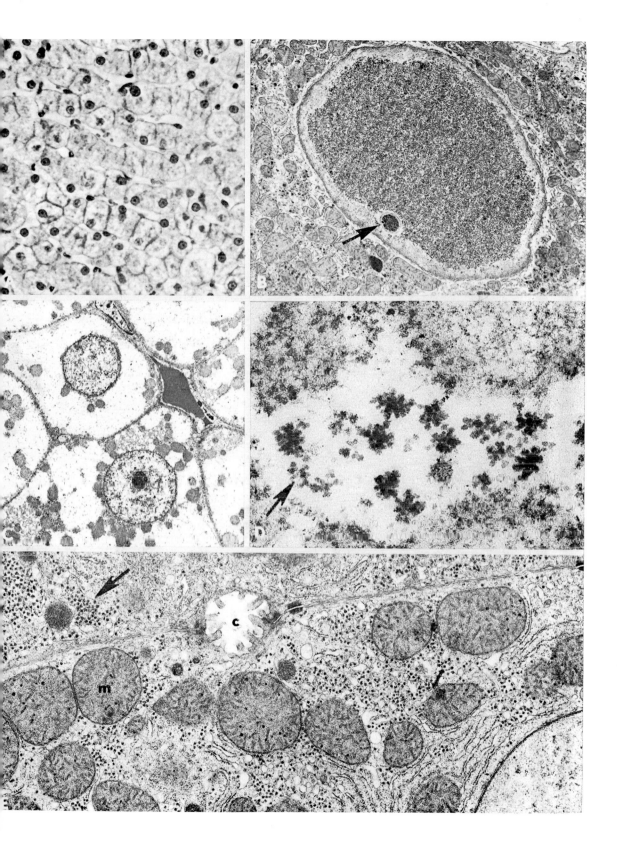

blood level for the entry and exit of glucose molecules into and out of the hepatocyte. That is, it acts as a "glucostat," setting the blood level at which the liver is to control plasma glucose. When there are high levels of both insulin and glucose in plasma (as after feeding), glucose rapidly enters the liver. When blood glucose becomes low in the face of high insulin levels, glucose exits from the hepatocyte with equal ease to produce normoglycemia.

Insulin binds to sites on the plasma membrane and markedly accelerates glucose transport. Flux of glucose across the plasma membrane of insulin-sensitive cells (adipocytes, hepatocytes, myocytes) occurs by passive transport and involves a carrier-mediated transport system. Insulin sensitivity is regulated by pituitary and adrenal hormones and other factors.

Within the glucose-consuming, insulin-sensitive cells, insulin also increases the rate of glucose transport and enhances utilization. It facilitates the entrance of glucose into the metabolic pool by stimulating phosphorylation of glucose molecules to glucose-6-phosphate and prevents the overproduction of glucose by inhibiting the action of glucose-6-phosphatase.

DIABETES MELLITUS

Diabetes mellitus is pathologic hyperglycemia, that is, the persistence of hyperglycemia during fasting. The excessive plasma glucose is eliminated by the kidney; glycosuria causes osmotic diuresis, polyuria, and polydipsia. Carbohydrate and lipid metabolism are abnormal and this leads to progressive emaciation and ketosis. In its total spectrum of pathologic metabolism, diabetes represents a set of complex syndromes of differing etiology but with one common denominator—hyperglycemia.

Naturally occurring diabetes in dogs is nearly always due to pancreatic islet β-cell destruction and resulting insulin deficiency. In diabetic dogs, insulin is undetectable in plasma by most assay techniques and does not increase after the stimulus of intravenous glucose infusion (Fig. 2.23). Glucose levels are high, for in the absence of insulin glucose cannot enter the hepatocyte. In rare cases, the islet β-cells are normal and diabetes results from the suppression of insulin activity by some nonpancreatic factor. Whatever the case, the pancreas is always involved in diabetes. If not as the primary cause (when β-cells are destroyed), the pancreas is affected secondarily by the elevated levels of blood glucose and has evidence of β-cell hyperplasia with exhaustion. In acute diabetes of dogs, however, vacuolation of β-cells is the classic and accepted lesion. The affected cells are devoid of β-granules and are filled with glycogen deposits and large, clear, membrane-bound vacuoles (Volk and Lazarus 1963).

PANCREATIC β-CELL TUMORS

The reverse situation develops in the presence of an *insulinoma*: a neoplasm of the pancreatic islet β-cell. Excess insulin is produced by the tumor cells and results in persistent hypoglycemia. The brain is most sensitive to the diminished blood levels of glucose and convulsions may occur. In tumor-bearing dogs, the convulsions are likely to occur in the early morning prior to feeding time; after eating, the production of hormones that promote elevations in blood glucose is stimulated (Capen and Martin 1969).

EPINEPHRINE AND OTHER HYPERGLYCEMIA-PRODUCING SUBSTANCES

Hyperglycemia results from the effects of epinephrine which activates latent hepatocyte phosphorylases to begin breakdown of the glycogen molecules. Factors such as excitement, convulsions, and other stresses will thereby tend to raise the blood glucose level. Hyperglycemia is also produced by glucagon and by the glucocorticoids. We will later study shock, in which a massive outpouring of adrenal corticoids develops in an effort to raise the drastically falling blood pressure. Hyperglycemia invariably accompanies this phase of the shock syndrome.

In adults, steady concentration of plasma glucose is maintained. Regulatory factors control production and release in the liver and the peripheral consumption by metabolizing cells. Normoglycemia is rapidly restored when glucose levels rise or fall to pathologic levels. The newborn animal has lower and more erratic plasma glucose levels. The control mechanisms have not

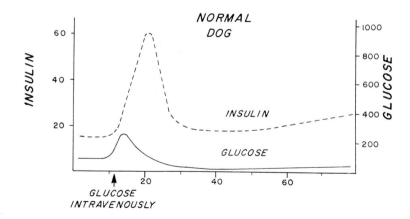

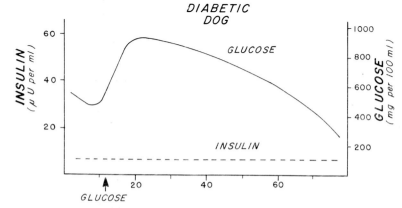

Fig. 2.23. Canine diabetes mellitus.

TIME IN MINUTES

developed sufficiently to deal with rapid changes in demands for glucose. The newborn of some species may be particularly prone to hypoglycemia because of a low glycogen content in the liver. This is true in pigs where signs of hyperglycemia (weakness, convulsions, and coma) develop when colostrum is withheld too long. In contrast, newborn chicks, lambs, calves, and foals usually resist starvation for several days.

GLYCOGENOLYSIS

Glycogenolysis, the degradation of glycogen to glucose, is the converse of glycogen formation and is the mechanism whereby blood glucose is replenished. In hepatocytes, it occurs in the cytoplasmic matrix. As molecules of glycogen are broken down, the α-particles disintegrate and disappear from the cell (Fig. 2.24).

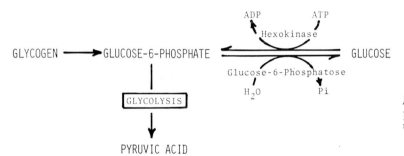

Fig. 2.24. Metabolic pathways of glycogen utilization.

Glycogenolysis in the normal animal is initiated by epinephrine which activates an inactive phosphorylase within the hepatocyte. A key role in regulating the speed of this reaction is played by cyclic-3'5'-adenosine monophosphate, more widely known as cyclic AMP (because the atoms in its phosphate group are arranged in a ring). Formation of cyclic AMP within the cell takes place when the plasma membrane–associated enzyme adenylate cyclase responds to the arrival of epinephrine. Epinephrine binds to sites on the hepatocyte plasma membrane where adenylate cyclase is located and increases the activity of this enzyme. Adenylate cyclase transforms the molecules of ATP, which are located on the inner side of the plasma membrane, into cyclic AMP (cAMP), which then diffuses throughout the cell, acting as a second messenger to convert glycogen to glucose.

Glycogen is degraded within lysosomes in several pathologic conditions. This especially occurs when glycogen is present in large amounts and when the glycogenolytic stimulus is intense. *Glycogenosomes* are large, membrane-bound aggregates of glycogen. They stain for acid phosphatase and are, by this definition, autolysosomes (Becker and Cornwall 1971; Kotoulas et al. 1971; Pfeifer 1972; Phillips et al. 1967).

Glucagon initiates breakdown of glycogen by causing lysosomes to become fragile and to increase in size. The glycogenosomes that develop provide for the rapid degradation of glycogen molecules (Deter and De Duve 1967).

TOXIC GLYCOGENOLYSIS

Depletion of tissue of glycogen and high levels of glycemia and glycosuria are characteristic of some intoxications. In clostridial enterotoxemia of lambs, extremely rapid hepatic glycogenolysis occurs. The mechanism involves the rapid mobilization of glycogen due to a lysosomal response to anaerobiasis. The severe endothelial cell destruction caused by the clostridial epsilon toxin is responsible for reduced transendothelial transfer between vascular lumen and hepatocyte with resultant stimulation of catabolic activity and breakdown of glycogen molecules (Gardner 1973).

Epinephrine and glucagon secretion play little role in this type of toxic glycogenolysis.

GLYCOGEN INFILTRATION

Glycogen infiltration is the abnormal accumulation of glycogen in cells. It is nearly always a reflection of hyperglycemia (blood glucose above normal) and is a common finding in diabetes mellitis. Glycogen infiltration is reversible and with control of hyperglycemia the glycogen content of cells returns to normal.

Glycogen is normally present in liver cells, usually as a-rosettes (in muscle, glycogen is generally monoparticulate). It is the function of liver glycogen to replace blood glucose, and glycogen is rapidly removed from hepatocytes under the influence of epinephrine. Glycogen disappears in starving, fasting, and cachectic animals and reappears when feed is given (Ericsson 1966). Blockade of glucose metabolism may be induced by feeding glucose analogs. Glycogenolysis is increased and as the analog accumulates in the cell, its utilization is blocked. The presence of excess analog leads to overhydration and rarefaction of the cytoplasm (Rosa 1971; Yu and Phillips 1971).

In the kidney, glycogen infiltration reflects excessive resorption of glucose from the glomerular filtrate (Maunsbach et al. 1962). Hyperglycemia results in spill of glucose into the glomerular filtrate and glycosuria. The proximal convoluted tubules are affected, for these are the nephron segments involved in glucose absorption. In diabetes mellitus, large glycogenosomes occur in these tubule cells (Orci and Stauffacher 1971). Under renal disease we will examine the experimental administration of sucrose intravenously, which produces vacuolar lesions in the kidney in which large amounts of glycogen accumulate ("sucrose nephrosis").

Glycogen occasionally is seen in nuclei which are swollen and vacuolated. Intranuclear glycogen occurs in hepatocyte nuclei during diabetes mellitus of dogs and in the livers of aged ruminants in which the cause is not known (Rajya and Rubarth 1967). Ultrastructural examination of affected bovine livers reveals large aggregates of β-particles in the nuclear inclusions of glycogen (Reid 1973b). Intranuclear glycogen also is seen in neoplastic cells (Weiss 1965) and appears to be synthesized in situ in the interchromatin regions of the nucleus (Karasaki 1971).

Small deposits of glycogen have been reported within mitochondria and other cellular organelles. Glycogen has even been described as being incorporated into viral particles as they bud from the plasma membrane (Kajima and Majde 1970).

GLYCOGEN STORAGE DISEASE

Glycogen storage diseases have been described in man and some animals. They involve the inability to process carbohydrates intracellularly by virtue of a genetic deficiency in the production of specific enzymes. Glucose-6-phosphatase and the glucosidases are among those enzymes known to be deficient. Lesions are characterized by the accumulation of massive amounts of normal-appearing glycogen in the cytosol of the cell and in the cytocavitary system (Baudhuin et al. 1964; Garancis et al. 1970; Reed et al. 1968; Sheldon et al. 1962). Glycogenosis of the central nervous system has been reported in the cat (Sandström et al. 1969). The cytopathology consists of large membrane-bound aggregates of glycogen rosettes in neurons and resembles Pompe's disease in man.

Abnormal, low-molecular weight glycogen has been reported in a generalized storage disease in man. The lucent aggregates of small fibrils are massed together among normal-appearing glycogen rosettes in the cytoplasm (Krivit et al. 1973).

CELL DEGENERATION INVOLVING LIPIDS

Normal adult adipose cells contain a single large locule of lipid (Cushman 1970; Napolitano 1963). The triglycerides that make up the adipocyte locule are formed from free fatty acids as they enter the cell. During lipolysis, triglycerides are again converted to fatty acids which leave the cell. The continuous deposition and mobilization of adipose cell triglycerides provide an important storage and utilization system for energy. Plasma fatty acids are deposited in or removed from adipose cells under various influences including blood lipid levels and genetic and endocrine factors. Insulin is known to stimulate triglyceride synthesis.

LIPID MOBILIZATION

Lipolysis is the derivation of free fatty acids from adipose cell triglycerides. It is promoted during starvation, short periods of fasting, and acute stress involving adrenal gland secretion. Within the cell, cyclic AMP is the chemical messenger that initiates and regulates the breakdown of stored triglycerides. In response to several hormonal stimuli (chiefly epinephrine and corticosteroids) the level of cyclic AMP rises in the adipose cell. This activates a kinase which in turn activates triglyceride lipase. The lipase then degrades the stored triglycerides into fatty acids. The adipose cell atrophies by the gradual segregation of the lipid locule into globules and eventually returns to a more primitive mesenchymal type.

Epinephrine is a potent lipid mobilizer and injection of this drug is accompanied by an increase of free fatty acids in the plasma. Lipolysis is also influenced by the sympathetic nervous system; when sympathetic nervous activity increases (due to stress, cold, emotional arousal, trauma, etc.), plasma lipids increase. Conversely, denervation of fat increases the adipose cell mass (Fredholm 1970).

ADIPOSE CELL TYPES

White adipose cells function chiefly as sites of lipid storage. They also provide insulation for muscle and viscera. The white adipose cells arise in the fetus from undifferentiated mesenchymal cells in which small lipid globules develop and coalesce (Wensvoort 1968). In contrast to these cells, *brown fat cells* function as heat generators. These large mitochondria-rich cells are present in fetuses, neonates, and in hibernating and cold-acclimated adults. They contain multiple, tiny lipid globules and small concentrated mitochondria (Suter 1969). The thermogenic role of brown fat cells is important as a protective mechanism in situations involving hypothermia (Heaton 1973).

CYTOLOGIC DETECTION OF LIPIDS

Solvents used in routine histologic techniques dissolve out fats, leaving clear spaces. To distinguish lipids from the clear spaces of hydropic or glycogen deposits, special techniques are used to detect fat: (1) osmic acid oxidizes unsaturated fats to black insoluble material and can be used in paraffin sections; (2) Sudan III and oil red O stain neutral fats (but require frozen sections); (3) polarized light is rotated by cholesterol and lecithins and the characteristic patterns of light transmission can be diagnostic; and (4) melting point determination on warmed microscope stages reveals characteristics of individual lipids. Cell lipids processed for ultrastructural studies with osmium remain intact. Lipoids such as cholesterol leave characteristic cleftlike spaces called "cholesterol clefts."

LIPIDS IN PLASMA

The four major chemical components of plasma lipids are cholesterol, cholesterol esters, triglycerides, and phospholipids. These are not soluble in aqueous solutions and in plasma they are not in free form but are bound to carrier proteins.

The heterogeneous macromolecules that result from this lipid-peptide association are called lipoproteins and have been classified into four families:

(1) *Chylomicrons* are of dietary origin and consist of over 90% triglycerides and very little cholesterol. They are present in plasma from 2–10 hrs after feeding but are normally absent in 10–15 hrs in most species.

(2) *Very low density lipoproteins* (pre-β-lipoproteins) are also triglyceride-rich with a triglyceride-cholesterol ratio of approximately 5:1.

(3) *Low density lipoproteins* (β-lipoproteins) are cholesterol-rich and triglyceride-poor. They are elevated in hypercholesteremia.

(4) *High density lipoproteins* (α-lipoproteins) are protein-rich and lipid-poor.

These classes are based upon electrophoretic migration and ultracentrifugation. For example, chylomicrons remain at the point of origin on paper or gel electrophoresis and float at a density of 0.95 in the ultracentrifuge. At the other extreme, the high density lipoproteins display greater alpha electrophoretic migration and float at a density of 1.06–1.20.

An absorptive lipemia occurs after feeding. In the intestinal lumen, dietary fat is fragmented by the detergent action of bile acids and by esterases and lipases in intestinal and pancreatic secretions. It is then taken up by intestinal obsorptive cells and complexed with protein, thus entering the bloodstream via the thoracic duct as chylomicrons. Smaller amounts of fatty acids enter the blood directly via the portal vein.

Chylomicronemia (hyperglyceridemia or elevation of neutral fats) is common after a fatty meal. In some animals such as cats, lipuria may result. In the liver or adipose tissue, chylomicrons pass through endothelial cells via the cytocavitary system where they are acted on by lipolytic lipases (Blanchette-Mackie and Scow 1971). The resulting lipids are extruded into the interstitial spaces and rapidly taken up by adipose cells or by hepatocytes (Stein and Stein 1967).

Many pathologic alterations in blood lipids are best analyzed by examining the lipoproteins. Factors influencing lipid levels of individuals include dietary lipids, age, energy requirements, endocrine balance, and time since last feeding. In starving and fasting animals, blood lipids are elevated. In chronic infectious diseases, such as tuberculosis, blood lipids are also altered.

LIPIDS IN THE HEPATOCYTE

Hepatocytes take up free fatty acids (Fig. 2.25). Fatty acids are esterified to triglycerides which appear in the cisternae of the endoplasmic reticulum as small (60–120 nm), lightly osmiophilic *liposomes* (Fig. 2.26). Liposomes are chemically heterogeneous for they incorporate phospholipids, cholesterol, and protein in the endoplasmic reticulum. They emerge (probably via the Golgi complex) as low density lipoproteins (Baglio and Farber 1965; Hamilton et al. 1967; Mahley et al. 1968; Schlunk and Lombardi 1971). Cholesterol, which enters the blood from the intestine, associates with chylomicrons and deposits in the liver. Here it takes advantage of the unique

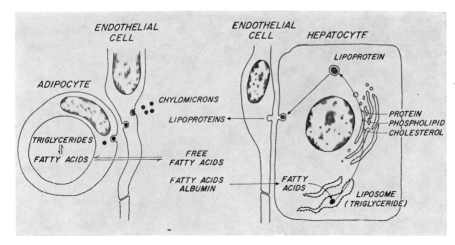

Fig. 2.25. Metabolic pathways of lipids. Triglycerides stored in adipose cells are constantly being mobilized and deposited.

capacity of hepatocytes to degrade sterol to bile acids, which are then excreted.

CLASSIFICATION OF ABNORMAL LIPID ACCUMULATION

Cellular changes involving lipids can be somewhat arbitrarily divided into four patterns of alteration: (1) *fat infiltration*, normal adipose cells in abnormal sites; (2) *fatty degeneration*, accumulation of lipids in cells which metabolize them normally but which have been damaged in some way; (3) *cytolipodystrophy*, paralysis of the lysosomal system by lipids which the cell cannot process by virtue of lacking appropriate lipases; and (4) *fat atrophy*.

FAT INFILTRATION

Fat infiltration (or stromal infiltration of fat) is the appearance of normal adipose cells (adipocytes) in the interstitium of organs not normally containing them. It occurs chiefly in the connective tissues of heart, pancreas, skeletal muscles, and lymph nodes (Fig. 2.26). In the heart, for example, the accumulation of adipose cells may extend through the wall, producing small deposits below the endocardium which can be seen grossly. Fat infiltration does not usually affect function. It is most common in aged and obese animals and probably reflects the incapacity of aging mesenchymal cells to deal with circulating lipids. It bears no causal relationship to fatty degeneration even though these may occur together.

"Fatty infiltration" was used by Virchow in a pathogenetic sense to differentiate the abnormal intracellular accumulation of fat in previously healthy cells (as a result of systemic metabolic derangements) from accumulation in injured cells. These are both properly considered fatty degeneration. The fatty liver of the market steer and the rat with experimental hypothalamic lesions and voracious appetite were considered examples of the overloading of otherwise healthy cells. This distinction is not useful, for it artificially divides the processes of fatty degeneration and leads to false interpretation of the pathogenesis of the lesion.

FATTY DEGENERATION

Fatty degeneration is the abnormal appearance of visible fat (of normal molecular structure) in the cell. Most degenerating cells contain lipid globules in the cytoplasmic matrix and, while this is technically fatty degeneration, the term is usually applied to massive accumulations that distort the cell (Fig. 2.27). Fatty degeneration is commonly seen in cells that normally metabolize lipids, those of the liver, kidney, and heart. Affected organs are soft, flabby, and friable, with a yellow mottled appearance.

Microscopically, the distribution and size of lipid globules is a reliable index of injury. Most of the lipids are present as globules of triglycerides or neutral lipids. They are not membrane-bound but exist free within the cytoplasmic matrix due to

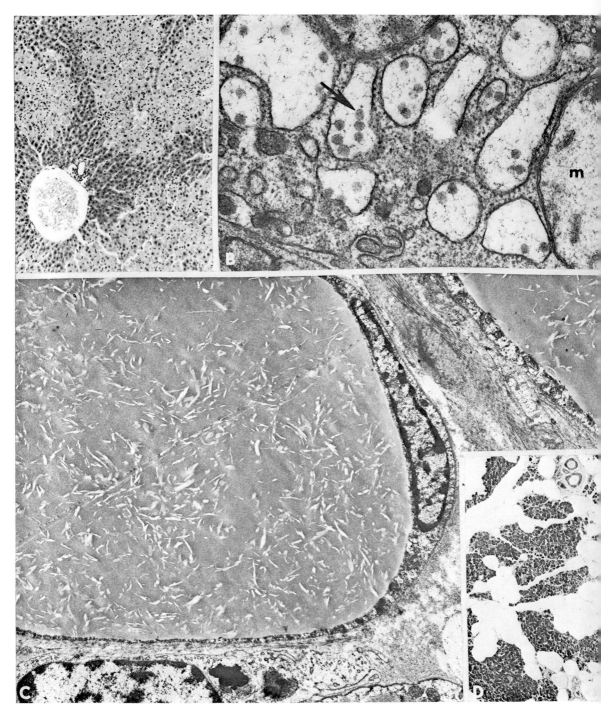

Fig. 2.26. Fatty changes. A. Acute carbon tetrachloride poisoning, mouse. Centrolobular necrosis with islands of viable cells around portal triads. B. Ultrastructure of viable cells with accumulation of liposomes (arrow) in endoplasmic reticulum cisternae and degeneration of mitochondria (m). C. Large lipid locule of triglycerides in fat infiltration of pancreatic stroma, aged dog. D. Histology of C.

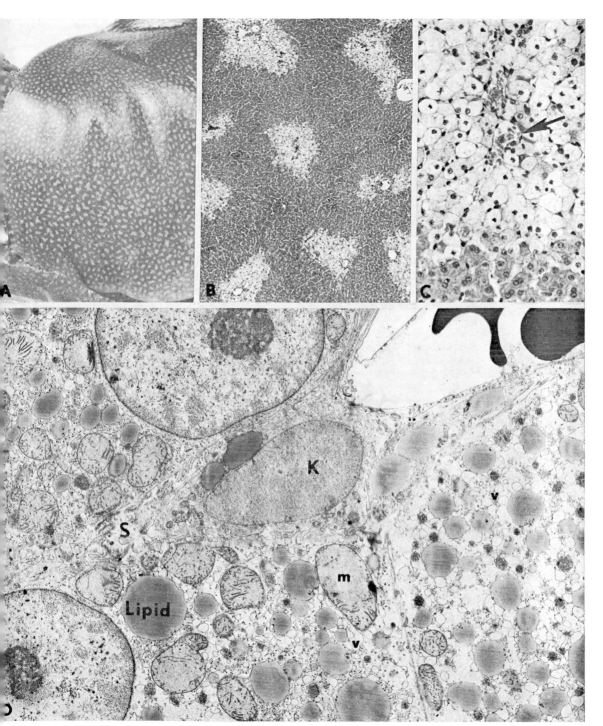

Fig. 2.27. Fatty degeneration, liver, dog with diabetes mellitus.
A. Gross appearance. B. and C. Histology. Central vein (arrow). D.
Ultrastructure. Mitochondria (m) are swollen and distorted,
Kupffer cells (K) also contain lipid globules. Nuclei are normal.
Globules dominate cytoplasm and glycogen is absent. Smooth
endoplasmic reticulum is fragmented and vesicular (v). Cytoplasmic
matrix is rarified. Sinus (S).

high surface tension of the external phospholipid monolayer surrounding the lipid. There is a close association of lipid globules and proliferating smooth endoplasmic reticulum, a process that has been called "paralipic topolysis." In severe fatty degeneration, lipid globules pass into the nucleus, probably through connections between the cytocavitary network and nuclear pores (Karasaki 1973).

Imbalance between supply, utilization, and synthesis of lipids by the cell results in fatty degeneration. Excessive fat-mobilizing lipolysis occurs when there is increased usage of fat for energy. This is common in defective carbohydrate utilization: during starvation and in diabetes. Lipids in adipose cells are degraded and excess fatty acids are delivered to the liver. Within hepatocytes, triglycerides may accumulate due to depletion of phospholipids required for synthesis of lipoproteins. Excess dietary fat with increased numbers of chylomicrons can cause fatty livers by much the same mechanism.

Choline is a lipotrophic factor necessary for the metabolism of triglycerides. Choline deficiency interferes with phospholipid synthesis and there are formation of abnormal lipoproteins and accumulation of triglycerides. The impaired release of low density lipoproteins is responsible for the accumulation of liposomes (Lombardi 1966).

Specific metabolic injuries to the metabolic flow of lipid intracellularly have been studied in hepatocytes and provide insight into mechanisms involving fatty degeneration. Direct mitochondrial injury, for example, results in decreased fatty acid oxidation with increases in the fatty acid pool and accumulation of triglycerides. Most models used in the study of fatty degeneration involve blockade in the conversion of triglycerides to lipoprotein within the endoplasmic reticulum.

MECHANISMS OF FATTY DEGENERATION

Here we investigate several models of liver cell damage that relate to naturally occurring liver disease. They produce their injury in the hepatocytes at different sites in the metabolic pathways. Carbon tetrachloride causes lipoperoxidation on membranes of the endoplasmic reticulum. Ethanol intoxication causes multiple de-

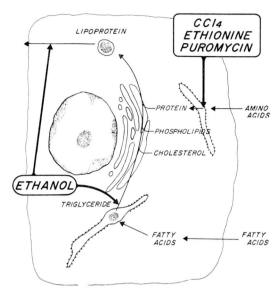

Fig. 2.28. Hepatocyte toxicity: sites of action of ethanol, carbon tetrachloride, ethionine, and puromycin.

fects in lipid metabolic pathways. Aflatoxin depresses RNA-polymerase-directed protein synthesis (Fig. 2.28). Despite these simplistic statements regarding mechanisms, all of the hepatotoxins produce destructive secondary changes in liver cells that tend to alter cell morphology progressively if the animal survives.

Hepatocellular damage is affected by molecular size and accessibility of a toxin to the liver cell. For example, the potent toxins of the poisonous Amanita toadstools readily cause hepatocyte necrosis, but leave the Kupffer cells and bile ductules intact. If the toxin is conjugated to albumin experimentally (resulting in much larger macromolecules) and then administered, the necrotic reactions begin in the sinusoid-lining Kupffer cells. Toxicity is markedly enhanced because the toxin is much more slowly eliminated in the renal glomerulus (Derenzini et al. 1973).

Carbon tetrachloride (CCl_4) poisoning occurs as a result of accidental ingestion of this solvent or when pets are left in airtight rooms where it has been used to clean upholstery or clothing. Acute necrosis of the liver is the result. The rough endoplasmic reticulum is the primary target of CCl_4. The free radicals of CCl_4 initiate lipoperoxidation of the endoplasmic reticulum membranes, inhibit protein synthesis, and depress enzyme activity. Structurally, one sees dilatation, loss of ribosomes, and fragmentation of the membrane into vesicles. In the final manifestation of necrosis, several related phenomena are critical. Triglycerides accumulate progressively as a consequence of failure to synthesize the lipoprotein moieties required to form lipoprotein. Triglycerides become inspissated in liposomes (Fig. 2.26) and globules of neutral lipids develop in the cytoplasmic matrix. Experimentally, if lipoperoxidation is prevented with antioxidants such as sulfaguanidine, liver damage from CCl_4 does not occur (Leduc 1973).

Excessive and chronic ingestion of alcohol in humans is associated with derangements in liver structure and function. The principal manifestation of toxicity is the accumulation of lipids in the liver. Hepatocytes are engorged with globules of neutral lipids and liposomes. Long-term alcohol consumption leads to cirrhosis and clinical evidence of liver disease.

Alcohol is absorbed from the anterior gastrointestinal tract and immediately metabolized in the liver. The conversion of alcohol to acetaldehyde, which is catalyzed by the liver enzyme alcohol dehydrogenase, rapidly removes alcohol from the blood. Acetaldehyde is further oxidized to acetate and then to the key intermediate acetyl CoA. At low blood levels (<10 mg/100 ml) the oxidizing enzyme alcohol dehydrogenase is not saturated with substrate and the alcohol-disappearance curve is exponential; at high levels, the oxidizing enzyme is saturated and the disappearance curve is linear (Isselbacher and Greenberger 1964). The action of alcohol dehydrogenase appears to be adaptive; that is, after prolonged intake of alcohol, levels of enzyme in the liver are elevated and the oxidation of substrate appears to be more efficient. Conversely, in severe parenchymal disease of the liver, enzyme levels are diminished and the susceptibility to alcohol toxicity is greater.

Alcohol has many effects on the hepatocyte (Fig. 2.28). Some are observed in acute toxicity, others in chronic toxicity. Some are direct (or toxic) and others are indirect, the result of overload of metabolic pathways. One of the most pronounced effects of alcohol is on the metabolism of lipids. It exerts direct and indirect effects on five major mechanisms: (1) increases in mobilization of fatty acids from peripheral adipose cells, (2) increased fatty acid synthesis by hepatocytes, (3) decreased utilization or oxidation of fatty acids, (4) increased esterification of fatty acids to triglycerides, and (5) decreased release of fat from the hepatocyte. There is no definitive answer on the relative importance of these mechanisms in alcohol toxicity but it is clear that in acute intoxication the mobilization of free fatty acids from adipose cells is a major mechanism. In contrast, in chronic alcohol intoxication increased esterification and decreased release of fat are quantitatively more important. In chronic intoxication, levels of plasma lipids are altered. In early phases the plasma triglycerides are increased, but later phases are characterized by decreasing levels of triglycerides which accompany increases of plasma free fatty acids.

When laboratory animals are poisoned experimentally with alcohol, one of the early ultrastructural changes is found in the endoplasmic reticulum. This organelle dilates, loses its ribosomes, and becomes fragmented (Iseri et al. 1966). Depressions in protein synthesis are detectable biochemically and correlate with this structural change.

Increasing structural and biochemical evidence has accumulated that chronic ethanol ingestion causes damage to mitochondrial membranes of hepatocytes in both humans and animals (Rubin et al. 1970; Svoboda et al. 1966). The alterations are a direct effect of ethanol consumption and not caused by deficiency of nutrition factors.

Nutritional deficiencies may be a complicating factor, but are not necessary for liver lesions to develop. In monkeys, fatty livers have been produced on a diet where 41% of calories were derived from alcohol (control animals which had 41% contributed by sucrose did not have lesions). Addition of choline did not prevent fatty degeneration, indicating that ethanol was solely responsible (Ruebner et al. 1972).

The aflatoxins are a group of hepatotoxic metabolites produced by certain strains of *Aspergillus flavus*. They are synthesized during growth of the fungus in feedstuffs and they poison animals when these feeds are ingested. Aflatoxins were first isolated from peanut (groundnut) meal that had been associated with ill-defined intoxications of trout, turkeys, pigs, and cattle. It is now known that most animals are susceptible and that the liver lesions depend upon the dosage and chronicity of exposure. Among the most susceptible animals are ducklings, dogs, and swine.

The primary effect of aflatoxin is on the liver where it causes, in most species, hepatocyte necrosis, fibrosis, and bile duct reduplication. Hepatomas occur in trout and hepatocarcinomas in rats when these species are placed on chronic feeding experiments.

Four major toxins (B_1, B_2, G_1, and G_2) have been identified by their chromatographic mobility and fluorescence under ultraviolet light. B_1 is the most toxic and has been widely used in experimental studies of aflatoxicosis. An accurate diagnosis includes the demonstration of the aflatoxin in the feed and urine of the intoxicated animal. Day-old ducklings are exquisitely sensitive to aflatoxin and are used for bioassay. The oral 7-day LD_{50} for aflatoxins in ducklings is (in μg): B_1, 18.2; B_2, 84.8; G_1, 39.2; and G_2, 172.5.

The site of action of aflatoxin is the nucleolus. There is a direct toxic effect on DNA-dependent RNA polymerase which in turn suppresses activity of RNA and protein synthesis. This action resembles the toxicity of actinomycin D. Ultrastructurally, disaggregation of the nucleolus can be detected soon after treatment with aflatoxin. The appearance of numerous helical polysomes has been reported within a few minutes of injection and these have been hypothesized to be a special type of transient transfer RNA (Bernhard et al. 1965; Monneron 1969; Svoboda et al. 1966).

DNA synthesis is affected by the affinity of aflatoxin to bind to the DNA molecule. Demonstrated in cell cultures, this inhibition allows cell survival at a nondividing stage but results in sporadic cytomegaly. Giant cells may be seen in livers of intoxicated animals (Svoboda et al. 1971). The inhibition of mitosis and nucleic acid synthesis is reflected in diminished incorporation of labeled precursors into cell DNA and proteins.

LIPODYSTROPHY

Cellular lipodystrophy results from the accumulation of abnormal lipid molecules within the cytoplasm. Lipid aggregates form because of paralysis of the enzymatic machinery involved in lipid metabolism. They may amass within parenchymal cells due to a primary enzyme deficit or within macrophages when these cells take up lipid debris. Large, foamy, fat-staining cells are the hallmark of this type of cellular change.

Ultrastructurally, the cytoplasm is filled with massive osmiophilic phagolysosomes or autophagosomes that distort the cell. The internal structure of these bodies varies from homogeneous material to dense aggregates of membranes. Differences in appearance depend upon the nature of the lipid and on the enzyme capacity of the lysosomes in the affected cell.

Cytolipidosis is seen in a wide variety of diseases where excessive or abnormal lipid accumulations cannot be processed by macrophages. Many of these are metabolic diseases and the type of lipid involved is not precisely known (Table 2.5). Lipids may accumulate at local sites or may be deposited within the reticuloendothelial system during hyperlipidemia.

The *genetic lipodystrophies* include a variety of rare diseases characterized by the accumulation of abnormal lipid complexes, usually within the nervous system. They have been described chiefly in dogs and cats and are important as models of the more widely studied human counterparts. The chemical nature of the abnormal lipids in animal diseases largely remains undefined, although it holds the key to the enzyme deficit responsible. Tay-Sachs disease of children is a neuronal lipodystrophy secondary to storage of gangliosides. There is absence or severe deficiency of a specific lysosomal glycohydrolase (hexosaminidase) which results in accumulation in the cytoplasm of gangliosides (O'Brien 1973).

Cytolipidosis commonly affects macrophages in tissue containing lipid debris. This change is an integral part of demyelination of the nervous system. Myelin sheaths unravel and are ultimately phagocytized. Large swollen macrophages, called

Table 2.5. Cell storage diseases

Deposit	Enzyme Defect	Site	Animal	Reference
Ganglioside GM$_1$	β-galactosidase	Neuron	Man Cow Cat	Donnelly, *J. Path.* 111:173, 1973 Blakemore, *J. Comp. Path.* 82:179, 1972 Farrell, *J. Neuropath. Exp. Neurol.* 32.1, 1973
GM$_2$	Hexosaminidase	Neuron	Man (Tay-Sachs dis.)	O'Brien, *Fed. Proc.* 32:191, 1973
Unknown	?	Neuron	Dog Cat Pig Cow	Bernheimer, *Acta Neuropath.* 16:243, 1970 Percy, *Arch. Path.* 92:136, 1971 Read, *Vet. Path.* 5:67, 1968 Read, *Vet. Path.* 6:235, 1969
Sphingomyelin	Sphingomyelinase	Macrophage	Man (Niemann-Pick dis.)	
Glucocerebroside	β-glucosidase	Macrophage	Man (Gaucher's dis.) Dog	Hartely, *Vet. Path.* 10:191, 1973
Galactocerebroside	β-galactosidase	Macrophage	Dog (globoid cell leukodystrophy) Man (Krabb's dis.)	Fletcher, *Am. J. Vet. Res.* 32:177, 1971 Suzuki, *Lab. Invest.* 23:612, 1970 Yunis, *Lab. Invest.* 21:415, 1969
Ceramide trihexoside	Ceremide trihexoside-cleaving enzyme	Vascular wall & endothelium	Man (Fabry's dis.)	Bagdade, *Lab. Invest.* 18:681, 1968
Glycoprotein	?	Neuron	Dog Man (Lafora's dis.)	Holland, *Am. J. Path.* 58:509, 1970
Oligosaccharide (mannose + glucosamine)	α-mannosidase	Neuron	Cow (pseudolipidosis)	Jolly, *Am. J. Path.* 74:211, 1973
Lipofuscin	?	Neuron	Dog (canine lipofuscinosis) Man	Patel, *Lab. Invest.* 30:366, 1974 Koppang, *J. Sm. An. Proc.* 10:369, 1970
Uncharacterized lipids	?	Vascular wall & macrophages	Man Dog Parakeet	Ferrans, *Am. J. Path.* 64:67, 1971 Leav, *Lab. Invest.* 18:433, 1968
Glycogen	?	Neurons & myocytes	Cat Dog Sheep	Sandstrom et al. *Acta Neuropath.* 14:196, 1969 Mostafa, *Acta Vet. Scand.* 11:197, 1970 Manktelow, *J. Comp. Path.* 85:139, 1975

Gitter cells, become filled with membrane-bound collections of dense myelin membranes (Lampert 1967; O'Daly 1967).

GLYCOLIPIDOSES

Glycolipids accumulate in cells in some familial diseases involving specific enzyme defects. Progressive neuronal glycoproteinosis occurs in dogs (Holland 1970) and its counterpart in humans is progressive familial myoclonus epilepsy (LaFora's disease). The neurologic dysfunction is due to accumulation in the neuronal cytoplasm of PAS-staining inclusions which have a dense core and are surrounded by a fibrillar periphery. Inclusions do not stain for glycogen, lipids, minerals, or nucleic acids.

FAT ATROPHY

When lipid mobilization is excessive and extended over long periods, lipolysis induces characteristic changes in adipose tissue. These lesions are commonly present in starving hypoproteinemic animals, particularly in the very young and very old. Fat around the coronary band of the heart is prominently affected (Oksanen and Osborn 1972). The watery and translucent appearance of atrophic fat in affected animals is responsible for the term "serous atrophy of fat."

Microscopically, lipid locules of the adipose cell break up and decrease in size when fat undergoes atrophy (Slavin 1972; Williamson 1964). Ultrastructural changes in adipose cells during starvation include marked irregularities in the cell surface with increases in pseudopodial projections and pinocytotic vesicles (Napolitano 1963). There is an increase in the basement membrane material of the surface lamina which becomes irregular and evaginated (Fig. 2.29). Increase in the smooth endoplasmic reticulum and development of autophagosomes also occur.

Significant changes occur in the interstitium of adipose tissue in starving animals. Large mesenchymal cells appear that actively synthesize and release large amounts of collagen and basement membrane material. Acid mucopolysaccharides are deposited and the interstitium stains intensely with alcian blue and the Hale procedure.

CYTOPLASMIC INCLUSIONS

During the examination of pathologic tissues, one commonly encounters large masses within abnormal cells which are not present in their normal counterparts. Pathologists are trained to recognize and differentiate these bodies in making an etiologic diagnosis.

The identification of inclusions is particularly helpful in viral infections where virion-bearing bodies tend to have characteristic stain affinities. By utilizing the Feulgen (for DNA) and acridine orange (for single- versus double-stranded nucleic acids) techniques, inclusion bodies can be identified histochemically as containing DNA and RNA. Viral inclusions can be specifically identified with the use of immunologic reagents such as fluorescent antibody techniques which can be applied to tissue sections. Ultrastructural examination, in most cases, unequivocally identifies the type of virus involved.

Many inclusion bodies consist of the aberrant formation of protein fibers or membranes which accumulate in the cell. Small strands of protein fibrils are common in injured cells and are usually distributed in a random, haphazard manner. Some of these fibers represent distinctly abnormal, reduplicating proteins (see amyloid). In most cases, however, the origin is unknown.

Crystalline protein inclusions are seen in (otherwise) normal cells of the liver, gonads, and kidneys of many species. They occur within cell organelles or free in the nucleoplasm or cytoplasmic matrix. The specific protein is rarely identified.

Protein-lattice inclusion bodies more commonly occur in abnormal cells and may form large, regular rhomboid structures (Fig. 2.30). Protein is laid down in repeating units and the inclusions have a linear structure with defined periodicity. Lattice-protein bodies are found in viral infections, metabolic diseases (Kjaerheim 1971), and as incidental, nonspecific changes in degenerating cells. They are particularly common in cells that normally contain fibers, such as myocytes and neurons (Masurovsky et al. 1970; Schochet et al. 1968; Seite et al. 1971). Large rhomboids of unknown origin are common in the nuclei of hepatocytes

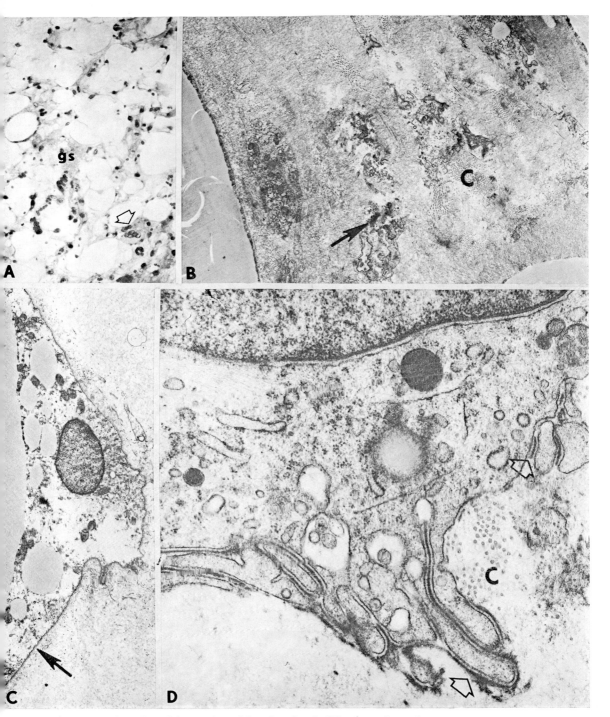

Fig. 2.29. Atrophy of fat, malnutrition in pig. A. Histology. Irregular adipose cells are interspersed with deposits of ground substance (gs) and plasma protein precipitates. Multinuclear cells (arrow). B. Ultrastructure. Ground substance between adipose cells contains collagen (C), granular deposits of acidic mucopolysaccharides and fibrin (arrow). C. Margin of adipose cell with breakdown of locule into small globules. Cell surface is surrounded by basement membrane (arrow). Granular precipitates in interstitial space. D. Mesenchymal cell with marked convolutions of the plasma membrane and reduplication of basement membrane material (arrow).

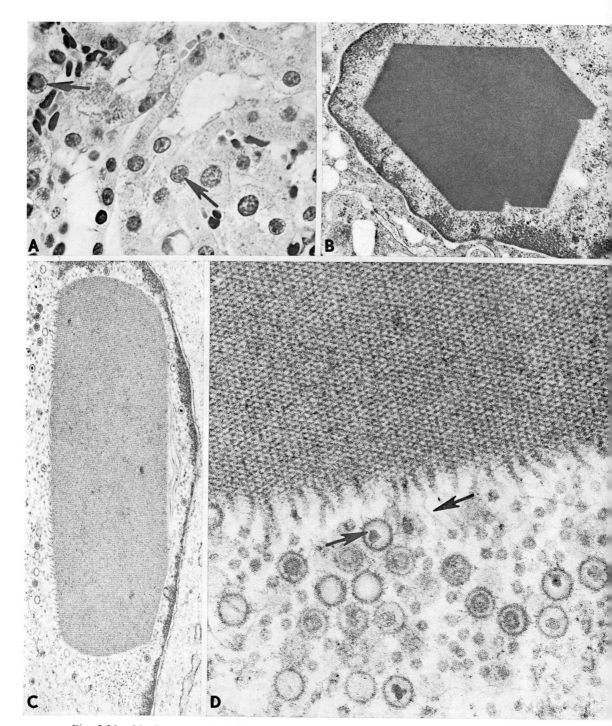

Fig. 2.30. Nuclear protein inclusions. A. Lead poisoning, renal tubule cell. Large amorphous lead-histone complexes (arrow). B. Protein filaments in crystal form, hepatocyte, aged dog. C. Protein crystal formed of helices of viral-induced ribonucleoprotein (bovine herpesvirus). Naked virions surround periphery. D. DNA strands (arrows) at forming edge of crystal and within immature virions (Micrograph, A. D. Boothe).

of aged dogs and have been seen in the cytoplasm of human liver cells.

HYALIN

"Hyalin degeneration" is a term used by light microscopists in reference to dense, amorphous, eosinophilic material. These heterogeneous changes have in common only the presence of uniform, structureless, proteinaceous material called hyalin. The term describes only physical appearance as seen by light microscopy and is not related to chemical composition or to a specific pattern of degeneration. Implicit in these lesions is the lifeless nature of the substances involved; that is, there has been a physical change in cells or their products whereby they have lost their identity and fused into a structureless, homogeneous mass.

The term hyalin is applied to intracellular and extracellular material. Hyalin substances located extracellularly may be specifically identified as: (1) collagen ("connective tissue" hyalin) in scars and tumors; (2) basement membrane reduplication in arteriosclerosis, renal glomerulosclerosis, and many subepithelial lesions; (3) plasma protein inspissation—albumin casts in renal tubules; and (4) amyloid.

MUCOSUBSTANCES

Mucosubstances (or mucin) are produced in excess in some mesenchymal tissues that undergo degenerative changes. Large amounts of glassy, homogeneous mucopolysaccharide-containing material, which stains intensely with the metachromatic stains toluidine blue and alcian blue, develop in the ground substance of the connective tissues. Ultrastructurally, mucosubstances appear as irregular foci of small granular material. We have already seen mucoid degeneration as a component of adipose atrophy (Fig. 2.29). It is also commonly seen in the prefibroplasia phases of inflammation and occurs in degeneration of mesenchymal cells in the skin, renal medulla, heart valves, and muscular arteries.

In some instances of mucoid degeneration, there is a definite connection with changes in the endocrine system. Two striking examples where mucosubstances are deposited are the "sex skin" of female monkeys that develops during estrus and the subcutis of animals with severe thyroid deficiency ("myxedema"). The connective tissues are greatly expanded by the deposition of acidic mucopolysaccharides and the exudation of fluid into the interstitium.

GOBLET CELL MUCIN

Mucosubstances are produced by goblet cells in the respiratory and gastrointestinal tracts but mucous cell hyperplasia (as it occurs in catarrhal exudates) is not mucinous degeneration despite the erroneous efforts of some pathologists to include it in this category.

PIGMENTS

In many diseases, colored substances are deposited in tissue. Other than being pigments, they have little in common even though they are considered together here. The *endogenous pigments* are produced within the body. Of these, we will examine the melanins, lipochromes, and hemoglobin derivatives in detail (Table 2.6).

EXOGENOUS PIGMENTS

Exogenous pigments enter via the skin, lung, and intestinal tract. These are most common and most serious in the lung where the diseases are known collectively as the pneumoconioses. Some, such as coal dust pigment (anthracosis), cause little tissue reaction. Others, including silicon dioxide (silicosis) and iron dust (siderosis), may produce extensive inflammation and fibrosis.

Exogenous pigments entering the intestinal tract are generally of less import to health. Metallic poisons such as lead (plumbism) and silver (argyria) may cause pigmentation following ingestion and absorption. Tetracyclines, used widely as broad spectrum antibiotics in antimicrobial therapy, are known to be incorporated into bone where they form a fluorescent compound and stain the tissue yellow in visible light. This characteristic is unre-

Table 2.6. Pigments

Pigments	Seen in
Melanin	Normal pigmentation
	Focal congenital pigmentary defects
	Tumors (melanomas)
Lipofuscin	Myocardium and neurons of aging animals
	Systemic metabolic disease (lipofuscinosis)
Bile pigments	Liver disease, congenital and acquired
Malarial pigments (hematin-polypeptide complex)	Malarial infection

lated to antibacterial effect and is used by experimental pathologists as a tool and specific label for calcifying tissues.

Only rarely do pigments enter through the skin. The best examples are Prussian blue, India ink, and mercuric sulfide (vermilion), which are used in tattooing.

MELANIN

Melanin is the brown pigment of skin, hair, leptomeninges, and choroid of the eye. In lower vertebrates it is widespread and occurs in the interstitium of many organs. Melanin is a high molecular weight biochrome bound to protein. It is formed and resides in characteristic granules called *melanosomes.* In mammals, the only known function of melanin is the protection against solar ultraviolet radiation. It is thought to capture injurious free radicals generated in the skin during injury.

In vertebrates there are two types of melanin-containing cells: *melanocytes,* which synthesize melanin; and *melanophages,* which accept and store melanin but do not synthesize it. Melanocytes stem from melanoblasts, nonpigmented precursor cells of neural crest origin. *Melanophores,* or contractile cells, are melanocytes of some lower vertebrates that participate in the rapid color changes by intracellular aggregation and dispersion of melanosomes. These pigmented cells also contain reflecting organelles. Compound melanosomes must be differentiated from multiple melanosomes being degraded within macrophage lysosomes.

The formation of melanin begins with the enzyme tyrosinase, a copper-protein substance that facilitates the oxidation of tyrosine to dioxyphenylalanine (dopa) and dopa to dopaquinone in the initial stages of synthesis. The detection of tyrosinase (the dopa reaction) is the basis of the histochemical identification of melanocytes and melanoblasts. Tyrosinase is synthesized on the ribosomes and is conveyed to the Golgi apparatus where it accumulates in small membrane-bound vesicles called *premelanosomes* (Novikoff 1968). During maturation of the melanosome, melanin develops into oriented protein strands and concentric lamellae. As melanization proceeds, melanin polymers are deposited on the protein framework and it is obscured.

In the process of pigmentation, melanosomes are transferred from the dendrites of the melanocytes into the keratinocytes. Increase in transfer activity causes increased pigmentation. Tanning of the human skin by UV radiation involves an increase in the length of dendrites and increases in melanosomes and tyrosinase activity. It does not involve increased numbers of melanocytes. Melanocytes in the skin lack the desmosomes and tonofilaments present on the keratinocytes.

PATHOLOGIC MELANIZATION

Lesions in the process of melanin pigmentation can result from changes anywhere in the pathway of development (Table 2.7). This may involve abnormalities in tyrosinase production of deficits in the transfer of melanosomes to keratinocytes. In chronic dermatitis, for example, the skin often shows pigmented defects which are due to failure of transfer to the hyperplastic keratinocytes. Keratinocytes are free of melanin and the melanocytes are filled with melanosomes and have blunted dendrites. The papillomas of black cattle are pale and white because the melanin does not transfer to the abnormal papilloma cells.

In the genetically determined lysosomal disease of mink, cattle, whales, mice, and humans called Chediak-Higashi syndrome, giant bizarre melanosomes are produced (Zelickson et al. 1967). The pigment-deficiency in the gray Collie syndrome is due

Table 2.7. Pathologic changes in melanization

Defect in	Occurs in	Pathologic Change
Differentiation of melanoblast	Focal congenital hypomelanosis Piebald mice Neoplastic melanocyte lesions	Melanosomes absent in local area of skin.
Tyrosine synthesis	Albinism	Melanocytes lack melanosomes; if present, they are normal and are transferred normally (genetically determined failure to synthesize sufficient tyrosine).
Melanosome formation	Chediak-Higashi syndrome Neoplastic melanocyte lesions	Abnormal aggregation of melanin molecules with bizarre sizes and shapes.
Transfer to keratinocyte	Chronic dermatitis Neoplastic melanocyte lesions	Melanocyte is normal but keratinocytes lack melanosomes. Melanin is not transferred to the abnormal keratinocyte.

to diminished formation of melanin from tyrosine. The number of melanocytes does not differ from that in normal Collies, but there are fewer melanosomes present (Lund and Barkman 1974).

HEMOGLOBIN-DERIVED PIGMENTS

Hemoglobin, the oxygen-carrying pigment of erythrocytes, is a combination of globin and the pigment complex heme. During normal and pathologic breakdown, different types of pigment complexes are formed. Most of these are heterogeneous and, except for ferritin, are not chemically defined. In rare (and probably artifactual) instances, hemoglobin has been reported to crystallize in the erythrocyte. Ferritin and hemosiderin are the principal iron storage compounds in animal tissue.

FERRITIN

Ferritin is an iron-laden aggregate of the protein apoferritin. It is water soluble and, because it is distributed throughout the cytoplasmic matrix of the cell, is not easily demonstrable histochemically (Kerr and Muir 1960). Ultrastructurally, ferritin is a dense spherical morula 9.5–12.5 nm in diameter (Massover et al. 1973). It is a hydrous iron oxide core surrounded by several subunits or proteinaceous micelles of 2.7 nm diameter that are arranged at the apices of a regular octahedron.

Ferritin is formed when iron is added to apoferritin in the cytoplasmic matrix. Intracellular transport may occur through the cytoplasmic matrix or in the cytocavitary network. These pathways converge in lysosomes where ferritin is converted to hemosiderin (Trump et al. 1973). Cell iron overload may result either from massive accumulation of iron pigments or a deficiency of lysosomal excretion of hemosiderin.

The microscopic estimation of iron in tissues must include an evaluation of ferritin. The histologist must bear in mind that a liver not demonstrating hemosiderin may nonetheless be overloaded with iron in the form of ferritin. In normal mammalian liver, iron is not readily demonstrable; yet, biochemically, the liver may contain up to 25 mg/100 gr. About two-thirds is ferritin and the remainder is hemosiderin.

HEMOSIDERIN

Hemosiderin is a brown, granular, iron-containing pigment which forms when erythrocytes are lysed. It develops within macrophages anywhere in the reticuloendothelial system but is particularly common in spleen, liver, and foci of hemorrhage. Hemosiderin appears as amorphous masses of densely packed micelles of hydrous iron oxide that are derived from degenerating units of ferritin. Biochemical analysis is hampered by lack of methods for isolation and the fact that hemosiderin is always contaminated by other cell proteins. The relation of ferritin to hemosiderin remains ambiguous. Differences appear to lie in the degees of denaturation of apoferritin and the incorporation of protein debris as ferritin aggregates in the iron-loaded cell.

BILIRUBIN

Bilirubin is a pigment formed from the breakdown of hemoglobin by macrophages of the reticuloendothelial system. It is conjugated in the liver and excreted in bile. This yellow-brown pigment accumulates because of excessive production or failure of removal by damaged hepatocytes.

MALARIAL PIGMENT

Brownish *malarial pigment* is formed by the excretion of catabolized hemoglobin from certain species of Plasmodia. Massive deposits of this pigment may be found in reticuloendothelial cells of the spleen and liver of infected animals. Ultrastructural examination reveals dense irregular granules with little characteristic structure. Analysis of malarial pigment indicates it represents various phases in the degradation of hemoglobin (Morselt et al. 1973).

LIPOFUSCIN

Lipofuscin is a golden brown pigment found in the cytoplasm of cells in the heart, brain, adrenal cortex, and gonads of older animals. The deposits fluoresce brown in ultraviolet light and stain with fat-soluble dyes. The inert aggregates of lipofuscin increase with advancing age and are believed to be derived from the progressive oxidation of lipids, hence the term "wear-and-tear" pigment.

Ultrastructurally, lipofuscin consists of membrane-bound aggregates of dense granules, vacuoles, and lipid droplets. They are highly heterogeneous and may exist as small spherical globules or as immense irregular structures (Brunk and Ericsson 1972).

Ceroid is an acid-fast variant of lipofuscin which is associated with disturbances of vitamin E and fatty acid metabolism. Ultrastructurally, it closely resembles lipofuscin (Hartroft and Porta 1965). Ceroid is occasionally encountered in vertebrates incidentally (with no indication of how it evolved) (Wood and Yasutake 1956).

NEURONAL CEROID-LIPOFUSCINOSIS

This disease is an autosomal recessive syndrome in English Setter dogs characterized by the intracellular accumulation of lipopigments (predominantly in neurons) and associated with progressive loss of cells and cerebral function. Autofluorescent pigments consist of about 50% acidic lipid polymers and the precise mechanism is a disturbance in detoxification of peroxides, based upon markedly decreased tissue levels of p-phenyldiamine-linked peroxidase.

CALCIFICATION

CALCIUM IN THE CELL

Calcium ion (Ca^{++}) is a critically important regulator of activity in the cell cytoplasm. The homeostatic mechanisms regulating Ca^{++} are complex and involve regulation of: (1) the passive influx into the cytosol from three compartments (extracellular space, mitochondrial matrix, and endoplasmic reticulum cisterna) and (2) the active extrusion of calcium from the cytosol back into these zones by calcium pumps in their membranes.

The plasma membrane, endoplasmic reticulum, and mitochondrial membranes are capable of energy-linked calcium transport and thereby regulate the concentration of Ca^{++} in the cytosol. Even though intracellular and extracellular amounts of calcium may be similar, in ionic form the extracellular Ca^{++} is over 100 times the Ca^{++} in the cytosol. Calcium transport across the plasma membrane and endoplasmic reticulum occurs by ATP hydrolysis and is not influenced by sodium or potassium ions. The mitochondrial calcium pump is different. Here, Ca^{++} uptake occurs also by substrate oxidation and is blocked by inhibition of electron transport. Mitochondrial injury is often manifested as the accumulation of large dense granules of calcium salts in the matrix area.

PLASMA CALCIUM

Plasma levels of calcium in mammals, birds, and reptiles are maintained by *para-*

thyroid hormone (PTH) which stimulates bone resorption and hypercalcemia, and by *calcitonin* which inhibits resorption and leads to hypocalcemia. In fish, secretions of the corpuscles of Stannius regulate plasma calcium. Factors that elevate or depress high-affinity, calcium-binding proteins in plasma may also influence calcium levels. For example, plasma calcium in laying hens is three times that in male birds. This is a result of estrogenic stimulation of synthesis and release of circulating phosphoproteins with a high affinity for calcium.

Calcium exists in plasma in ionic form (Ca^{++}) and bound to plasma proteins. It is required for maintenance of skeletal and cardiac muscle contractility, blood coagulation, neural transmission, capillary endothelial junctions, and bone marrow. When low levels of plasma calcium develop and persist, disturbances in these systems result. Ca^{++} is a general requirement for secretory activity in cells storing their secretory products in membrane-bound granules. Inhibition of Ca^{++}-activated exocytosis influences most endocrine glands.

PLASMA CALCIUM AND BONE RESORPTION

PTH mobilizes calcium from the skeleton, increases renal excretion of phosphorus, and augments the rate of absorption and excretion of calcium from the intestine. It is synthesized by ribosomes on the endoplasmic reticulum of the parathyroid chief cell as a larger precursor termed proparathyroid hormone and is occured in response to low levels of calcium in plasma (hypocalcemia). It causes calcium ions to be removed from bone matrix to replenish the circulating calcium pool (see Fig. 10.7).

PTH acts upon bone and produces *osteolysis,* the absorption and destruction of bone in which bone matrix is modified and bone calcium salts are lost. It causes increased osteolysis both by osteoclasts and osteocytes. Osteoclasts located on bone trabecular surfaces are stimulated in some unknown way to increase in numbers and activity. When PTH is given to cows, bone resorption is increased fivefold by osteoclastic activity (Rowland et al. 1971). Bone-absorbing osteoclasts have active, ruffled plasma membranes where they abut the bone matrix. The active and vigorous pinocytotic action of this border has been demonstrated in time-lapse motion picture studies of bone in vitro. Ultrastructurally, the plasma membrane consists of repeating units along the cytoplasmic surface which contain fine bristlelike structures of 15–20 nm that project perpendicularly into the cytoplasm (Kallio et al. 1971). These specialized areas of the plasma membrane, which are involved in active ion exchange, are structurally different from those that border the nonbone-related surfaces of the osteoclast.

Deep in bone, the osteoblasts are also transformed into osteocytes which may secrete proteases and collagenases that resorb bone. In osteocytic osteolysis, the surrounding matrix of bone becomes less dense and is nearly devoid of mineral (Matthews and Martin 1971).

CALCIUM IN TISSUE

When in postmortem dissection tissue is encountered that feels gritty and scrapes against the knife, it is probable that calcium deposits are present. They appear in routine histologic preparations as granular or amorphous blue-black deposits. The von Kossa stain, which detects phosphates associated with calcium, is considered proof that the substance in question is calcium.

Ultrastructurally, calcium appears as amorphous granules and needles superimposed upon an homogeneous focus of mucopolysaccharide or other connective tissue component. In some circumstances, calcium is deposited in linear fashion along basement membranes or in concentric circles around a central matrix (Fig 2.31). X-ray diffraction studies reveal that the mineral is most often deposited as units of hydroxyapatite (Parsons 1968).

Two forms of pathologic tissue calcification are recognized: *dystrophic calcification,* in which calcium salts are deposited in degenerating cells; and *metastatic calcification,* wherein they are deposited in normal tissues in the presence of hypercalcemia. This dichotomy is not entirely satisfactory since the role of cellular factors is difficult to assess.

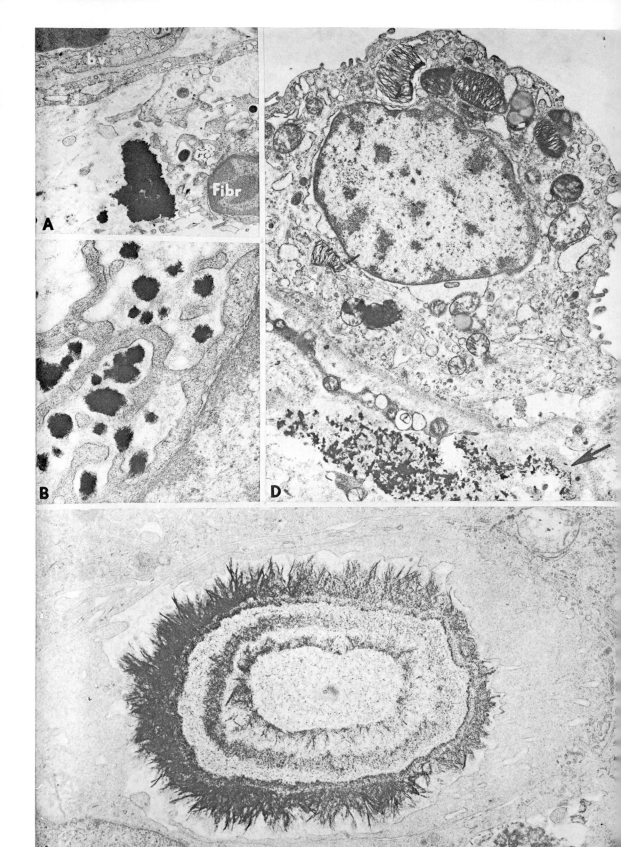

DYSTROPHIC CALCIFICATION

Dystrophic calcification is seen at sites of scarring, hemorrhage, and old infections. Lesions of tuberculosis, trichinosis, histoplasmosis, and caseous lymphadenitis are frequently mineralized. Calcium salts develop in association with necrotic debris. One of the most serious sites of dystrophic calcification is the degenerating smooth muscle layer of arteries. Calcium is deposited on the altered microfibrillar portions of elastic tissue and calcification spreads to involve large portions of the artery (Haust and Geer 1970).

Calcific metaplasia represents a variant of dystrophic calcification wherein tissues are converted into masses of calcium and in some cases into bone. These hard, circumscribed deposits, called tumorous calcinosis or calcinosis circumscripta, are most often seen in the conversion of the tendons of some birds to bone. In turkeys, between the twelfth and sixteenth weeks of life, the collagenous tendons of the leg become ossified. The change is initiated by alterations in the connective tissue. As the tendons mature, their extracellular connective tissue matrix loses water and collagen becomes highly aggregated and cross-linked. Fibroblasts become cuboidal and develop fatty changes; lipids and mucopolysaccharides accumulate in the extracellular matrix. The resulting disturbance of ions leads directly to the accumulation of calcium deposits (Engel and Zerlotti 1967).

METASTATIC CALCIFICATION

Metastatic calcification occurs in living tissue as a result of high levels of calcium in circulating blood. Excessive vitamin D and hyperparathyroidism are the most common causes. The fundamental abnormality is the pathologic entry into cells of large amounts of ionic calcium which precipitate in organelles, chiefly in the mitochondria. Certain tissues such as muscle, intestine, and lung are commonly affected although these lesions may be seen in any tissue (Yu and Blumenthal 1963).

The kidney calcified by hypervitaminosis D has been a widely studied model of metastatic calcification (Giacomelli et al. 1964; Scarpelli 1966). Cytologic lesions include pinocytosis and uptake of calcium in the proximal convoluted tubule. Calcific deposits develop in cytoplasmic vacuoles, mitochondria, and epithelial basement membrane. Vitamin D causes a progressive uncoupling of oxidative phosphorylation in mitochondria; it is suggested that these are the organelles first involved in the pathogenesis of metastatic calcification.

Widespread soft-tissue calcification occurs in a variety of diseases for which the mechanism of calcification is not established. Dietary deficiency of magnesium, chronic renal disease, and plant toxicities are known factors in some of these. In cattle and sheep, certain geographical areas are known for the occurrence of calcifying diseases. Among these are Manchester Wasting Disease of Jamaica, *enteque seco* in Brazil, and *Naalehu* disease in Hawaii.

Calciphylaxis is the process whereby calcium precipitates in tissues in response to a challenging agent such as iron. The term was coined during studies of an experimental model utilizing a sensitizing calcifier such as vitamin D or parathyroid hormone, a critical waiting period of 24 hrs, and challenge with mineral salts such as ferric chloride (Selye et al. 1969). Calciphylaxis is a rarely used term although it has been applied to local calcific deposits due to the injection of iron and vitamin D in baby pigs (Penn 1970) and to calcification following iron injection in humans (Rees and Cole 1969). The reaction as an experimental model may also produce systemic calcification and the lung and spleen are heavy sites of deposition. Calciphylaxis has been considered a defensive reaction for sequestering pathogens and chemicals that would otherwise do harm by circulating in blood.

Fig. 2.31. Calcification. A. Amorphous perivascular calcium deposits in interstitium of alveolar wall, lung of dog with uremia. Blood vessel (bv), fibroblast (Fibr.). B. Filopodia of fibroblast surrounding foci of mineral. C. Laminar deposition of calcium salts around an organic matrix (Schaumann's body), lymph node, hamster with paratuberculosis. D. Calcification of the basement membrane of the alveolar wall (arrow), dog with uremia and "pumice lung." Alveolar epithelial cell is granular pneumocyte.

REFERENCES

Afzelius, B. A. The occurrence and structure of microbodies. *J. Cell Biol.* 26:835, 1965.

Allen, J. R. et al. Ultrastructural and biochemical changes associated with pyrrolizidine-induced hepatic megalocytosis. *Cancer Res.* 30:1857, 1970.

Allison, A. C. and Nunn, J. F. Effects of general anaesthetics on microtubules. A possible mechanism of anaesthesia. *Lancet* 2:1326, 1968.

Allison, A. C., Magnus, I. A. and Young, M. R. Role of lysosomes and of cell membranes in photosensitization. *Nature* 209:874, 1966.

Aoki, T. et al. An immunoferritin study of the occurrence and topography of H-2', θ and TL alloantigens on mouse cells. *J. Exp. Med.* 130:979, 1969.

Arstila, A. V. Studies on cellular autophagocytosis. *Lab. Invest.* 24:162, 1971.

Arstila, A. V. and Trump, B. F. Ethionine induced alteration in the Golgi apparatus and in the endoplasmic reticulum. *Virch. Arch. B* 10:344, 1972.

Axline, S. G. and Cohn, Z. A. In vitro induction of lysosomal enzymes by phagocytosis. *J. Exp. Med.* 131:1239, 1970.

Baglio, C. M. and Farber, E. Reversal by adenine of the ethionine-induced lipid accumulation in the endoplasmic reticulum of the rat liver. *J. Cell Biol.* 27:591, 1965.

Bassi, M. and Bernelli-Zazzera, A. Ultrastructural cytoplasmic change in liver cells after reversible and irreversible injury. *Exp. Mol. Path.* 3:332, 1964.

Baudhuin, P., Hers, H. G. and Loeb, H. An electron microscopic study of type II glycogenosis. *Lab. Invest.* 13:1139, 1964.

Becker, F. F. and Cornwall, C. C. Phlorizin-induced autophagocytosis during hepatocytic glycogenolysis. *Exp. Mol. Path.* 14:103, 1971.

Behnke, O. and Forer, A. Evidence for four classes of microtubules in individual cells. *J. Cell Sci.* 2:169, 1967.

Bernhard, N. et al. Lésions nucléolaires précoces provoquées par l'aflatoxin dans le cellules hepatiques du rat. *Compt. Rend.* 261:1785, 1965.

Björkerud, S. The isolation of lipofuscin granules from bovine cardiac muscle with observations on the properties of the isolated granules on the light and electron microscopic levels. *J. Ult. Res. Suppl.* 5, 1963.

Blanchette-Mackie, E. J. and Scow, R. O. Sites of lipoprotein lipase activity in adipose tissue perfused with chylomicrons: Electron microscopical cytochemical study. *J. Cell Biol.* 51:1, 1971.

Bluemink, J. G. Cortical wound healing in the amphibian egg: An electron microscopical study. *J. Ult. Res.* 41:95, 1972.

Bolender, R. P. and Weibel, E. R. A morphometric study of the removal of phenobarbitol-induced membranes from hepatocytes after cessation of treatment. *J. Cell Biol.* 56:746, 1973.

Brandes, D., Anton, E. and Barnard, S. Lysosomes and cellular regressive changes in rat mammary gland involution. *Lab. Invest.* 20:465, 1969.

Brooks, R. E. and Siegel, B. V. Nuclear bodies of normal and pathological human lymph node cells: An electron microscopic study. *Blood* 29:269, 1967.

Brunk, U. and Ericsson, J. L. E. Electron microscopical studies on rat brain neurons. Localization of acid phosphatase and mode of formation of lipofuscin bodies. *J. Ult. Res.* 38:1, 1972.

Burger, P. C. and Herdson, P. B. Phenobarbital-induced fine structural changes in rat liver. *Am. J. Path.* 48:793, 1966.

Capen, C. C. and Martin, S. L. Hyperinsulinemia in dogs with neoplasia of the pancreatic islets. *Vet. Path.* 6:309, 1969.

Caramia, F. et al. A glycogen body in liver nuclei. *J. Ult. Res.* 19:573, 1967.

Claude, A. Growth and differentiation of cytoplasmic membranes in the course of lipoprotein granule synthesis in the hepatic cell. *J. Cell Biol.* 47:745, 1970.

Crocker, B. P., Saladino, A. J. and Trump, B. F. Ion movements in cell injury. *Am. J. Path.* 59:247, 1970.

Cushman, S. W. Structure-function relationships in the adipose cell. *J. Cell Biol.* 46:326, 1970.

D'Agnostino, A. N. An electron microscopic study of cardiac necrosis produced by 9 alpha-fluorocortisol and sodium phosphate. *Am. J. Path.* 45:633, 1964.

Davis, C. L. and Gorham, J. R. The pathology of experimental and natural cases of yellow fat disease in swine. *Am. J. Vet. Res.* 15:55, 1954.

de Bruijn, W. C. Glycogen, its chemistry and morphologic appearance in the electron microscope. *J. Ult. Res.* 42:29, 1973.

De Duve, C. and Baudhuin, P. Peroxisomes. *Physiol. Rev.* 46:323, 1966.

De Duve, C. and Wattiaux, R. Functions of lysosomes. *Ann. Rev. Physiol.* 28:435, 1966.

Derenzini, M. et al. Pathogenesis of liver necrosis produced by amanitin-albumin conjugates. *Lab. Invest.* 29:150, 1973.

Deter, R. L. and De Duve, C. Influence of glucagon as inducer of cell autophagy in some properties of rat liver lysosomes. *J. Cell Biol.* 33:437, 1967.

Drochmans, P. Morphologie du glycogene. *J. Ult. Res.* 6:141, 1962.

Dumont, A. and Robert, A. Ultrastructure of complex nuclear bodies produced experimentally in hamster peritoneal macrophages. *J. Ult. Res.* 36:483, 1971.

Dupuy-Coin, A. M. and Bouteille, M. Developmental pathway of granular and beaded nuclear bodies from nucleoli. *J. Ult. Res.* 40:55, 1972.

Engel, M. B. and Zerlotti, E. Changes in cells, matrix and water of calcifying turkey leg tendon. *Am. J. Anat.* 120:489, 1967.

Ericsson, J. L. E. and Glinsman, W. H. Focal degenerative cytoplasmic alterations in liver cells induced by hypoxia. *Acta Path. Micro. Scand.* 64:151, 1965.

Ericsson, J. L. E., Orrenius, S. and Holm, J. Alterations in canine liver cells induced by protein deficiency. Ultrastructural and biochemical observations. *Exp. Mol. Path.* 5:329, 1966.

Essner, E. Endoplasmic reticulum and the origin of microbodies in fetal mouse liver. *Lab. Invest.* 17:71, 1967.

Essner, E. and Oliver, C. Lysosome formation in hepatocytes with Chediak-Higashi syndrome. *Lab. Invest.* 30:596, 1974.

Estes, L. and Lombardi, B. Effect of choline deficiency on the Golgi apparatus in rat hepatocytes. *Lab. Invest.* 21:374, 1960.

Fahimi, H. D. and Cotran, R. S. Permeability studies in heat-induced injury of skeletal muscle using lanthanum as fine structural tracer. *Am. J. Path.* 64:143, 1971.

Finegold, M. J. and Green, L. E. Mitochondrial damage in experimental and congenital adrenal hyperplasia. *J. Cell Biol.* 45:455, 1970.

Fox, H. Degeneration of the tail notocord of *Rana temporaria* at metamorphic climax. Examination by electron microscopy. *Zt. Zellf.* 138:371, 1973.

Fredholm, B. B. Studies on the sympathetic regulation of circulation and metabolism in isolated canine subcutaneous adipose tissue. *Acta Physiol. Scand. Suppl.*, p. 354, 1970.

Garancis, J. C. et al. Type III glycogenosis. *Lab. Invest.* 22:468, 1970.

Gardner, D. E. Pathogenesis of *Clostridium welchii* type D enterotoxemia. III. Basis of the hyperglycemic response. *J. Comp. Path.* 83:525, 1973.

Geuskens, M. and Bernhard, W. Cytochimie ultrastructurale du nucléole. *Exp. Cell Res.* 44:579, 1966.

Giacomelli, F., Spiro, D. and Wiener, J. A study of metastatic renal calcification at the cellular level. *J. Cell Biol.* 22:189, 1964.

Goldfischer, S. et al. Peroxisomal abnormalities in metabolic diseases. *J. Histochem. Cytochem.* 21:972, 1973.

Goldman, R. D. and Follett, E. Birefringent filamentous organelle in BHK-21 cells and its possible role in cell spreading and motility. *Science* 169:286, 1970.

Gorius, J. B. and Houssay, D. Auer bodies in acute promyelocytic leukemia. *Lab. Invest.* 28:135, 1973.

Goyer, R. A. et al. Lead and protein content of isolated intranuclear inclusion bodies from kidneys of lead-poisoned rats. *Lab. Invest.* 22:245, 1970.

Greenwalt, J. W., Rossi, C. S. and Lehninger, A. L. Effect of active accumulation of calcium and phosphate ions on the structure of rat liver mitochondria. *J. Cell Biol.* 23:21, 1964.

Gustafsson, R. G. and Tata, J. R. Skeletal muscle mitochondria of rat in experimental hyperthyroidism. *J. Ult. Res.* 9:396, 1963.

Haddad, A. et al. Radioautographic study of in vivo and in vitro incorporation of fucose-^{3}H into thyroglobulin by rat thyroid follicular cells. *J. Cell Biol.* 49:850, 1971.

Hamilton, R. L. et al. Lipid transport in liver. I. Electron microscopic identification of very low density lipoprotein in perfused rat liver. *Lab. Invest.* 16:305, 1967.

Harris, R. A., Harris, D. L. and Green D. E. Effect of Bordetella endotoxin upon mito-chondrial respiration and energized processes. *Arch. Biochem. Biophys.* 128:219, 1968.

Hartroft, W. S. and Porta, E. A. Ceroid. *Am. J. Med. Sci.* 250:324, 1965.

Haust, M. D. and Geer, J. C. Mechanism of calcification in spontaneous aortic arterio-sclerotic lesions of the rabbit. *Am. J. Path.* 60:329, 1970.

Hays, R. M., Singer, B. and Malamed, S. The effect of calcium withdrawal on the structure and function of the toad bladder. *J. Cell Biol.* 25:195, 1965.

Heaton, J. M. A study of brown adipose tissue in hypothermia. *J. Path.* 110:105, 1973.

Heggtveit, H. A., Herman, L. and Mishra, R. I. Cardiac necrosis and calcification in experimental magnesium deficiency. *Am. J. Path.* 45:757, 1964.

Henderson, D. W., Goll, D. E. and Stromer, M. H. A comparison of shortening and Z line degradation in postmortem bovine, porcine, and rabbit muscle. *Am. J. Anat.* 128:117, 1970.

Holland, J. M. et al. Lafora's disease in the dog. *Am. J. Path.* 58:509, 1970.

Hruban, Z., Slesers, A. and Hopkins, E. Drug-induced and naturally occurring myeloid bodies. *Lab. Invest.* 27:62, 1972.

Hruban, Z. et al. Effects of some hypocholesteremic agents on hepatic ultrastructure and microbody enzymes. *Lab. Invest.* 30:474, 1974.

Iseri, O. A., Lieber, C. S. and Gottlieb, L. S. The ultrastructure of fatty liver induced by prolonged ethanol ingestion. *Am. J. Path.* 48:535, 1966.

Isselbacher, K. J. and Greenberger, N. J. Metabolic effects of alcohol on the liver. *New Engl. J. Med.* 270:351, 1964.

Jacob, J. Involvement of the nucleolus in viral synthesis in cells of primary renal tumors of leopard frogs. *Cancer Res.* 28:2126, 1968.

Jezequel, A. M., Shreeve, M. M. and Steiner, J. W. Segregation of nucleolar components in Mycoplasma infected cells. *Lab. Invest.* 16:287, 1967.

Jolly, R. D., Alley, M. R. and O'Hara, P. J. Familial acantholysis of Angus calves. *Vet. Path.* 10:473, 1973.

Kajima, M. and Majde, J. LCM virus as a carrier of non-viral cellular components. *Naturwissenschaften* 2:1, 1970.

Kallio, D. M., Garant, P. R. and Minkin, C. Evidence of coated membranes in the ruffled border of the osteoclast. *J. Ult. Res.* 37:169, 1971.

Karasaki, S. Cytoplasmic and nuclear glycogen synthesis in Novikoff ascites hepatoma cells. *J. Ult. Res.* 35:181, 1971.

———. An electron microscopic study of intranuclear canaliculi in Novikoff hepatoma cells. *Cancer Res.* 30:1736, 1970.

———. Passage of cytoplasmic lipid into interphase nuclei in preneoplastic rat liver. *J. Ult. Res.* 42:463, 1973.

Kent, S. P. Diffusion of plasma proteins into cells: A manifestation of cell injury in rabbit skeletal muscle exposed to lecithinase C. *Arch. Path.* 88:407, 1969.

Kerr, D. N. and Muir, A. R. A demonstration of the structure and disposition of ferri-tin in the human liver cell. *J. Ult. Res.* 3:313, 1960.

Kessel, R. G. Annulate lamellae. *J. Ult. Res. Suppl.* 10:1, 1968.

Kisilevsky, R. et al. Ribosomal alterations following ethionine intoxication. *Lab. Invest.* 28:8, 1973.

Kjaerheim, A. Crystals in skeletal muscle in congenital hyperlacticacidemia. *J. Ult. Res.* 36:538, 1971.

Kotoulas, O. B. et al. Fine structural aspects of the mobilization of hepatic glycogen. *Am. J. Path.* 63:23, 1971.

Krishan, A., Uzman, B. G. and Hedley-Whyte, E. T. Nuclear bodies: A component of cell nuclei in hamster tissues and human tumors. *J. Ult. Res.* 19:563, 1967.

Krivit, W. et al. Fine structural aspects of the mobilization of hepatic glycogen. *Am. J. Path.* 63:23, 1971.

Lampert, P. W. A comparative electron microscopic study of reactive, degenerating and dystrophic axons. *J. Neuropath. Exp. Neurol.* 26:345, 1967.

Lavin, P. and Koss, L. G. Effects of a single dose of cyclophosphamide on various organs in the rat. *Am. J. Path.* 62:169, 1971.

Leduc, E. H. Sulfaguanidine protection of mouse liver from carbon tetrachloride-induced necrosis. *Lab. Invest.* 29:186, 1973.

Loewenstein, W. R. Permeability of membrane junctions. *Ann. N.Y. Acad. Sci.* 137:441, 1966.

Lombardi, B. Consideration of the pathogenesis of fatty liver. *Lab. Invest.* 15:1, 1966.

Lund, J. E. and Barkman, D. Color dilution in the gray Collie. *Am. J. Vet. Res.* 35:265, 1974.

Lutzner, M. A. and Hecht, F. Nuclear anomalies of the neutrophil in a chromosomal triplication. *Lab. Invest.* 15:597, 1966.

Mahley, R. W. et al. Lipid transport in the liver. *Lab. Invest.* 19:358, 1968.

Majno, G., La Gattuta, M. and Thompson, T. E. Cellular death and necrosis. *Virch. Arch. Path. Anat.* 333:421, 1960.

Malmqvist, E. et al. Pathologic lysosomes and increased urinary glycosylceramide excretion in Fabry's disease. *Lab. Invest.* 25:1, 1971.

Marinozzi, V. and Fiume, L. Effects of α-amanitin on mouse and rat liver cell nuclei. *Exp. Cell Res.* 67:311, 1971.

Massover, W. H., Lacaze, J.-G. and Durrieu, L. The ultrastructure of ferritin macromolecules. *J. Ult. Res.* 43:460, 1973.

Masurovsky, E. B. et al. Origin, development and nature of intranuclear rodlets and associated bodies in chicken sympathetic neurons. *J. Cell Biol.* 44:172, 1970.

Matthews, J. L. and Martin, J. H. Intracellular transport of calcium and its relationship to homeostasis and mineralization. *Am. J. Med.* 50:589, 1971.

Maunsbach, A. B., Madden, S. C. and Latta, H. Light and electron microscopic changes in proximal convoluted tubules of rats after administration of glucose, mannitol, sucrose or dextran. *Lab Invest.* 11:421, 1962.

Meldolesi, J. et al. Effect of carbon tetrachloride on the synthesis of liver endoplasmic reticulum membranes. *Lab. Invest.* 19:315, 1968.

Miller, J. M. et al. Incidence of lymphocytic nucleolar projections in bovine lymphosarcoma. *J. Nat. Cancer Inst.* 43:719, 1969.

Miller, O. L., Jr. and Hamkalo, B. A. Visualization of RNA synthesis on chromosomes. *Int. Rev. Cytol.* 33:1, 1972.

Monneron, A. Experimental induction of helical polysomes in adult rat liver. *Lab Invest.* 20:178, 1969.

Morrison, A. B. and Panner, B. J. Lysosome induction in experimental potassium deficiency. *Am. J. Path.* 45:295, 1964.

Morselt, A. F. W., Glastra, A. and James, J. Microspectrophotometric analysis of malarial pigment. *Exp. Parasit.* 33:17, 1973.

Mottet, N. K. and Hammer, S. P. Ribosome crystals in necrotizing cells from the posterior zone of the developing chick limb. *J. Cell Sci.* 11:403, 1972.

Moulé, Y. Effects of aflatoxin B₁ on the formation of submicrosomal particles in rat liver. *Cancer Res.* 33:514, 1973.

Napolitano, L. M. The differentiation of white adipose cells. An electron microscope study. *J. Cell Biol.* 18:663, 1963.

Napolitano, L. M. and Gagne, H. I. Lipid-depleted white adipose cells. *Anat. Rec.* 147:273, 1963.

Nass, M. M. K., Nass, S. and Afzelius, B. A. The general occurrence of mitochondrial DNA. *Exp. Cell Res.* 37:516, 1965.

Neutra, M. and Leblond, C. P. Synthesis of the carbohydrate of mucus in the Golgi complex as shown by electron microscope radioautography of goblet cells from rats injected with glucose-H³. *J. Cell Biol.* 30:119, 1966.

Novikoff, A. B. and Novikoff, P. M. Microperoxisomes. *J. Histochem. Cytochem.* 21:963, 1973.

Novikoff, A. B., Albala, A. and Biempica, L. Ultrastructural and cytochemical observations on B-16 and Harding-Passey mouse melanomas. *J. Histochem. Cytochem.* 16:299, 1968.

O'Brien, J. S. Tay-Sachs disease from enzyme to prevention. *Fed. Proc.* 32:191, 1973.

O'Connor, T. M. and Wyttenbach, C. R. Cell death in the embryonic chick spinal cord. *J. Cell Biol.* 60:448, 1974.

O'Daly, J. A. and Imaeda, T. Electron microscopic study of Wallerian degeneration in cutaneous nerves caused by mechanical injury. *Lab Invest.* 17:74, 1967.

Oksanen, A. and Osborn, H. G. Fatty tissue in starved lambs. *Acta Vet. Scand.* 13:340, 1972.

Orci, L. and Stauffacher, W. Glycogenosomes in renal tubular cells of diabetic animals. *J. Ult. Res.* 36:499, 1971.

Orrenius, S., Ericsson, J. and Ernster, L. Phenobarbital-induced synthesis of the microsomal drug-metabolizing enzyme system and its relationship to the proliferation of endoplasmic membranes. *J. Cell Biol.* 25:627, 1965.

Panabok'ke, R. G. An experimental study of fat necrosis. *J. Path.* 75:319, 1958.

Parsons, D. T. The examination of mineral deposits in pathological tissues by electron diffraction. *Int. Rev. Exp. Path.* 6:1, 1968.

Penn, G. B. Calciphylactic syndrome in pigs. *Vet. Rec.* 86:718, 1970.

Pfeifer, U. Zur Stellung des lysosomalen Glykogenabbaues im hepato cellulären Glykogentoffwechsel. *Virch. Arch. B* 10:108, 1972.

Pham, T. D., Luse, S. A. and Dempsey, E. W. A unique form of endoplasmic reticulum in endocardial endothelia of the desert iguana. *J. Ult. Res.* 39:149, 1972.

Phillips, M. J. et al. Glycogen depletion in the newborn rat liver. *J. Ult. Res.* 18:142, 1967.

Prieur, D. J., Davis, W. C. and Padgett, G. A. Defective function of renal lysosomes in mice with the Chediak-Higashi syndrome. *Am. J. Path.* 67:227, 1972.

Pucci, I. Mitochondrial changes induced by fluoroacetate in chick embryo myocardium in vivo. *Exp. Cell Res.* 35:412, 1964.

Rajya, B. S. and Rubarth, S. Vacuolation and glycogen deposition in the hepatic cell nuclei of ruminants. *Acta Vet. Scand.* 8:201, 1967.

Read, W. K. and Bay, W. W. Basic cellular lesion in chloroquine toxicity. *Lab. Invest.* 24:246, 1971.

Reddy, J. and Svoboda, D. Further evidence to suggest that microbodies do not exist as individual entities. *Am. J. Path.* 70:421, 1973a.

——. Microbody (peroxisome) matrix: Transformation into tubular structures. *Virch. Arch. B* 14:83, 1973b.

——. The relationship of nucleolar segregation to ribonucleic acid synthesis following the administration of selected hepatocarcinogens. *Lab. Invest.* 19:132, 1968.

Reed, G. B., Jr., Dixon, J. F. P. and Neustein, P. B. Type IV glycogenosis. *Lab. Invest.* 19:546, 1968.

Rees, J. K. and Cole, G. A. Calciphylaxis in man. *Brit. Med. J.* 2:670, 1969.

Regan, J. D. et al. Xeroderma pigmentosum. *Science* 174:147, 1971.

Reid, I. M. Hepatic nuclear glycogenosis in the cow: A light and electron microscope study. *J. Path.* 110:267, 1973a.

——. Nuclear bodies in bovine mammary gland in different physiologic states. *Exp. Cell Res.* 78:25, 1973b.

Reid, I. M. and Isenor, R. N. Effect of starvation on nuclear bodies and rough endoplasmic reticulum in the bovine hepatocyte. *Exp. Cell Res.* 75:282, 1972.

Reid, I. M., Shinozuka, H. and Sidransky, H. Polyribosomal disaggregation induced by puromycin and its reversal with time. *Lab. Invest.* 23:119, 1970.

Resibois, A. et al. Lysosomes and storage diseases. *Int. Rev. Exp. Path.* 9:93, 1970.

Rosa, F. Electron microscope study of the in vivo effect of 2-deoxy-d-glucose on the rat hepatocyte. *J. Ult. Res.* 35:66, 1971.

Rowland, G. N. et al. Microradiographic evaluation of bone and ultrastructure of C-cells and parathyroid glands of cows receiving parathyroid extract. *Beitr. Path. Bd.* 144:360, 1971.

Rubin, E., Beattie, D. S. and Lieber, C. S. Effects of ethanol on the biogenesis of mitochondrial membranes and associated mitochondrial function. *Lab. Invest.* 23:620, 1970.

Ruebner, B. H. et al. Production of fatty liver by ethanol in Rhesus monkeys. *Lab. Invest.* 27:71, 1972.

Sahaphong, S. and Trump, B. F. Studies of cellular injury in isolated kidney tubules of the flounder. *Am. J. Path.* 63:277, 1971.

Salomon, J. C., Salomon, M. and Bernhard, W. Modification des cellules du parenchyme hepatique du rat sous l'effect de la thioacetamide. *Bull. Cancer* 49:139, 1962.

Sandström, B., Westman, J. and Öckerman, P. A. Glycogenosis of the central nervous system in the cat. *Acta Neuropath.* 14:194, 1969.

Scaletta, L. J. and MacCallum, D. K. A fine structural study of divalent cation-induced epithelial union with connective tissue. *Am. J. Anat.* 133:431, 1972.

Scarpelli, D. G. Experimental pathology of vitamin-D induced nephrocalcinosis. *Meth. Achiev. Exp. Path.* 1:560, 1966.

Schaff, Z., Barry, D. W. and Grimely, P. M. Cytochemistry of tubuloreticular structures in lymphocytes from patients with systemic lupus erythematosus and in cultured human lymphoid cells. *Lab. Invest.* 29:577, 1973.

Schlaepfer, W. W. Experimental alteration of neurofilaments and neurotubules by calcium and other ions. *Exp. Cell Res.* 67:73, 1971.

Schlunk, R. R. and Lombardi, B. C. Liver liposomes. I. Isolation and chemical characterization. *Lab. Invest.* 17:30, 1971.

Schochet, S. S., Lampert, P. W. and Earle, K. M. Neuronal changes induced by intrathecal vincristine sulfate. *J. Neuropath. Exp. Neurol.* 27:645, 1968.

Seite, R., Escaig, J. and Covineau, S. Microfilaments et microtubules nucléaires et organisation ultrastructurale des batonnets intranucléaires des neurones sympathiques. *J. Ult. Res.* 37:449, 1971.

Selye, H. et al. Clinical implications of calciphylaxis. *Union Med. Can.* 98:1467, 1969.

Shelbourne, J. D., Arstila, A. V. and Trump, B. F. Studies on cellular autophagocytosis. *Am. J. Path.* 72:521, 1973.

Sheldon, H., Silverberg, M. and Kerner, L. On the differing appearance of intranuclear and cytoplasmic glycogen in liver cells in glycogen storage disease. *J. Cell Biol.* 13:468, 1962.

Simoni, P. et al. Ribosome crystallization in normal and in Marek's disease affected chickens. *Exp. Cell Res.* 78:433, 1973.

Slavin, B. G. The cytophysiology of mammalian adipose cells. *Int. Rev. Cytol.* 33:297, 1972.

Smuckler, E. A. and Benditt, E. P. The early effects of actinomycin on rat liver. *Lab. Invest.* 14:1699, 1965.

Stein, O. and Stein, Y. The role of the liver in the metabolism of chylomicrons studied by electron microscopic autoradiography. *Lab. Invest.* 17:436, 1967.

Stenger, R. J. Regenerative nodules in carbon tetrachloride-induced cirrhosis. A light and electron microscopic study of lamellar structures encountered therein. *J. Ult. Res.* 14:240, 1966.

Stenram, U. Electron microscope study on liver cells of rats treated with actinomycin D. *Zt. Zellf.* 65:211, 1965.

Stromer, M. H., Goll, D. E. and Rice, R. V. Morphology of rigor-shortened bovine muscle and the effect of trypsin on pre- and post-rigor myofibrils. *J. Cell Biol.* 34:431, 1967.

Suter, E. R. The fine structure of brown adipose tissue. III. The effect of cold exposure and its mediation in newborn rats. *Lab. Invest.* 21:259, 1969.

Svoboda, D. J. and Reddy, J. Microbodies in experimentally altered cells. *Am. J. Path.* 67:541, 1972.

Svoboda, D. J., Grady, H. J. and Higginson, J. Aflatoxin B₁ injury in rat and monkey liver. *Am. J. Path.* 49:1023, 1966.

Svoboda, D. J., Reddy, J. K. and Liu, C. Multinucleate giant cells in liver of marmosets given aflatoxin B₁. *Arch. Path.* 91:452, 1971.

Tandler, B., Hutter, R. V. P. and Erlandson, R. A. Ultrastructure of oncocytoma of the parotid gland. *Lab. Invest.* 23:567, 1970.

Tandler, B. et al. Riboflavin and mouse hepatic cell structure and function. *J. Cell Biol.* 41:477, 1969.

Thake, D. C., Cheville, N. F. and Sharp, R. K. Ectopic thyroid adenomas at the base of the heart of the dog. Ultrastructural identification of dense tubular structures in endoplasmic reticulum. *Vet. Path.* 8:421, 1971.

Trump, B. F. and Ginn, F. L. The pathogenesis of subcellular reaction to lethal injury. *Meth. Achiev. Exp. Path.* 4:1, 1969.

Trump, B. J. et al. The relationship of intracellular pathways of iron metabolism to cellular iron overload and iron storage diseases. *Am. J. Path.* 72:295, 1973.

Vogt, M. T. and Farber, E. On the molecular pathology of ischemic renal cell death. *Am. J. Path.* 53:1, 1968.

Volk, B. W. and Lazarus, S. S. Ultramicroscopic evolution of B-cell ballooning degeneration in diabetic dogs. *Lab. Invest.* 12:697, 1963.

Volk, T. L. and Scarpelli, D. G. Mitochondrial gigantism in the adrenal cortex following hypophysectomy. *Lab. Invest.* 15:707, 1966.

Weber, A. et al. Occurrence of nuclear pockets in lymphocytes of normal, persistent lymphocytotic and leukemic adult cattle. *J. Nat. Cancer Inst.* 43:1307, 1969.

Weber, A. F. and Fromme, S. P. Nuclear bodies: Their prevalence, location, and ultrastructure in the calf. *Science* 141:912, 1963.

Weber, R. Ultrastructural changes in regressing tail muscles of Xenopus larvae at metamorphosis. *J. Cell Biol.* 22:481, 1964.

Weiss, E. Intranukleäre und intrazytoplasmatische Glykogenablagerungen im Mastzellentumoren des Hundes. *Vet. Path.* 2:514, 1965.

Weiss, L. The cell periphery. *Int. Rev. Cytol.* 26:63, 1969.

Weiss, M. and Meyer, J. Comparison of the effects of Coxsackievirus A9 and of actinomycin D on the nucleolar ultrastructure of monkey kidney cells. *J. Ult. Res.* 38:411, 1972.

Weissman, G. and Thomas, L. Studies on lysosomes. *J. Exp. Med.* 116:433, 1962.

Wensvoort, P. Adipose tissue in calves and lambs. *Vet. Path.* 5:270, 1968.

Wiener, J., Spiro, D. and Loewenstein, W. R. Ultrastructure and permeability of nuclear membranes. *J. Cell Biol.* 27:107, 1965.

Williamson, J. R. Adipose tissue. Morphological changes associated with lipid mobilization. *J. Cell Biol.* 20:57, 1964.

Williamson, J. R., Lacy, P. E. and Grisham, J. W. Ultrastructural changes in islets of the rat produced by tolbutamide. *Diabetes* 10:460, 1961.

Wischnitzer, S. The annulate lamellae. *Int. Rev. Cytol.* 27:65, 1970.

Wisniewski, H. and Terry, R. D. Experimental colchicine encephalopathy. I. Induction of neurofibrillary degeneration. *Lab. Invest.* 17:577, 1967.

Wood, E. M. and Yasutake, W. T. Ceroid in fish. *Am. J. Path.* 32:591, 1956.

Young, R. W. The role of the Golgi complex in sulfate metabolism. *J. Cell Biol.* 57:175, 1973.

Yu, D. T. and Phillips, M. J. Hepatic ultrastructural changes in acute fructose overload. *J. Ult. Res.* 36:222, 1971.

Yu, S. Y. and Blumenthal H. T. The calcification of elastic fiber. *Lab. Invest.* 12:1154, 1963.

Zelickson, A. S. et al. The Chediak-Higashi syndrome: Formation of giant melanosomes and the basis of hypopigmentation. *J. Invest. Derm.* 49:575, 1967.

CHAPTER THREE

Blood and Vascular System

PATHOLOGY OF THE CAPILLARY BED

The circulatory system culminates in the capillary bed. The enormous luminal volume of this bed and its even greater capacity to expand or enlarge under the influence of vasoactive substances is not always appreciated. Capillaries are not innervated and they do not have encircling muscular layers. The distinction of differing types of capillaries ultrastructurally is based upon the completeness of their three layers: endothelium, basement membrane, and pericytes. Three major capillary types are distinguished: continuous, fenestrated, and discontinuous (Fig. 3.1.). Further systematic breakdown of these groups seems unnecessary, for it appears that there are as many different capillary types as there are organs (Majno 1965). Precapillary arterioles contain a small myocyte sheath and end at a lower limit of approximately 14μ in the capillary network. Postcapillary venules range from $10–100\mu$ in diameter. In the absence of intraluminal erythrocytes, the postcapillary venules may be confused with lymph vessels (Leak 1971).

COMPONENTS OF THE CAPILLARY WALL

ENDOTHELIUM

The flattened endothelial cells of capillaries are joined together by specialized cell junctions which have macula occludens with 4 nm gaps. The luminal sides adhere tightly but the junction is looser at the outer surface. The apposing material of the intercellular junction contains mucopolysaccharides (Luft 1966) which allegedly

CONTINUOUS — Muscle / Nerve / Adipose / Dermis

FENESTRATED — Intestinal villi / Endocrine glands / Renal Glomerulus

DISCONTINUOUS — Liver / Bone marrow / Spleen

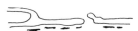

Fig. 3.1. Classification of capillaries.

represent the fused external layers of the endothelial cell membranes. Fenestrae are present in capillaries of the intestinal mucosa, endocrine glands, and renal glomeruli and are important in the regulation of permeability.

Endothelial cells contain myofibrils and if these function in contractility, they may explain many alterations involving constriction and expansion of the capillary in response to vasoactive chemicals. Dense granules are present in endothelial cells (most prominently in lower vertebrates) and in all species granules tend to be commoner in pathologic states characterized by increased transportation of macromolecules across the cell. They may be the source of the clotting factors contained in the endothelium.

Portions of reactive endothelial cells may protrude into the capillary lumen as intraluminal flaps. True pseudopodia, rarely present normally, are commonly seen in injured and inflamed endothelium. They are associated with phagocytosis. Capillary endothelium is phagocytic but is the most sluggish member of the reticuloendothelial system. In the renal glomerulus, phagocytes located outside the capillary protrude through the endothelium. Their activity is termed *transendothelial phagocytosis* (Farquhar and Palade 1961).

BASEMENT MEMBRANE

The *capillary basement membrane* is a fibrillary-structured membrane of approximately 50 nm thickness. Chemically, it is similar to collagen, but the presence of a mucopolysaccharide component is obvious from its staining with the periodic acid-Schiff (PAS) reaction and its resistance to hyaluronidase. The membrane is composed of dense and clear layers both of which thicken with age. The basement membrane functions as a filter, allowing passage of water and small molecules of less than 10 nm size but not colloids. It also serves as a cytoskeleton for endothelial regeneration following injury to the capillary.

PERICYTES

The *pericytes* surround capillaries of continuous and fenestrated types and are modified smooth muscle cells. The branching stellate processes grasp the capillary and may occasionally extend to other vessels. Pericytes may become phagocytic in the processes of edema and inflammation. Transitional forms between pericytes and smooth muscle cells occur and are difficult to differentiate.

PATHWAYS ACROSS THE ENDOTHELIUM

Substances are transported across the capillary endothelium in the following ways: (1) direct diffusion; (2) entrance and exit via cell junctions; and (3) active transport via plasmalemmal vesicles (caveolae, pinocytotic vesicles). In fenestrated endothelium, the slit pores impart a special transporting character to the vessel wall.

TRANSPORT BY DIFFUSION

Although not demonstrable microscopically, diffusion is the important means of capillary transport under normal circumstances. Water, electrolytes, gases, and molecules of low molecular weight diffuse through the luminal plasma membrane, into the cytoplasmic matrix, and out the opposing surface. Cell swelling of even small magnitude effectively diminishes the capacity of the endothelial cell to transport substances by diffusion.

CELL JUNCTION TRANSPORT

Normally, some macromolecular materials are transported through intercellular junctions. Molecules the size of horseradish peroxidase (40,000 MW), when utilized as tracers, can be shown to permeate the intercellular clefts (Karnovsky 1967). The restricted transport in capillaries of the brain (the "blood-brain-barrier") is due to very tight intercellular junctions caused by the presence of zonula occludens at endothelial cell junctions.

In inflammation, transportation of fluids and macromolecules through altered cell junctions is a highly significant mechanism. Injury to the endothelial cell appears to loosen its intercellular attachments. This has been clearly shown in experimental cadmium poisoning in which the testicle is markedly affected by edema. The first discrete evidence of capillary injury is seen as separation of endothelial cells and the development of small spaces and cavities in intercellular junctions (Gabbiani et al. 1974). Fluid loss through intercellular junctions is prominent in acute viral injury to endothelium. Equine viral arteritis virus replicates in endothelial cells causing severe cell swelling and vacuolation. The initial changes involve degeneration and loosening of intercellular junctions followed by passage of large amounts of plasma into the perivascular spaces.

PLASMALEMMAL VESICULAR TRANSPORT

This as a basis for rapid transcapillary exchange of fluid and small molecules is questionable but vesicles probably do function effectively for larger molecules. They take in small gulps of particles on one surface and expel them at the other. The first phase is "cell drinking" (endocytosis) and the second its reverse (exocytosis). Although plasmalemmal vesicles are termed pinocytotic, the process involved differs from true pinocytosis for there is no subsequent digestion or fusion with lysosomes.

The early stages of endothelial damage induced by some of the bacterial toxins are characterized by increases and irregularities in plasmalemmal vesicles. Fusion can result in channels that extend from the luminal to the basal surface of the endothelial cells and these channels behave as fenestrae for the transport of fluid (Hashimoto et al. 1974).

Active transport by plasmalemmal vesicles has been widely studied in experiments with tracer particles such as ferritin and horseradish peroxidase. Two minutes after intravenous injection of ferritin, particles appear in the vesicles near the cell membrane. Subsequently, they progressively occur in all vesicles, in microvesicular bodies, in the basement membrane, and in pericapillary spaces. These experiments clearly demonstrate the capacity to transport macromolecules (Simionescu et al. 1974). Plasmalemmal vesicles contain enzymes associated with ATP systems but their role in active transport is not established (Marchesi and Barrnett 1963).

While the proof of capillary transport lies with tracer experiments, other criteria provide circumstantial evidence that vesicles transport particulate material and solutes. For example, there is an agreement between the number of vesicles and the biological activity of the endothelial cell. In endothelial hypertrophy, which occurs in capillaries of the heart during cardiac hypertrophy, there are marked increases in vesicles associated with the plasma membrane (Figs. 3.2, 3.3, and 3.4).

VARIANCE IN CAPILLARY PERMEABILITY

Regional differences in the permeability of capillaries can be explained on the basis of structural variations in the vascular wall. Transport kinetics indicate that permeability to macromolecules increases in the order: limbs, intestine, liver sinusoids, brain. Superimposed upon anatomical differences are systemic factors which alter permeability.

Cyclic changes occur in vessels of some organs that are endocrinologically controlled. For example, endothelial cells of the capillaries of the uterine mucosa are flattened and relatively structureless in sexually inactive females. They become markedly enlarged and filled with ribosomes upon stimulation with progesterone during the mating season (Friederici 1967).

Blood pressure exerts some effect on the passage rate of low molecular proteins through endothelium. When hypertension is induced experimentally in rats, there is evidence that the protein tracers such as horseradish peroxidase pass into tissue in massive amounts and this implies a loss of molecular barrier in the endothelial cell (Hüttner et al. 1973).

Research on the activity of capillaries is hampered by the failure of these structures to survive intact in vitro. Endothelial cells have recently been grown in cell culture and it is hoped this system will be useful in experimental pathology (Lewis et al. 1973).

SPECIALIZED STRUCTURES THAT INFLUENCE THE VASCULAR WALL

NEUROLOGIC CONTROL

Neurologic control of blood vessels is clearly demonstrable by directly stimulating perivascular nerve fibers with microelectrodes. Unmyelinated nerve axons ramify along the exterior layers of the

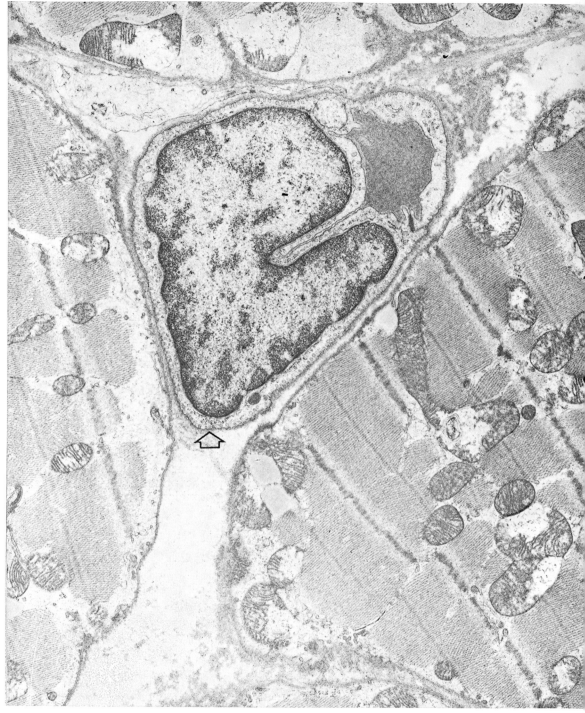

Fig. 3.2. Endothelial cell hypertrophy. Capillary, interfiber space, left ventricular myocardium, aged hypoxic dog with marked cardiac hypertrophy. Basal membrane (arrow) is lined with plasmalemmal vesicles which are organized and uniform in size.

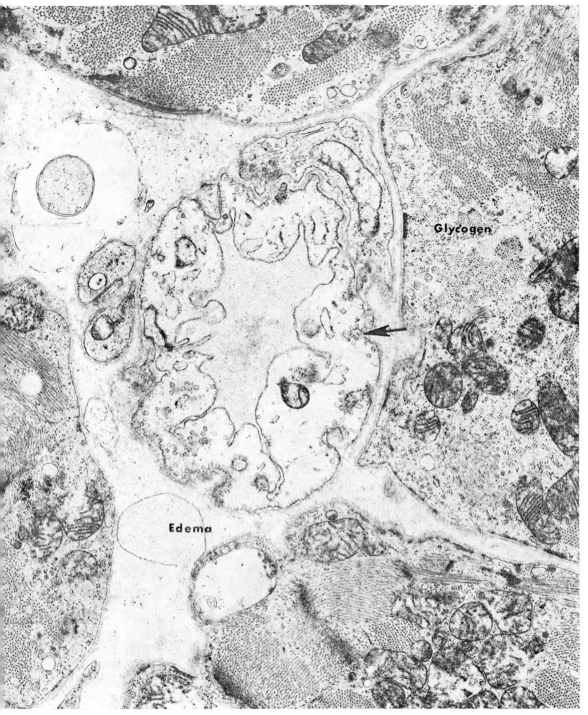

Fig. 3.3. Endothelial cell swelling. Capillary in edematous inter-
fiber space, left ventricular myocardium, cat, cardiac failure with
dilatation. Plasmalemmal vesicles (arrow) at the plasma membrane
are enlarged and disoriented. The cytoplasm is swollen and
numerous infoldings are present in the luminal plasma membrane.

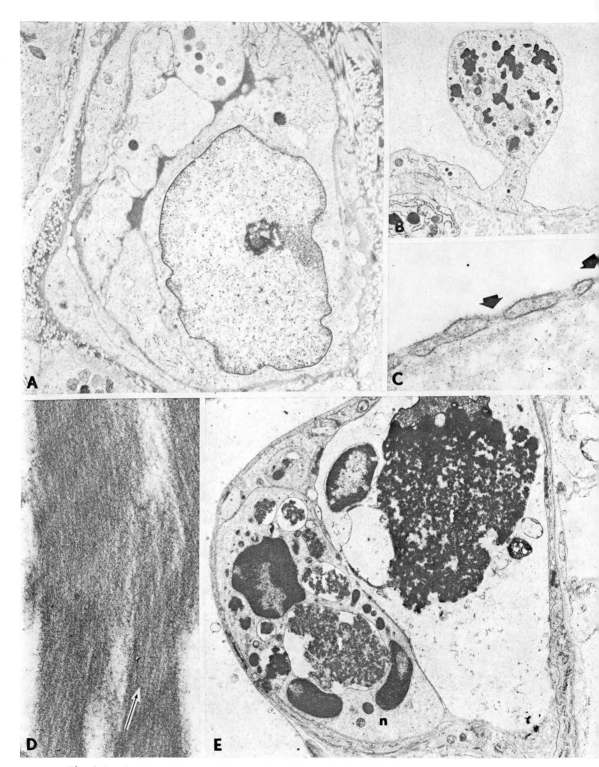

Fig. 3.4. A. Granule-containing endothelium of the high type present in an equine mast cell lesion. B. Hemosiderin granules in an endothelial bleb. C. Fenestrated epithelium in the pituitary sinus, fenestrae (arrows). D. Ultrastructure of fibrin strands; note faint periodicity (arrow). E. Fibrin (f) in neutrophilic leukocytes (n) blocking the capillary bed of lung. Intravascular coagulation, sheep, anaphylactic shock.

terminal arterioles and penetrate the tunica media to lie in close apposition to vascular myocytes. Only those vessels in the terminal vascular bed with smooth myocytes receive direct motor innervation. There is no evidence that the nonmuscular capillaries have either efferent or motor innervation.

CAROTID SINUS AND AORTIC ARCH BAROCEPTORS

Vagal sympathetic stimulation to blood vessels causes vasoconstriction of the terminal arterioles. This vasomotor discharge arises in the medulla oblongata and produces a systemic pressor (tending to increase blood pressure) effect. The vagal response is initiated by baroceptors in the carotid sinus and aortic arch which sense a drop in blood pressure due to lessened cardiac action. Decreased stimulation of the aortic arch and carotid sinus baroceptors decreases the afferent vasodilatory and cardioinhibitory neutral discharges.

JUXTAGLOMERULAR APPARATUS: A RENAL PRESSOR SYSTEM

The juxtaglomerular apparatus is activated by lowering of blood pressure and blood sodium. Arterial pressure drop, as sensed by the arteriole, is transmitted to the granular cells and action is initiated by their release of the enzyme renin into plasma (Fig. 3.5). Renin acts on an unidentified plasma protein substrate converting it to a polypeptide, angiotensin I. The latter is converted to the potent vasoactive polypeptide angiotensin II by another converting enzyme.

also seen in dogs having cardiac failure with edema and sodium retention (Spielman et al. 1973).

The secretory nature of the cytoplasmic granules was first established in experiments showing increased cell content of granules in renal ischemia, adrenalectomy, and low sodium intake (Hartroft 1963). Hyponatremia (decreased plasma sodium) increases renin synthesis and release, and hypernatremia diminishes them (Nichols and Hennigar 1964; Wegmann 1970). High plasma renin values may be predicted, therefore, in low sodium diets and during the use of diuretics. It appears that the amount of sodium absorbed at the macula densa determines renin release (Gomba et al. 1972).

CAROTID AND AORTIC BODIES AND CHEMORECEPTION

These bodies function as chemoreceptors by virtue of connection with the central nervous system. Although no secretion is demonstrable physiologically, they contain dense secretory-type granules within their parenchymal cells and histochemical techniques indicate that they are sites for synthesis, storage, or secretion of substances such as serotonin or epinephrine. It is generally accepted that these bodies are chemoreceptors for CO_2 concentration in blood, and degranulation in response to changes in CO_2 is visible. Afferent innervation of the parenchymal cells is prerequisite to the chemoreceptor hypothesis (Adams 1958). Although synapses are closely associated with normal parenchymal cells, the nature of the flow has not been established.

The carotid and aortic bodies are small

$$\text{Substrate} \xrightarrow{\text{Renin}} \text{Angiotensin I} \xrightarrow{\text{Converting enzyme}} \text{Angiotensin II}$$

The lungs are a major site of conversion. Angiotensin II, concerned with raising blood pressure by peripheral vasoconstriction, is effective in hypovolemic shock. When large amounts of blood are lost in the dog, the blood pressure begins to drop. Levels of plasma renin rise as a compensatory reaction (Hembrough et al. 1974) (Fig. 3.6). Elevated renin levels are

and difficult to locate and are rarely examined in pathologic states. Carotid bodies of animals maintained at high altitudes allegedly undergo hyperplasia with increased numbers of and vacuolation in the light chief cells (Edwards et al. 1972). Tumors occur in the aortic and carotid bodies but well-documented cases of naturally occurring hyperplasia are rare (Cheville 1972).

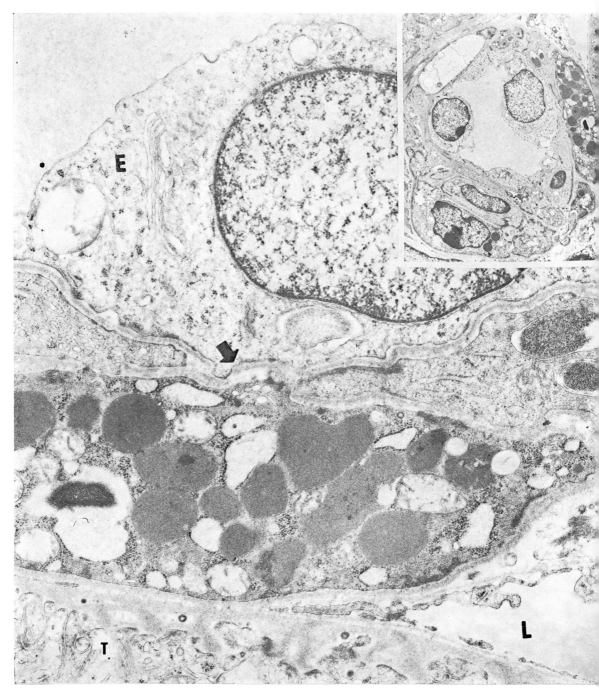

Fig. 3.5. Juxtaglomerular cells, afferent arteriole of renal glomerulus, mouse. Note association of granular juxtaglomerular cell and endothelial cell (E) at arrow. Lymphatic vessel (L) and tubule cell (T). *Inset:* Low-power electron micrograph.

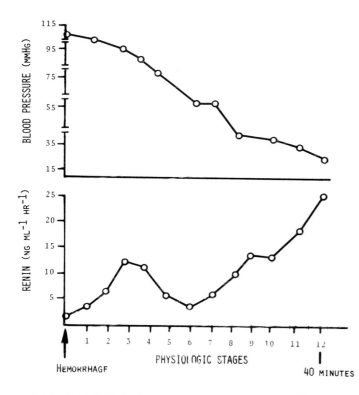

Fig. 3.6. Renin levels in serum in relation to blood pressure during hemorrhage in the dog (modified from Hembrough).

PLASMA PROTEINS

The plasma membrane of endothellal cells, compared to that of other cell types, is remarkably unselective in its permeability. Large water-soluble molecules such as glucose, sucrose, and inulin rapidly pass out of capillaries into the tissue. Only in the case of molecules such as the plasma proteins can capillary permeability be considered as a primary factor in limiting exchange.

PLASMA PROTEIN CONCENTRATION

The concentration of proteins in plasma differs considerably among species and can be determined by a small hand refractometer or by chemical methods such as the biuret reaction. Most adult mammals have values within a range of 6 to 7.5 gms per 100 ml. *Hypoproteinemia,* a decrease in the total plasma protein concentration, occurs in diseases that decrease protein synthesis or promote loss by exudation. The liver is the site of synthesis of albumin, fibrinogen, and some of the globulins, and in liver disease hypoproteinemia may lead to loss

of colloidal osmotic pressure in the plasma. In severe burns, large amounts of all plasma proteins are lost and measurements during this type of injury may indicate the severity of the tissue damage (Ritzmann 1973).

DIFFERENTIATION OF PLASMA PROTEINS

Plasma albumin, fibrinogen, and globulins each have distinctive physical and chemical characteristics that separate them from the others. Their individual net charges are utilized to separate them by electrophoretic migration. In the electrophoresis unit a small sample of plasma is placed on paper wetted with buffer and migration is induced by opposing electrical charges at the ends of the paper strip. The proteins on the paper are then stained and the pattern is transposed to graphic form, the electrophoretogram, by a densitometer (Fig. 3.7). The percent of each plasma protein can be calculated by partitioning the peaks on the electrophoretogram and calculating the various percentages from the total plasma protein concentration. For practical purposes, the protein that is

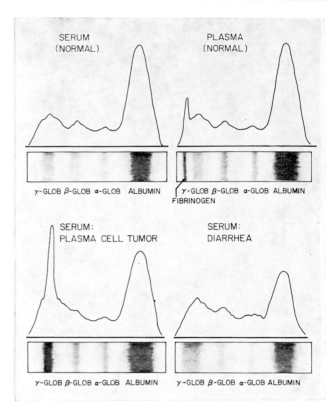

Fig. 3.7. Electrophoretograms of normal serum and plasma, and serum from dogs with plasma cell tumor and severe diarrhea.

most often affected in hypoproteinemia is albumin.

ALBUMIN

The albumin molecule has a molecular weight of 69,000 and is the smallest of the major plasma proteins. Its functions in plasma are: (1) To regulate the exchange of water between blood and tissue. Albumin is the major factor in maintaining osmotic regulation: each gm % of serum albumin exerts osmotic pressure of 5.5 mm Hg. (2) To act as a buffer. Albumin is amphoteric and can combine with both acids and bases. (3) To act as a reserve of protein in the body. Albumin levels in blood do not rise above normal except during hemoconcentration or dehydration. Hypoalbuminemia is a common finding in acute diseases such as edema, glomerulonephritis, and protein-losing diarrhea where the albumin molecules escape from the vascular system (Marsh et al. 1969; Reynolds et al. 1971). The reduced plasma protein concentration is reflected in the lower peak of albumin in the electrophoretogram.

Albumin polymorphism, the presence of two different albumin types in sera, occurs in hybrid animals produced from inter-species crosses. Mules (Amin and Shamloo 1963) and bird hybrids such as chicken-turkey crosses (Phillips et al. 1973) have electrophoretic patterns with two distinct peaks of albumin in electrophoretograms. In the chicken-turkey cross, the faster migrating albumin is identical to that in normal chicken serum; the slower is identical to turkey albumin. Inherited polymorphism of serum albumin has also been reported to occur in fowl, cattle, and humans.

FIBRINOGEN

Fibrinogen is the precursor of fibrin, the substance of the blood clot. It is removed during the clotting process and leaves serum containing albumin and globulins. The fibrinogen molecule is large, elongate, and asymmetric and is synthesized in the liver. It is nodose and consists of three beads (6.5 nm diameter) held together by a thin strand. Plasma levels of fibrinogen may be markedly decreased in diseases that are accompanied by intravascular clotting.

GLOBULIN

The globulin portion of serum protein is a very complex mixture. It includes the gamma globulins, the molecules produced by the lymphoid system that have antibody activity (see Chapter 5). The alpha and beta globulins are produced by the liver and function in various ways; many are active in the transport of other substances in blood. One globulin (transferrin) combines stoichiometrically with iron and is responsible for iron transport. In iron deficiency anemia there is a significant increase in transferrin in plasma. In some chronic infections this globulin may be decreased, leading to less efficient transport of iron. Another globulin, ceruloplasm, combines with copper for purposes of transport. The plasma lipoproteins consist of combinations of lipids with alpha globulins.

EDEMA

Edema is the abnormal accumulation of fluid in interstitial spaces or body cavities. It results when the forces that move fluid from the vascular lumen to the interstitium are augmented over those producing the reverse effect. Starling's law states that hydrostatic pressure in the vascular system (aided slightly by perivascular osmotic pressure) moves fluid out of the system (Fig. 3.8). The forces holding the fluid within the blood are the osmotic pressure of the plasma proteins and, to a lesser extent, tissue pressure around blood vessels.

Edema fluid closely resembles lymph. It is characterized as a transudate by having a low protein content and a specific gravity below 1.012. Microscopically, tissue spaces are distended by albuminous fluids and lymph vessels are dilated. The fluid appears in electron micrographs as uniform, lightly granular precipitates. In most instances the structural changes in the vascular wall that occur in edema are too subtle to be meaningful.

Experimentally, the abnormal passage of fluid and macromolecules through damaged capillaries has been demonstrated using electron-dense tracers. After the intravenous injection of ferritin in animals whose brain vasculature has been damaged by *E. coli* endotoxin, it is seen ultrastructurally that ferritin particles are not transported normally but appear throughout the endothelial cell cytoplasm and in the perivascular spaces (Drommer 1973).

LOCAL EDEMA

Edema may be general or local. Local edema (that is, noninflammatory) is nearly always due to lymphatic blockade. The normal flow of interstitial fluid into the lymphatics is prevented and edema fluid accumulates locally. This type of edema is associated with lymphatics damaged by surgery, neoplasms, and intravascular parasites. Rare hereditary malformations of the lymphatic vessels have been reported in dogs and calves (Luginbuhl et al. 1967; Morris et al. 1954). Because of the blockade in the lymph vessels, the diseases are mani-

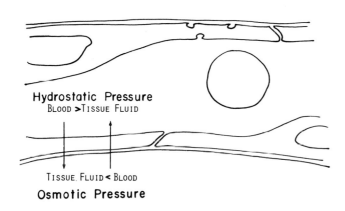

Hydrostatic Pressure
BLOOD >TISSUE FLUID

TISSUE FLUID < BLOOD
Osmotic Pressure

Fig. 3.8. Forces draining fluid from and into the capillary.

fested as local subcutaneous edema of the limbs.

Local edema is also an early and significant part of inflammation. Inflammatory edema, which is due to damage of the endothelium with increased capillary permeability, is rapidly converted to an exudate that is high in protein and specific gravity. The massive edema of the subcutis and serous surfaces that develops in equine viral arteritis is characterized by the deposition of large amounts of albumin and fibrinogen (see Chapter 4).

GENERALIZED EDEMA

Generalized edema occurs most often in one of two basic mechanisms: increased hydrostatic pressure of the blood or decreased colloid osmotic pressure of plasma protein. Decreased levels of plasma proteins are seen in chronic blood-loss anemia, in chronic renal disease (with loss of albumin in the urine), and in starvation. When protein levels in plasma fall below 5%, the potential for edema is present. Fluid is usually found in the subcutis in the cervical areas and around the legs.

The sites of edema are important factors in both diagnosis and prognosis. In most tissues, fluid does not have immediate clinical significance to the patient. In the lungs and brain, however, edema may rapidly produce severe disease and even death. Fluid in locations which relate to severe clinical affection often have special designations: anasarca, swelling of the subcutis due to severe generalized edema; hydrothorax, fluid in the thoracic cavity (also hydropericardium); and ascites (hydroperitoneum), fluid in the peritoneal cavity.

ANASARCA AND CARDIAC FAILURE

In progressive cardiac failure, generalized edema is nearly always present. Fluid is present in the body cavities and in subcutaneous tissues, particularly in the limbs. Because the heart cannot pump the amount of blood received from the veins, venous pressure rises and is transmitted to the capillary bed where fluid exudes. Endothelial cells of capillaries and veins involved in stasis are usually swollen and the cell organelles disoriented (Tedder and

Shorey 1965). Fluid and protein precipitates disrupt the basement membrane and pericapillary spaces. In the end stage of cardiac failure, capillaries of the myocardium are involved in edema. Pinocytotic vesicles, markedly increased in the earlier phase of cardiac hypertrophy, are generally enlarged, coalesced, and disoriented (Fig. 3.3). In these final stages of cardiac failure, other secondary problems are superimposed upon the capillaries. The retention of chlorides by the kidney aggravates the already existing edema. The continued escape of protein lowers the osmotic pressure of blood and raises that of tissue, enhancing fluid exudation.

ASCITES

Ascites is the intraperitoneal accumulation of fluid. The genesis of ascites is complex and probably involves retention of sodium ions and water, hypoalbuminemia, and decreased colloid osmotic pressure. It is not mediated solely by increased hydrostatic pressure in all species, because experimental ligation of the portal vein in dogs does not cause remarkable accumulation of fluid in the peritoneal cavity.

Any rise in intrahepatic portal venous pressure (as seen in congestive cardiac failure, constrictive pericarditis, cirrhosis, or occlusion of hepatic veins) may lead to ascites. The pathogenesis begins with increased pressure in the liver sinusoids, which alters the fenestrated endothelial cells and promotes the escape of plasma into the subendothelial spaces of Disse. This excess extracellular fluid is removed by the hepatic lymphatics. That which cannot be handled leaks through the capsule of the liver into the peritoneal cavity. If the quantity of fluid is large, the absorptive capacity of the peritoneal lymphatics is exceeded and ascites results. The liver capsule becomes edematous and pools of fluid develop under the surface mesothelium. Ultrastructurally, mesothelial cells are hypertrophic and vesicular, with evidence of phagocytic activity.

PULMONARY EDEMA

Pulmonary edema is the accumulation of edema fluid in the alveolus of the lung.

It is brought about by excessive amounts of plasma exuding from the capillary bed of the lung into the alveoli. In the earliest phases, fluid accumulates in the interstitium of the alveolar wall, where it disrupts the basement membranes of the endothelial cells and membranous pneumocytes. The first evidence of edema occurs perivascularly and it is believed that fluid is rapidly drained along connective tissue fibers to perivascular cuffs which lead to lymph vessels (Cottrell et al. 1967; Pietra et al. 1971). Electron microscopy has not revealed the presence of lymphatics within the alveolar wall, but only in tissues surrounding the bronchioles and arterioles.

Two major mechanisms are involved in the causation of pulmonary edema: (1) circulatory failure-induced changes in pulmonary hemodynamics, which result in a slow exudation of fluid into alveoli and (2) any sudden diffuse and direct damage to the pulmonary capillary endothelium. The latter is usually a peracute stage of inflammation and if the animal survives is followed by pneumonitis. Both of the above conditions are associated with marked capillary dilation; the distinction between extreme hyperemia and pulmonary edema is often arbitrary.

Pulmonary edema associated with cardiac failure is inevitably chronic. Lymph flow increases, lymphatics enlarge, and the alveolar walls become thickened. Granular pneumocyte hyperplasia is common and these cells may line the alveoli (Ortega et al. 1970). In long-standing pulmonary edema, collagen is deposited in the alveolar wall and the resiliency of the respiratory lobules is diminished (Fig. 3.9).

SHOCK

Shock is the syndrome resulting from hypotension caused by acute generalized circulatory failure of the capillary bed. It is a state of acute peripheral circulatory failure caused by sudden severe injury. The fundamental disturbance is that blood volume is too small to fill the vascular system. The common denominator is a fall in blood pressure; the accompanying cell damage is due to hypoxia. Death may occur at any phase of shock due to acute circulatory failure and its attendant damage to the central nervous system, the myocardium, and other organs.

Shock is seen in conditions that produce: (1) loss of blood volume and (2) peripheral pooling of blood in the capillary bed or veins. Normal arterial blood pressure is maintained by cardiac output and by total vascular peripheral resistance. Shock may follow marked depression of either of these mechanisms. It is an ominous sign and often terminates in death despite treatment.

Animals with shock are lethargic and unresponsive to external stimuli. Muscle weakness is a prominent sign. Body temperature is apt to be subnormal (because of lowered metabolism) and there is pallor and coolness of the skin. Heart rate is increased in most types of shock but may be slow and irregular. Depression of renal function and urine production often occur. Because shock can be caused by diverse types of injury, the clinical appearances cannot be rigidly defined. Factors such as pain, cold, general anesthesia, hypoproteinemia, dehydration, and exhaustion do not cause shock directly but certainly augment the mechanisms which cause circulatory collapse. Trauma impairs thermoregulation, and in the presence of a cold environment falls in body temperature and oxygen consumption occur (Stoner 1969). These suppress the mechanisms that operate to overcome the shock state.

Cytopathology in shock is a result of hypoxia. As a consequence of inadequate peripheral circulation there is decreased oxygen delivery (Crowell 1970). Hypoxia leads to decreased oxidative phosphorylation and ATP production. Lesions occur in mitochondria. Pyruvate cannot enter the Krebs cycle and cells are forced to obtain energy by anaerobic glycolysis. Lactate accumulates and leads to metabolic acidosis. Thus, in the terminal stages of shock, a metabolic disease accompanies the circulatory deficit. Although hyperglycemia is characteristic of early shock (related to catecholamine release), hypoglycemia occurs in the later stages due to depletion of liver glycogen and hyperinsulinemia. During shock there is a prolongation of insulin half life due to reduced peripheral utilization.

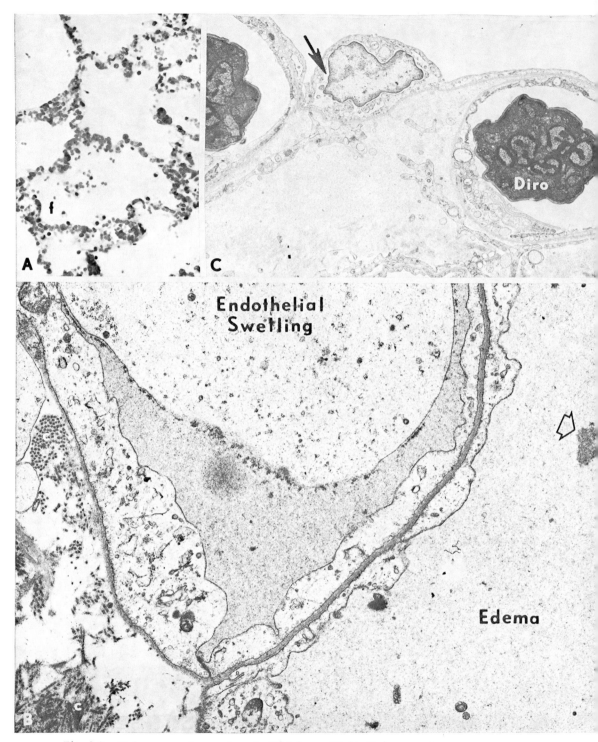

Fig. 3.9. Pulmonary edema, dog. A. Histology. Fluid (f) is present in alveoli. Capillaries are hyperemic and erythrocytes have extravasated into the alveoli. B. Plasma proteins (of edema fluid) fill the alveolus. Note fibrin deposits (arrow), swollen endothelium and interstitial collagen fibers (c). C. Edema of the alveolar wall (interstitial edema) due to shedding of microfilaria of *Dirofilaria immitis* (Diro) into the pulmonary capillary bed from heart. Membranous pneumocyte (arrow) is swollen and projects into alveolus.

Table 3.1. Lesions of shock in the dog

Organ	Gross Appearance	Microscopic Lesions	Mechanism
Liver	Congested Swollen	Hyperemia of sinusoids Serous exudation (in spaces of Disse)	Constriction of myocytes of hepatic vein and increase in venous portal pressure
Intestine	Hyperemia Hemorrhage (blood in feces)	Hyperemia of villi Subepithelial edema Necrosis and sloughing of villous tips	Elevated portal venous pressure
Heart	Hyperemia Subendocardial hemorrhage	Focal necrosis of cardiac myocytes	Hypoxia (also medial necrosis of aorta)
Lung	Hyperemia Edema (rare)	Hyalin thrombi in capillaries	Vascular stasis, intravascular platelet aggregation or coagulation
Adrenal	Hyperemia Hemorrhage (rare)	Foci of necrosis and hemorrhage	?

Differences in the manifestation of shock are related to the cause of shock and to the species of animal affected. Great species differences exist (Chang and Hackel 1973; Zweifach 1961). The brain and heart are highly susceptible to hypoxia generated by a fall in blood pressure; foci of necrosis and hemorrhage develop in these organs in most species. Tissues vary in the amount of oxygen removed during blood flow. While the average is approximately 25%, the myocardium removes 75% of the oxygen of the blood flowing through the capillary system of the heart. When cardiac output is diminished by one-quarter and blood oxygenation is reduced, as happens during shock, the total oxygen transported to the heart cannot meet the requirements of myocardial metabolism.

Shock in the dog has been widely studied and we use this animal as a model (Table 3.1). The liver is the prominent organ affected (Hackel et al. 1964; Ramsey et al. 1972). Constriction of veins raises the portal venous pressure and causes stasis in the liver and intestine. Hepatocytes undergo degeneration and necrosis (Blair et al. 1968) and this results in their failure to effectively detoxify harmful substances. The Kupffer cells fail to remove macromolecules. Split products of fibrinolysis, bacteria, and endotoxins, which arrive in the liver from the portal venous system, are allowed to pass into the general circulation.

Vascular dilatation in shock leads to a lower flow rate which favors the aggregation and sludging of erythrocytes. Platelets tend to aggregate and, in the presence of generalized hypercoagulability, this leads to microthrombus formation (Drommer 1972; Schulz and Rabanus 1965). Thrombosis augments the vascular damage and the cycle is repeated (Sandritter and Lasch 1967). Disastrous effects may occur in the lung where platelet microemboli block the capillary bed. Release of hydrolytic enzymes by disintegrating platelets and neutrophils causes swelling of endothelium and membranous pneumocytes (Connell et al. 1975).

Counterregulatory mechanisms are initiated in shock regardless of the cause. These are evoked by low blood pressure and diminished cardiac output (via pressure receptors) and stimulate the sympathetic nervous system to produce peripheral vasoconstriction and tachycardia. Hemodynamic alterations of the lung circulation reduce the active ventilatory surface and result in hypoxic stimulation of the central respiratory centers.

HYPOVOLEMIC SHOCK

Hypovolemic shock is shock due to loss of blood volume. It is a common effect of massive loss of whole blood during hemorrhage ("hemorrhagic shock"). Loss of blood volume can also occur, deceivingly, when large amounts of plasma exude into tissue, as happens in severe burns and crush injuries.

Extensive blood loss is required before animals develop hypovolemic shock. Healthy animals may lose one-quarter of their blood volume without showing immediate clinical signs and loss of one-half may be required to produce death. When much blood is lost, the arterial blood pressure drops and venous return to the heart decreases. The heart rate may increase, but stroke volume and cardiac output are diminished.

Arterial vasoconstriction is a rapid response to drop in blood pressure and produces increased peripheral resistance, which shunts blood from the skin and viscera to the heart and brain. The interacting mechanisms that enhance vasoconstriction include: (1) lessened stimulation of baroceptors in the aortic arch and carotid sinus which decreases the afferent vasodilatory and cardioinhibitory neural discharges, (2) vagal and vasomotor discharge from the medulla oblongata, and (3) release of catecholamines from the adrenal medulla. Norepinephrine constricts peripheral vascular beds; epinephrine constricts most of these and dilates the coronary arteries (Walker et al. 1959).

The effects of extensive loss of blood volume produce profound changes in the kidney. Renal vasoconstriction reduces perfusion and causes the juxtaglomerular cells to degranulate. Plasma renin concentrations rise and activate the angiotensin system. Angiotensin tends to raise the falling blood pressure by causing peripheral vasoconstriction. It also stimulates the secretion of antidiuretic hormone (vasopressin) by the pituitary which acts to conserve water normally lost from the lower nephron. Aldosterone secretion by the adrenal cortex is augmented and leads to increased resorption of salt and water by the renal tubule. All of these mechanisms conserve fluid and support blood volume.

If arterial blood pressure is measured during and after extensive blood loss, two plateaus in the pressure curve are seen (Fig. 3.10). The first of these, which begins during the blood loss, is due to pressoreceptor reflexes. These produce strong sympathetic stimulation (and parasympathetic inhibition) to blood vessels when the arterial pressure begins to fall. The response is vasoconstriction and contraction of the spleen, spewing erythrocytes and platelets

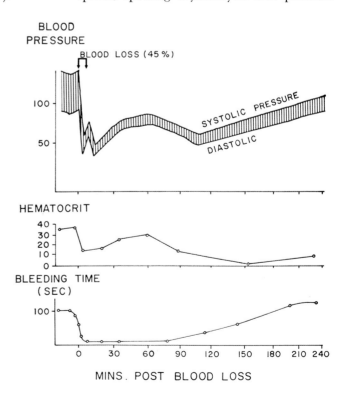

Fig. 3.10. Hematologic changes during acute hemorrhage.

into the blood (Hatcher et al. 1954). These compensatory mechanisms are blocked by general anesthesia and animals whose reflexes have been so removed lose arterial pressure from the onset of blood loss. A second, later, and more powerful plateau is the CNS ischemic reflex. It is activated when arterial pressure becomes sufficiently low to cause brain ischemia.

Progressive deterioration of the circulatory system occurs in massive burns and blood loss despite the above compensatory mechanisms. The designation *irreversible shock* implies the refractory state of circulatory failure with inability to clinically control the disease. When blood is removed from a dog in sufficient quantity to produce shock and is not replaced for 4 hrs, the dog will enter a shock state that cannot be reversed despite total restoration of the blood volume. The infused fluid or blood seems to be sequestered in the peripheral capillary beds, suggesting that there is vasomotor paralysis of the microcirculation caused in part by hypoxia.

HYPOVOLEMIC SHOCK IN INFECTIOUS DISEASE

The loss of plasma volume is a critical factor in several infectious diseases, notably in simian hemorrhagic fever, epidemic hemorrhagic disease of deer, and equine viral arteritis. We have examined the vascular changes and edema that occur in severe equine viral arteritis. The collapse and death that characterize the terminal stages of this disease are due to a fatal sequence of events: capillary necrosis, increased vascular permeability, loss of intravascular plasma volume, hemoconcentration, and hypotension. Other factors such as thrombocytopenia, decreased prothrombin levels, adrenal necrosis, and lymphocyte depletion play roles in the process but the hypovolemic shock is most responsible for the fatalities that occur.

SHOCK DUE TO POOLING OF BLOOD

The expansion of the capillary bed beyond the capacity of blood to fill it results in the shock state. Vasodilation is a potent mechanism for reducing arterial blood pressure. When the splanchnic blood vessels are fully dilated, they have the capacity to accommodate nearly the total blood volume. If this occurred, blood pressure would drop to zero. Normally, continual vasoconstriction of the terminal arterioles prevents this from happening. However, toxins and other substances that cause peripheral vasodilation may lead to the shock state. This type of shock is common in animals and is seen particularly in toxic and septic conditions.

Toxic shock is mediated by toxins released from damaged tissue, venoms (Ramsey et al. 1972), or microbial endotoxins that cause vascular paralysis. It commonly accompanies severe burns and intestinal gangrene. The mechanism is decreased cardiac output and arterial pressure secondary to sequestration of venous blood in the hepatosplanchnic bed. Severe injuries may be accompanied by release of hepatic lysosomal hydrolytic enzymes in a free, active form; elevation of acid phosphatase may accelerate the appearance of shock (Janoff et al. 1962).

One of the most studied examples is *endotoxic shock,* produced by the cell wall lipopolysaccharide (endotoxin) of gram negative bacilli such as *E. coli.* Endotoxin injures the capillary endothelium, inducing vasodilation and fluid loss (Coalson et al. 1970; Drommer 1972). After the experimental intravenous injection of endotoxin, there is a precipitous decline in arterial blood pressure, with simultaneous elevation in portal venous return and cardiac output. Examination of the splanchnic veins 1 hr later reveals marked congestion and dilatation. Venous pooling plays a highly significant role in endotoxin shock. In dogs, pooling in the hepatic-portal system is responsible for a significant decrease in venous return of blood to the heart. Perfusion of blood through the kidney is markedly diminished and oliguria may occur. The platelet count drops precipitously; there may be platelet aggregation and coagulation within the vascular system.

Septic shock (exotoxic shock) occurs in overwhelming infections by cocci and other gram positive bacteria. It is therefore essential that blood pressure is maintained in severe systemic infections. Blood viscosity increase is a factor that may reduce blood flow to the capillary bed. The pathways leading from bacterial sepsis to shock are not known and it is difficult to separate the presence of shock from such other phenomena as bacteria-induced vascular diseases and disseminated intravascular coagulation.

OTHER TYPES OF SHOCK

In addition to the two principal patterns of shock, there are less important (and less understood) ways in which shock syndromes occur. The varying adjectives applied to shock indicate the complexity of reactions leading to the final common pathway.

Neurogenic shock may occur in animals with severe fright, pain, and trauma (without hemorrhage). They enter a shock state mediated by the nervous system which induces peripheral vasodilation and loss of effective circulating blood. The mechanism appears to be vasodilation of the peripheral circulation. The study of shock which accompanies severe crush injuries is revealing. If tourniquets are applied to limbs crushed experimentally, external fluid loss is prevented but circulatory collapse is not (if nerves remain intact). In contrast, sectioning of the nerves, even without the tourniquet, prevents shock. Neurogenic shock is true circulatory collapse and should not be confused with fainting. Neurogenic shock is commonly seen in restrained wild birds and mammals, especially in cold weather.

Cardiac shock may occur due to sudden decrease in cardiac output which accompanies sudden extensive damage to the heart. Most animals succumb directly to myocardial inadequacy. In those rare animals that do not, shock may ensue because of pooling of the blood in the capillary beds.

Anaphylactic shock is the circulatory collapse that accompanies the binding of antigens to cell-bound antibodies. It is mediated through the massive intravascular release of histamine which induces increased arteriolar and venous dilatation. The clinical signs of shock that appear are due to greatly reduced arterial pressure and venous return of blood to the heart. The syndrome is dominated by immune-complex–induced platelet aggregation, trapping of aggregates in the lung, and increased pulmonary vascular resistance.

HEMORRHAGE

Hemorrhage is due most commonly to trauma. The blood vessel is torn and whole blood escapes. Most injuries associated with hemorrhage are external and may deprive the animal of blood (exsanguination). When blood escapes into tissue, that is, not through broken surfaces, it accumulates as a blood-filled space or *hematoma*. Accumulation of blood in the body cavities is called *hemothorax, hemopericardium,* or *hemoperitoneum,* depending on which cavity is involved.

Very tiny hemorrhages into the skin, mucous membranes, and serosal surfaces are designated *petechiae*. Their presence often indicates a severe generalized process. Petechiae are commonly seen in septicemia, where the endothelium is destroyed by bacterial toxins, and in viral infections, in which the virus replicates in the vascular endothelium. The viral diseases hog cholera, equine viral arteritis, Newcastle disease of chickens, and epidemic hemorrhagic disease of deer are all characterized by multiple petechiation caused, in part, by necrosis of endothelial cells.

Hemorrhages slightly larger than petechiae are called *purpura*. These are associated most commonly with disturbances of the clotting mechanism allowing more extensive escape of blood due to failure of blockage of the injured vessel. *Ecchymoses* are large hemorrhages (over 1 cm in diameter). Large bruises are ecchymoses.

The significance of lost blood depends upon the acute or chronic nature of the hemorrhage and how much blood has been lost. The consequence of acute blood loss may be hypovolemic shock; that of chronic loss is seen as anemia.

When hemorrhage occurs within tissue, erythrocytes are lysed or are phagocytized by macrophages (erythrophagocytosis). Hemoglobin is released and is degraded into bilirubin and hemosiderin. These impart their characteristic colors to the appearance of the tissues involved. Bilirubin may form yellow crystals called hematoidin in tissue.

HEMOSTASIS

In vertebrates, blood circulates in a closed vascular system and elaborate devices have evolved to prevent blood loss following injury. Despite species differences, the basic mechanisms of hemostasis are remarkably similar (Archer 1970; Doolittle and Surgenor 1962; Hackett and Hann 1967; Rowsell 1968; Stopforth 1970). *Vasoconstriction,* an immediate, transient response, is effective in reducing blood flow to the site of injury. Thrombocyte or *platelet adherence* to injured endothelium occurs and is capable of stopping blood loss in small vascular breaks. *Coagulation,* the polymerization of fibrin from fibrinogen, is the highly effective mechanism in stanching blood flow. This is particularly true when coagulation is combined with platelet aggregation in the formation of thrombi. When blood loss occurs in an enclosed space, the back pressure of blood accumulating extravascularly is also a factor in the prevention of further extravasation.

BLOOD COAGULATION

Clotting (blood coagulation) results when blood is removed or escapes from the vascular system. It also occurs within vessels during life as an integral part of thrombosis. Coagulation is initiated when thrombin, a proteolytic enzyme, acts on plasma fibrinogen converting it to fibrin:

$$\text{Fibrinogen} \xrightarrow{\text{Thrombin}} \text{Fibrin monomer} \xrightarrow{\text{Thrombin Ca}^{++}} \begin{array}{c}\text{Fibrin polymer}\\ \text{(insoluble)}\end{array}$$

The end result is the red clot, a tangled meshwork of fibrin strands with entrapped blood cells (Fig. 3.4).

Fibrinogen is a soluble plasma protein with a molecular weight of nearly 340,000. The molecule is nodose and consists of three beads (6.5 nm diameter) held together by a thin strand of protein (Hall 1963). *Fibrin,* which polymerizes from fibrinogen molecules, forms long fibrils. In thin sections regular crossbanding can occasionally be seen, separated by 5 nm spacing. The periodicity of the bands is approximately 23 nm (Still and Boult 1957).

Prothrombin is synthesized in the liver (Anderson and Barnhart 1964). The *prothrombin complex* which initiates thrombin production may be formed in two ways: (1) Extrinsic clotting occurs when shed blood contacts tissue debris lipopro-

teins (collectively called *thromboplastin);* thrombin is generated in seconds. (2) Intrinsic (or cell-free) clotting is brought about by contact of negatively charged surfaces with factor XII (Hageman factor). Intrinsic coagulation involves a cascade of complex enzymic reactions, each of which activates the next until the thrombin is formed (Fig 3.11). When the vessel wall is disrupted, subendothelial collagen, basement membrane material, and other connective tissue elements are exposed to plasma. Free carboxyl groups of the exposed collagen activate factor XII. When activated, factor XII initiates the rapid, complex sequence of clotting that terminates in fibrin polymerization (Table 3.2). Factor XII also allegedly may initiate the complement, kinin, and plasmin systems.

COAGULATION DISORDERS

Absence of any of the substances involved in the clotting sequence may result in inadequacy of blood coagulation, as also may defects in any factor. Alternatively, coagulation may be impaired by inhibitors or by the proteolytic action of plasmin. The clinical signs of these diseases involve hemorrhaging, and the differential diagnosis is entirely a laboratory exercise. It is usually necessary that the coagulation time, bleeding time, partial thromboplastin time, prothrombin time, and platelet count be determined (Table 3.3).

When an abnormal clotting mechanism is suspected because of prolonged clotting times and abnormal partial thromboplastin and prothrombin times, the specific coagulation factor deficit can be determined. Commercial reagent kits are available for the identification of these factors.

HEREDITARY DEFICIENCIES

Hereditary coagulation disorders have been described for most of the coagulation factors in man. In animals, only a few are known and some of these are not manifested as disease. Congenital deficiencies in fibrinogen have been reported in humans and goats (Breukink et al. 1972).

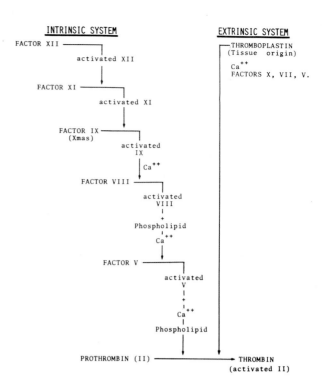

INTRINSIC SYSTEM   EXTRINSIC SYSTEM

Fig. 3.11. Reaction sequences of coagulation factors.

Table 3.2. Blood coagulation factors (a = activated; Factor VI is not now used)

Factor	Common Name	Comment
I	Fibrinogen (Ia = fibrin)	Produced by the liver. Congenital afibrinogenemia seen in goats and humans.
II	Prothrombin (IIa = thrombin)	Produced by the liver. Vitamin K dependent. Acquired deficiencies are common.
III	Tissue thromboplastin	Component of tissues. Brain & lungs certain high concentrations.
IV	Calcium	Must be unbound. If plasma calcium is bound by oxalates or citrates, clotting is prevented.
V	Proaccelerin (plasma accelerator globulin)	Labile. Required in the activation of prothrombin.
VII	Proconvertin	Involved in the activation of prothrombin. Vitamin K dependent. Hereditary deficiency occurs in Beagles.
VIII	Antihemophilic factor A	Classic hemophilia. Seen in Irish Setters. Deficiencies seen as an hereditary sex-linked disorder in males. Also occurs in cats, cattle, swine, horses.
IX	Antihemophilic factor B (Christmas factor)	Hereditary deficiencies seen in Cairn Terriers. Can be depressed by coumarin-type drugs.
X	Stuart factor	Deficiencies can be hereditary or acquired. Depressed by coumarin drugs.
XI	Plasma thromboplastin antecedent	Involved in the early sequences of clot formation. Activated by Factor XII.
XII	Hageman factor	Deficiencies asymptomatic.
XIII	Fibrin stabilizing factor	Strengthens clot network once fibrin is formed.

Table 3.3. Coagulation tests

Test	Definition	Normal Value for Dogs	Levels in[a] Hemorrhage	Hemophilia	Hypoprothrombinemia	Thrombocytopenia
Coagulation time	Time for blood to coagulate in vitro after being withdrawn from a vein	1–5 sec	n	n	+	n
Bleeding time	Time for bleeding to stop after a puncture wound with periodic removal of blood with filter paper	<6 min	n	n	n	+
Prothrombin time	Time required for clotting of oxalated plasma by addition of calcium (in presence of excess thromboplastin)	to 15 sec	n	n	+	n
Platelet count	Number of circulating thrombocytes	200,000 per cmm	n	n	n	+
Partial thromboplastin time	Measurement of intrinsic and common coagulation systems	45 sec	n	+	+	n

[a] n = normal, + = increased

ular clearance and fibrinolysis. If the second injection is given within 20 hrs, the reticuloendothelial system is sufficiently blockaded that the classic reaction develops with thrombi in the kidney, lung, adrenal, and other viscera.

FIBRINOLYSIS

The fibrinolytic mechanism is the physiologic converse of the coagulation mechanism. The end product of coagulation, fibrin, is the substrate for the fibrinolytic enzyme plasmin (fibrinolysin). Fibrinolysis is a defense against overactivity of the coagulation system, which otherwise would lead to the disastrous accumulation of fibrin within the blood vessels that characterizes disseminated intravascular coagulation. Vascular patency appears to depend, therefore, upon an equilibrium between coagulation and fibrinolysis (Hawkey 1970).

PLASMIN

Plasmin is formed from an inactive precursor (plasminogen) which is a β-globulin normally present in plasma. Activators of plasminogen are commonly present in blood and allegedly originate in capillary and venous endothelium:

PLASMINOGEN ACTIVATOR

Plasminogen activator is distributed in tissues unevenly and is detected by a quantitative extraction and assay method (Astrup and Buluk 1963) or by a histochemical fibrin (substrate)-slide technique (Kwaan and Astrup 1967; Myhre-Jensen 1971). In the latter, a section of frozen tissue is placed on a slide containing a thin layer of fibrin rich in the fibrinolytic proenzyme, plasminogen. Holes develop in the fibrin showing where fibrin has been digested by activated plasminogen and these sites of digestion can be related to tissue structures in the section.

Fibrinolytic activity is particularly associated with vascular endothelium and fibrin can be shown to be dissolved when placed over surface endothelium (Warren and Kahn 1974). Activity is also present in leukocytes and some epithelial cells. Mesothelial and synovial membrane cells are quite active in some species. In the kidney, fibrinolytic mechanisms are strong in medullary areas but weak in the renal cortex. Intracellular localization, as determined by subcellular fractionation techniques, indicates that the plasminogen activator is associated with the microsomal (endoplasmic reticulum) and lysosomal fractions.

Plasminogen (β-globulin in serum)
$\downarrow$ Plasminogen activator (in tissue)

$$\text{Fibrin} \xrightarrow{\text{Plasmin}} \text{Breakdown products}$$

The practical detection of plasmin is not clinically meaningful in animal blood, because the stress of collection tends to give invalid data and because detection in plasma is difficult due to the immense amount of antiplasmin present in plasma. This, unfortunately, leaves us with limited knowledge of how plasmin functions in disease processes.

Increased plasma levels of activators of plasminogen are associated with ischemia, acute bacterial infection, anaphylactic shock, and fear states. There is a direct relationship between vasoactive change and fibrinolytic activity. Injections of histamine and adrenalin also induce enhanced fibrinolysis in dogs (Holeman 1965). Exogenous activators of plasminogen include the bac-

Fig. 3.12. Platelets. A. Platelets attached to a defect in capillary endothelium (e). Adrenal cortical cell, sheep, anaphylactic shock. Mitochondria (m), smooth endoplasmic reticulum (ser). Note breaks in endothelial wall. Platelet pseudopods in cross section (arrow) cover endothelial defect. B. Scanning electron micrograph of platelet aggregation. Note pseudopod formation in early agglutination (arrow) and dense platelet aggregates (asterisk). C. Intravascular pseudopod formation, platelets of deer with high fever and inflammatory disease (epidemic hemorrhagic disease). D. Enlarged micrograph of deer platelet with long pseudopod (p).

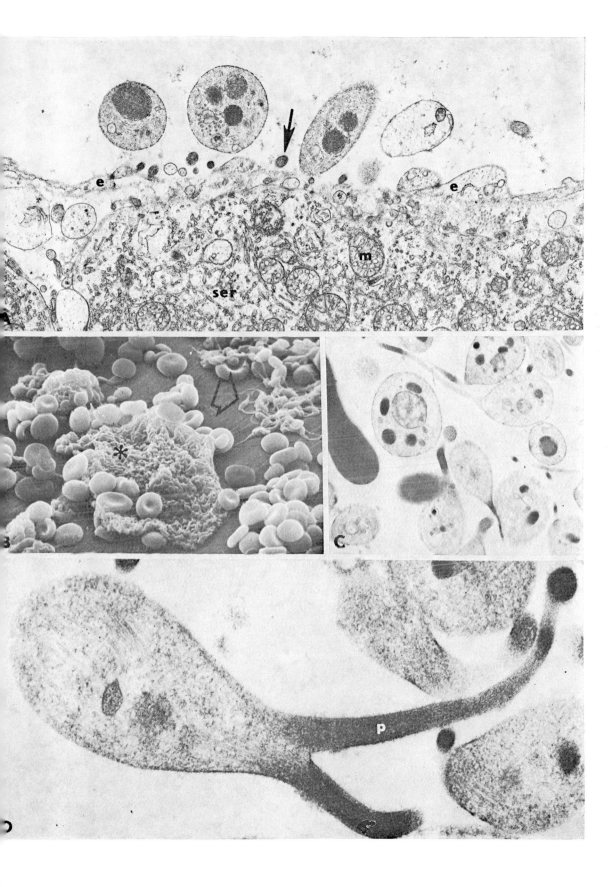

terial products streptokinase and staphylokinase. Vampire bat saliva is a potent source of fibrinolytic activity and enables these predators to feed on the blood of cattle and other mammals.

PLATELET AGGREGATION

Thrombocytes or platelets are necessary for maintenance of vascular integrity. When endothelium is injured, platelets attach to the site of damage, cover the defect, and prevent loss of blood (Figs. 3.12 and 3.13). Platelets are marvelously designed to function in hemostasis. They do so by extending long pseudopods that attach to endothelial defects, by aggregating with themselves, and by releasing factors that initiate blood coagulation. When mammalian blood is devoid of platelets, the vascular system is extraordinarily susceptible to hemorrhage.

PLATELET STRUCTURE

Mammalian platelets originate from bone marrow megakaryocytes which fragment along fissure lines that develop in the cisternae of their endoplasmic reticulum.

The demarcation is initiated by focal invaginations of the megakaryocyte plasma membrane which rapidly spread inward to dissect the cell (MacPherson 1972). Disintegration following fusion of the fissure lines results in the production of 3000–4000 platelets per megakaryocyte (Behnke 1968).

The external membrane of the platelet represents the cisternal surface of membranes of the endoplasmic reticulum. It is responsible for the intense activity and highly negative charge of the platelet surface. The platelet surface is covered by an amorphous glycocalyx with radiating threads which represent a plasma halo of carbohydrates bound in the form of glycoprotein. The halo readily absorbs clotting factors and fibrinogen, giving platelets an extreme tendency to aggregate when in contact with rough surfaces.

The distinctive components of the platelet interior are the large *alpha granules*. They contain acid hydrolases (such as acid phosphatase) and smaller amounts of cationic proteins, cathepsins, and fibrinogen. They also appear to be the source of adenine nucleotides (ADP and ATP), Ca^{++}, and serotonin; the release of these substances by platelets when measured chemi-

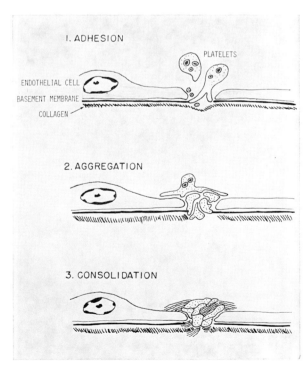

Fig. 3.13. Phases of hemostatic plug formation.

cally correlates with the degranulation of α-granules. The small highly osmiophilic membrane-bound *dense bodies* that are occasionally encountered in platelets are also a potent source of nucleotides and serotonin.

The lentiform shape of the platelet is maintained by the *marginal band* composed of bundles of microfilaments and microtubules at the periphery. Under various stressful conditions the microtubules depolymerize and reassemble and are important in the formation of pseudopods. Abnormal platelets are commonly found in bone marrow neoplasms, especially myeloproliferative disease (Maldonado 1974).

PLATELET RELEASE REACTION

The *platelet release reaction* is the secretion of adenine nucleotides, Ca++, lysosomal enzymes, serotonin, and fibrinogen into the surrounding environment. It occurs when platelets contact injured endothelial surfaces and initiates the process of platelet aggregation.

The release reaction begins when platelets contact connective tissues of the damaged vascular wall. The components of subendothelial connective tissue, in order of their affinity for platelets, have been ranked: collagen fibers, noncollagen fibrils, basement membrane material, and elastin. Of these, collagen and its breakdown products are most significant.

Platelets undergo a remarkable transformation once they adhere to collagen. They change shape from disks to swollen spheres, extend spikelike pseudopods, and progress through a series of changes that collectively are called the platelet release reaction. The marginal band contracts forcing organelles to the cell center. The contents of dense bodies and α-granules are forced into the canaliculi and extruded from the platelet; the released substances promote aggregation of other platelets. Ultrastructurally, the granules disappear from the cell interior and fibrous substances resembling fibrin appear in the cisternae (Droller 1974; White 1972).

Of the released substances, adenosine diphosphate (ADP) is the most powerful inducer of platelet aggregation. Circulating platelets which contact the reactive site swell, stick together, and undergo a release reaction. The process accelerates until large masses of platelets have formed. ADP, and many other promoters of the reaction, do so by decreasing the level of cAMP in the platelet. The prostaglandins, which are effective promoters of aggregation, also act via this mechanism.

Platelet aggregation may also occur without defects in endothelium. When circulating platelets contact bacteria, bacterial mucopeptides, or cell debris, they become phagocytic and degranulation and aggregation occur (Clawson 1973; Rašková et al. 1971). This commonly occurs in the terminal stages of severe systemic infectious diseases. Abnormal platelets are seen with distorted granules and intracellular microorganisms.

When platelets interact with collagen (allegedly involving an enzyme, collagen glucosyltransferase, on the platelet surface) in the presence of plasma proteins, factor XI is activated. This mechanism for activation of the coagulation system bypasses factor XII and may explain the observation that animals with factor XII deficiency do not show bleeding tendencies.

PLATELET DEFICIENCY

Thrombocytopenia, a drop below normal in the number of circulating platelets or thrombocytes, is accompanied by abnormal bleeding tendencies and aptly demonstrates the perpetual function of these cells in maintaining a closed vascular system (Sorenson 1960; Van Horn and Johnson 1966). Studies of dog thyroids perfused with platelet-rich or platelet-poor plasma clearly demonstrate the protection offered by platelets against the development of endothelial damage, edema, and purpura (Gimbrone et al. 1969).

The diagnosis of platelet deficiency is based chiefly on three criteria: bleeding in the history, low platelet count, and increased bleeding time. The history should include a tendency for bleeding because it is impossible for platelet deficiency to exist for even brief periods without affecting hemostasis. The platelet or thrombocyte count should be low, but platelet deficiency can also exist when platelets themselves are abnormal. (The count may be normal and even elevated but the platelets present do not function normally.) To confirm the diagnosis of platelet deficiency, the establishment of an abnormal bleeding time is essential.

Acquired thrombocytopenia may occur in systemic infectious diseases, in acute radiation injury, during drug treatment, and as part of some immunologic diseases involving antiplatelet antibodies. Viruses are known to replicate within platelets; this is responsible for thrombocytopenia and hemorrhage (Laird et al. 1968; Margolis and Kilham 1972). For example, the hemorrhagic diathesis characteristic of the terminal phases of acute hog cholera is due, in part, to viral-induced thrombocytopenia (Heene et al. 1971). Bleeding into submucosal and subserosal areas is characteristic of severe infectious canine hepatitis; the virus destroys megakaryocytes and other cells in the bone marrow. The occurrence of erythrocyte extravasation correlates with the lowest points in the thrombocyte count curve (Fig. 3.14.) Although the liver is injured and decreased prothrombin and fibrinogen levels in plasma have been detected, these factors appear to be far less significant in promoting bleeding. They merely exaggerate the tendency.

Thrombocytes are diminished during aspirin intake by virtue of aspirin's effect in depressing cyclic AMP activity. Platelets and thrombocytes utilize cAMP in important synthetic pathways. They are excellent systems for cAMP assay. During depression by large doses of aspirin, the platelet count may drop precipitously (Mielke et al. 1973).

A decrease in circulating platelets accompanies some physiologic changes, particularly changes in body temperature. Significant depressions in platelets, coagulation factors, and leukocytes occur in dogs made hypothermic by surface body cooling. These alterations serve as a protective mechanism that inhibits thrombosis under conditions of retarded blood flow. Thrombocytopenia and prolonged clotting time (due to deficiency of coagulation factors VIII and IX) occur during hibernation. The striking decrease in platelet numbers is due to sequestration in the cords and red pulp of the spleen. It is alleged that lowered body temperature induces the marginal microtubules to contract, which changes the shape of the platelet and promotes its retention during passage through the spleen (Reddick et al. 1973).

Hereditary deficiencies in platelets have

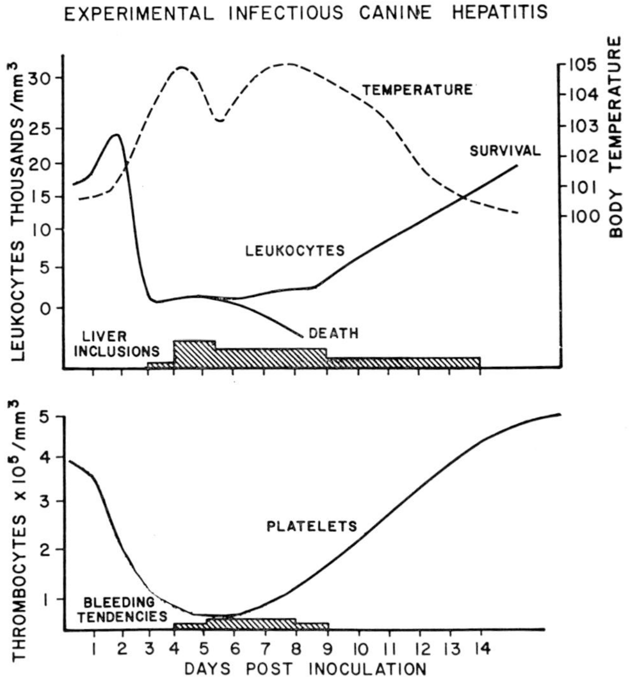

EXPERIMENTAL INFECTIOUS CANINE HEPATITIS

Fig. 3.14. Pathogenesis of infectious canine hepatitis: relation of platelet deficiency to bleeding.

been reported in humans involving: (1) deficiency of ADP within platelet granules and (2) defective ADP release mechanisms (an "aspirinlike" defect). In the first category, the platelets lack dense osmiophilic granules. They will undergo primary aggregation when ADP is added in vitro but will fail to secondarily aggregate when collagen is added (Mourer et al. 1972; Weiss and Ames 1973).

THROMBOSIS

When vascular endothelium is injured, the process of thrombosis is initiated in an attempt to repair the defect in the endothelial wall and to prevent loss of blood from the vascular system. The two usually inseparable mechanisms that bring this about are platelet agglutination and fibrinogen polymerization. The solid mass made up of blood constituents which forms within the vessels (or endothelium of the heart cavities) is called a *thrombus* (Fig. 3.15) and the process of its formation, *thrombosis*. Morphologically, thrombi must be differentiated from clots that form extravascularly, from clots that form in vessels after death (postmortem clotting), and from disseminated intravascular coagulation.

When an injury to endothelium occurs, circulating platelets adhere to the subendothelial connective tissue of the defect by the extension of pseudopodia (Sheppard and French 1971). Contact with collagen, bacteria, basement membrane, and injured endothelial cells induces platelets to adhere and to release ADP. Adhering platelets swell and extend multiple dendritic pseudopodia over the endothelial defect in an attempt to bridge the gap (Ashford and Freiman 1967; Tranzer and Baumgartner 1967). The rapidly advancing pseudopodia become enmeshed in the defective areas of the endothelium. Ultrastructural studies have also revealed the development of membranous sacs on the surface of the platelet that may be associated with release of ADP upon adherence (Warren and Vales 1972).

Under the influence of ADP, platelets aggregate and form an unstable platelet plug. Fusing platelets discharge granules and thromboplastin into the surrounding

defect. Platelet plugs are not sufficient to stanch blood flow from any but the smallest wounds. The second mechanism of hemostasis, fibrin polymerization, is found in all vertebrates and provides a solid gel-fibrin complex which plugs larger vascular defects. Although platelet aggregates break up easily, reformation occurs and thrombin begins to form. Thrombin (originating from platelet thromboplastin) efficiently converts fibrinogen to fibrin. This provides the framework for further platelet adhesion and the establishment of a stable thrombus (French et al. 1964; Honour et al. 1971; Jørgensen et al. 1967a; Mustard et al. 1962; Stehbens and Biscoe 1967) (Fig. 3.11).

Experimental thrombosis has been studied by placing a silk suture in the carotid artery of pigs (Jørgensen et al. 1967b). Within 1 hr, a thrombus of densely packed platelets is present. The subsequent formation of alternating bands of fibrin and platelets may impart a laminated appearance to the thrombus. With time, the platelets disintegrate and the thrombus appears as a friable, heterogeneous-colored mass of fibrin. Anticoagulant drugs such as heparin have little effect on the platelet component but can effectively depress the deposition of fibrin.

Thrombi are heterogeneous structures and their heterogeneity is a reflection of both the site where they are formed and their age. Thrombi that develop in slow zones of blood flow such as veins are composed of fibrin strands with entrapped erythrocytes since the dominant mechanism of formation is coagulation. In contrast, arterial thrombi are generally due to endothelial injury and the initial thrombus is composed of aggregated platelets. As arterial thrombi grow, however, flow patterns adjacent to the thrombi cause fibrin to be deposited and the platelet mass that persists is transformed into a fibrin mass. Fibrin strands polymerize between the separating and degenerating platelets.

When the fibrin around a platelet thrombus becomes fully polymerized, circulating platelets no longer adhere to it readily. Neutrophils stick to the fibrin-platelet mass by virtue of chemotactic factors produced by plasmin-fibrin interaction and the release of platelet factors that in-

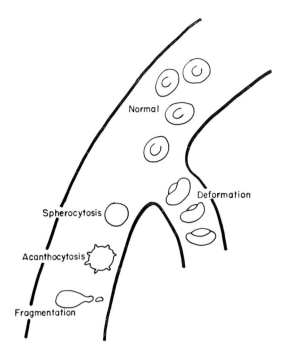

Fig. 3.17.   Deformation of erythrocytes.

and the pathologically rigid cell which cannot change shape predisposes an animal to intravascular disease. Deformity is especially required for the passage of erythrocytes through the spleen and other sinuses (Wennberg and Weiss 1968). There is marked distortion of the cell as it passes through the endothelial fenestrae with resumption of normal shape as the cell enters the sinus. In hemorrhage, diapedesis of erythrocytes through endothelium is also characterized by deformation and resumption of normal shape (Skalak et al. 1970).

PLASMA MEMBRANE

The reactive surface of the erythrocyte consists of the structural components of its plasma membrane and the mucopeptides and globulins that are adsorbed to it. The cell surface possesses a large net negative charge that prevents cell-to-cell contact. These anionic sites (chiefly neuraminic acid termini on the mucopeptides) can be altered by chemical and viral agents (Nicolson 1973). The erythrocytic plasma membrane is also injured by secondary effects that are induced by pathologic hemoglobin. The pathologic response of the injured erythrocytic plasma membrane may

be manifested as surface pitting, pseudopod formation, pinocytosis, membrane reduplication, and cellular fragmentation (Figs. 3.18, 3.19, 3.20, and 3.21).

PITTING

Ultrastructurally, foci of molecular damage to the plasma membrane can be seen as tiny pits or craters on the erythrocyte surface. Pitting is characteristic of erythrocyte toxins and is due, in most cases, to the migration of precipitated abnormal hemoglobin in contact with the plasma membrane (Fig. 3.18). Pitting also occurs as portions of the defective membrane are removed in the spleen. Pits and craters have been photographed on the surfaces of erythrocytes of chickens with lymphosarcoma and are allegedly due to the action of enzymes released from necrotic tumor tissue (Chandler and Fletcher 1973).

PSEUDOPOD FORMATION

Irregular, pleomorphic, club-shaped processes on the cell surface are common findings in blood of severely ill animals. Foci of pseudopodia or blebs are particularly common in uremia, heat stroke, plasma electrolyte imbalance, the chemical toxici-

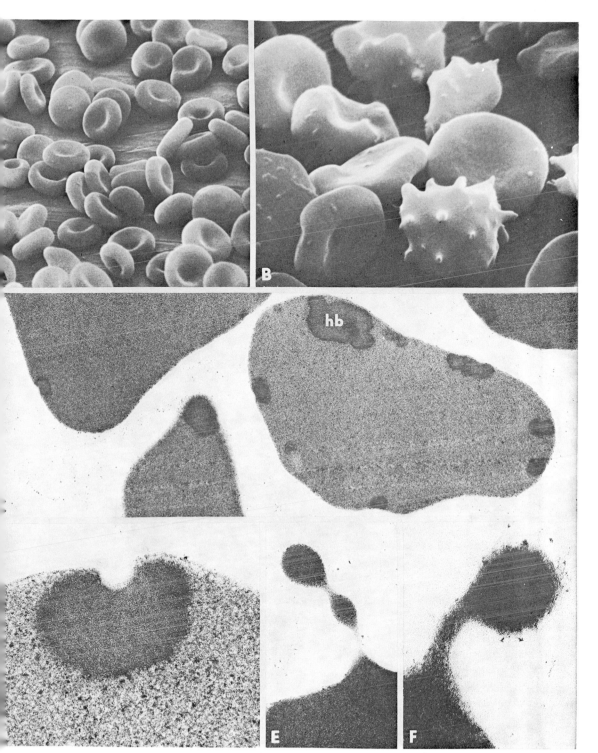

Fig. 3.18. Erythrocyte pathology, phenylhydrazine poisoning,
sheep. A. Normal erythrocytes, scanning electron micrograph. B.
Affected toxic erythrocytes (poikilocytes) with knobby protuberances
on their surfaces. C. Ultrastructure of erythrocytes in cross section
showing precipitation of hemoglobin (hb, Heinz bodies). D.–F.
Enlargement illustrating defects in plasma membrane. Surface
knobs comparable to those in B.

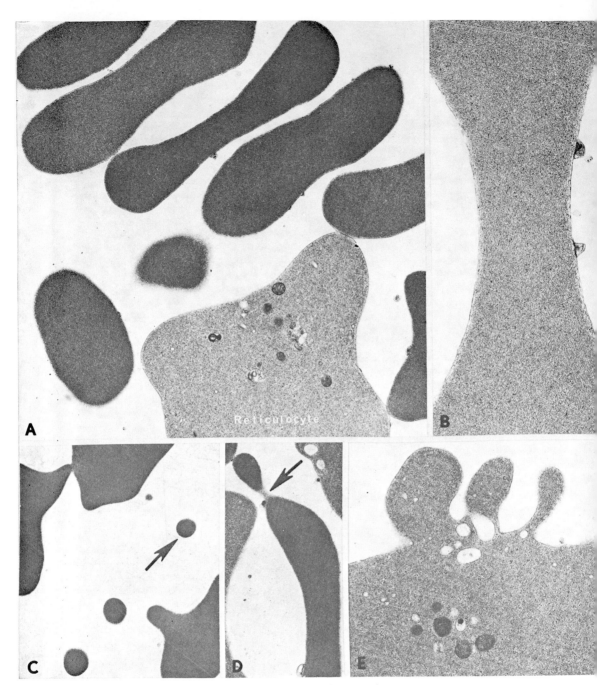

Fig. 3.19. Erythrocyte surface pathology. A. and B. Surface
membrane bodies, Basenji dog, pyruvate kinase deficiency. C. and D.
Fragmented erythrocytes from terminal stages of uremia in a dog.
Portions have pinched away from the cell (arrows). E. Pseudopod
formation with vesicles and internalization, cat, cortisone therapy
for lymphosarcoma.

Fig. 3.20. A. Spherocytes (s), nucleated erythrocytes (n), and
leptocytes (l), dog with autoimmune hemolytic anemia. B. Normal
erythrocyte (top) and early and late phases of spherocytosis. C.
Extensive erythropoiesis (erythroid hyperplasia), aged dog, progressive
heart failure. Hyperplasia is due to anoxia (in attempt to compensate for decreased cardiac output). D. atrophy of bone marrow,
aplastic anemia, dog. E. Erythrocyte precursors and neutrophil (n).

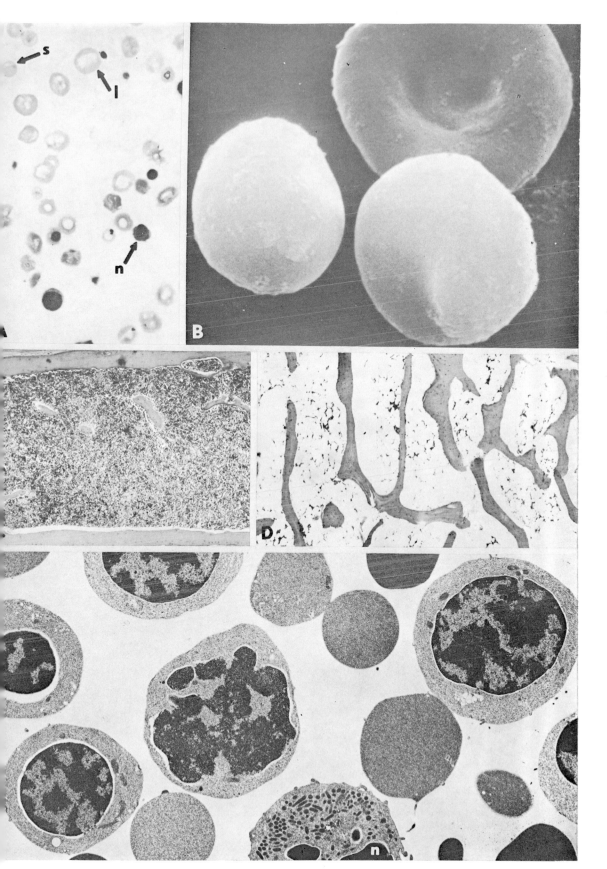

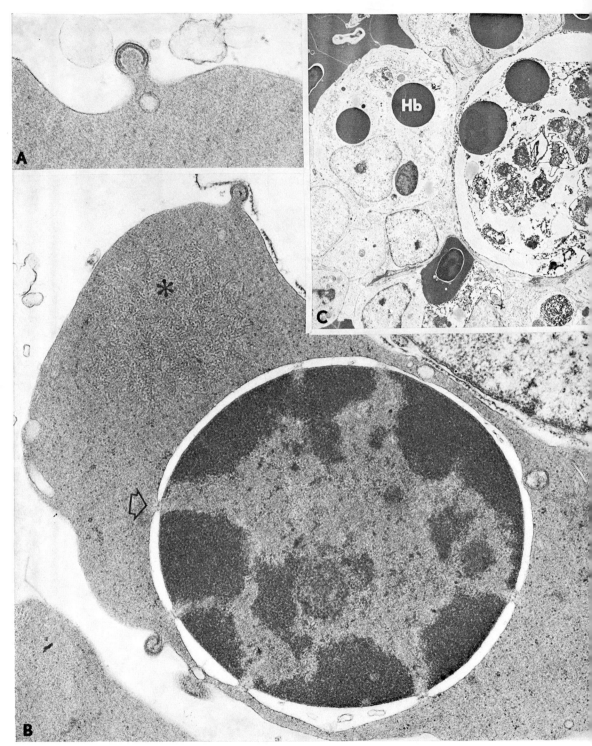

Fig. 3.21. A. and B. Newcastle disease virus budding from the surface of chicken erythrocytes in spleen. Foci of viral nucleocapsids (asterisk) distort the cytoplasm. Note chromatin pattern in erythrocyte nucleus and open channels leading from nuclear pores (arrow). C. Erythrophagocytosis in splenic red pulp, Newcastle disease. Macrophages are filled with dense spherical globules of hemoglobin (Hb).

ties, and generalized, malignant neoplasms (Skinnider and Ghadially 1973).

SPICULATION

Spiculocytes are erythrocytes deformed by a relatively uniform distribution of surface spicules. Other terms (echinocytes, burr cells, acanthocytes, and spiculated cells) have originated in human hematology and are related to damage in specific diseases. The change illustrates a severe defect in the plasma membrane and is seen in serious toxic injury. A defect in plasma membrane permeability to ions is the fundamental lesion in some types of muscular dystrophy of mice and men, and erythrocyte spiculation is seen here (Matheson and Howland 1974). Experimentally, when ATP levels in erythrocytes are decreased, the cells develop spicules on the surface; with the addition of glucose and regeneration of ATP they assume their normal discoid shape (Hochmuth and Mohandas 1972).

FRAGMENTATION

The separation of portions of the erythrocyte is a consequence of the diseases which also cause blebbing. Fragmentation of erythrocytes is seen in the blood from animals with these diseases and is due to a shearing effect which occurs due to intravascular "trauma" of excessively fragile erythrocytes (Brain et al. 1967; Nevaril et al. 1968). The most severe examples of fragmentation have been described in uremia.

SURFACE MEMBRANE BODIES

Reticulocytes and other immature erythrocytes, when spewed into the circulation during anemia, are predisposed to plasma membrane defects. These cells contain effete organelles such as degenerate mitochondria, amorphous granular bodies, nuclear remnants, small opaque vesicles, and autophagic vacuoles (Kent et al. 1971). In the process of their expulsion from the maturing erythrocyte, these structures may remain attached to the plasma membrane (Campbell 1972; Gasko and Danon 1972; Seelig 1972) (Fig. 3.19).

PINOCYTOSIS

Erythroblasts take up iron for hemoglobin synthesis by *pinocytosis*. This capacity is retained by mature erythrocytes and, in some forms of anemia, pinocytotic vesicles may be seen remaining on or near the cell surface. This appears to occur in immunologically induced anemia, in which the pinocytotic vacuoles are induced by antibodies on the erythrocyte surface (Blanton et al. 1968). A pathologic variant of pinocytosis is membrane internalization, the focal irregular invagination of portions of the plasma membrane which forms small submembranous vacuoles by endocytosis. This commonly occurs in diseases where abnormal intracellular metabolism alters the plasma membrane. It also is a usual pathway of injury in aging and toxic hemolysis. Membrane internalization is induced by several drugs including primaquine, hydrocortisone, vinblastine, and chlorpromazine (Ben-Bassat et al. 1972; Ginn et al. 1969) It occurs in relation to the dose administered and is dependent upon the ATP-energized state of the plasma membrane. Membrane reduplication may occur in some toxic diseases. Dense aggregates of tightly whorled membranes are present on the erythrocyte surface.

HEMOGLOBIN

Hemoglobin is a combination of a simple histone protein *globin* with *heme,* a porphyrin molecule containing an iron atom in its center. All vertebrate hemoglobins have the same molecular configuration. The globin, which is about 97% of the molecule, is a tetramer of two pairs of dissimilar polypeptide chains: two a- and two β-chains ($a_2\beta_2$). The molecule dissociates into two symmetrical dimers: $a_2\beta_2 \rightleftarrows 2$ $a\beta$. The tendency to dissociate varies among species. Cat hemoglobin forms subunits much more readily than dog hemoglobin. Much of our detailed knowledge of the tertiary structure of the hemoglobin molecule (the fold of the chains within the molecule) comes from x-ray crystallographic studies of horse hemoglobin.

Erythrocyte survival demands that intracellular hemoglobin remain in solution. To do so, the hemoglobin molecule must maintain its rigid, tertiary structure with little conformation change. Each coiled chain of hemoglobin must have an external polar, charged layer of hydrophilic amino acids and an internal layer of nonpolar, noncharged hydrophobic amino acids. Disruption of the α-helix, replacement of polar with nonpolar amino acids, or disruption of the binding to heme results in the hemoglobin molecule becoming insoluble within the erythrocyte.

The precipitation of unstable hemoglobin within the erythrocyte is manifested as aggregates of dense, irregular, granular structures called *Heinz bodies* (Fig. 3.18). These bodies may be heterogeneous, for, during precipitation, hemoglobin may entrap other erythrocyte organelles such as mitochondria, ribosomes, siderosomes, and free ferritin. Heinz bodies attach to the cell membrane which becomes deformed; this renders the cell susceptible to erythrophagocytosis. Increased erythrocyte fragility may also be reflected in the deleterious effect of abnormal hemoglobin on the cation pump. Fluid intake, spherocytosis, and osmotic lysis can occur (Rifkind 1965).

Hemoglobin differs sufficiently among species that its substructure has been used as a guideline of phylogenetic development. Ontogenetically, several types of hemoglobin are produced. Mammalian erythrocytes change rapidly at birth from a content of fetal type hemoglobin (Hb-F) to an adult type (Hb-A) which differ in β-chain amino acid sequence. The transition from Hb-F to Hb-A is abrupt and fetal hemoglobin does not recur except in some specific types of anemia. In fetal sheep and goats, an intermediate hemoglobin type occurs called Hb-C. In blood loss anemia, Hb-C is again produced. The change from Hb-A to Hb-C is mediated by an active globin-mRNA in the reticulocyte (Nienhuis and Anderson 1972).

INTRAERYTHROCYTIC METABOLIC PATHWAYS

The normal erythrocyte is defended against colloid osmotic lysis because its membrane is relatively impermeable to free ion movement. To balance the slow, continual, passive leak of potassium and the intake of sodium, an energy-utilizing pump operates to actively push sodium out and pull potassium in. Energy in the form of ATP is supplied by oxidation of glucose to lactic acid (glycolysis). The erythrocyte has no Krebs cycle and 90% of glucose enters the anaerobic glycolysis pathway which converts glucose to lactic acid generating ATP. Deficiencies in this scheme lead to water intake and osmotic hemolysis. When the pump is destroyed, there is equalization of cell and plasma cations, intake of water, cell swelling, and lysis. In summary, cell swelling (hydrocytosis) involves sodium accumulation and potassium loss with associated water intake and shift towards critical cell volume. Cell contraction (desiccytosis) occurs with the excess potassium loss without corresponding sodium gain.

As the erythrocyte ages, the enzyme components which maintain energy production gradually wane. There is concomitant decrease in ATP. Membrane function is affected, the normal biconcave shape becomes spheroidal, and the cells have an increased susceptibility to osmotic lysis. In passage through the splenic filter, aged erythrocytes are removed from the circulation and the component parts are processed by splenic macrophages. Any space-occupying defect in the cell membrane makes the erythrocyte less flexible and highly liable to erythrophagocytosis. Pitting, the removal of defective portions of the cell, may occur as it squeezes through the endothelial lining of the splenic venous sinus (Schnitzer et al. 1972). The mechanical trauma of excessively fragile erythrocytes may also result in intravascular fragmentation and hemolysis (Bull et al. 1967).

ERYTHROPOIESIS

Mature erythrocytes originate from a pool of self-perpetuating bone marrow stem cells (Fig. 3.20). These dormant reserves are triggered into action by humoral substances called erythropoietin. The erythrocytes develop from large nucleated stem cells by almost imperceptible gradations of an orderly sequence. Different cells in this series are arbitrarily divided on the basis of structure and staining into pronormoblasts, normoblasts (basophilic, polychromatic, and orthochromatic), reticulocytes, and mature erythrocytes (Weiss 1965; Windqvist 1954).

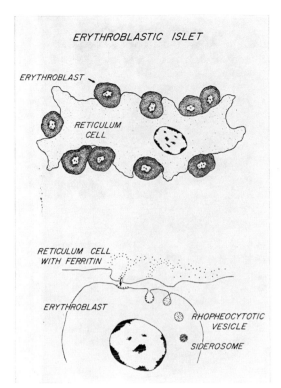

Fig. 3.22. Transfer of iron from reticulum cell to erythroblast. Nurse reticulum cell surrounded by erythroblasts (top). Transfer of ferritin particles (bottom).

During maturation the nucleus increasingly contracts, becomes pyknotic, and (in mammals) is ejected from the cell. *Erythroblastic islets* in the bone marrow are large central pleomorphic reticulum cells surrounded by a ring of developing erythroblasts (Fig. 3.22). The reticulum cells serve as nurse cells and transfer their cytoplasmic ferritin to the erythroblasts which accept it by endocytosis (rhopheocytosis). They are known to phagocytize expelled erythroblast nuclei. Iron is also transferred to developing erythroblasts by *transferrin,* the plasma glycoprotein that transports iron in its ferric state. Transferrin attaches to immature red cells and gives up its iron to them but is not incorporated itself into the cell.

In anemia characterized by intense erythropoiesis, nucleated erythrocytes appear in the blood prematurely and can be seen to denucleate (Simpson and Kling 1967; Skutelsky and Danon 1970). *Howell-Jolly*

bodies, which are dense remnants of nuclear chromatin, may persist in the cell. They stain intensely with nuclear dyes and are characteristic of some specific types of anemia. Erythroblast pathology has also been reported in bone marrow suppression caused by nutritional deficiencies such as vitamin E (Nafstad and Nafstad 1968).

When animals become deficient in erythrocytes, they respond by releasing these cells from storage sites in the spleen and bone marrow, by increasing cardiorespiratory function, and by changing the hemoglobin-oxygen association. The most significant long-term effects, however, are the induction of bone marrow hyperplasia and, in severe anemia, of extramedullary hematopoiesis in spleen and liver. When these events occur, they are reflected in changes in some important clinical pathologic tests. There are increases in (1) serum iron levels, (2) plasma iron turnover measured using Fe^{59}, (3) reticulocyte count (except in horses), and (4) bone marrow erythroid cells (decrease in myeloid:erythroid ratio). In the bone marrow, erythroblastic "islands" increase in number. These are developing erythrocytes surrounding a macrophage which provides ferritin for hemoglobin synthesis in the erythroblast (Ben-Ishay and Yoffey 1972). Bone marrow hypoplasia and the production of abnormal erythroblasts are seen in nutritional deficiencies, chemical toxicities, and viral diseases (Brodsky and Kahn 1969; McGuire et al. 1969; Schnitzer et al. 1972). Bone marrow defects and deficiency of erythropoietin may also be due to hereditary disease (Bateman et al. 1972; Wong et al. 1972).

ERYTHROPOIETIN

Erythropoietin is the term applied to soluble, chemically undefined factors that enhance erythropoiesis. They are produced or activated in response to low tissue oxygen levels. Transient elevations of plasma erythropoietin are detectable during hypoxia while sustained levels are often present in severe anemia.

Erythropoietin can be measured by bioassay methods and, with purification, by a radioimmunoassay technique. To date, these are insufficiently sensitive to measure erythropoietin in plasma (without concentration) and have not been applied to clinical evaluation. A hemagglutination-inhibition test appears to be more specific and may prove valuable (Lange et al. 1970).

The kidney is recognized as the chief site of erythropoietin production. Renal ablation in rats markedly inhibits their capacity to respond to hypoxia. Other sites of formation exist, because anephric animals continue to form erythropoietin. Erythropoietin has been localized in the epithelial cells of the renal glomerulus in anemic sheep (Fisher et al. 1965; Frenkel et al. 1968) and several other species. It is not readily extractable from kidney tissue, for it allegedly exists there in precursor form. This form, erythrogenin, is extractable from the microsomal (endoplasmic reticulum) elements and reacts with serum to give erythropoietin (Fig. 3.23).

POLYCYTHEMIA

Increased numbers of erythrocytes per cubic mm of blood are seen in animals that are dehydrated. This *relative polycythemia,* which is also called hemoconcentration, is due to a diminution of the quantity of plasma in the blood. The erythrocyte count, hemoglobin, and hematocrit are elevated but the total erythrocyte volume is normal. Hemoconcentration occurs because water is lost from the blood beyond the capacity of the interstitial fluids to replace it. It is seen in water deprivation, vomiting, diarrhea, and excessive fluid loss in fever. It is often a serious sign and should be followed by fluid therapy.

Absolute polycythemia exists whenever the total erythrocyte volume is elevated above normal. Absolute erythrocytosis secondary to low oxygen content in the atmosphere is fairly common. It occurs in mammals at high altitudes and in fish in very warm waters (Georgiev 1972). Absolute erythrocytosis may also accompany cardiac failure and diffuse pulmonary disease.

Familial primary polycythemia occurs as a simple autosomal recessive condition in Jersey cattle (Tennant et al. 1967). Affected calves are weak, lethargic, and dyspneic and usually die by 6 months of age with hyperemia of the pulmonary capillary bed. Isolated cases of primary polycythemia have also been reported in dogs and cattle (Donovan and Loeb 1959; Fowler et al. 1964).

ANEMIA

Anemia, the deficiency of circulating erythrocytes, may be a reduction of erythrocyte numbers or of hemoglobin-erythrocyte cell mass. The consequence is the same, impaired delivery of oxygen to cells. The decrease in oxygen-carrying capacity of blood (hypoxemia) results when the erythrocytes are lost beyond the ability of storage sites in the spleen and bone marrow to replace them.

When insufficient numbers of erythrocytes are present, the blood becomes thin and watery. As a result the mucous membranes around the eyes, mouth, and genitals become noticeably pale. The compensatory mechanisms which operate to combat the decreased oxygen-carrying capacity of the blood are: (1) hyperventilation of the lungs, (2) increased cardiac output, and (3) reduction of hemoglobin-oxygen affinity. The decreased affinity of hemoglobin for oxygen allows the increased release of oxygen to tissues. These are but borderline adjustments. They may allow the anemic animal to appear normal at rest but cannot overcome the demands of exertion.

Anemia is caused either by increased loss of erythrocytes or by abnormal erythropoiesis with insufficient production (Table 3.4). In practice, many anemias are not that simple. Anemia due to chronic hemorrhage (for example, infestation with many bloodsucking parasites) is primarily

```
HYPOXIA  →  KIDNEY  →  ERYTHROGENIN
                          +
                     SERUM FACTOR
                          ‖
          ERYTHROPOIETIN  →   ⌠STEM CELL
                              ⌡ERYTHROBLAST
```

Fig. 3.23. Erythropoietin.

Table 3.4. Mechanisms of anemia

Blood loss: hemorrhage
  Acute
  Chronic
Erythrocyte destruction: hemolytic (intravascular)
  or erythrophagocytic
  Cell membrane damage
  Osmotic lysis
  Hemoglobin abnormality
Abnormal production of erythrocytes (quantity or
  quality)
  Deficiency disease: iron, copper, folic acid, vitamins B-6 and B-12
  Bone marrow toxicity: irradiation, chemical suppression
  Myelophthisic (replacement of bone marrow by other tissue)

---

caused by the slow loss of erythrocyte numbers. Superimposed upon this mechanism, however, is a progressively developing iron deficiency which depresses erythropoiesis. Anemia which accompanies Ostertagiosis of calves results chiefly from blood loss but hypoplasia of the bone marrow also occurs and is allegedly due to toxic products of the parasite. Similarly, infection with leptospires causes a destructive hemolytic anemia which is augmented by a toxic effect of the organism on the bone marrow. It is therefore difficult in anemia which accompanies complex diseases such as uremia, hypothyroidism, chronic infectious diseases, and terminal cancer to sort out the dominant cause.

Even though erythrocyte destruction occurs in many infectious diseases due to the direct effects of microbes, anemia may also be a nonspecific side effect of fever. Transient periods of high fever are followed by short periods of decreased packed cell volume values and increased reticulocyte counts. The mechanism is not known but appears related to elevated body temperature rather than to the primary cause of the fever itself (Karle 1969).

ANEMIA DUE TO HEMORRHAGE

ACUTE

Following extensive hemorrhage there are immediate and remarkable increases in hemoconcentration and blood coagulability. Coagulation becomes highly efficient and erythrocytes are rapidly spewed into the circulation by release from storage sites in the spleen and bone marrow. This is manifested as a rise in the packed cell volume that develops immediately after the transitory drop which accompanies actual blood loss. These stored erythrocytes are normal cells; no pathologic changes are detectable when blood is examined microscopically. The volume of lost blood is compensated for by the drawing of interstitial fluid into the vascular system and hemodilution slowly begins to restore the PCV to normal. The neural and humoral factors that affect cardiac output and blood pressure are activated and, in spite of the loss of large amounts of blood, animals may remain conscious and appear normal clinically.

Most animals can lose one-third of their total blood volume without evidence of disease. The consequence of acute blood loss is not anemia but hypovolemic shock. If increased heart rate, hyperventilation, peripheral vasoconstriction, and the shift of water from tissue to blood are unable to compensate, shock develops and death follows.

CHRONIC

Slow insidious hemorrhage is a frequent cause of death in animals. Bloodsucking intestinal parasites and external parasites such as fleas are frequent causes. These anemias are associated with a hypocellular but functionally hyperactive bone marrow.

Internal bleeding (such as intraperitoneal blood loss) may also cause chronic anemia but blood components, especially iron, are recoverable. Bleeding into the intestine or to the exterior causes loss of iron and iron-deficiency anemia is superimposed upon chronic blood loss.

ERYTHROCYTE DESTRUCTION

Lysis of erythrocytes results when the plasma membrane is ruptured. This occurs because of direct damage to the membrane or it may occur indirectly due to abnormalities of hemoglobin or of the mechanisms that maintain osmotic equilibrium (Table 3.5). If extensive damage produces overt lysis of cells intravascularly, hemoglobin is liberated into the circulating blood (hemolytic anemia). During a

Table 3.5. Mechanisms of erythrocyte destruction

Mechanism	Type	Caused by
Cell membrane damage	Enzyme digestion	Rattlesnake venom (phospholipase)
		Clostridial toxins (lecithinase)
	Viral replication	Newcastle disease
		Murine leukemia
		Colorado tick fever
	Bacterial attachment	*Haemobartonella* spp.
		Eperythrozoon spp.
	Immunologic lysis	Autoimmune hemolytic anemia
		Isoimmune hemolytic anemia
	Lipid deficiency	Vitamin E deficiency
	Mechanical damage	Uremia
Osmotic lysis	Enzyme abnormality	Pyruvate kinase deficiency, hereditary
		Aspirin poisoning
	Bacterial replication	*Anaplasma* spp.
	Protozoal replication	*Plasmodium* spp. (malaria)
		Babesia spp.
	Hypotonic solutions	(in vitro)
Hemoglobin abnormality	Denaturation	Phenylhydrazine toxicity
		Copper toxicity
	Abnormal globin synthesis	Hemoglobinopathy
	Abnormal heme synthesis	Porphyria
	Methemoglobinemia	Nitrite poisoning

hemolytic crisis, the binding power of plasma haptoglobulin is exceeded and hemoglobin is excreted by the renal glomerulus. The molecule dissociates $(a_2\beta_2 \rightleftharpoons 2\ a\beta)$ and the dimer (32,000 MW) is readily excreted by the renal filter. Hemoglobin is absorbed by the proximal convoluted tubule but when the absorptive capacity is exceeded, hemoglobinuria results (Bunn and Jandle 1969).

Hemolytic anemia is observed in drug-induced anemia of several animals, leptospirosis in the cow and dog, clostridial infections of sheep and cattle, copper poisoning of sheep, immunologic hemolysis in suckling newborn animals, and some of the intracellular parasites such as *Anaplasma* spp. Affected erythrocytes are seen ultrastructurally as being less dense and in various stages of collapse. The extent of hemoglobinemia and subsequent hemoglobinuria are indices of the severity of the disease process.

Less explosive types of erythrocyte damage may not induce lysis but sufficiently alter the erythrocyte so as to induce erythrophagocytosis of large numbers of cells in the spleen, liver, and bone marrow. Diseases associated with anemia of this type include those infections where microorganisms replicate within the erythrocyte,

uremia, some of the immunologic types of anemia, and metabolic diseases.

BACTERIAL INFECTION

Two important groups of bacteria in the order Rickettsiales infect erythrocytes of vertebrates. *Hemobartonella* spp. (family Bartonellaceae) do so by attaching to the cell surface. *Anaplasma* spp. (family Anaplasmataceae) enter the erythrocyte and replicate. As with other bacteria, these prokaryotic organisms lack nuclei and defined organelles such as mitochondria and endoplasmic reticulum.

The Hemobartonellae are pleomorphic membrane-delimited organisms that contain an undulate plasma membrane and a granular matrix of variable density. Organisms are attached to the host erythrocyte's plasma membrane but do not enter the cell. They exist in deep, grooved infoldings on the erythrocyte surface (Demaree and Nessmith 1972; Jain and Keelon 1973; Simpson and Love 1970; Venable and Ewing 1968) and may appear to be intracellular on casual examination (Fig. 3.24). The rod forms measure 0.2 by 1.0 to 5.0μ. Larger ring-shaped forms develop due to indentations in the cytoplasmic zones.

Most infections with Hemobartonellae

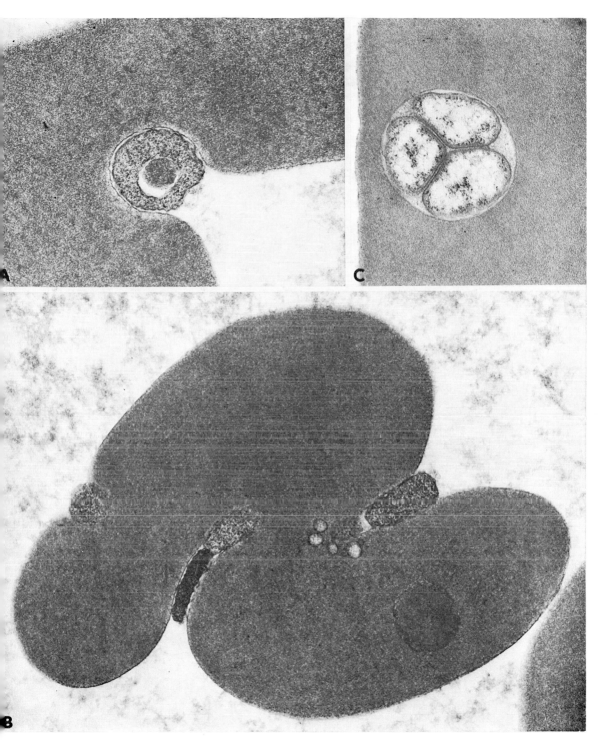

Fig. 3.24. A. and B. *Hemobartonella canis* indented into the surface of canine erythrocytes (Micrographs, J. Venable). C. *Anaplasma marginale* within a bovine erythrocyte (Micrograph, C. Simpson).

are asymptomatic. The exceptions are very young animals or those with acquired immunologic deficits. Splenectomy is an established method for inducing parasitemia and clinical disease in individuals with inapparent infections. Anemia, the only known manifestation of infection, is due to increased erythrophagocytosis and not to overt damage to the erythrocyte.

Eperythrozoon spp. are closely related members of the family Bartonellaceae that exist indented into the surface of the erythrocyte (McKee et al. 1973). Organisms occur in coccoid, rod, or ring forms with diameters of 0.3–0.4μ.

Anaplasma spp. are transmitted by ticks and other insects and enter the erythrocyte by becoming invaginated into its surface. After penetration they are found as single initial bodies bound by a membrane at the erythrocyte periphery. Replication of the initial body by binary fission leads to 2–8 bodies within the membrane-bound vacuole (Fig. 3.24) and this structure represents the marginal body or "inclusion body" which is the dense, Giemsa-staining body found in blood smears of infected animals. Erythrocyte metabolism is not markedly altered in infected cells but because of the damaged cell surface, erythrocytes are rapidly removed by the reticuloendothelial cells of the spleen. Anemia peaks at 1–6 days after the peak of parasitemia (Fig. 3.25). In the latter stages of anemia it is also alleged that an autoimmune process contributes to red cell destruction. In chronic infection, bone marrow exhaustion may contribute to severe disease and death. The excess bilirubin formed by erythrocyte destruction is excreted, but animals dead of anaplasmosis are icteric and have splenomegaly and gall bladder enlargement.

Other bacteria associated with erythrocyte destruction are the leptospires and clostridial species (whose potent exotoxins digest the lecithins in the red cell plasma membrane) (Simpkins et al. 1971).

PROTOZOAL INFECTION

Plasmodium spp., the malarial protozoan parasites of reptiles, birds, and mammals, require two hosts for survival: an invertebrate in which sexual reproduction occurs and a vertebrate in which they multiply asexually. A bite by an infected female mosquito introduces sporozoites into the vertebrate host.

An exoerythrocytic phase is initiated by infection of different tissues: in birds, usually the reticuloendothelial system; in mammals, the liver. During the exoerythrocytic phase the organism goes through several asexual reproductions. Sporozoites transform to trophozoites, to multinucleate schizonts, and finally to mature schizonts. The end result is an immense host cell containing unicellular merozoites (Fig. 3.26). Upon their release, the extracellular

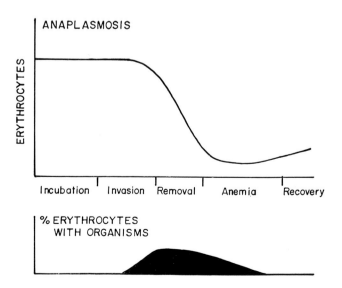

Fig. 3.25. Relation of parasites to anemia in bovine anaplasmosis.

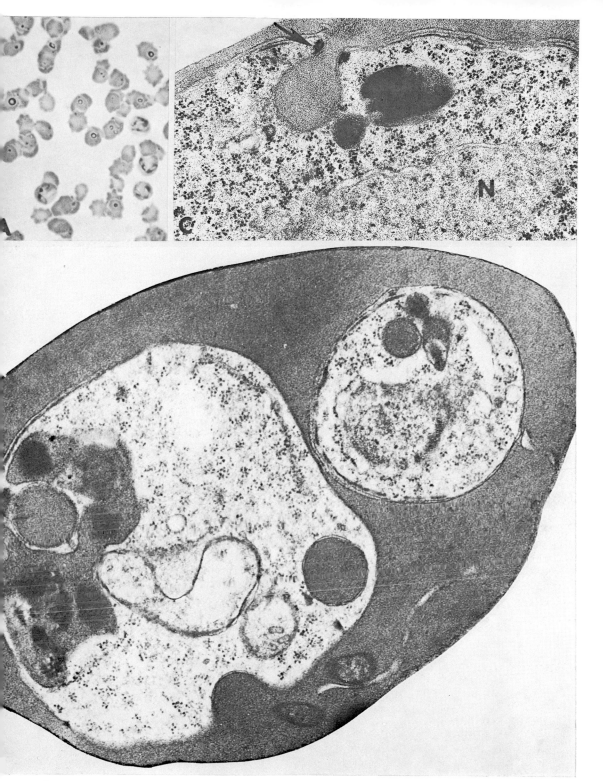

Fig. 3.26. A. *Babesia equi* in erythrocytes, horse. B. Erythrocytes
bearing protozoa (*Plasmodium* sp.). C. Note the nuclear zones (N)
and the specialized feeding apparatus of the malarial parasite (arrow)
(Micrographs B and C, M. Aikawa).

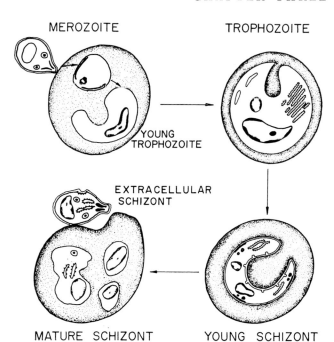

Fig. 3.27. Pathogenesis of the intraerythrocytic replication of Plasmodia.

merozoites then either invade new cells and repeat the extraerythrocytic cycle or infect erythrocytes.

Merozoites and sporozoites, the infective forms, possess a *conoid,* a specialized structure used for attachment. Penetration is initiated on contact of the conoid with the erythrocytic plasma membrane. A depression is created and develops into a cavity that eventually encloses the parasite without disrupting the plasma membrane. Within the red cell, the membrane-bound merozoite promptly begins its transformation and dedifferentiation. The parasite becomes rounded and its pellicle loses the thick inner membrane. The conoid and paired organelles disappear, initiating the development of the trophozoite. Trophozoites are capable of feeding and growth and they begin the asexual replicative cycle (Fig. 3.27). Schizogony occurs and ends when new merozoites bud from the mother schizont (Aikawa et al. 1969; Bodammer and Bahr 1973).

Plasmodial parasites feed on hemoglobin; malarial pigment (hemozoin) represents the residue of hemoglobin digestion. Hemoglobin is taken into the organism by phagocytosis and enters its food vacuole directly. Some species have a specialized cy-tostome on the pellicular membrane that actively ingests host cell cytoplasm. It is remarkable how long infected erythrocytes survive. As new merozoites bud from mother schizonts, however, the erythrocyte becomes irregular and pale. Dense debris, ferritin, and pigment are strewn around the cell. Daughter merozoites feed by lysis of the erythrocyte, probably by secreting a lytic substance that disrupts the electrolyte-maintaining mechanisms of the plasma membrane.

Babesia spp. are members of the suborder Piroplasmidea and destroy vertebrate erythrocytes by intracellular replication. Organisms are limited by a plasma membrane and contain endoplasmic reticulum, Golgi complexes, and food vacuoles (Simpson 1974; Simpson et al. 1967). They replicate by a modified form of schizogony; the pleomorphic offspring range from round to cigar-shaped forms with central or peripheral nuclei. Erythrocyte destruction occurs by the direct action of the parasite but anemia is often out of proportion to the number of parasitized red cells and it is believed that a late destructive immunologic reaction occurs.

Bovine babesiosis (Texas cattle fever) due to *B. bigemina* was the first protozoan parasite infection shown to be arthropod-transmitted. Control of the tick vector eliminated the disease from the United States. This is a severe hemolytic disease accompanied by fever and hemoglobinuria. Infected female ticks feed on cattle, injecting sporozoites into the bloodstream. These enter erythrocytes and change into ring-shaped structures, then progressively transform into ameboid trophozoites. They multiply by budding to produce two pyriform bodies that are attached at one end but later separate. Parasitemia occurs when organisms break out of red cells. They infect others to initiate succeeding asexual cycles of schizogony. Parasitemia and relapse occur at irregular and unpredictable intervals. During the relapses, phagocytosis of erythrocytes and trophozoites by monocytes occurs, but this does not significantly affect the life cycle of the parasite.

VIRAL DISEASE

Virions of several kinds bud from the surface of erythrocytes. In Newcastle disease of chickens, viral nucleocapsids are formed within hemoglobin. They are transported to the plasma membrane and, by modifying it, are incorporated into virions that bud from the surface of the red cell (Fig. 3.21). The murine oncornaviruses have been shown to replicate and assemble at the erythrocytic plasma membrane (Bächi and Howe 1972; Oshiro et al. 1972; Snodgrass et al. 1973; Wollmann 1970). Herpesviruses have been photographed within vacuoles in splenic erythrocytes in fatal cases of duck plague; Colorado tick fever viruses have been seen embedded in erythrocyte hemoglobin (Emmons et al. 1972).

IMMUNOLOGICALLY MEDIATED INJURY

The plasma membrane of the erythrocyte is injured by antibodies specifically reacting to antigens within or attached to the cell surface (see Chapter 5). The action of antibody and complement upon the red cell results in the formation of discrete holes in the plasma membrane and eventual lysis (Dourmashkin and Rosse 1966; Rosse et al. 1966). One hole is necessary and sufficient for hemolysis (Muller-Eberhard

et al. 1966). Some drug reactions are caused by immune mechanisms. Penicillin in large doses may coat the erythrocyte surface which is subsequently acted on by anti-penicillin antibodies. Other drugs are known to induce an autoimmune reaction by changing the makeup of the plasma membrane which then becomes immunogenic (Croft et al. 1968).

HEREDITARY ENZYME DEFICIENCY

The observation that the antimalarial drug primaquine produced strange hemolytic effects on erythrocytes of certain human patients led to the discovery of the inherited glucose-6-phosphate dehydrogenase deficiency, the most common red cell enzyme deficiency in humans. Many specific defects are now identified in man and some, although rare, occur in animals.

Pyruvate kinase deficiency in erythrocytes of Basenji dogs is responsible for recurring episodes of hemolytic anemia. Affected pups are detected at about 8 weeks of age and have PCV and hemoglobin values that are 60–70% of normal. There is a 10–20-fold increase in circulating reticulocytes and the erythrocyte half-life is greatly shortened during the anemic phases. Pyruvate kinase deficit disrupts the glycolytic cycle resulting in altered plasma membrane energy sources; affected cells develop ionic abnormalities (Nathan et al. 1965; Searcy et al. 1971).

There is a plasma membrane defect involved in a mild hereditary hemolytic anemia with stomatocytosis which occurs in Alaskan Malamute dogs affected with chondrodysplasia. The enlarged erythrocytes have a diminished mean corpuscular hemoglobin (30%) that is responsible for the reduced hemoglobin concentration, low red cell count, and normal PCV. Erythrocytes have increased Na^+ and water. Their survival time is shortened and both red cell osmotic pressure and fragility are increased. The genetic defect responsible is not known (Pinkerton et al. 1974).

A simplified pathway of glucose metabolism is shown in Fig. 3.28. Some of the enzymes for which hereditary deficiencies have been reported are indicated in view of the precise point at which the metabolic defect is produced.

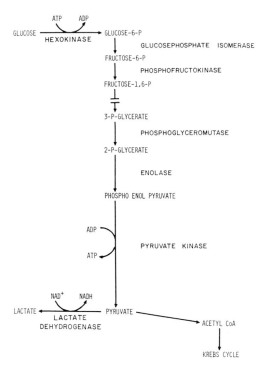

Fig. 3.28. Simplified pathway of glucose metabolism.

DEFECTIVE HEMOGLOBIN

Acquired defects in the hemoglobin molecule are only rarely responsible for erythrocyte destruction. Drugs such as phenylhydrazine induce oxidative denaturation of hemoglobin that precipitates as Heinz bodies. The aggregates of insoluble hemoglobin render erythrocytes susceptible to lysis and erythrophagocytosis by altering the plasma membrane (Rifkind 1965) (Fig. 3.17).

Erythropoietic porphyria is a rare congenital disease of cattle (Kaneko et al. 1971) and man in which abnormal porphyrin is formed in the immature developing erythrocyte. The defect of the heme part of hemoglobin involves overproduction of type I porphyrins due to an enzymatic defect in the conversion of porphobilinogen to uroporphyrinogen. These porphyrins cannot be used for hemoglobin synthesis and interfere with erythropoiesis. Porphyrins accumulate in electron-lucent crystal-shaped spaces in some of the human forms of porphyria (Waldo and Tobias 1973).

HEMOGLOBINOPATHY

This implies a genetically determined alteration of the globin portion of the hemoglobin molecule. The abnormal variants are due to substitution or deletion of one or more amino acids in the globin chains which are detected by altered electrophoretic mobility. In humans, hemoglobinopathies are manifested as abnormal oxygen affinity, as hemoglobin instability, or as polymerization of the hemoglobin molecule into Heinz bodies.

Modern research on the hemoglobinopathies was stimulated by the discovery by Linus Pauling of the molecular basis of sickle cell anemia of humans. The defect involves the substitution of a single amino acid in the abnormal hemoglobin (Hb-S). Sickle cell anemia is a serious genetic affection of black races; 10% carry the sickle trait (their erythrocytes contain about half Hb-S), but only 0.2% develop anemia (90–100% of their hemoglobin is Hb-S). The synthesis of Hb-S is due to a mutation in the globin gene that causes replacement of one pair of amino acid residues in the β-chain. This drastically reduces the solubility of the hemoglobin molecule in its deoxygenated state, so that it precipitates into fibers within erythrocytes and causes them to become elongated and rigid (Döbler and Bertles 1968; Finch et al. 1973). The rigid rods (14–17 nm diameter with 6.4 periodicity) distort and wrinkle the cell surface and cause increased fragility and erythrophagocytosis.

No counterpart to sickle cell anemia exists in animals although erythrocytes of deer sickle with oxygenation (rather than deoxygenation). Sickling is reversible and returns upon deoxygenation. The plasma membrane becomes stretched around a long central hemoglobin rod. Deer sickling is an in vitro phenomenon which occurs in the laboratory under high pH and oxygen tension and has no apparent pathologic consequences (Kitchen et al. 1967; Simpson and Taylor 1974).

INSUFFICIENT ERYTHROCYTE PRODUCTION

Underproduction of erythrocytes may result from primary bone marrow failure or from diminished humoral stimulation of marrow erythropoiesis. Put more simply, the mechanism of the deficit may be a stem cell defect or a normal stem cell within an abnormal environment. Deficiency of the environment (chiefly of erythropoietin) is not clearly established in clinical veterinary medicine. Erythropoietin is implicated in anemia which accompanies chronic renal disease, disseminated metastatic tumors, and hepatic failure. Even though sufficient erythropoietin is synthesized, it may be inactivated or ineffective in reaching the site of erythropoiesis.

The commoner causes of insufficient erythrocyte production relate to suppression of bone marrow stem cell production. Within the marrow, red cell precursors are highly susceptible to chemical agents that suppress metabolism. Extremely large numbers of erythrocytes are formed continually and in some mammals as many as 3 million per second are released into the circulating blood. Because of this high rate of cell division, erythropoietic cells are rapidly destroyed by radiation and immunosuppressive drugs. The bone marrow becomes hypocellular and filled with plasma and fibroblasts. Chloramphenicol is a notorious bone marrow toxin that kills by producing aplastic anemia.

Because of the high rate of erythropoiesis, the marrow is also susceptible to deficiencies of several essential dietary factors. Some of these are iron, folic acid, vitamins B_{12} and B_6, and protein. The most important dietary deficiency factor causing anemia is that of iron.

IRON-DEFICIENCY ANEMIA

Deficiencies of iron may be observed in a short time as the formation of small erythrocytes with decreased hemoglobin content. The hypochromic red cells develop chiefly because of the lack of sufficient iron for the formation of heme molecules; erythrocytes are released into the circulation before receiving their full levels of hemoglobin. Other minor mechanisms also operate in defective iron-deficiency erythrocytes. The plasma membrane is overly susceptible to oxidative damage due to what appear to be enzymic defects. Experimentally, glutathione peroxidase activity is markedly diminished in affected cells and

it is hypothesized that this enzyme normally acts upon peroxides, preventing them from oxidizing sulfhydryl groups in the plasma membrane (Loria et al. 1967; Rodvien et al. 1974).

Iron-deficiency anemia is seen as a dietary disorder in newborns, as part of chronic blood loss due to intestinal parasites, and as part of intestinal malabsorption diseases of adult animals. The factors that affect iron metabolism are: (1) dietary content—whether iron is present in sufficient amounts and form for absorption, (2) presence of normal gastric HCl and pancreatic juice for action, (3) sufficient percent absorption by intestinal absorptive epithelial cells, (4) adequate transport proteins in plasma, and (5) the amount excreted or lost in blood and sloughed epithelial cells.

In plasma, iron is complexed to the protein transferrin which has the electrophoretic mobility of a β_1-globulin and which serves as an iron carrier. Plasma iron represents the balance between iron of hemoglobin breakdown and iron absorbed from the intestine minus iron removed by heme synthesis, cell metabolism, and storage.

Iron deficiency is commonly seen in baby pigs born with low levels of iron in tissue. Their extraordinarily rapid rate of growth coupled with low levels of iron found in sow's milk require that they obtain large amounts of dietary iron. The plasma iron, which is normally 100–300 μg/100 ml may drop to 50 μg in anemic piglets. Iron binding capacity of plasma is increased and when iron is given it is rapidly complexed to transferrin and accepted by erythroblasts. In affected pigs, the mucous membranes are pale and systemic signs of anemia such as dyspnea and cardiac abnormalities occur. Mechanistically, the sequence of events is as follows: dietary iron deficiency, depletion of iron stores, decreased saturation of transferrin, decreased delivery to erythroid cells, impaired hemoglobin synthesis, and anemia. The bone marrow is hypercellular but an estimate of iron deficiency can be made in marrow smears by observing hemosiderin granules stained with Prussian Blue. The continued division of erythroblasts produces excessive numbers of small pale erythrocytes with a shortened life span (hypochromic, microcytic anemia).

Two models of iron-deficiency hypochromic anemia in the mouse involve defects of iron absorption and transfer by the intestinal mucosa. In regard to the intestinal absorptive cell, mice with *microcytic anemia* (mk mice) have an iron entry defect; mice with *"sex-linked anemia"* (sla mice) have a defect in exit of iron (Bannerman and Pinkerton 1967; Pinkerton 1968; Russell et al. 1970).

In normal mice, as in other mammals, iron passes through the intestinal epithelial cell in two phases. The early phase, in which iron goes through the microvilli, terminal web, and cytoplasmic matrix to reach the endoplasmic reticulum, is rapid. The later phase is longer and involves the transitory storage of iron in the cisternae and slow transfer of iron out the lateral surfaces of the cell. In mk mice, iron never reaches the intestinal absorptive cell. In sla mice, large amounts of stainable iron are present in the ileal mucosa but cannot be transferred to the lamina propria and into the bloodstream (Bédard 1973).

OTHER MODELS OF ANEMIA WITH
HEREDITARY DEFECTIVENESS

An erythropoietic stem cell defect occurs in gray Collies with cyclic neutropenia (see Chapter 4). The most overt manifestation of the stem cell defect is the disappearance of neutrophilic leukocytes from the circulation every 10–12 days. Reticulocytes also undergo this curious cyclic depression and there is reduction of the formation of erythrocytes. The cycle reflects competition of differing hemic populations (granulocytes, platelets, and erythroblasts) for the limited number of stem cells produced Patt et al. 1973).

A genetically determined macrocytic anemia due to defective cellular environment for differentiating erythropoietic cells occurs in inbred Sl/Sl mice. The absence of some unidentified splenic factor causes erythrocyte formation to be depressed. The condition is not corrected by the transplantation of bone marrow stem cells from normal donor mice. It is improved by the transplantation of intact spleens. The failure of splenic factors is demonstrated by the failure of Sl/Sl spleens to support hemopoiesis when given to lethally x-radiated mice.

In contrast to the above murine model,

the hereditary macrocytic anemia in W/W mice is due to a defect in stem cell population. The transplantation of normal stem cells (or even Sl/Sl stem cells) to W/W mice corrects the defect. Although the parent strain of mice are black, homozygous (WW) mice are white due to a defect in melanoblasts. Heterozygous (Ww) mice are black with a white bellyspot, the latter being due to failure of melanoblasts to migrate fully from the neural crest cells. Gonadal defects also are present and WW mice are sterile.

ERYTHROPHAGOCYTOSIS

Removal of damaged or senescent erythrocytes is a function of the macrophages of the reticuloendothelial system. Enormous numbers of erythrocytes are destroyed each day and it is estimated that in normal humans 9 million cells die each hour. In most normal mammalian species, phagocytosis is most effective in the spleen, but in anemia it may reach significant proportions in the liver, bone marrow, lung, and lymph nodes. In birds and lower vertebrates the liver and bone marrow are highly effective in erythrophagocytosis (Aikawa and Sprinz 1971; Simpson 1971).

When the erythrocyte is phagocytized, hemoglobin is released within the macrophage and induces lysosomal enzymes specific for erythrocyte degradation (Gemsa et al. 1973). The hemoglobin molecule is rapidly broken down and its component parts are metabolized separately. Protein and iron are returned to their respective "pools" and the porphyrin fraction is not reused. Bilirubin is formed in macrophages of the reticuloendothelial system from ruptured heme and is shed into the plasma, where it is transported to the liver for conjugation with glucuronic acid. Bilirubin glucuronide is secreted by the biliary system into the duodenum, and it is degraded by intestinal bacteria to several compounds termed collectively fecal urobilinogen. The differentiation of free (unconjugated) and conjugated bilirubin is important because during hemolysis free bilirubin is elevated.

Ultrastructurally, the phagocytes are filled with dense bodies containing erythrocyte fragments (Fig. 3.21). Erythrocytes are taken up by phagosomes which fuse with acid phosphatase-containing lysosomes that initiate enzymic degradation (Collet and Petrik 1971; Morselt et al. 1973; Schnitzer and Smith 1966). Ferritin granules progressively accumulate in the dissolving hemoglobin within the phagosome and allegedly escape to exist free in the macrophage cytoplasm. Separated ferritin is completely reutilized. Rhomboid crystals of hematoidin and amorphous dense aggregates of hemosiderin characterize later stages of erythrophagocytosis (Richter 1960). Lamellar structures (remnants of erythrocyte cell membranes) are occasionally observed and remain for long periods within the macrophage.

SPLEEN

The spleen selectively removes abnormal erythrocytes from circulation (Rifkind 1965; Simon and Burke 1970). It is anatomically adapted to this role, as erythrocytes must pass from the arterial to the venous system through reticular cell networks beset by macrophages and must finally squeeze through the endothelial lining cells of the venous sinuses. Phagocytosis along this route may involve removal of the erythrocyte intact, fragmentation, or pitting (Schnitzer et al. 1973). Nuclei of erythroblasts are also selectively removed during passage through the endothelium of the marrow sinuses (Tavassoli and Crosby 1973). Macrophages in the red pulp, lymphoid sheath marginal zones, and peripheral white pulp are involved in phagocytosis; endothelial cells do not take part (Edwards and Simon 1970).

To enter the venous sinuses, erythrocytes, which in most mammals measure approximately 7μ in diameter, must pass through endothelial gaps of no more than 3μ. To do so, considerable deformation of the erythrocyte must be possible. Splenic blood is highly viscous. Its hematocrit is high and levels of oxygen and glucose are low. These factors favor spherocytosis, the formation of less biconcave and more spheroid erythrocytes. Abnormal erythrocytes, which lose flexibility, cannot pass the splenic filter. They are retained in the splenic sinuses and impede circulation through this organ (Chen and Weiss 1973). In the passage of abnormal cells through the endothelial gaps, selective pitting may occur. Small abnormal portions of the erythrocyte are removed.

Hypersplenism is a vague syndrome of splenomegaly, anemia, and bone marrow hyperplasia which may accompany a highly overactive spleen. Blood flow in the enlarged spleen is markedly retarded ("congestive splenomegaly"), allowing excessive sequestration of erythrocytes. Changes in the blood are the result of excessive erythrophagocytosis.

Slowing and stasis of blood in the spleen are major factors in enhancing erythrophagocytosis. Radiographic examination of the spleen following Cr^{151}-labeling of erythrocytes reveals two compartments (Pictet et al. 1969). Rapid flow of 98% of the blood goes directly to venous sinuses from the arteriole. A small percent, however, is slowed and percolates through the biliary cords. Redistribution of this flow in disease effectively promotes splenic erythrophagocytosis.

LEUKOCYTES

Evaluation of the number and quality of white blood cells provides reliable and often striking evidence of disease. An evaluation of circulating granulocytes gives particularly valuable information on the nature and progress of infectious diseases. The significant change occurs in the population of neutrophilic leukocytes (hereafter referred to as neutrophils). Analogous cells in lower vertebrates are termed heterophils and in insects, amebocytes. The precise function of these aggressively phagocytic cells varies but in all species they exert potent phagocytic and bactericidal effects. Neutrophils also function normally to remove small amounts of tissue debris and fibrin polymers from the vascular system. In systemic febrile diseases these functions are markedly increased.

In the developing mammalian fetus, the maturation of the neutrophil population heralds the capacity to react with an inflammatory process. This occurs in the later phases of gestation and provides the fetus with a newly acquired capacity to resist some infectious agents. In fetuses of most species, phagocytic capacity develops slightly before bactericidal activity. Both mechanisms reach adult levels in the pig fetus at or near 100 days of gestation, that is, at about three-fourths of the time spent in utero (Holmes et al. 1972).

Pathologic changes in neutrophils may be evaluated as: (1) number per cubic millimeter of blood; (2) structure, which involves the evaluation of the number and size of cytoplasmic granules by microscopy; and (3) chemotactic index, which is the capacity to attract, phagocytize, and digest determined quantities of bacteria and is a measure of granulocyte function. Other less utilized tests include those for degranulation and for the detection of specific enzymes.

Leukocytosis is the increase in the number of circulating white blood cells. Although it may occur during digestion and pregnancy, its value lies in the striking increases that accompany inflammation and necrosis. One may indicate a more specific diagnosis after examining stained blood smears: neutrophilic leukocytosis, monocytosis, etc. The degree of leukocytosis is related not only to the inciting agent but to the capacity of storage and synthesis sites in the spleen and bone marrow.

Leukopenia is a decrease in the total number of circulating white blood cells. This is most commonly seen in systemic viral diseases in which viruses replicate in and destroy circulating leukocytes and organs that produce them. It also occurs due to destruction of leukocytes in the terminal stages of overwhelming bacterial infections, during the sequestration of neutrophils in the pulmonary capillary bed in septic shock and anaphylaxis, and in any disease involving the depression of granulocytopoiesis.

Mature leukocytes, like erythrocytes, originate from a pool of self-perpetuating bone marrow stem cells. The kinetics of abnormal leukopoiesis in animals have been adequately examined in only a few instances (Prasse et al. 1973; Valli et al. 1971). Granule elaboration is the distinctive feature of maturation (Wetzel et al. 1967). The number of granules is a rough index of cell maturity (Fig. 3.29).

Neutrophilic leukocyte granules are of two types. Azurophil (primary) granules are small, primary lysosomes. In most species, they contain lysosomal digestive hydrolases (such as β-glucuronidase), a sulfated mucosubstance, and peroxidase which functions at pH optima in the acid range. The larger and more numerous specific (secondary) granules contain alkaline phosphatase, cationic proteins, lactoferrin, and most of the leukocyte's lysozyme. Specific granules do not contain acid phosphatase or other acid hydrolases and are, by definition, not lysosomes (Bagglioni et al 1970; Farquhar et al. 1972). Specific granules also contain proteolytic enzymes that act on collagen (Lazarus 1972) and elastin (Janoff 1972). They also allegedly contain some lipases which are lacking in macrophages.

REFERENCES

Adams, W. E. *The Comparative Morphology of the Carotid Body and Carotid Sinus.* Charles C Thomas, Springfield, 1958.

Aikawa, M. and Sprinz, H. Erythrophagocytosis in the bone marrow of canary infected with malaria. *Lab. Invest.* 24:45, 1971.

Aikawa, M. et al. The fine structure of malarial parasites. *Exp. Paras.* 30:284, 1971.

Amin, A. and Shamloo, K. D. Occurrence of paralbuminemia in mule. *Can. J. Biochem. Physiol.* 41:2025, 1963.

Archer, R. K. Blood coagulation in non-human vertebrates. *Symp. Zool. Soc. Lond.* 27:121, 1970.

Ashford, T. P. and Freiman, D. G. The role of the endothelium in the initial phases of thrombosis. *Am. J. Path.* 50:257, 1967.

Fig. 3.29. Immature neutrophilic leukocytes. A. In bone marrow, normal horse. Granules are peripheral and large Golgi complexes central. Cell at right is more immature as indicated by nucleus. B. Immature neutrophils in the lung capillary of a dog with acute pneumonia. Alveolar wall (aw) is at bottom; neutrophil is adjacent to the capillary endothelial cell.

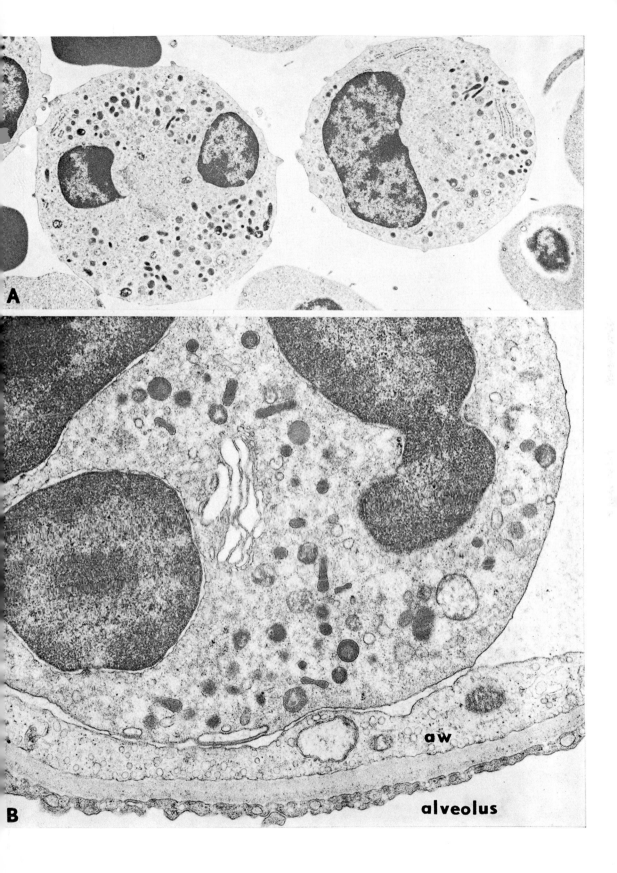

Astrup, T. and Buluk, K. Thromboplastic and fibrinolytic activities in vessels of animals. *Circ. Res.* 13:253, 1963.

Bächi, T. and Howe, C. Fusion of erythrocytes by Sendai virus studies by electron microscopy. *Proc. Soc. Exp. Biol. Med.* 141:141, 1972.

Bagglioni, M., Hirsch, J. G. and De Duve, C. Further biochemical and morphological studies of granule fractions from rabbit heterophil leukocytes. *J. Cell Biol.* 45:586, 1970.

Bannerman, R. M. and Pinkerton, P. H. X-linked hypochromic anaemia of mice. *Brit. J. Haem.* 13:1000, 1967.

Bateman, A. E. et al. The role of erythropoietin in prenatal erythropoiesis of congenitally anaemic flex-tailed (f/f) mice. *Brit. J. Haem.* 22:415, 1972.

Bédard, Y. C., Pinkerton, P. H. and Simon, G. T. Radioautographic observations on iron absorption by the duodenum of mice with iron overload, iron deficiency and x-linked anemia. *Blood* 42:131, 1973.

Behnke, O. An electron microscopic study of the megakaryocyte of the rat bone marrow. *J. Ult. Res.* 24:412, 1968.

Ben-Bassat, I., Bensch, K. G. and Schrier, S. L. Drug-induced erythrocyte membrane internalization. *J. Clin. Invest.* 51:1833, 1972.

Ben-Ishay, Z. and Yoffey, J. M. Ultrastructural studies of erythroblastic islands of rat bone marrow. II. The resumption of erythropoiesis in erythropoietically depressed rebound marrow. *Lab. Invest.* 26:637, 1972.

Blair, O. M. et al. Hepatocellular ultrastructure in dogs with hypovolemic shock. *Lab. Invest.* 18:172, 1968.

Blanton, P. L., Martin, J. and Haberman, S. Pinocytotic response of circulating erythrocytes to specific blood group antibodies. *J. Cell Biol.* 37:716, 1968.

Bodammer, J. E. and Bahr, G. F. The initiation of a "metabolic window" in the surface of host erythrocytes by *Plasmodium berghei* NYU-2. *Lab. Invest.* 28:708, 1973.

Brain, M. C., Esterly, J. R. and Beck, E. A. Intravascular hemolysis with experimentally produced vascular thrombi. *Brit. J. Haem.* 13:868, 1967.

Brecher, G. and Bessis, M. Present status of spiculated red cells and their relationship to the discocyte-echinocyte transformation: A critical review. *Blood* 40:333, 1972.

Breukink, H. J. et al. Congenital afibrinogenemia in goats. *Zentr. Vetmed. A* 19:661, 1972.

Brodsky, I. and Kahn, S. B. Effect of leukemia virus on erythropoiesis. *J. Nat. Cancer Inst.* 42:39, 1969.

Bull, B. S. et al. Red blood cell fragmentation in microangiopathic haemolytic anemia: In Vitro studies. *Lancet* 2:1123, 1967.

Bunn, H. F. and Jandle, J. H. The renal handling of hemoglobin. *J. Exp. Med.* 129:925, 1969.

Campbell, F. R. Electron microscopic studies on the fate of erythroblast ribosomes. *Anat. Rec.* 174:513, 1972.

Chandler, F. W. and Fletcher, O. J., Jr. Erythrocyte membrane defects associated with a transplantable lymphoid tumor. *J. Nat. Cancer Inst.* 51:1351, 1973.

Chang, J. and Hackel, D. B. Comparative study of myocardial lesions in hemorrhagic shock. *Lab. Invest.* 28:641, 1973.

Chen, L.-T. and Weiss, L. The role of the sinus wall in the passage of erythrocytes through the spleen. *Blood* 41:529, 1973.

Cheville, N. F. Ultrastructure of canine carotid body and aortic body tumors. *Vet. Path.* 9:166, 1972.

Clawson, C. C. Platelet interaction with bacteria. III. Ultrastructure. *Am. J. Path.* 70:449, 1973.

Coalson, J. J., Hinshaw, L. B. and Guenter, C. A. The pulmonary ultrastructure in septic shock. *Exp. Mol. Path.* 12:84, 1970.

Collet, A. J. and Petrik, P. Electron microscopic study of the in vivo erythrophagocytosis by alveolar macrophages of the cat. *Zt. Zellf.* 116:464, 1971.

Connell, R. S., Swank, R. L. and Webb, M. C. The development of pulmonary ultrastructural lesions during hemorrhagic shock. *J. Trauma* 15:116, 1975.

Cornell, C. N. and Muhrer, M. E. Coagulation factors in normal and hemophiliac-type swine. *Am. J. Physiol.* 206:926, 1964.

Cottrell, T. S. et al. Electron microscopic alterations at the alveolar level in pulmonary edema. *Circ. Res.* 21:783, 1967.

Croft, J. D. et al. Coombs test positivity induced by drugs. Mechanisms of immunological reaction and red cell destruction. *Ann. Int. Med.* 68:176, 1968.

Crowell, J. W. Oxygen transport in the hypotensive state. *Fed. Proc.* 29:1848, 1970.

Debbie, J. G. and Abelseth, M. K. Pathogenesis of epizootic hemorrhagic disease. I. Blood coagulation during viral infection. *J. Inf. Dis.* 124:217, 1971.

Demaree, R. S. and Nessmith, W. B. Ultrastructure of *Haemobartonella felis* from a naturally infected cat. *Am. J. Vet. Res.* 33:1303, 1972.

Döbler, J. and Bertles, J. F. The physical state of hemoglobin in sickle cell anemia erythrocytes in vivo. *J. Exp. Med.* 127:711, 1968.

Dodds, W. J. Canine von Willebrand's disease. *J. Lab. Clin. Med.* 76:713, 1970.

Donovan, E. F. and Loeb, W. F. Polycythemia rubra vera in the dog. *J.A.V.M.A.* 134: 36, 1959.

Doolittle, R. F. and Surgenor, D. M. Blood coagulation in fish. *Am. J. Physiol.* 203:964, 1962.

Dourmashkin, R. R. and Rosse, W. F. Morphologic changes in membranes of red blood cells undergoing hemolysis. *Am. J. Med.* 41:699, 1966.

Droller, M. J. An electron microscope study of the time course of platelet nucleotide, calcium, and acid phosphatase secretion. *Lab. Invest.* 31:197, 1974.

Drommer, W. Feinstrukturelle Alterationen an den Capillaren und Venulen im zentralen Nervensystem des Schweines nach experimentellem Colitoxinschock. *Acta Neuropath.* 22:13, 1972.

———. Permeation von Ferritin an normalen und durch Colitoxin geschädigten Gefässen im zentralen Nervensystem des Schweines. *Acta Neuropath.* 24:30, 1973.

Edwards, C., Heath, D. and Harris, P. Ultrastructure of the carotid body in high alti tude guinea pigs. *J. Path.* 107:131, 1972.

Edwards, V. D. and Simon, G. T. Ultrastructural aspects of red cell destruction in the normal rat spleen. *J. Ult. Res.* 33:187, 1970.

Emmons, R. W. et al. Intraerythrocytic localization of Colorado tick fever virus. *J. Gen. Virol.* 17:185, 1972.

Farquhar, M. G. and Palade, G. E. Glomerular permeability. II. Membrane transfer around the glomerular capillary wall in nephrotic rats. *J. Exp. Med.* 114:699, 1961.

Farquhar, M. G. et al. Cytochemical localization of acid phosphatase in granule fractions from rabbit polymorphonuclear leukocytes. *J. Cell Biol.* 54:141, 1972.

Field, R. A., Rickard, C. G. and Hutt, L. J. Hemophilia in a family of dogs *Cornell Vet.* 36:283, 1946.

Finch, J. T. et al. Structure of sickled erythrocytes and of sickle cell hemoglobin fibers. *Proc. Nat. Acad. Sci.* 70:718, 1973.

Fisher, J. W., Taylor, G. and Porteous, D. Localization of erythropoietin in glomeruli of sheep kidney by fluorescent antibody technique. *Nature* 205:611, 1965.

Fowler, M., Cornelius, C. and Baker, N. Clinical and erythrokinetic studies on a case of bovine polycythemia vera. *Cornell Vet.* 51.159, 1964.

French, J. E., MacFarlane, R. G. and Sanders, A. G. The structure of haemostatic plugs and experimental thrombi in small arteries. *Brit. J. Exp. Path.* 45:467, 1964.

Frenkel, E. D., Suki, W. and Baum, J. Some observations on the localization of erythropoietin. *Ann. N.Y. Acad. Sci.* 149:292, 1968.

Friederici, H. H. R. The early response of uterine capillaries to estrogen stimulation. An electron microscopic study. *Lab. Invest.* 17:322, 1967.

Gabbiani, G. et al. Acute cadmium intoxication. *Lab. Invest.* 30:686–95, 1974.

Gasko, O. and Danon, D. Deterioration and disappearance of mitochondria during reticulocyte maturation. *Exp. Cell Res.* 75:159, 1972.

Gemsa, D. et al. Erythrocyte catabolism by macrophages in vitro. *J. Clin. Invest.* 52:812, 1973.

Georgiev, G. Untersuchungen über das Blut der Regenbogenforellen *(Salmo irideus Gibb). Arch. Exp. Vet.* 26:733, 1972.

Gimbrone, M. A. et al. Preservation of vascular integrity in organs perfused in vitro with a platelet rich medium. *Nature* 222:33, 1969.

Ginn, F. C., Hockstein, P. and Trump, B. J. Membrane alteration in hemolysis: Internalization of plasmalemma induced by primaquine. *Science* 164:843, 1969.

Gomba, S. et al. An electron histochemical study on the distribution of sodium ions in the juxtaglomerular apparatus. *Virch. Arch. B* 11:284, 1972.

Graham, J. B. et al. Canine hemophilia. *J. Exp. Med.* 90:97, 1949.

Guest, M. M. Red blood cells: Change in shape in capillaries. *Science* 142:1319, 1963.

Hackel, D. B. et al. Hemorrhagic shock in dogs. *Arch. Path.* 77:575, 1964.

Hackett, E. and Hann, C. Slow clotting of reptile bloods. *J. Comp. Path.* 77:175, 1967.

Hall, C. E. Electron-microscopy of the fibrinogen molecule and the fibrin clot. *Lab. Invest.* 12:998, 1963.

Hartroft, P. M. Juxtaglomerular cells. *Circ. Res.* 12:525, 1963.

Hashimoto, P. H. et al. Vascular leakage through intraendothelial channels induced by cholera toxin in the skin of guinea pigs. *Am. J. Path.* 75:171, 1974.

Hatcher, J. D. et al. The circulatory adjustments to posthemorrhagic anemia in dogs. *Circ. Res.* 2:499, 1954.

Hawkey, C. M. Fibrinolysis in animals. *Symp. Zool. Soc. Lond.* 27:133, 1970.

Heene, D. et al. Gerinnungsstörungen bei akuter Schweinepest. *Beitr. Path. B* 114:259, 1971.

Hembrough, F. B. et al. Renin activity of canine plasma during controlled hemorrhage. *Am. J. Vet. Res.* (in press), 1976.

Hochmuth, R. M. and Mohandas, N. Metabolic dependence of red cell shape: Observations with the scanning electron microscope. *Microvasc. Res.* 4:295, 1972.

Holeman, R. Enhancement of fibrinolysis in the dog by injection of vasoactive drugs. *Am. J. Physiol.* 208:511, 1965.

Holmes, B. et al. Development of bactericidal capacity and phagocytosis-associated metabolism of fetal pig leukocytes. *Inf. Immun.* 5:232, 1972.

Honour, A. J., Pickering, G. W. and Sheppard, B. L. Ultrastructure and behavior of platelet thrombi in injured arteries. *Brit. J. Exp. Path.* 52:482, 1971.

Hovig, T. et al. Experimental hemostasis in normal dogs and dogs with congenital disorders of blood coagulation. *Blood* 30:636, 1967.

Hüttner, I. et al. Studies on protein passage through arterial endothelium. *Lab. Invest.* 29:536, 1973.

Jain, N. C. and Keelon, K. S. Scanning electron microscopic feature of *Haemobartonella felis*. *Am. J. Vet. Res.* 34:697, 1973.

Janoff, A. Human granulocyte elastase. *Am. J. Path.* 68:579, 1972.

Janoff, A. et al. Pathogenesis of experimental shock. *J. Exp. Med.* 116:451, 1962.

Jørgensen, L. et al. Adenosine diphosphate-induced platelet aggregation in myocardial infarction in swine. *Lab. Invest.* 17:616, 1967a.

Jørgensen, L. et al. Resolution and organization of platelet-rich mural thrombi in carotid arteries of swine. *Am. J. Path.* 51:681, 1967b.

Kaneko, J. J., Zinkl, J. G. and Keeten, K. S. Erythrocyte porphyrin and erthrocyte survival in bovine erythropoietic porphyria. *Am. J. Vet. Res.* 32:1981, 1971.

Karle, H. The mechanism of erythrocyte destruction induced by injection of bacterial pyrogen. *Acta Path. Micro. Scand.* 77:318, 1969.

Karnovsky, M. J. The ultrastructural basis of capillary permeability studied with peroxidase as a tracer. *J. Cell Biol.* 35:213, 1967.

Kayden, H. J. and Bessis, M. Morphology of normal erythrocyte and acanthocyte using Nomarski optics and the scanning electron microscope. *Blood* 35:427, 1970.

Kent, G. et al. Autophagic vacuoles in human red cells. *Am. J. Path.* 48:831, 1971.

Kitchen, H., Putnam, F. and Taylor, W. J. Hemoglobin polymorphism in white-tailed deer. Subunit basis. *Blood* 29:867, 1967.

Kwaan, H. C. and Astrup, T. Demonstration of cellular fibrinolytic activity by the histochemical fibrin slide technique. *Lab. Invest.* 17:140, 1967.

Laird, H. M. et al. Replication of leukemogenic-type virus in cats inoculated with feline lymphosarcoma extracts. *J. Nat. Cancer Inst.* 41:879, 1968.

Lange, R. D., Jordan, T. A. and McDonald, T. P. Partial characterization of an antiserum to erythropoietin. *Israel J. Med. Sci.* 7:877, 1970.

Lazarus, G. S. Role of granulocyte collagenase in collagen degradation. *Am. J. Path.* 68:565, 1972.

Leak, L. V. Studies on the permeability of lymphatic capillaries. *J. Cell Biol.* 50:300, 1971.

Lee, L. and McCluskey, R. T. Immunohistochemical demonstration of the reticuloendothelial clearance of circulating fibrin aggregates. *J. Exp. Med.* 116:611, 1962.

Lewis, L. J. et al. Replication of human endothelial cells in culture. *Science* 181:453, 1973.

Loria, A. et al. Red cell life span in iron deficiency anemia. *Brit. J. Haem.* 13:294, 1967.

Luft, J. H. Fine structure of capillary and endocapillary layer as revealed by ruthenium red. *Fed. Proc.* 25:1771, 1966.

Luginbuhl, H. et al. Congenital hereditary lymphocdema in the dog. *J. Med. Gen.* 4: 153, 1967.

MacPherson, G. G. Origin and development of the demarcation system in megakaryocytes of rat bone marrow. *J. Ult. Res.* 40:167, 1972.

Majno, G. Ultrastructure of the vascular membrane. *Handbook of Physiology,* Vol. 3, John Field, ed., p. 2293. Williams and Wilkins, Baltimore, 1965.

Maldonado, J. E. Dysplastic platelets and circulating megakaryocytes in chronic myeloproliferative disease. *Blood* 43:811, 1974.

Marchesi, V. T. and Barrnett, R. J. The demonstration of enzymatic activity in pinocytotic vesicles of blood capillaries with the electron microscope. *J. Cell Biol.* 17: 547, 1963.

Margaretten, W., Csavossy, I. and McKay, D. G. An electron microscopic study of thrombin-induced disseminated intravascular coagulation. *Blood* 29:169, 1967.

Margolis, G. and Kilham, L. Rat virus infection of megakaryocytes: A factor in hemorrhagic encephalopathy. *Exp. Mol. Path.* 16:326, 1972.

Marsh, C. L. et al. Loss of serum protein via the intestinal tract in calves with infectious diarrhea. *Am. J. Vet. Res.* 30:163, 1969.

Matheson, D. W. and Howland, J. L. Erythrocyte deformation in human muscular dystrophy. *Science* 184:165, 1974.

Mauier, H. M. et al. "Impotent" platelets in albinos with prolonged bleeding times. *Blood* 39:490, 1972.

McGuire, T. C., Henson, J. B. and Quist, S. E. Impaired bone marrow response in equine infectious anemia. *Am. J. Vet. Res.* 30:2099, 1969.

McKay, D. G., Margaretten, W. and Csavossy, I. An electron microscope study of the effects of bacterial endotoxin on the blood-vascular system. *Lab. Invest.* 15:1815, 1966.

McKee, A. E., Ziegler, R. F. and Giles, R. C. Scanning and transmission electron microscopy of *Haemobartonella canis* and *Eperythrozoon ovis. Am. J. Vet. Res.* 34:1196, 1973.

Mielke, C. H., Ramos, J. C. and Britten, A. F. H. Aspirin as an antiplatelet agent. *Am. J. Clin. Path.* 59:236, 1973.

Morris, B. et al. Congenital lymphatic edema in Ayrshire calves. *Austr. J. Exp. Biol. Med. Sci.* 32:265, 1954.

Morselt, A. F. W., Cambier, P. H. and James, J. Electron microscopical and microphotometric studies on the breakdown of erythrocytes by macrophages. *Histochemie* 37:161, 1973.

Muller-Eberhard, H. J. et al. A molecular concept of immune cytolysis. *Arch. Path.* 82: 205, 1966.

Mustard, J. F. et al. Canine factor-VII deficiency. *Brit. J. Haem.* 8:43, 1962a.

Mustard, J. F. et al. Canine hemophilia B (Christmas disease). *Brit. J. Haem.* 6.259, 1960.

Mustard, J. F. et al. Factors influencing thrombus formation in vivo. *Am. J. Med.* 33: 621, 1962b.

Myhre-Jensen, O. Localization of fibrinolytic activity in the kidney and urinary tract of rats and rabbits. *Lab. Invest.* 25:403, 1971.

Nafstad, I. and Nafstad, P. H. J. An electron microscopic study of blood and bone marrow in vitamin E-deficient pigs. *Vet. Path.* 5:520, 1968.

Nathan, D. G. et al. Extreme hemolysis and red-cell distortion in erythrocyte pyruvate kinase deficiency. *New Engl. J. Med.* 272:118, 1965.

Nevaril, C. G. et al. Erythrocyte damage and destruction due to shearing. *J. Lab. Clin. Med.* 71:784, 1968.

Nichols, J. and Hennigar, G. Effects of pulmonary hypertension on adrenal and kidneys of dogs infected with heart worms *(Dirofilaria immitis). Lab. Invest.* 13:800, 1964.

Nicolson, G. L. Anionic sites of human erythrocyte membrane. *J. Cell Biol.* 57:373, 1973.

Nienhuis, A. W. and Anderson, W. F. Hemoglobin switching in sheep and goats. *Proc. Nat. Acad. Sci.* 69:2184, 1972.

O'Leary, D. S. et al. Experimental infection with *Plasmodium falciparum* in Aotus monkeys. III. The development of disseminated intravascular coagulation. *Am. J. Trop. Med. Hyg.* 21:282, 1972.

Ortega, P. et al. Serial light and electron microscopic studies on the dog lung in chronic experimental pulmonary edema. *Am. J. Path.* 60:57, 1970.

Oshiro, L. S. et al. Replication of feline C-type virus at the plasma membrane of erythrocytes. *J. Nat. Cancer Inst.* 48:1419, 1972.

Patt, H. M., Lund, J. E. and Maloney, M. A. Cyclic hematopoiesis in grey Collie dogs: A stem cell problem. *Blood* 42:873, 1973.

Phillips, M., Olsen, M. W. and Stone, S. S. Bisalbuminemia in the serum of chicken-turkey hybrids. *Comp. Biochem. Physiol.* 46:533 (B), 1973.

Pictet, R. et al. An electron microscope study of the perfusion-fixed spleen. *Zt. Zellf.* 96:372, 1969.

Pietra, G. G. et al. Histamine and interstitial pulmonary edema in the dog. *Circ. Res.* 29:329, 1971.

Pinkerton, P. H. Histological evidence of disordered iron transport in the x-linked hypochromic anemia of mice. *J. Path. Bact.* 95:155, 1968.

Pinkerton, P. H. et al. Hereditary stomatocytosis with hemolytic anemia in the dog. *Blood* 44:557, 1974.

Pinkiewiez, E. Die Blutgerinnungsfakloren der 1. Phase bei gesunden und Kranken Pferden. *Wien. Tierarztl. Mntsh.* 48:791, 1961.

Prasse, K. W. et al. Factor V deficiency and thrombocytopenia in a dog with adenocarcinoma. *J.A.V.M.A.* 160:204, 1972.

Prasse, K. W. et al. A model of granulopoiesis in cats. *Lab. Invest.* 28:292, 1973.

Prathap, K. Surface lining cells of healing thrombi in rat femoral veins: An electron-microscope study. *J. Path.* 107:1, 1972.

Prose, P. H., Lee, L. and Balk, S. Electron microscopic study of the phagocytic fibrin-clearing mechanism. *Am. J. Path.* 47:403, 1967.

Ramsey, N. W. et al. Mechanism of shock produced by an elapid snake *(Micrurus f. fulvius)* venom in dogs. *Am. J. Physiol.* 222:782, 1972.

Rašková, H. et al. Release of 5-hydroxytryptamine and morphological changes in blood platelets induced by mucopeptides of streptococcal cell walls. *J. Inf. Dis.* 123:587, 1971.

Reddick, R. L., Poole, B. L. and Penick, G. D. Thrombocytopenia of hibernation mechanism of induction and recovery. *Lab. Invest.* 28:270, 1973.

Reynolds, H. Y. et al. Serum immunoglobulin levels in grey Collies. *Proc. Soc. Exp. Biol. Med.* 136:574, 1971.

Richter, G. W. The nature of storage iron in idiopathic hemochromatosis and hemosiderosis. *J. Exp. Med.* 112:551, 1960.

Rifkind, R. A. Heinz body anaemia: An ultrastructural study. II. Red cell sequestration and destruction. *Blood* 26:433, 1965.

Ritzmann, S. E. Diagnostic interpretation of serum protein abnormalities in thermal burns. *Am. J. Clin. Path.* 60:135, 1973.

Rodvien, R., Gillum, A. and Weintraub, L. K. Decreased glutathione peroxidase activity secondary to severe iron deficiency. *Blood* 43:281, 1974.

Rosse, W. F., Dourmashkin, R. and Humphrey, J. H. Immune lysis of normal human and paroxysmal nocturnal hemoglobinuria (PNH) red blood cells. *J. Exp. Med.* 123:969, 1966.

Rowsell, H. C. The hemostatic mechanism of mammals and birds in health and disease. *Adv. Vet. Sci.* 12:337, 1968.

Rowsell, H. C. et al. A disorder resembling hemophilia B (Christmas disease) in dogs. *J.A.V.M.A.* 137:247, 1960.

Russell, E. S. et al. Characterization and genetic studies of microcytic anemia in the house mouse. *Blood* 35:838, 1970.

Salmon, J. and Lambert, P. H. Determination of fibrinogen derivative by immunofluorescence in experimental and clinical kidney disorders. *Scand. J. Haem.* 8:351, Suppl. 13, 1971.

Sandritter, W. and Lasch, H. G. Pathologic aspects of shock. *Meth. Achiev. Exp. Path.* 3:86, 1967.

Schnitzer, B. and Smith, E. B. Observations of phagocytized red cells containing Heinz bodies. A light and electron microscope study. *Am. J. Clin. Path.* 46:538, 1966.

Schnitzer, B., Aikawa, M. and Spencer, H. H. Pernicious anemia: An ultrastructural study of the bone marrow before and after vitamin B_{12} therapy. *Am. J. Clin. Path.* 58:1, 1972.

Schnitzer, B. et al. Pitting function of the spleen in malaria: Ultrastructural observations. *Science* 177:175, 1972.

Schnitzer, B. et al. An ultrastructural study of the red pulp of the spleen in malaria. *Blood* 41:207, 1973.

Schulz, H. and Rabanus, B. Die Kapilläre Plättchenthrombose im elektronenmikroskopischen. *Bild. Beitr. Path. Anat.* 131:290, 1965.

Searcy, G. P., Miller, D. R. and Tasker, J. B. Congenital hemolytic anemia in the Basenji dog due to erythrocyte pyruvate kinase deficiency. *Can. J. Comp. Med.* 35:67, 1971.

Seelig, L. L. Surface multivesicular structures associated with maturing erythrocytes in rats. *Zt. Zellf.* 133:181, 1972.

Sheppard, B. C. and French, J. E. Platelet adhesions in the rabbit abdominal aorta following the removal of endothelium: A scanning and transmission electron microscopic study. *Proc. Roy. Soc. Lond. B* 176:427, 1971.

Simionescu, M., Simionescu, N. and Palade, G. E. Morphometric data on the endothelium of blood capillaries. *J. Cell Biol.* 60:128, 1974.

Simon, G. T. and Burke, J. S. Electron microscopy of the spleen. III. Erythro-leukophagocytosis. *Am. J. Path.* 58:451, 1970.

Simpkins, H. et al. Structural and compositional changes in the red cell membrane during *Clostridium welchii* infection. *Brit. J. Haem.* 21:173, 1971.

Simpson, C. F. Fate of erythrocytes containing Heinz bodies in the spleen and liver of dogs and turkeys. *Vet. Path.* 8:118, 1971.

———. Phagocytosis of *Babesia canis* by neutrophiles in the peripheral circulation *Am J. Vet. Res.* 35:701, 1974.

Simpson, C. F. and Kling, J. M. The mechanism of denucleation in circulating erythroblasts. *J. Cell Biol.* 35:237, 1967.

Simpson, C. F. and Love, J. N. Fine structure of *Haemobartonella bovis* in blood and liver of splenectomized calves. *Am. J. Vet. Res.* 31:255, 1970.

Simpson, C. F. and Taylor, W. J. Ultrastructure of sickled deer erythrocytes. *Blood* 43:899, 1974.

Simpson, C. F., Kirkham, W. W. and Kling, J. M. Comparative morphologic features of *Babesia caballi* and *Babesia equi Am. J. Vet. Res.* 28:1093, 1967.

Simpson, C. F., Kling, J. M. and Neal, F. C. The nature of bands in parasitized bovine erythrocytes. *J. Cell Biol.* 27:225, 1965.

Skalak, R., Brancmark, P I. and Ekholm, R. Erythrocyte adherence and diapedesis. *Angiology* 21:224, 1970.

Skinnider, L. F, and Ghadially, F N. An ultrastructural study of ropalocytosis in human blood and bone marrow. *J. Path.* 109:1, 1973.

Skutelsky, E. and Danon, D. Comparative studies of nuclear expulsion from the late erythroblast and cytokinesis. *Exp. Cell Res.* 60:427, 1970.

Slappendel, R. J. et al. Response to heparin of spontaneous disseminated coagulation in the dog. *Zentr. Vetmed. A* 19:502, 1972.

Snodgrass, M. J., Yuhas, J. M. and Hanna, M. G. J. Histoproliferative effect of Rauscher leukemia virus on lymphatic tissue. *J. Nat. Cancer Inst.* 50:735, 1973.

Sorensen, D. K. An effective therapeutic regimen for the hemopoietic phase of the acute radiation syndrome in dogs. *Radiat. Res.* 13:669, 1960.

Spielman, W. S., Davis, J. O. and Gotshall, R. W. Hypersecretion of renin in dogs with a chronic aortic-caval fistula and high-output heart failure. *Proc. Soc. Exp. Biol. Med.* 143:479, 1973.

Spurling, N. W. et al. Hereditary factor-VIII deficiency in the Beagle. *Brit. J. Haem.* 23:59, 1972.

Stehbens, W. E. and Biscoe, T. S. The ultrastructure of early platelet aggregation in vivo. *Am. J. Path.* 50:219, 1967.

Still, W. J. S. and Boult, E. H. Electron microscopic appearance of fibrin in thin sections. *Nature* 179:868, 1957.

Stoner, H. B. Studies on the mechanism of shock. The impairment of thermoregulation by trauma. *Brit. J. Exp. Path.* 50:125, 1969.

Stopforth, A. A study of coagulation mechanisms in domestic chickens. *J. Comp. Path.* 80:525, 1970.

Swanton, M. C. Hemophilic arthropathy in dogs. *Lab. Invest.* 8:1269, 1959.

Tavassoli, M. and Crosby, W. H. Fate of the nucleus of the marrow erythroblast. *Science* 79:912, 1973.

Tedder, E. and Shorey, C. D. Intimal changes in venous stasis. *Lab. Invest.* 14:208, 1965.

Tennant, B. et al. Familial polycythemia in cattle. *J.A.V.M.A.* 150:1493, 1967.

Tranzer, J. P. and Baumgartner, H. R. Filling gaps in the vascular endothelium with blood platelets. *Nature* 216:1126, 1967.

Valli, V. E. O. et al. The kinetics of haematopoiesis in the calf. *Res. Vet. Sci.* 12:535, 1971.

Van Horn, D. L. and Johnson, S. A. The mechanism of thrombocytopenic bleeding. *Am. J. Clin. Path.* 46:204, 1966.

Vassalli, P. and McCluskey, R. T. The pathogenic role of fibrin in deposition in immunologically induced glomerulonephritis. *Ann. N.Y. Acad. Sci.* 116:1052, 1964.

Venable, J. H. and Ewing, S. A. Fine structure of *Haemobartonella canis (Rickettsiales bartonellaceae)* and its relation to the host erythrocytes. *J. Paras.* 54:259, 1968.

Waldo, E. D. and Tobias, H. Needle-like cytoplasmic inclusions in the liver in porphyria cutanea tarda. *Arch. Path.* 96:368, 1973.

Walker, W. F. et al. Adrenal medullary secretion in hemorrhagic shock. *Am. J. Physiol.* 197:773, 1959.

Warren, B. A. and Khan, S. The ultrastructure of the lysis of fibrin by endothelium in vitro. *Brit. J. Exp. Path.* 55:138, 1974.

Warren, B. A. and Vales, O. The release of vesicles from platelets following adhesion to vessel walls in vitro. *Brit. J. Exp. Path.* 53:206, 1972.

Wegmann, W. Die juxtaglomerulare Apparat der Niere bei primaren und sekundaren Hyperaldosteronismus. *Virch. Arch. A* 349:21, 1970.

Weiss, H. J. and Ames, R. P. Ultrastructural findings in storage pool disease and aspirin-like defects of platelets. *Am. J. Path.* 71:447, 1973.

Weiss, L. The structure of bone marrow. *J. Morphol.* 117:467, 1965.

Wennberg, E. and Weiss, L. Splenic erythroclasia. *Blood* 31:778, 1968.

Wetzel, B. K., Horn, R. G. and Spicer, S. S. Fine structural studies on the development of heterophil, eosinophil, and basophil granulocytes in rabbits. *Lab. Invest.* 16:349, 1967.

White, J. G. Exocytosis of secretory organelles from blood platelets incubated with cationic polypeptide. *Am. J. Path.* 69:41, 1972.

Windqvist, G. Morphology of the blood and hemopoietic organs in cattle under normal and some experimental conditions. *Acta Anat. (Suppl.)* 22:1, 1954.

Wollmann, R. L. Virus-induced hemolytic anemia in mice. *Cancer Res.* 30:1003, 1970.

Wong, K. Y., Hug, G. and Lampkin, B. C. Congenital dyserythropoietic anemia. Type II. Ultrastructural and radioautographic studies of blood and bone marrow. *Blood* 39:23, 1972.

Zucker-Franklin, D., Nachman, R. L. and Marcus, A. J. Ultrastructure of thrombosthenin. The contractile protein of human blood platelets. *Science* 157:945, 1967.

Zweifach, B. W. Aspects of comparative physiology of laboratory animals relative to the problem of experimental shock. *Fed. Proc. (Suppl.)* 9:18, 1961.

CHAPTER FOUR

Inflammation and Repair

Inflammation is the continuum of vascular exudative changes in tissue that is elicited by the effect of irritants on blood vessels. It begins with increased capillary permeability and ends with revascularization and repair. The inflammatory process encompasses exudation of fluid, the chemotactic accumulation of leukocytes, phagocytosis, vascularization, and fibroplasia. In essence, it extends the defense mechanisms existing in circulating blood into the interstitium.

In acute inflammation, the vascular wall is altered and plasma factors such as albumin, fibrinogen, antibody, complement, and lysozyme pour into the tissues. This is followed by the exudation of phagocytic cells, chiefly neutrophils and monocytes, and inflamed tissues become distended with fluids and cells. Although severe lesions can be life-threatening when they occur in vital organs such as lung and brain, the inflammatory process is essentially curative. It is designed to dilute, inactivate, and remove irritants.

Inflammatory lesions as seen microscopically vary in intensity and in dominance of a particular component. Differences depend upon the type of irritant and upon the animal species involved. Despite phylogenetic variables, inflammation is a remarkably uniform biological reaction against a wide variety of physical, chemical, and biological irritants. It is an evolutionary, adaptive response enhancing survival for those animals that possess vascular systems. Individuals of vertebrate species that lack the capacity to produce a vigorous inflammatory response do not survive.

The age of an animal influences the character of the reaction. The adult has a greater capacity to react than the neonate and the neonate a greater capacity than the fetus. Fetal inflammatory reactions, like those of lower animals, are largely histiocytic; pluripotential cells respond by becoming phagocytic. The inability of the fetus to respond relates to inert or retarded vascular responses, the presence of only immature, slowly reacting pregranulocytes in the circulation, and low levels of complement and other chemoattractants in serum (Schwartz and Osburn 1974).

Celsus, a Greek philosopher and a contemporary of Christ, enunciated four cardinal signs which are observed grossly in acute inflammation: redness, swelling, heat, and pain ("rubor, tumor, calor, and dolor"). Galen (about A.D. 180) added a fifth: loss of function.

With the application of the light microscope to pathology in the middle 1800s, Cohnheim, a German experimental pathologist, revealed the vascular alterations that are the basis of the inflammatory response. By examining mesentery from a loop of intestine pulled through an abdominal incision of a curarized frog, he observed the early changes in blood flow and vascular permeability. Cohnheim recognized that increased capillary permeability was due to direct injury to endothelium and that this explained the initiating reaction in inflammation. Hyperemia and the exuding fluid obviously give rise to redness and swelling.

The cardinal signs were further illustrated by Lewis's (1927) observations of the "triple response" of skin to a linear stroke produced by a marker (Fig. 4.1). A few seconds after injury, the stroke line was red-

keep intimate company with fibroblasts, especially in perivascular locations, and initiate or enhance the acute stage of inflammation by liberation of granules containing potent vasoactive factors. Histamine, the predominant factor, acts directly on capillary endothelium to cause hyperemia and increased permeability (Rowley and Benditt 1956). In acute inflammatory lesions, mast cells are diminished in number due to degranulation and lysis (Clark and Higgenbotham 1968).

Mast cell granules are the source of the vasoactive amines histamine and serotonin (5-hydroxy tryptamine) as well as the acid mucopolysaccharide heparin. Other less defined alkaline proteolytic enzymes are also present. Tissue samples can be assayed for their content of these substances. Specific histochemical techniques have been developed for histamine, and stains for acidic mucopolysaccharides are used as presumptive evidence of heparin content. Differences in granule content, concentration, and molecular configuration account for the heterogeneity of granule morphology.

Mast cell granules are round, metachromatic, membrane-bound, and structurally heterogeneous (Fig. 4.2). The most mature granules are homogeneous, amorphous, and dense (Combs 1966). Granules with concentrically arranged cords are allegedly younger. Occasional compound granules are seen which also contain crystalloids of protein. When granules are artificially ruptured, ultrastructural examination reveals small beaded filaments which are interpreted as heparin-protein complexes (Serafini-Fracassini et al. 1969). Histamine is allegedly stored in ionic linkage to the heparin-protein complex and is released as the result of a simple ion exchange between histamine in the granule and cations in the extracellular fluid (Röhlich et al. 1971).

Degranulation of mast cells is an immediate reaction in tissue injury. It releases massive quantities of histamine and serotonin locally and these cause the early transient dilation and disunion of postcapillary venules. The resultant leakage of plasma is limited to the small and medium-sized (20–30 nm) venules rather than to the capillary bed proper (Fig. 4.3). Histamine, sero-tonin, and bradykinin induce the formation of intercellular gaps in vascular endothelium, due in part to endothelial cell contraction. Heparin is also released. Its anticoagulant effect prevents the polymerization of fibrin from the exuding fibrinogen and thereby sustains exudation.

Mast cells are exceptionally vulnerable and reactive to irritants (Smith and Lewis 1961). Exposure to trauma, ultraviolet light, heat, or cold, as well as to a variety of chemical and bacterial toxins, causes degranulation. Immunologic degranulation occurs when special types of antibodies bind to mast cell membranes and are subsequently complexed with the specific antigen (Roberts 1970). Explosive systemic degranulation may lead to anaphylactic shock.

Degranulation involves structural changes in the cell membrane. Granule membrane and plasma membrane join, fuse, and lyse with extrusion of intact granules into the periphery. On exit from the cell, the granule loses its density and becomes pale and granular. Granules appear to be joined in a common membrane-bound cisterna which opens at the cell surface (Padawer 1970, 1971). In the final stages of degranulation, the cell is filled with anastomosing cavities (which represent coalescing granule membranes) and the cell membrane is shredded by the release of many granules (Röhlich et al. 1971).

The location of mast cells in lung, brain, and intestine helps to explain some of the clinical signs seen in these organs. By their action on the capillary bed, mast cells play important pathogenetic roles in pulmonary edema, brain edema, and diarrhea. Species differences in mast cell numbers and granule size may be important in differences in inflammatory reactions. They are numerous in the dog, cat, cow, and hamster while being rare in the rabbit and guinea pig.

The basophil and the globule leukocyte have the structure and staining affinities of tissue mast cells. Despite some differences, we will proceed with the concept that these cells belong together as a related population, differing according to cell age and tissue location.

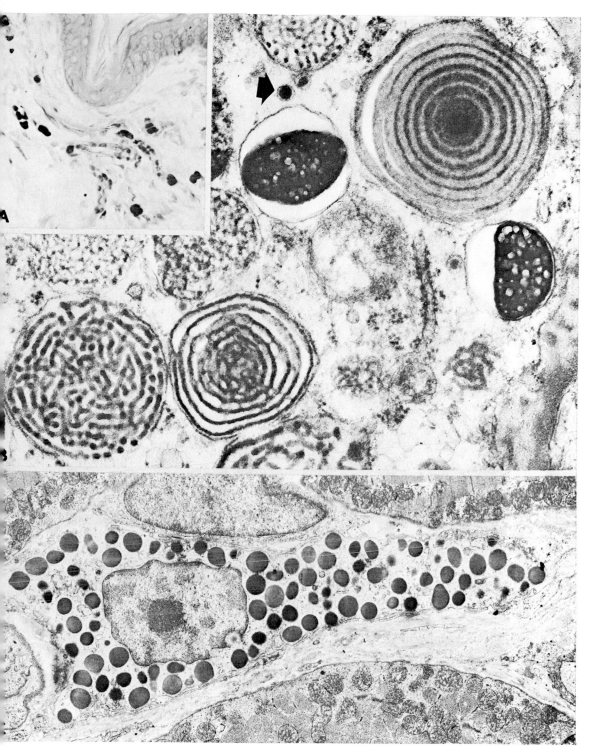

Fig. 4.2. Mast cells. A. Around blood vessels, healing skin incision, cat. B. Ultrastructure of mast cell granules and small dense granules (arrow). Note target forms, membrane-bound aggregates of rodlets and large dense granules. C. Intact, stellate-shaped mast cell, interstitium of heart.

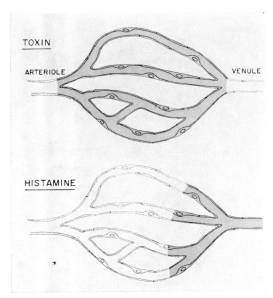

Fig. 4.3. Comparison in site of effect of histamine and toxin in capillaries.

LARGE MOLECULE MEDIATORS OF INFLAMMATION

KININ SYSTEMS

Endogenous humoral mediators of inflammation other than histamine are released by injured or stimulated cells. *Kinins* are polypeptides in circulating blood that arise from globulin fractions. They are implicated as mediators because of their presence at sites of tissue injury and their capacity to reproduce inflammatory lesions experimentally. Lysis of cells, particularly leukocytes, releases enzymes that generate kinins which then sustain and enhance the early transitory capillary alterations begun by histamine. Bradykinin, which can be synthesized in the laboratory, serves as the prototype kinin. In sensitive tissues such as skin, it is alleged to have activity above 10 times that of histamine.

Kinins are potent mediators of vasodilation, pain, and increased capillary permeability, that is, of major signs of acute inflammation. Action on arterioles and venules is mediated through contraction of smooth muscle. Smooth muscle contraction is also stimulated elsewhere and may result in bronchoconstriction. The role of kinin systems in inflammation is not well defined, for analysis is made difficult by the short life span of kinin molecules and by the instability of their precursors (Cochrane et al. 1971; Margolis and Bishop 1963; Movat and Anwar 1971). The kinins are destroyed by kinin inhibitors almost immediately upon being generated in serum. Inactivation has been attributed to a carboxypeptidase B enzyme in serum that removes the C-terminal arginine residue on the peptide molecule.

Kinins are released from a plasma α_2-globulin substrate by a plasma enzyme system called kallikrein. These kinin-generating enzymes are present in neutrophils and these cells, when lysed, thereby sustain the inflammatory reaction (Movat et al. 1973). *Kallikreins* then are the poorly understood proteolytic enzymes of plasma that generate the vasoactive kinins from globulin substrates. They are extracted by chemical precipitation of plasma protein, purified by chromatography, and identified by rat uterus bioassay (the recording of muscle contractions of the isolated rat uterus suspended in bath solutions). Kallikreins have also been localized intracellularly in secretory granules of the pancreas and other exocrine organs (Bhoola and Dorey 1971).

$$\text{KININOGEN} \xrightarrow[\;]{\text{Kallikrein}} \text{KININ} \longrightarrow \begin{array}{l} \text{Vasodilation} \\ \text{Capillary permeability} \\ \text{Nerve end stimulation} \\ \text{Smooth muscle contraction} \end{array}$$

$(\alpha_2\text{-globulin})$

CHEMOTACTIC FACTORS

Chemotactic factors are derived from complement by enzymic cleavage of portions of the complement molecules. Cleavage occurs by enzymes intrinsic to complement and also by extrinsic enzymes such as plasmin, thrombin, trypsin, and neutral tissue proteases. The chemotactic factors act on circulating neutrophils and probably also on other leukocytes, inducing them to migrate through the vascular wall into inflammatory tissue. A chemotactic factor inhibitor has been identified in serum of humans which irreversibly inactivates complement-derived chemotactic factors (Ward and Berenberg 1974).

PROSTAGLANDINS

These 20-carbon chain unsaturated cyclic fatty acids exert enhancing or depressant effects on nearly every biologic process. Minor changes in molecular structure may lead to reversal of activity. E-type prostaglandins are potent bronchodilators whereas the F-type compounds are bronchoconstrictors. Prostaglandin action mimics the action of cAMP. Aspirin and indomethacin, which inhibit cAMP, are also active inhibitors of prostaglandins. Although the prostaglandins exert some effect on the inflammatory process, the significance of this activity has not been assessed adequately. Intradermal injection of prostaglandin E_1 causes sustained erythema and altered vascular permeability. Whether these actions occur directly or are mediated through histamine is not clear (Arora et al. 1970; Horton 1963; Zurier 1974). There are elevations in the levels of prostaglandins in inflamed tissues that correlate with cellular exudation. It has been hypothesized that infiltrating monocytes and macrophages are the source of these substances (Velo et al. 1973).

ARTERIOLAR DILATION

Local tissue injury induces an immediate axon reflex arc; that is, one not traversing the spinal cord of the CNS. This arc is the cause of arteriolar dilation, manifested as the pale red flare of the triple response. Following stimulation of sensory nerve endings at the site of injury, a nerve impulse passes centrally along the axon to its division and then peripherally to the arteriole supplying the injured area. Synaptic vesicles within the adrenergic synapse liberate adrenalin which dilates the peripheral blood vessels. In Lewis's experiments, sectioning of cutaneous nerves prior to producing skin injury abolished the flare of the triple response (but not the injury line or wheal). Futhermore, the flare was retarded in direct correlation with the presence of Wallerian degeneration and death of the nerves sectioned. Although the cen-

tral nervous system can also affect the inflammatory response by action of vasodilator and vasoconstrictor nerves, all the essential elements of inflammation can occur without these central influences (Chapman and Goodell 1964; Devine and Simpson 1967; Richardson and Beaulnes 1971).

ENDOTHELIAL CELL DISUNION

The discovery of histamine in 1919 revived Cohnheim's announcement that acute inflammation involved increased vascular permeability resulting from direct injury to endothelium (Rich 1921). Classically, the earliest signs of damage to endothelial cells had been depicted at the intercellular junction. Carbon particles, when injected intravenously, were found outlining intercellular junctions of endothelial cells where inflammatory lesions had been produced by Arnold in 1875. Histologic examination of this experimental model revealed dilatation of capillaries and venules (hyperemia). Small, granular, pale, eosinophilic precipitates of albumin were present in perivascular spaces and carbon was identified in the vessel wall (Florey et al. 1959; Spector 1956).

When the early stages of spontaneous inflammatory lesions are examined by electron microscopy, one sees subtle changes in the capillary endothelial cells. Fenestrae are enlarged (in vessels that contain them), plasmalemmal vesicles are increased in number at the luminal surface, and endothelial cell junctions are irregular. These changes were examined previously in edema (Chapter 3). In inflammation, however, the endothelial cell is injured and cytopathic changes in the intercellular junctions of the damaged cells dominate the picture. The massive amounts of fluid that exude do so through gaps and cavities between endothelial cells (Cotran 1967; Cotran and Majno 1964). Loose-type junctions are enlarged. Changes in tight junctions (zonula occludens), which occur in the brain, involve changes in the mucopolysaccharide layer that is present between endothelial cells (and extends from the luminal surface into the basement membrane).

As fluid leakage progresses in the later stages of inflammatory lesions, endothelial cell plasma membrane changes indicate a highly active cell surface. Endothelial cell swelling develops and is manifested as a decrease in electron opacity and dispersement of cell organelles. Blebs of cytoplasm bulge into tissue spaces through breaks in the basement membrane. Swollen endothelial cells protrude into the vessel lumen (Fig. 4.4). They markedly retard blood flow in larger capillaries and cause stasis in smaller vessels. In the normal bloodstream of arterioles, cells are concentrated in the central "axial zone" as opposed to the peripheral cell-free "plasmatic zone." With slowing and stasis, leukocytes marginate, attach to the vessel wall, and begin to emigrate through it.

Similar changes are seen in the endothelial cells of lymph vessels (Casley-Smith 1964; Leak and Kato 1972). The anchoring filaments which surround lymphatic vessels and play a major role in opening cell junctions disappear in inflammatory lesions. Lymph vessels are markedly dilated as a result of the removal of exuding fluid. Fluid drains to regional lymph nodes which are adapted to trap and localize irritants by macrophage phagocytosis.

A simple method to demonstrate local fluid exudation is used to assay mediators of inflammation. Dyes such as trypan blue, when injected intravenously, bind to plasma albumin. Albumin-dye complexes do not pass the endothelial barrier except at sites where it has been altered. When histamine is injected subcutaneously followed by intravenous trypan blue, albumin begins to leak, allowing the site of histamine injection to become blue. It does so in relation to the extent of the histamine-induced endothelial injury and the reaction can be measured and quantitated. This dye test can be used to characterize a variety of mechanisms that produce vascular injury: toxins that directly damage endothelium, immunologic mechanisms such as the Arthus and passive anaphylaxis reactions which involve antigen-antibody

on the vascular wall (Chapter 5), and injuries caused by endotoxin sensitization such as the Shwartzman reaction.

Ultrastructural examination of experimental lesions produced by local injection of histamine followed by carbon intravenously reveals the serial changes in inflammation (Majno and Palade 1959; Marchesi 1962). Carbon leaks through the intercellular spaces with fluid and is trapped by basement membranes which allow exudation of plasma but not particulate material. Topographically, histamine exerts its injurious effect on the postcapillary venules. As the process goes on, other mechanisms induce permeability changes in the capillary bed. Injuries produced by heat or turpentine injection show similar leakage of carbon except that they indiscriminately injure the capillary bed (Movat and Fernando 1963).

The intravenous injection of water-soluble molecules of differing sizes has provided a more specific determination of vessel permeability. After injection of ferritin (10 nm diameter) and horseradish peroxidase (4 nm) following local injury, both substances exude through intercellular spaces and fenestrae. Peroxidase, due to its smaller size, shows earlier and more extensive localization. Plasmalemmal vesicles (caveolae) appear to contribute little to peroxidase transport but ferritin readily crosses the endothelial cell within these structures.

In summary, the most crucial factor in the pathogenesis of inflammation is the integrity of the endothelial cell. Whether the cell is injured directly (by endogenous histamine or exogenous toxins) or affected indirectly (by hypoxia), endothelial cell changes determine the extent of the plasma protein-containing fluid that escapes to the extravascular spaces. The differing molecular weights of the plasma proteins (albumin 69,000; globulin 150,000; and fibrinogen 500,000) are responsible for the type of exudation and thus reflect the degree of

Fig. 4.4. Vasculitis, lymph node capillary, horse with acute viral arteritis. A. Histology. Hyperemia with exudation of fluid, fibrin (arrow), and neutrophils. B. Ultrastructure. Swelling of endothelial cells with vacuolation and development of virions (heavy arrow) in cytoplasm. Lumen occluded with platelets and neutrophil. Fibrin (thin arrow). C. Virions.

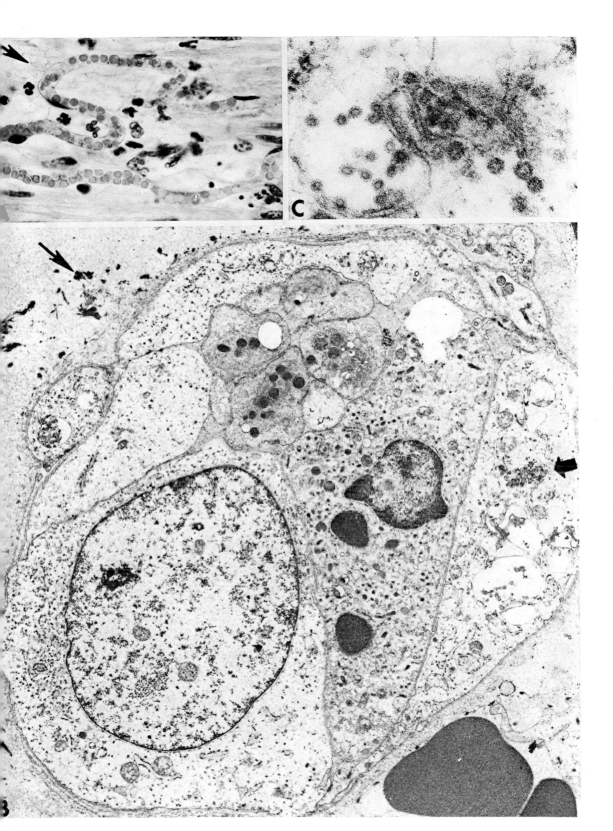

C

endothelial injury. Albumin, the smallest and fastest migrating protein on electrophoresis, is the first plasma protein to leak through the vessel wall. When severe injury allows free passage of plasma proteins, the equilibrium between hydrostatic pressure of the blood and osmotic pressure of the tissue fluid is altered. Extravascular protein abolishes the osmotic suck of the plasma proteins and more fluid exudes. Increased hydrostatic pressure in dilated arterioles augments fluid loss. The tissue swells, giving rise to pain—two of the five cardinal signs of inflammation.

SEROUS EXUDATE

The initial exudate in most early inflammatory lesions is chiefly serous; that is, leakage has been confined largely to fluid and albumin. Albumin appears histologically as homogeneous eosinophilic granular material. Ultrastructurally, it is seen as a granular precipitate of varying density outside the lumen of the vessel. Globulin molecules are larger than albumin but also exude. The globulin fractions of serum (a, β, and γ) contain a wide variety of specifically active substances which are highly important in defense. Some of the humoral factors that appear in serous exudates include the following:

ANTIBODIES

Antibodies are γ-globulins synthesized to combine specifically with protein antigens which induced their production. Produced by protein synthesis in plasmacytes, antibody molecules circulate in plasma and exude into foci of inflammation. They neutralize viruses, inactivate toxins, enhance (as "opsonins") the phagocytosis of bacteria, and lyse bacterial cells. In lytic processes, antibody functions to recognize specific invading organisms and to attract complement which actually does the work of lysis.

COMPLEMENT

Complement (C) is a self-assembling, extracellular system of serum enzymes that occurs in body fluids in association with membranes. The C sequence is activated by antigen-antibody (immune) complexes and by some other large molecules. All of the functions of C are plasma membrane oriented. These include: (1) irreversible damage to cells (both host and bacterial), (2) activation of release mechanisms (histamine from mast cells, procoagulants from platelets, etc.), and (3) chemotaxis. Complement plays significant roles in inflammation in both the mediation of the chemotactic attraction of leukocytes and in killing of bacterial cells. It is essential for immunologic bacteriolysis and hemolysis in which it functions as a nonspecific effector of specific antibody activities (Ellman 1971; Willoughby et al. 1969).

At least 9 different enzyme components of C combine to form the final reactive molecular complex. Action is initiated by antibody which activates C1, the first component. The early acting components, C1, C2, and C4, react in sequence to generate an enzyme C3 convertase that induces the late acting components C3, C5, and C9 to aggregate. The terminal components form doughnut-shaped aggregates within the plasma membranes of bacteria. The central hole penetrates the membrane and allows electrolytes and water to leak from the cell. The bacterial cells then swell and the plasma membrane may rupture. The tiny holes produced in plasma membranes by C are uniform in size.

Under chemotaxis we shall examine how the terminal components of C participate in inflammation by attracting neutrophils, by causing them to release hydrolytic enzymes, and by playing roles in increasing vascular permeability.

Complement systems are found in most vertebrate species and primitive C-like systems exist in some lower animals (Colten et al. 1968; Gigli and Austen 1971; Lachman et al. 1962). It has not been possible to demonstrate a classic C system in the lamprey but the serum of elasmobranch fishes serves as a potent source (Legler and Evans 1967). Some species have C that does not lyse erythrocytes: e.g., pig, horse, dog, and mouse.

Naturally occurring inhibitors of C may depress the C-enzyme sequence. Exogenous substances such as cobra venom fractions, hydrazine, and zymosan are used experimentally because of their capacity to inactivate C3. Hereditary deficiencies of individual components of C have been reported: C5 deficiency of mice, C6 deficiency of rabbits, and C1-inactivator deficiency of humans (which results in angioneurotic edema).

PROPERDIN

Properdin is a serum protein distinct from the immunoglobulins and C. It provides an alternate pathway for initiating C-dependent processes. Properdin bypasses the early acting C components and activates the terminal C sequence. It is active on gram-negative bacteria and, like C, plays a role in immunologic tissue injury (Westberg et al. 1971).

INTERFERONS

Interferons are proteins of cell origin that arise during viral and other microbial infections, circulate, and exude into inflamed tissue to aid in nonimmune defense. Interferons induce, in host cells, a state of refractoriness to the takeover of cell systems by the invading organism (a state preventing intracellular replication). The interferons are thus most effective against viral infections (see viruses, Chapter 12).

LYSOZYME

Lysozyme (muramidase) is a small cationic enzyme that catalyzes the hydrolysis of the linkage between N-acetyl-muramic acid and N-acetylglucosamine, substances abundant in the cell walls of bacteria. The antibacterial role of lysozyme is of less significance than other enzymes of lysosomes but it appears to function in digesting glycopeptide cell wall debris of bacteria killed by other mechanisms. An inherited lysozyme deficiency occurs in rabbits, and affected individuals provide a model for study of this enzyme (Prieur et al. 1974).

ROLE OF IRON-BINDING PROTEINS IN INFLAMMATION

The concentration of ionic iron and iron-transferrin complexes in plasma usually declines in severe acute inflammation. This has been proposed as a biologic mechanism of the host to withhold an essential nutrient from microorganisms. Iron in plasma and tissues is considerably less than that required for bacterial growth and siderosomes in the bacterial cell are organelles designed to withdraw iron from the host's transferrin.

Hyposideremia in acute inflammation occurs in animal tissue due to release of low molecular weight proteins from leukocytes. Iron-free lactoferrin (an iron-binding protein similar to transferrin) is released from neutrophil granules and removes iron from circulating iron-transferrin complexes. This occurs especially in an acidic environment which causes transferrin to release iron and lactoferrin to accept it. Iron-lactoferrin complexes are then taken up by macrophages of the reticuloendothelial system (van Slick et al. 1974). Other uncharacterized neutrophil-associated proteins appear to increase hepatic uptake of iron, further depleting circulating transferrin.

Animals with hypoferritinemia and hypotransferrinemia are more susceptible to some bacterial infections, a situation that may apply to hemolytic crises, liver stasis, and excessive dietary iron. Experimentally, it has been shown that the number of bacterial cells (injected intraperitoneally) required to kill mice is lowered 3–5 log units by a concurrent injection of iron. The number of *Clostridium perfringens* growing in guinea pig muscle increases 6000-fold after iron injection; the number of *E. coli* in rat kidney increases 1000-fold (Weinberg 1974). The injected iron saturates both transferrin and lactoferrin and causes increased fatalities by blocking the inhibitory effect of these iron-binding proteins (Bullen et al. 1974).

PATHOGENESIS OF SEROUS EXUDATION

In *serous exudates,* cells in tissue are spread apart by edema fluid. This serves to ease the rapid migration of exuding phagocytes (Fig. 4.5). In the skin, serous exudates are commonly seen in blisters caused by excessive friction, burns, or chemical toxins. Epithelium reacts to injuries with a general loosening of cell attachments due to intercellular fluid accumulation. Keratinocytes pull apart, remaining attached only at desmosomes ("inter-

and action of antibacterial cationic proteins (Zeva and Spitznagel 1968).

Hydrogen peroxide (H_2O_2) is formed by oxidative reactions in the neutrophil during the initial burst of activity that follows phagocytosis. When neutrophils are maintained in vitro, unidentified oxidases consume oxygen from, and form H_2O_2 into, the medium. Hydrogen peroxide is microbicidal for most organisms in the absence of a catalyst but high concentrations are required. It is most effective in association with neutrophil peroxidase. Hydrogen peroxide formed by some microorganisms (e.g., Streptococci) may contribute significantly to antimicrobial activity. Conversely, microbial catalase inhibits H_2O_2 function and may protect some bacteria. Catalase-rich strains of Staphylococci are more virulent for mice than are strains of low catalase content.

Superoxide anion (O_2^-), a free radical form of O_2, is generated in the early autooxidative processes in the phagosome. This highly reactive radical is probably toxic to microorganisms (Johnson et al. 1975) but it is not clear whether it is active in itself or only after conversion to H_2O_2. Two molecules interact as: $2O_2^- + 2H^+$—(superoxide dismutase)$\rightarrow O_2 + H_2O_2$. Superoxide dismutase (SOD) protects the cell from O_2^- toxicity but may also inhibit bactericidal activity. Superoxide anion and H_2O_2 accumulate in the phagosome where they interact with bacteria and also generate other oxidants such as $\cdot OH$ and O_2. Within the vacuole they are not interfered with by SOD or catalase, yet these enzymes protect the remainder of the cell from destruction. Subsequent fusion of phagosome with lysosome introduces digestive hydrolytic enzymes, cationic proteins, and peroxidase into the vacuole which enhance and accentuate antimicrobial action.

Myeloperoxidase (MPO), the name applied to the peroxidase of neutrophils, is localized in the primary azurophile granules. It is present in large amounts and is responsible for the green color of pus. Like other peroxidases, MPO catalyzes the oxidation of substances by H_2O_2. Myeloperoxidase, H_2O_2, and an oxidizable cofactor such as halide combine to form a highly potent antimicrobial system. This *MPO-mediated system* is effective against microbes at pH 4.5 to 5.0 and is inhibited by catalase. Myeloperoxidase reacts with H_2O_2 to form an enzyme-substrate complex with strong oxidative capacity. The cofactor is converted from a weak to a strong antimicrobial agent. When iodide is the cofactor, iodination of bacteria occurs by direct halogenation of bacterial proteins and other groups in or on the bacterium (cofactor function has not been demonstrated with certainty in vivo).

DEGRANULATION

Although neutrophil lysosomal enzymes are released into tissues by cell death and by regurgitation during phagocytosis, they are also released directly by exocytosis (Hirsch and Cohn 1960; Zucker-Franklin and Hirsch 1964; Zucker-Franklin et al. 1971). Exocytosis of granules and hydrolytic enzymes appears to be particularly important when the neutrophil is in contact with very large particles or with surfaces coated with antigen-antibody complexes (Henson 1971). In the latter case, the complement component C5 may interact with neutrophils to provoke the extracellular release of lysosomal enzymes without altering cell viability. Ultrastructurally, affected neutrophils exhibit transient aggregation of microfilaments, lyosomal fusion, and degranulation (Goldstein et al. 1973). After degranulation, the neutrophil appears denser. When the granules have diminished in number, the cytosol becomes filled with free ribosomes and cytoplasmic areas are denser and more basophilic.

The process of exocytosis (reverse endocytosis) appears to depend upon functional microtubules and microfilaments. High intracellular levels of cyclic AMP activate a protein kinase which in turn initiates microfilament action. Exocytosis is inhibited by substances that inhibit cyclic AMP or alter microfilaments.

Unfortunately, extruded neutrophil lysosomal substances may also damage normal tissue. In tissue undergoing acute inflammation, neutrophils have been shown to generate kinins, cleave complement components, initiate clot formation, and synthesize and release substances that cause fever. They may activate mast cells and platelets to liberate histamine and directly attack endothelial cells and basement membranes to sustain increased capillary permeability (Cochrane and Aikin 1968).

Destruction of tissue is initiated by at least two groups of substances found in the neutrophil lysosomes (Ranadive and Cochrane 1968): (1) proteolytic enzymes capable of degrading basement membranes, collagen, and elastin and (2) basic proteins that increase capillary permeability. Four basic proteins that affect permeability have been obtained by purification of neutrophil granules followed by gel electrophoresis. One of these also induces mast cell degranulation and histamine release and is inhibited by antihistamine in vivo.

Therapy is occasionally needed to control the deleterious effects of inflammation. Drugs such as corticosteroids which stabilize lysosomal membranes are potent inhibitors of neutrophil granule activity and intracellular digestion. Corticosteroids also inhibit chemotaxis of neutrophils, a fact that implicates lysosomal enzyme systems in response to chemoattractants. In view of the dosages required to inhibit chemotaxis, corticosteroids are not likely to be effective therapeutically.

FEVER

During severe local inflammatory lesions or in generalized infections, neutrophils are lysed intravascularly (Schumacher and Agudelo 1972). The release of protein components of their lysosomes is chiefly responsible for the signs of fever: increases in body temperature, respiration, and heart rate.

Normal body temperature is maintained by hypothalamic regulation of the production and dissipation of heat (Atkins and Huang 1958). Stimuli originate from superficial thermoreceptors in skin and deep receptors near the hypothalamus that respond to changes in temperature. During fever, the hypothalamic "thermostat" is elevated by endogenous pyrogens of neutrophil origin (Berlin and Wood 1964; Wood 1970). Monocytes and macrophages are also credited with pyrogen release.

Endogenous pyrogens appear to act as a final common pathway affecting the CNS for the development of fever induced by exogenous pyrogens such as microbial substances (Atkins et al. 1964), antigen-antibody complexes (Atkins and Heijn 1965), adrenocorticosteroids, and other chemicals (Chusid and Atkins 1972). This is illustrated by the experimental intravenous injection of exogenous pyrogens such as bacterial endotoxin, whole bacteria, or viruses. The fever that results correlates not with the amounts of exogenous pyrogen injected but with the level of leukocyte pyrogens generated during the reaction.

It is possible experimentally to distinguish between the two basic kinds of pyrogens. Repeated intravenous injections of bacterial endotoxin (an exogenous pyrogen) induce a state of refractoriness termed *tolerance* (Beeson 1947). The animal no longer responds to further doses of endotoxin by increasing body temperature, for its own endogenous pyrogenic mechanism has become exhausted. Repeated injections of granulocytic pyrogens, however, continue to cause a full response, for they act directly on the hypothalamus. Furthermore, rabbits made tolerant to exogenous substances by exhaustion remain fully responsive to endogenous pyrogens.

Some systemic changes accompany fever regardless of cause. Slight, transient drops in erythrocyte and leukocyte numbers are two of these (Fig. 4.10). When fever is produced experimentally with purified extracts of bacterial cells, the rise in body temperature is accompanied by a fall in circulating erythrocytes. The reaction is rapid and transient; it probably relates to trapping of erythrocytes in the spleen.

In summary, the progression of events leading to fever involves leukocytes, circulating plasma, the hypothalamus, and the effector end organs that disseminate body heat (by cutaneous vasoconstriction, sweat production, and shivering). Antipyretic drugs can therefore (in theory) act by (1) interfering with synthesis or release of endogenous pyrogen by leukocytes and other cells, (2) inactivating circulating endogenous pyrogen, (3) interfering with the action in the brain of endogenous pyrogen, or (4) interfering with the effector pathways. Aspirin, the commonest antipyretic substance, antagonizes the action of endogenous pyrogen within the hypothalamus.

TOXIC NEUTROPHILS

In severe bacterial infections, neutrophilic leukocytosis is the usual finding. The increase in leukocytes is due to expulsion

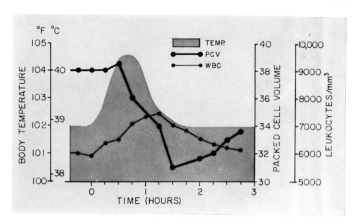

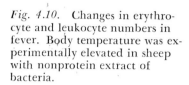

Fig. 4.10. Changes in erythrocyte and leukocyte numbers in fever. Body temperature was experimentally elevated in sheep with nonprotein extract of bacteria.

of neutrophils from sites of formation and to enhanced leukopoiesis. Because demand often exceeds supply, these new cells are usually immature. The development of increasing numbers of immature neutrophils in the circulation is called a "shift to the left" (based on the Schilling index of neutrophil maturity) and indicates a relatively severe disease process. Very large neutrophils (over 22μ in diameter) are sometimes found in blood smears (especially in the cat and horse) and are the result of inhibition of mitotic activity in precursor cells.

Many leukocytes show pathologic changes during circulation and are called *toxic neutrophils* by the hematologist. Characteristics of the toxic neutrophil include cytoplasmic vacuolation, the presence of Döhle bodies, and toxic granules (dense heavy-staining azurophil granules). *Döhle bodies* are light blue amorphous regions in the cytoplasm that ultrastructurally are lamellar aggregates of rough endoplasmic reticulum (McCall 1969). The chemotactic activity of toxic neutrophils is markedly reduced and their bactericidal effect is less than that of normal neutrophils.

DEFICIENCIES OF NEUTROPHILIC LEUKOCYTES

The importance of neutrophils in the inflammatory exudate and defense can be seen when infectious diseases occur in animals that have insufficient numbers of cells and cannot mount a neutrophilic response. Microbial inhibition of neutrophils is a major factor in determining the virulence of bacteria and viruses. The polysaccharide components of the cell walls of Anthrax

bacilli, Pneumococci, and some Streptococci have a marked inhibitory effect on the phagocytic function of neutrophils. Cryptococcal polysaccharides inhibit both neutrophils and macrophages, and lesions caused by this fungus are notorious for their lack of cellular exudation.

SUPPRESSION OF GRANULOCYTOPOIESIS

Chemical and radiologic suppression of granulocytopoiesis predisposes animals to infectious agents. Drugs termed "metabolic antagonists" have molecular structures so similar to the proteins utilized in metabolism that they are incorporated into pathways in the cell. The molecular structure is sufficiently dissimilar, however, to cause blocks in the metabolic machinery of the cell, and rapidly proliferating hematopoietic stem cells are among the first to be depressed by such treatment (Fig. 4.11). Animals so treated, for immunosuppression or for anticancer therapy, are highly susceptible to fungi and bacteria. Large doses of x-radiation cause depression of all white blood cells (panleukopenia).

CONGENITAL ABNORMALITIES IN NEUTROPHILS

Some rare but intriguing genetic abnormalities in neutrophils exist in animals. These "experiments in nature" readily illustrate the essential role of the neutrophil in continual monitoring of the blood for microbes and tissue products. The three models described below illustrate defects in neutrophil production, in neutrophil lysosome-phagosome fusion, and in bactericidal content of lysosomes.

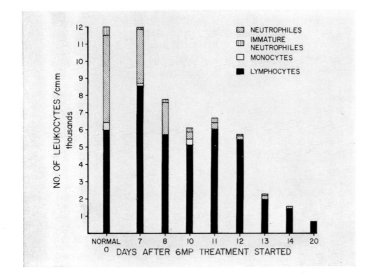

Fig. 4.11. Total and differential leukocyte counts on a monkey receiving the antimetabolite 6-mercaptopurine.

Cyclic neutropenia, which occurs in gray Collie pups, involves cyclic depression of neutrophil maturation in the bone marrow with consequential disappearance of mature neutrophils from the blood stream every 11 days. The disease occurs also in human infants in cycles of 28 days. The nature of the defect involves insufficient stem cell production rather than a control of hematopoiesis. Transplantation of marrow stem cells from normal to neutropenic dogs corrects the periodic depression of granulocytopoiesis (Dale and Graw 1974). The transplanted cells mature normally in the defective recipient dogs. The precise mechanism involved in cyclic neutropenia is unknown. Attempts to incriminate antineutrophil antibodies, elevated estrogen or gonadotropin levels, or hypersplenism have not been convincing. Pathologic changes occur in neutrophils and, although indicative of toxin-induced degeneration (Scott et al. 1973), this probably represents secondary damage in a chronically ill animal. Affected dogs develop periodic bacterial infections that coincide with phases of neutropenia (Fig. 4.12). Despite supportive clinical treatment, they eventually develop and succumb to lymphoid exhaustion, reticuloendothelial hyperplasia,

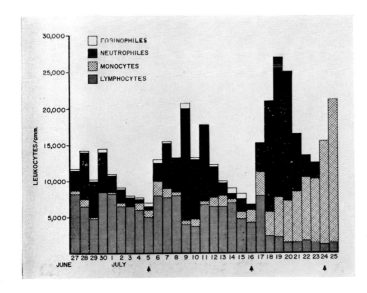

Fig. 4.12. Total and differential leukocyte counts on a gray Collie with cyclic neutropenia.

and amyloidosis (Cheville 1968; Lund et al. 1967).

The *Chediak-Higashi syndrome*, a second genetic neutrophil disease, is characterized by anomalous giant granules in neutrophils, increased susceptibility to infections, and defective pigmentation. It occurs in mink, partially albino Hereford cattle, killer whales, mice (beige strain), and humans (Lutzner et al. 1965; Renshaw et al. 1974; White 1967). Similar syndromes have also been reported in bison, white mutant tigers, and Persian cats (Kramer et al. 1975). The primary granules of the neutrophil are defective and although phagocytosis occurs normally, bactericidal activity is diminished.

The giant granules in neutrophils and other cells of affected animals arise from abnormal fusion of primary granules during development (Davis et al. 1971). In cattle, the defect involves abnormal bactericidal activity associated with the hexose monophosphate shunt and delayed degranulation. The essential mechanism in beige mice is allegedly the failure of neutrophil granules to migrate to phagosomes, causing delayed intracellular killing of bacteria (Gallin et al. 1974). Recurrent infections lead to early death. Affected animals also have defective pigmentation, thrombocytopenia, and lymphadenopathy. The giant cytoplasmic inclusions have been reported in many types of granule-forming cells including neurons (Sung and Okada 1971). The C-H syndrome that characterizes the Aleutian mutant strain of mink is the basis for the remarkable susceptibility of these animals to the chronic viral-induced plasmacytosis known as Aleutian disease.

Chronic granulomatous disease is a third neutrophil disease found only in humans. Affected children suffer severe recurrent infection caused by Staphylococci and gram-negative rods due to the impaired bactericidal activity of their neutrophil lysosomes (Eschenbach and Seebach 1971; Quie et al. 1967). Monocytes are similarly deficient. Despite vigorous neutrophil responses, normal degranulation, and adequate antibody formation, the neutrophils are unable to kill bacteria (Kauder et al. 1968; Mandel et al. 1970). The major metabolic defect is failure to produce sufficient hydrogen peroxide and patients are susceptible to catalase-positive organisms such as Staphylococci and Serratia. Their defective lysosomes readily kill catalase-negative bacteria such as Streptococci and *E. coli* which produce endogenous hydrogen peroxide that can be utilized by the bactericidal system of the neutrophil lysosome.

Pathologic changes in neutrophils have been reported in several genetic diseases (Jenis et al. 1971). Their significance has not been adequately investigated.

EOSINOPHILS

These large, ameboid, sluggishly phagocytic cells of blood have unique granules which hold the key to their specialized functions (Fig. 4.13). Like neutrophil lysosomes, the granules function in phagocytosis by membrane fusion with phagosomes. Changes in the structure and refractive index of the granule occur as enzymes infiltrate and destroy the phagocytosed particles (Archer and Hirsch 1963; Cotran and Litt 1969).

Normal eosinophil granules consist of a limiting membrane of single unit structure surrounding a cortical zone with high enzyme content. They are particularly rich in peroxidases; sulfatases and phosphatases are also present (Bainton and Farquhar 1970). In many mammals, a central crystalloid is present consisting of dense cubic protein lattices that are high in arginase. The basic protein of the eosinophil granule appears to be a homogeneous one (Gleich et al. 1973).

LEUKOTAXIS

Eosinophilic leukotaxis takes place in a variety of inflammatory lesions: in parasitic infections of the intestine, in the nasopharynx of animals with some allergic diseases, and, curiously, in salt-induced meningoencephalitis of pigs. Specific chemotactic factors for eosinophils have been established. Histamine, for example, will cause their accumulation; mast cells are often associated with eosinophil exudates (Mann 1969). Mast cell tumors and cutaneous mast cell lesions usually have large numbers of eosinophils. Eosinophils are prominent around degenerate mast cells and are known to phagocytize mast cell granules.

Eosinophils have a curious appetite for

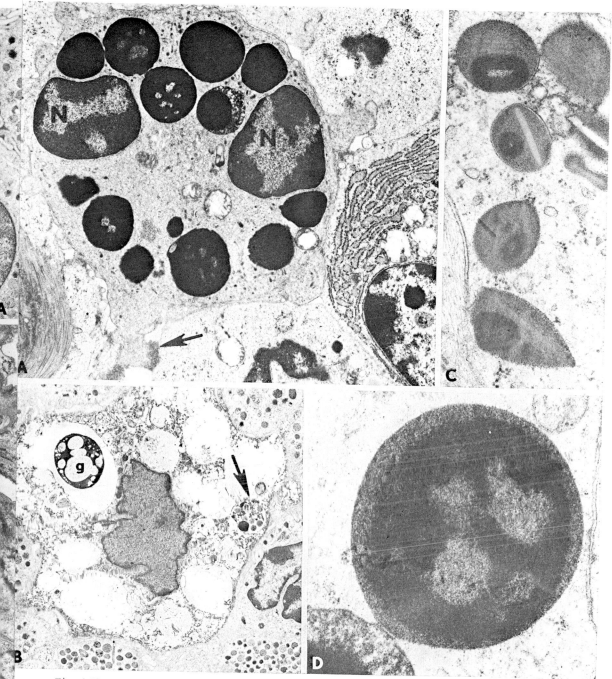

Fig. 4.13. Eosinophils. A. Eosinophil, intestinal submucosa, horse
with chronic parasitic enteritis. Granules are large, dense, and heterogeneous. Note the granular deposits at ends of filopodia (arrow)
which are interpreted as affinity of eosinophil for antigenic material.
Mature plasmacyte at right. Nucleus (N). B. Degranulate eosinophil
surrounded by mast cells, equine cutaneous mastocytosis. One large
pleomorphic granule (g) remains. Phagosome (arrow) contains mast
cell granules. C. Ultrastructure of sheep eosinophil granules.
D. Ultrastructure of horse eosinophil granules.

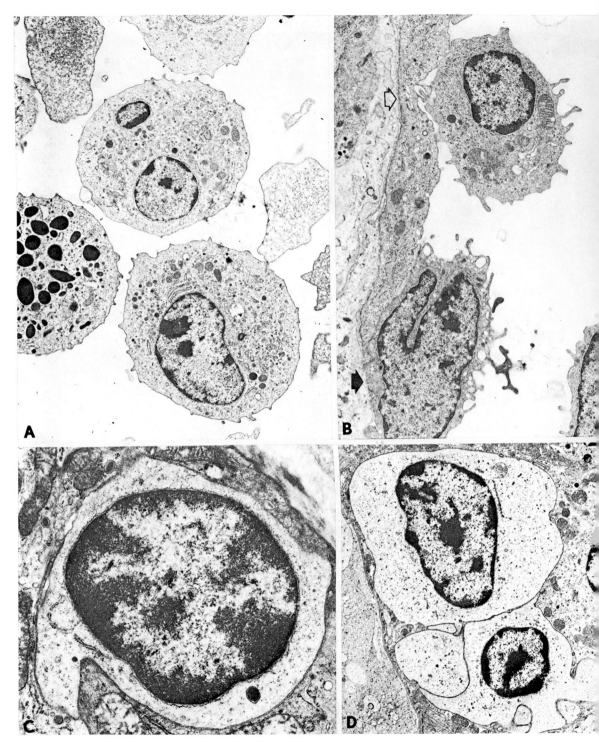

Fig. 4.15. A. Monocytes from circulating blood, tuberculosis. B. Circulating monocytes in process of emigration through capillary wall during inflammation. Note long processes on the cell surface and their interdigitation with processes on endothelial cell (arrow). C. Small lymphocyte fixed during migration between epithelial cells (peripolesis) in mammary gland epithelium. D. Small lymphocytes with rarified cytoplasm in process of migrating through renal tubular epithelium.

4.15). Their enumeration is difficult, for they cannot be differentiated from the larger lymphocytes with certainty. In general, the cytoplasm is more abundant and the larger nucleus is eccentric and bean-shaped. The plasma membrane of the monocyte imparts special functions to these cells (Weiss et al. 1966). It is thrown into many surface filopodia which, in the process of emigration through the vascular wall, are important in the initial contact of endothelium.

Monocytosis is the elevation of monocyte numbers in circulating blood beyond the range considered normal. It is seen in the recovery phases of bacterial infections (Fig. 4.12) and is characteristic of the acute stages of certain diseases. Only under severe conditions do monocytes phagocytize while in the bloodstream to become circulating macrophages. In some forms of severe intravascular hemolysis, monocytes become phagocytic, absorb erythrocytes, and degrade hemoglobin. Their role in erythrophagocytosis is related to the capacity of the plasma membrane to attach to immunoglobulins and complement on the erythrocyte surface (Abramson et al. 1970). Abnormal, inclusion body–containing monocytes are seen in some viral infections.

Monocytes emigrate into inflammatory lesions and promptly transform into macrophages (Ebert and Florey 1939; Nichols et al. 1971). Using tritiated thymidine as a DNA marker, blood monocytes (but not quiescent fibrocytes) become radioactively labeled. If an inflammatory lesion is produced (in an animal which has labeled monocytes), its macrophages will contain the label. It is thereby assumed that they are hematogenous in origin (Kosunen et al. 1963; Spector et al. 1967). Small lymphocytes have a low rate of labeling and appear unlikely as precursors of macrophages.

Monocytes enter an inflammatory lesion simultaneously with neutrophils. They do not appear in large numbers in the early stages of acute inflammation because: (1) substances chemotactic for neutrophils have no specific effect on monocytes, (2) they are not as aggressively ameboid as neutrophils, and (3) their numbers in circulating blood are much lower than neutrophils and their reproduction is stimulated at a much slower rate (Bennett and Cohn 1966; Spector

et al. 1967). It has been reported that large numbers of neutrophils in exudates tactically enhance monocyte migration.

The source of most blood monocytes appears to be the bone marrow, that is, the bone marrow promonocyte (van Furth and Cohn 1968). The sequence of promonocyte, monocyte, and histiocyte has been shown experimentally by the difference in isotope labeling of mononuclear phagocytes of bone marrow, blood, and peritoneal cavity. Volkman and Gowans observed (in damaged skin of rats injected with labeled cells of bone marrow or lymph node origin) that only bone marrow cells appeared as macrophages. Furthermore, radiation prevented the appearance of macrophages and radiation-suppressed monocyte development was prevented by shielding marrow sites during radiation.

LYMPHOCYTES

In most mammals, *lymphocytes* constitute 20–40% of the leukocytes in blood and over 90% of the cells in thoracic duct lymph. *Lymphocytosis,* the increase of numbers of lymphocytes in circulating blood, is seen in transient responses to severe muscular exercise, fear, and other stress. Lymphocytosis of long duration is less commonly encountered and is usually associated with malignant lymphoma (as lymphatic leukemia). Idiopathic lymphocytosis also occurs as a poorly understood condition which in cattle is thought to precede malignant lymphoma. *Lymphopenia,* a decrease in numbers of lymphocytes, occurs in viral diseases wherein the virus attacks the lymphoid system (canine distemper, hog cholera, and bovine viral diarrhea) and during therapy with such lympholytic agents as cortisone, radiation, and immunosuppresive drugs. Cytopathologic changes in lymphocytes are common in these conditions (Payne et al. 1971).

Small lymphocytes are tiny round cells with a narrow rim of cytoplasm containing free ribosomes (Fig. 4.15). Their Golgi zone is small and only rarely are lysosomes seen. Dense "azurophil" granules (5–15 per cell) and clear vacuoles are usually present. Nuclear chromatin is densely packed, particularly at the periphery of the nucleus. For these reasons (and because in most cell reactions the morphology of lymphocytes is altered to more active forms) the small lymphocyte as it occurs in the blood is thought of as a "resting cell." Its reactions of ameboid movement, phagocytosis, and chemotactic response are weak or absent (Carr 1970).

DIFFERENT SMALL LYMPHOCYTE POPULATIONS

Circulating small lymphocytes represent at least two different functional populations of lymphoid cells, although they cannot be distinguished structurally. These groups are differentiated on the basis of life span, their response to mitosis-inducing drugs, and the reactivity of their cell membranes in immunologic reactions. In the developing fetus, small lymphocytes originate in the bone marrow. It appears that differences in reactivity that are present in lymphocytes of adults are due to subsequent residence of the bone marrow stem cells in lymphoid organs such as the thymus and intestinal Peyer's patches (see Chapter 5). These organs confer special reactivity on the bone marrow cell, which then has the capacity to seed lymph nodes and provide clones of lymphocytes with specific reactivity.

One population of small lymphocytes (B cells) represents the precursors of the plasmacyte series of cells that form antibody. Following contact with the appropriate antigen, these cells transform into large blast cells (plasmablasts) with intensely basophilic ("pyroninophilic") cytoplasm. Ultrastructurally, they have evidence of a rapidly developing system of endoplasmic reticulum, which is the source of globulins with antibody activity.

To a second population of small lymphocytes (T cells) is attributed the function of reacting in cell-mediated reaction involving the direct interaction of small lymphocyte and foreign protein (Able et al. 1970). The immunologic reaction is represented in tissues as lymphocytic "exudates" (more often termed perivascular lymphocyte cuffs) in encephalitis, hepatitis, and other viral diseases. These cells are particularly important in immunologically cell-mediated diseases (graft rejection, contact hypersensitivity, lymphocytic choriomeningitis). They transform into large lymphocytes (activated T cells) that act by secreting lymphotoxins directly into target cells and lymphokines which attract nonspecific monocytes to lesions.

RECIRCULATION

In adult mammals, the small lymphocytes originate by lymphopoiesis in the cortex of lymph nodes (and other sites) where they are shed into the lymphatic circulation and enter the bloodstream via the thoracic duct. They recirculate. By hematogenous distribution to the lymph nodes, they migrate through the endothelium of postcapillary venules in the paracortical regions and reenter the lymphatic circulation (Gowans 1966). By cannulation of the thoracic duct and periodic examination of cells in lymph, it is clearly seen that enormous numbers of small lymphocytes enter the blood daily by this route. If lymph is continuously drained away in the cannula, an animal will become depleted of small lymphocytes. Gowans showed that thoracic duct lymphocyte flow can be restored in these animals by the intravenous injection of lymphocytes obtained from a closely related donor animal. By autoradiographic labeling, he demonstrated that the donor lymphocytes entering the lymphatics migrated through the postcapillary venules with high endothelium in the lymph nodes.

LYMPHOCYTES IN CULTURE

Lymphocytes obtained from the buffy coat of centrifuged blood will survive when placed in cell cultures. Some of these cells can be transformed into blast-type cells in vitro by mitogens such as phytohemagglutinin and concanavalin A. The small lymphocyte, normally repressed from mitosis, becomes derepressed and proliferates.

It is also alleged that small lymphocytes are pluripotential and can transform into macrophages in inflammatory lesions. Following his discovery of phagocytosis, Metchnikoff described the blood lymphocyte as an important source of macrophages responding to tubercle bacilli. Recent histologic studies utilizing ear chambers in rabbits also indicate that lymphocytes can transform to macrophages in inflammatory lesions. As an important biologic reaction, however, such lymphocyte transformation should be regarded with suspicion.

It is now reasonably certain that the small lymphocyte is the purveyor of immunologic memory. That is, a segment of the small lymphocyte population is immunologically committed to antigens previously contacted. When triggered by that specific antigenic stimulus, these are capable of transforming into large basophilic blast cells. For example, small lymphocytes taken from animals immunized with tetanus toxoid will transform to blast cells when placed in contact with tetanus antigen in the same culture.

The large lymphocytes seen in smears of normal circulating blood represent transformed small lymphocytes. They are large blast cells with intensely basophilic cytoplasm. Increased numbers of these large lymphocytes are commonly seen in the recovery stages of pyogenic infections and some viral diseases and are, in fact, immature plasmacytes (Spriggs and Jerrome 1967).

PLASMACYTES

Plasmacytes are synthesizers of gamma globulins with antibody activity. Their cytoplasm is filled with rough endoplasmic reticulum; the cisternae are distended with lightly granular material representing the globulin. The plasmacyte nucleus has a peripheral pattern of chromatin clumping around a central nucleolus that gives a "cartwheel" appearance to the cell (Fig. 4.16).

Pathologists have long associated plasmacytes with tissues in stages of recovery from infectious diseases. An example is chronic diffuse plasmacytic metritis of dogs. Continual endocrine stimulation of the uterus results in prolonged cystic hyperplasia of the endometrium with failure to discharge exudates. The uterine wall is infected repeatedly. Heavy plasmacyte infiltration occurs in the endometrium and in the medullary sinuses of the lymph nodes draining the uterus.

Plasmacytes develop from large blastic cells and these in turn originate from small lymphocytes. It is now clear that, when an antigenic stimulus (in the form of a microorganism) is given an animal, antibody formation begins in the most immature plasmacytes. The plasmacyte series of cells, going from precursor to maturity, are designated as hemocytoblast, plasmablast, and plasmacyte (see Fig. 5.1).

The localization of specific antibody in plasmacytes was first demonstrated by the indirect fluorescent antibody technique. Antibody-producing plasmacytes were stimulated in lymph nodes by injecting purified albumin intramuscularly and then were detected by specific staining with fluorescein-conjugated (antialbumin) antibodies. Shortly after the first electron micrographs revealed large amounts of protein-synthesizing endoplasmic reticulum in plasmacytes, the antibody molecules were localized in the cisternae by a similar immunologic technique. Ferritin was injected into rabbits, causing plasmacytes to develop in the medullary cords of lymph nodes. When sections of lymph node were overlaid with solutions of ferritin and then examined in the electron microscope, the dense ferritin molecules were visible in the cisternae of the endoplasmic reticulum (DePetris et al. 1963).

Electron microscopic techniques have revealed that antibody is first detected in the perinuclear space in newly developing hemocytoblasts. Antibody-forming splenic cells of rabbits immunized with horseradish peroxidase as an antigen were examined. A solution of peroxidase was applied (which attached to the antibody) and then a cytochemical test to detect the peroxidase (Leduc et al. 1968). Antibody appeared in the cisternae of the progressively enlarging endoplasmic reticulum concomitant with maturation of the hemocytoblasts.

Plasmacytes appear to secrete immunoglobulins by merocrine secretion. Transfer from storage in the cisternae of the endoplasmic reticulum appears to be direct. Antibody may be released at local sites of infection or directly into the bloodstream. Circulating antibody is highly efficient in combating systemic infection and in preventing infection of target cells at sites distant from the primary infection. It also appears that plasmacytes migrate to in-

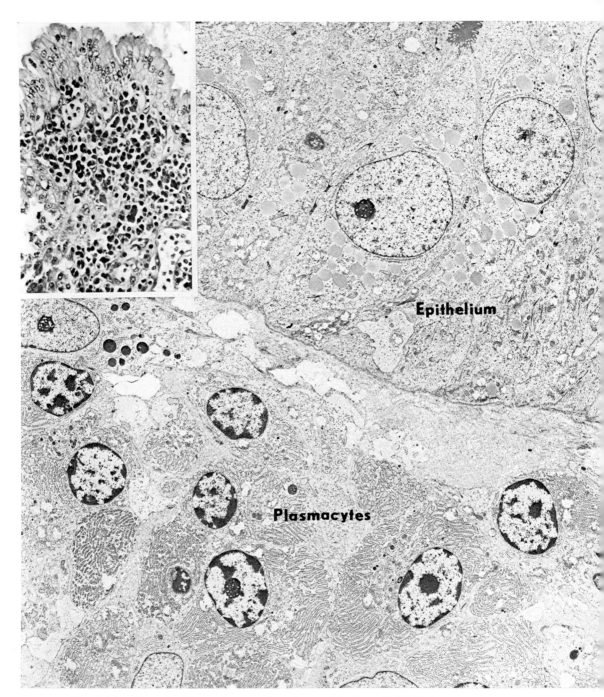

Fig. 4.16. Chronic diffuse plasmacytic endometritis, dog. Epithelial hyperplasia due to continual endocrine stimulation. Lumen of uterus is at top. Note large amounts of rough endoplasmic reticulum, cisternae of which are filled with globulin precipitates. Nuclei of plasmacytes have a characteristic "cartwheel" appearance with large nucleoli. *Inset:* Histology.

fected cells and become attached to their plasma membranes. In some, the membranes fuse; direct entry (empiripolesis) of the plasmacyte into antigen-containing cells has been observed. Plasmacytes are committed to antibody production and following excretion of globulin most lyse and die. They are incapable of dividing to increase the number of antibody-producing cells.

CLASSIFICATION OF INFLAMMATION

The pathologist sums up his evaluation of an inflammatory lesion at the necropsy. Although the etiologic diagnosis may not be possible, the pathologic diagnosis transmits to the clinician the basic facts of abnormal anatomy. Lesions may be classified according to their extent, duration, distribution, type of exudate, and location. The proper pathologic diagnosis should therefore include some of the following information.

Adjectives such as "ulcerative," "abscessing," "sclerosing," and "necrotic" often help to clarify the lesion. Like all things biological, inflammatory lesions are seldom precisely classifiable. Most purulent lesions are also fibrinous, i.e., fibrinopurulent. Many chronic lesions also contain foci of acute inflammation and can be appropriately called acute and chronic. Those exudates that infiltrate organs while not affecting the parenchymal cells are termed "interstitial" (Table 4.2).

CHRONIC INFLAMMATION

As the exudation of acute inflammation subsides in damaged tissue the processes concerned with repair begin. These involve: (1) alterations in ground substance,

(2) phagocytosis of necrotic cells and debris by macrophages, (3) invasion by and reorganization of capillaries to facilitate blood-tissue interchange, and (4) fibroblast invasion with deposition of collagen, which provides a scaffold for future parenchymal regeneration if that is possible. As these processes begin to dominate the inflammatory lesion, it is termed chronic.

If the irritant does not persist, the chronic phase is transitory. Clinicians generally apply "chronic" to those lesions that are prolonged by persistence of the irritant; that is, those that involve extensive production of fibroblasts and collagen. The use of "acute" and "chronic" thereby becomes somewhat arbitrary, a situation enhanced by modern chemotherapy in the treatment of inflammatory conditions.

GROUND SUBSTANCE

Wound fluids, mixtures of plasma proteins and ground substance, provide the milieu in which tissue reconstruction takes place. *Ground substance* is the amorphous, mucoid, gel-like material separating cells and fibers. It is composed of acidic mucopolysaccharides (hyaluronic acid and chondroitin sulfate) bound to protein. The long-chain polymers which impart the gel consistency to ground substance are broken by depolymerization in inflammation and the gel becomes fluid. Some bacterial enzymes, such as clostridial hyaluronidase, hasten this process.

As acute inflammation progresses in mesenchymal tissue, there is rapid formation of hyaluronic acid (Dunphy and Udupa 1955; Jackson 1958; White et al. 1959). Ground substance becomes exceedingly rich in acid mucopolysaccharides and regeneration of connective tissue is initiated. Fibroblasts appear to be the source of ground substance glycoproteins (Aleo et al. 1967; Peterson and Leblond 1964) but

Table 4.2. Classification of inflammation

Extent	Duration	Distribution	Exudate	Inflammation
Slight	Peracute	Focal	Serous	Gastritis
Moderate	Acute	Multifocal	Catarrhal	Tracheitis
Severe	Subacute	Diffuse	Fibrinous	Pericarditis
			Purulent	Epididymitis
	Chronic		Proliferative	Cholangiitis
			Granulomatous	Lymphadenitis

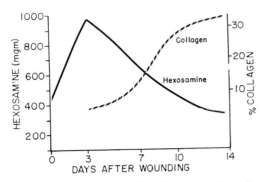

Fig. 4.17. Rise and fall of mucopolysaccharides in an experimental healing wound (after Dunphy 1955).

mast cells probably contribute in some way. Hyaluronic acid and hexosamine begin to disappear as fibroblasts produce collagen (Fig. 4.17). Amino acids such as glycine, lysine, and proline are also present and eventually become incorporated into the collagen molecule. Large amounts of basement membrane material accumulate in some chronic inflammatory lesions (Kurtz and Feldman 1962; Pierce and Nakane 1969).

MACROPHAGES

In inflammation *macrophages* constitute a second line of defense by phagocytizing particulate material and digesting it intracellularly. They are not rapidly attracted by the chemotactic substances that attract neutrophils, and they are less discriminating in the material they accept. Phagocytosis is slower and degradation less complete. In contrast to neutrophils, a large part of macrophage uptake occurs by pinocytosis. Digested debris accumulates in large membrane-bound residual bodies (secondary lysosomes) which may, by exocytosis, deposit their contents outside the cell (Fischer et al. 1970; Hard 1969).

The unequaled ability of macrophages to process foreign proteins in a slow, limited manner (that is, without enzymatically destroying them completely and being destroyed themselves in the process) allows them to fulfill a vital role in processing and retaining antigens for immunologic reactions.

In normal tissue, macrophages are con-

tinually involved in the phagocytosis and degradation of substances such as cholesterol, fibrin polymers, pulmonary alveolar secretions, and aged erythrocytes and leukocytes. In necrobiosis, they must clear and process dead cells and debris. In the atrophy of the involuting uterus following pregnancy, for example, macrophage lysosomes are filled with collagen fibrils (Parakkal 1972) which are removed for the return of the uterus to normal size.

Macrophages are large pale cells with highly developed Golgi zones. They are the phagocytic cells of the reticuloendothelial system, a functional classification proposed by Aschoff which encompasses macrophages of the lymphoid tissues, liver, lung, and other organs (Table 4.3).

Blood monocytes are the source of tissue macrophages in necrosis and inflammation. Monocytes giving rise to tissue macrophages can be observed in hanging drop preparations of blood. It is alleged that blood lymphocytes also give rise to macrophages, but the biologic importance of this transformation has not been established.

Activation of macrophage precursors occurs in the presence of particulate material and is influenced by increased body temperature and other factors. Activated (stimulated) macrophages are distinguished from the nonactive form by increased numbers of lysosomes, mitochondria, and pinocytotic vesicles. The Golgi complex is enlarged. In vitro these cells can be seen to spread and attach more rapidly to glass; they have increased levels of hydrolases in their lysosomes and hypermobility of the cell membrane.

Experimentalists define macrophages in terms of phagocytosis, supravital staining with neutral red or acridine orange, and

Table 4.3. Macrophages of the reticuloendothelial system

Macrophage Type	Cell of Origin
Tissue macrophage (histiocyte)	Blood monocyte
Serosal macrophage (peritoneum)	Mesothelial cell
Alveolar macrophage (lung)	Monocyte, Kupffer cell
Littoral macrophage (liver, spleen)	Reticular cell
Endothelial macrophage	Endothelial cell

the ability to fix rapidly to glass when placed in cell cultures. After injecting a few ml of culture media into the peritoneal cavity of a mouse and massaging the abdomen, the fluid when removed contains large numbers of peritoneal macrophages. The cells stick rapidly to the surface of culture tubes and although they do not replicate, they survive for several weeks and can be used for studies involving macrophages and lysosomes. Macrophages can also be obtained by "washing" the lungs of animals. Alveolar macrophages are slightly more active than peritoneal cells, probably because of continual exposure to particulate material in air.

The functional capacity of the macrophage system, or collectively the reticuloendothelial system, can be calculated from the clearance of carbon particles injected intravenously. The *phagocytic index* (PI) can be formulated where C_0 and C_t are the concentration of carbon in the blood at 0 time and at time t. Sophisticated use of the computer has been used in these procedures (Nelson 1969).

$$PI = \frac{\log C_0 - C_t}{t}$$

Blockade of the reticuloendothelial system can be transiently induced by overloading its macrophages with substances such as thorotrast or colloidal carbon. The macrophages are temporarily unable to phagocytize additional particulate material. Paralysis of macrophages accompanies some severe infectious diseases. Substances such as the capsular material of Anthrax bacilli appear to inhibit the cell membrane of macrophages, thus rendering them incapable of phagocytosis (Fig. 4.18).

FIBROBLASTS AND COLLAGEN DEPOSITION

Fibroplasia begins early after injury. Existing fibrocytes are the source of fibroblasts in healing wounds, although the pluripotentiality of vascular endothelium, pericytes, and lymphocytes indicates that these cells may provide other sources. *Fibroblasts* are differentiated from their mature counterparts by their basophilia, the presence of large amounts of rough endoplasmic reticulum, and prominent nucleoli, all evidence of active protein synthesis

(Cliff 1963; Goldberg and Green 1964; Ross et al. 1970).

In uninfected, uncomplicated skin wounds, fibroblasts multiply and collagen is laid down until the wound is completely bridged at about 5 to 7 days. In the subsequent 2 to 3 wks, scar tissue is organized and the progressive process of wound contraction develops. By 4 wks, when collagenization is largely completed, short dense elastic fibers begin to appear (Williams 1970). They consist of linearly arranged amorphous globules of elastin, a protein complexed with a hydrated mucopolysaccharide. The elastin components are interconnected, surrounded, and penetrated by bundles of microfibrils. The fibrillar-globular elastic fibers weave among collagen fibers, giving the newly formed connective tissue stretchability and elasticity (Ross 1973). Large amounts of basement membrane material are often deposited in wounds. Reticulin, a fibrous array of this material, is demonstrable by special histologic stains for argyrophilia. Ultrastructurally, reticulin is not a uniform substance but represents linear arrays of amorphous masses of granules (Matakas et al. 1972).

The process of wound contraction appears to depend upon specialized types of fibroblasts. After about 1 wk of wound growth, peculiar modifications of fibroblast structure occur. Nuclear membrane irregularities, surface attachment sites, and cytoplasmic microfilaments develop and are indications of a change to smooth musclelike cells (Gabbiani et al. 1972). These *myofibroblasts* have large arrays of microfilaments from which actomyosin is extractable and which stain with antismooth-muscle antisera. They appear to be responsible for the contraction of strips of granulation tissue that occurs in experimental pharmacologic testing and for the contraction and postinflammatory stricture of naturally occurring wounds (Ryan et al. 1973).

Collagen and other substances are not deposited to lie as inert bridging material. They exist in a dynamic state in which synthesis and removal of collagen is slowly occurring and collagenases, the enzymes degrading collagen, have been demonstrated in wounds several years old. Collagen fibers become progressively stronger

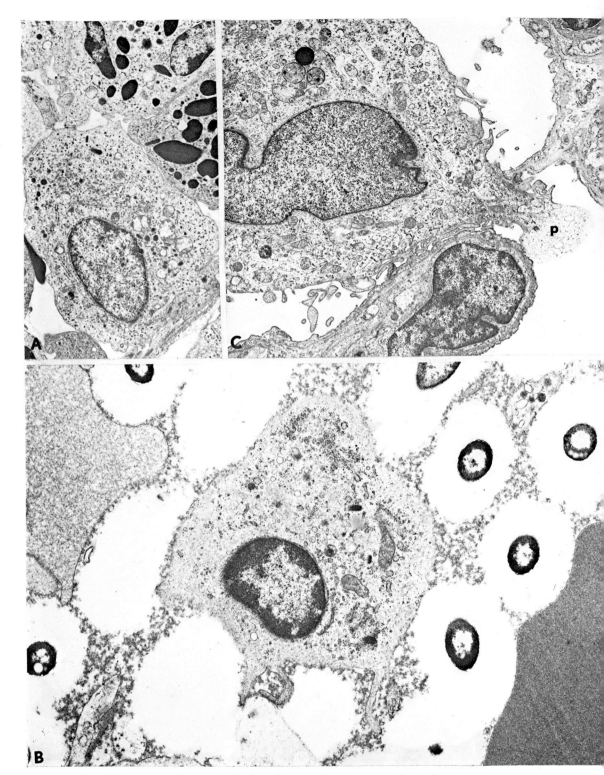

Fig. 4.18. Macrophages. A. Activated macrophage, venous sinus of spleen, tuberculosis. Granulocytes at top. B. Degenerate, paralyzed macrophage in splenic venous sinus surrounded by encapsulated anthrax bacilli. Macrophage is filled with ribosomes but few lysosomes are present (contrast with upper left). C. Alveolar macrophage in lung of a pig which has inserted a pseudopodium (p) through pore in alveolar wall (pore of Kohn).

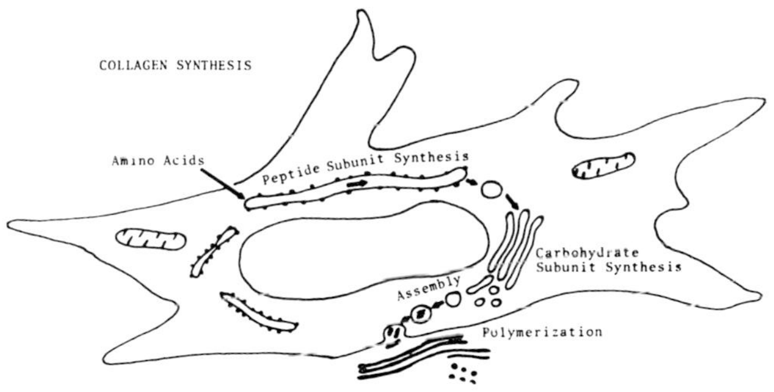

COLLAGEN SYNTHESIS

Amino Acids

Peptide Subunit Synthesis

Carbohydrate Subunit Synthesis

Assembly

Polymerization

Fig. 4.19. Synthesis of components of collagen in the fibroblast.

by increased bonding among fibrils. Even though wounds may be completely healed, they may break down if the animal experiences a severe systemic disease that represses collagen synthesis for long periods.

To understand how fibroplasia in wound healing is inhibited, it is necessary to review the biology of collagen production (Figs. 4.19 and 4.20). Collagen fibers are formed in the intercellular spaces by the polymerization of tropocollagen molecules which are released at the cell surface of the fibroblast. Synthesis of tropocollagen molecules begins with the production of polypeptide chains on the ribosome. These α-chains (analogous to α-chains of fibrinogen and other fibrillar proteins) have a simple amino acid constitution: about $\frac{1}{3}$ glycine, $\frac{1}{3}$ proline and hydroxyproline, and $\frac{1}{3}$ other amino acids.

Hydroxylation of proline causes the chains to become entwined to form a complex triple helix. These are transported to the Golgi complex where carbohydrate subunits are synthesized and procollagen molecules are assembled. Protropocollagen molecules are secreted extracellularly where they are oriented in an end-to-end and side-to-side manner. The stability of the collagen fiber is due to the formation of firm covalent intermolecular cross-linkages between the tropocollagen molecules (Olsen and Prockop 1974; Weinstock and Leblond 1974).

Fibroplasia in wounds is inhibited by tissue debris and bacterial infection. Other, less important local factors may include decreased temperature, irradiation, and foreign bodies such as talcum powder granules. Clinically, fibroplasia may be enhanced by elevated temperature and by debridement, the removal of necrotic tissue. Delayed wound healing due to suppression of fibroplasia accompanies many severe systemic diseases.

General factors that inhibit healing include old age, protein deficiency, vitamin C deficiency, and several endocrine effects. Ascorbic acid deficit markedly retards fibroplasia, for this vitamin is required as a cofactor for proline hydroxylase. In animals, scurvy is seen only in guinea pigs that have been fed on old stale feeds. Characteristics of scurvy include extensive formation of fibroblasts and synthesis of ground substance but very little deposition of collagen. Fibroblasts do not form in parallel arrangements and the resulting signs of disease are related to delayed wound healing and abnormalities of bone. In classic medical literature, human scurvy patients were often afflicted with the breakdown of very old scars, a fact that emphasizes the active metabolism that occurs even in dense collagen.

The heritable collagen dysplasias that occur in cattle, dogs, mink, and humans provide naturally occurring models for defective collagen formation and delayed wound healing (Gething 1971; Hegreberg et al. 1970). Newborn calves with dermatosparaxis, a deficiency of procollagen peptidase, have extremely fragile skin with large numbers of flat twisted unbanded collagen fibrils in disordered patterns. The striking deficiency of mature collagen fibers is demonstrable by their lack of birefringence under polarized light (O'Hara et al. 1970). The dermis accumulates large amounts of procollagen and is hyperelastic, fragile, and slow to heal.

Aging inhibits the healing of wounds. Fibroplasia, which is extremely active in neonates, is delayed in the aged animal and this perpetuates the chronicity of the healing process. Elastic fiber degenera-

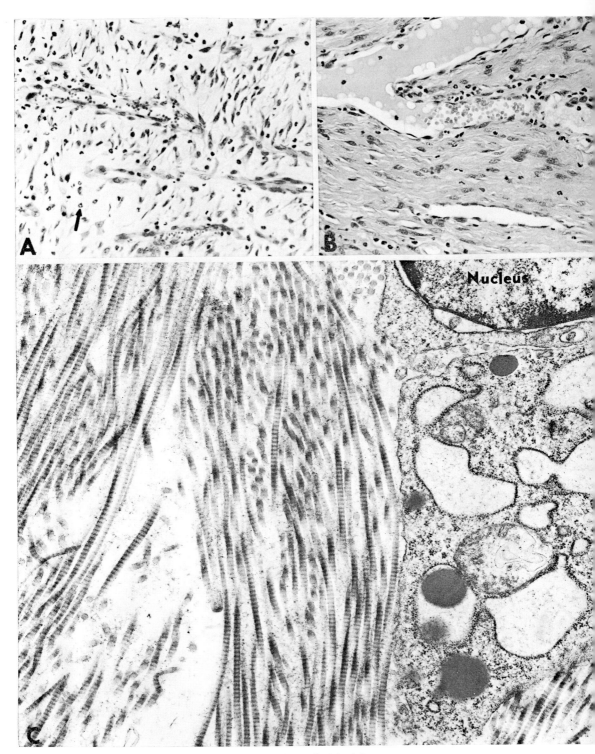

Fig. 4.20. Fibroplasia in healing wound, surgical incision, cat.
A. Endothelial cell invasion with extension of fibroblasts parallel to
the endothelial cell buds (1 wk after incision). Early deposition of
collagen has started and a few neutrophils (arrow) can be seen. B.
Advanced fibroplasia, connective tissue scar in healed wound (4 wks
after incision). C. Electron micrograph of collagen-producing fibroblast. Large group of collagen fibrils in center make up collagen fiber.
Fibroblast contains ribosomes and rough endoplasmic reticulum.
Inspissated material present within cisternae.

Table 4.4.   Steps in the normal and defective formation of collagen fibers

Activity and Location in the Cell	Defect	Reference
1. Translation of mRNA, amino acid assembly into polypeptides (pro-α chains) on the ribosomes of the fibroblast.	*Protein deficiency:* (1) Starvation	Gross, *J. Exp. Med.* 107:265, 1958
2. Hydroxylation of proline (and other amino acids) by *proline hydroxylase* on ribosomes of the rough endoplasmic reticulum (ER).	*Inhibition of proline hydroxylation:* (1) Ascorbic acid deficit (scurvy) (2) Corticosteroid therapy (3) Dilantin therapy (iron tie-up)[a]	Bates et al., *Biochim. Biophys. Acta* 278:610, 1972 Manthrope et al., *Acta Endo.* 77:310, 1974 Liu and Bhatnagar, *Proc. Soc. Exp. Biol. Med.* 142:253, 1973
3. Helix formation: aggregation of pro-α chains into triple helix of procollagen in ER cisternae and Golgi complex.		
4. Release of soluble procollagen by secretory granules at the cell surface.		
5. Extracellular alignment of tropocollagen molecules from protropocollagen (pro-α chains converted to α chains by *procollagen peptidase* which cleaves away an NH_2 terminal peptide).	*Procollagen peptidase deficiency:* lack of procollagen to collagen conversion (1) Collagen dysplasia of calves (dermatosparaxis) (2) Ehlers-Danlos (type VII) disease[a]	O'Hara et al., *Lab. Invest.* 23: 307, 1970

6. Formation of aldehyde end groupings in tropocollagen. *Lysyl oxidase* converts peptidyl lysine to allysine (aldehyde). *Lysyl hydroxylase* converts hydroxylysine to hydroxvallysine.	*Lysyl oxidase deficit:*
	(1) β-aminoproprionitrile poisoning (inhibition of lysyl oxidase)
	(2) Copper deficit
	  a. dietary deficiency
	  b. Menke's kinky hair syndrome[a]
	(3) Genetic enzyme deficiency in mottled (blotchy) mice
		Bornstein, *Am. J. Med.* 49:429, 1970
		
		Andrews et al., *Am. J. Path.* 78: 199, 1975
		Rowe, et al., *J. Exp. Med.* 139; 180, 1974

7. Cross linkage of tropocollagen.	*Lysyl hydroxylase deficiency:* (1) Ehlers-Danlos (type VI) disease[a] *Blockade of aldehyde groups:* (1) D-penicillamine toxicity (2) Homocystinuria[a] (3) Marfans syndrome[a] (?)	Pinnell et al., *New Engl. J. Med.* 286:1013, 1972 Deshmukh and Nimni, *J. Biol. Chem.* 244:1787, 1969 Kang and Trelstad, *J. Clin. Invest.* 52:2571, 1973

[a] Reported only in humans.

179

tion can be identified as splitting and granulation of the fibers in aged animals (senile elastosis). The deposition of collagen and of matrix material is also restricted in cartilage and bone of aged animals and seriously affects the healing process.

VASCULAR HYPERPLASIA AND INGROWTH

At the surviving vascular border of injured tissue, vascular sprouts appear. Endothelial cells throw out filopodia and migrate toward the stimulus. Curiously, they do not separate, but remain fused as an advancing endothelial sheet. The factors responsible for migration may include hypoxia, products from injured tissue, blood pressure differentials, or changes in the connective tissue stroma. Whatever the cause, vascular syncytia (cords of cells) form which rapidly differentiate and canalize. These vascular syncytia fuse and gradually establish a network of patent capillaries (Clark and Clark 1939).

Mesenchymal cells peripheral to vascular buds have the potential to differentiate to fibroblasts. They extend seemingly directly outward from new capillaries and give the newly forming granulation tissue an organized framework on which to function. Pericytes develop around new capillaries and appear to originate from undifferentiated mesenchymal cells, which become incorporated into the basement membrane of the newly formed capillaries (Crocker et al. 1970).

Fibrin, which provides a scaffold for migrating cells, is absorbed during vascular ingrowth. Fibrin persists beyond the disappearance of neutrophils and is not entirely removed until vascular invasion is accomplished. The newly formed endothelial cells are fibrinolytic (Astrup 1968). Unlike fibroblasts, they contain an activator of plasminogen. The removal of fibrin polymers is necessary as capillary buds migrate into the wound.

New blood vessels are highly permeable, as seen by their fragility in rabbit ear chambers. Trypan blue and blood-borne lipids pass freely through the walls (Friedman and Byers 1962; Schoefl 1963). Increased permeability is due, in part at least, to absence of basement membrane. More proximally the basement membrane is developed, and particulate material is sifted out at this barrier.

Vascularization is retarded in conditions of nutritional deficiency or other severe systemic diseases. In scurvy, as with fibroblasts, endothelial cells are abnormal (Friederici et al. 1966) and do not enter wounds at rates considered normal.

New lymphatics develop in healing wounds by sprouting from the endothelium of preexisting lymphatics (Pullinger and Florey 1937). Formation is slower and more capricious than that of blood vessels.

GRANULOMATOUS INFLAMMATION

Granulomatous inflammation is a special subtype of chronic inflammation. The inflammatory reaction in tissue is dominated by immense numbers of activated monocytes and macrophages. The hypertrophied, vacuolar, and foamy macrophages which one often encounters in these lesions are called *epithelioid cells* and are the hallmark of granulomatous inflammation (Spector 1969).

Granulomatous inflammation is associated with substances that macrophage lysosomes cannot adequately process. Mycobacteria, fungi, aberrant parasites, and inert particles such as asbestos and silica are notorious initiators of granulomatous lesions. The polysaccharides of bacterial cell walls are also important (Page et al. 1974). Streptococcal mucopeptides, when extracted chemically, are capable of inducing granulomatous inflammation experimentally.

The initial phagocytosis of the above bacterial substances is followed by "digestive failure," degeneration, and death of the macrophage. Blood monocytes emigrate to the location, transform to macrophages, and rephagocytize the agent and its associated cell debris. New macrophages collect in progressively enlarging foci called *granulomas*. Although the material may not be destroyed, the granuloma provides an effective means of localizing it and allowing other inflammatory and immunologic mechanisms to act for longer periods of time. Granulomas are a certain sign of chronicity and involve multiple episodes of necrosis, lymphocyte infiltration, and fibrosis.

INDUCTION PHASE OF GRANULOMATOUS
INFLAMMATION

Ultrastructurally, the macrophages in progressively expanding granulomas are seen to have enlarged and to have developed enormous increases in lysosomes, Golgi complexes, and vesicles. Striking undulations and pseudopods can be seen in the plasma membrane (Fig. 4.21). Specific organisms and protein crystals can sometimes be seen within phagosomes and phagolysosomes. As a result of degenerative processes initiated by phagocytized materials, autophagy is conspicuous in these macrophages.

IMMUNOLOGIC PHASE OF GRANULOMATOUS
INFLAMMATION

The induction phase of infectious granulomas is a macrophage response to toxic material and the tissue reaction is purely inflammatory. For example, Streptococcal cell wall polysaccharides induce granulomas with no immunologic basis; neither antibody nor cell-mediated immunoreactivity plays a role in the evolution or resolution of the lesions (Page et al. 1974). As infectious granulomas expand, however, they become increasingly complex. Although the dominant cell type remains the macrophage, many other cells invade. The pattern of immigrating cells is altered considerably by the agent involved and by the immunologic response it induces in the host. The lesion becomes, in a sense, an immunologically induced granuloma (Epstein 1967).

In some lesions, plasmacytes are a common component of the granuloma, and this indicates a role, even though ineffective, of these antibody-containing cells in attempting to overcome the organism involved. Antibodies may develop in the serum of the host, but these are not credited with significance either in recovery of the host or in resolution of the lesion. A few days after the injection of antigens mixed in an oily substance, severe granulomatous lesions develop in chickens at the site of injection. When the chicken is deprived of its capacity to form antibodies by bursectomy, there is no effect on granuloma formation; lesions develop in the same size and quality as in normal chickens (White 1970). In contrast, when the chicken is deprived of its thymus, the granulomatous reaction is abolished, a fact that implicates cell-mediated immunologic mechanisms.

Cell-mediated immune mechanisms have been associated with granulomatous inflammation because of the histologic character and time-course of development of the granuloma. Small lymphocytes are known to invade granulomas. The role of cell-mediated immunity has been established in an experimental model in which plastic beads linked to various haptens are injected intravenously into guinea pigs (Unanue and Benacerraf 1973). In normal animals, the beads are trapped in the lung and induce only a mild inflammatory response. In guinea pigs previously immunized with the specific hapten, severe granulomas develop upon recognition of the carrier determinants of the hapten-protein conjugates. This immunologically induced granuloma differs from its nonimmune counterpart only in intensity. The effect of cell-mediated immunity in producing and increasing the severity and duration of the lesions is attributed to the involvement of small lymphocytes. Lymphocyte mediators are released in the reaction and induce not only the infiltration of macrophages, but also pronounced structural changes in the macrophages themselves.

GIANT CELLS

Fusion of monocytes and macrophages can give rise to giant cells. Historically, the formation of these huge, multinucleate cells from monocytes has been established in vitro by observing the fusion of monocytes in cultures or in hanging drop preparations. Ultrastructural studies on tissue reveal extensive alterations in the plasma membranes of adjacent monocytes and macrophages. Fusion occurs in regions of extensive plasma membrane interdigitation. Cells with multiple nuclei result. The nuclei may be clustered in the center of the cell or arranged in ring form around the periphery (Davis 1963; Silverman and Shorter 1963; Sutton and Weiss 1966).

The finding of giant cells in lesions suggests the possibility of diseases involving fungi, mycobacteria, and some foreign bodies and is a valuable aid in diagnosis (Fig. 4.22). How giant cells are induced has been examined in aspergillosis. The fungal metabolite cytochalasin produced by some Aspergilli affects cell movement by altering microtubules of macrophages. Cell membranes are also affected and fusion results in large multinuclear giant cells (Krishan 1971).

Cytochalasin inhibits cytokinesis (cytoplasmic division) without affecting karyokinesis (nuclear division) by drug-induced changes in microfilaments. Cell movement and granule secretion are also inhibited, allegedly by the same mechanism. Depression of glucose metabolism and the incorporation of uridine and thymidine into nucleic acids has also been described, but a logical translation into cytopathologic change has not been reported.

Giant cells may also form by division of nuclei without cytoplasmic division. This mechanism is seen in congenital dysplasias (Percy and Hulland 1968) and neoplasms; it rarely occurs in granulomatous inflammation.

REPAIR

Repair of tissues involves both fibrous reconstruction and hyperplastic regeneration (Edwards and Dunphy 1958; Schilling 1968). It is a fundamental process of all living things. The enormous differences in repair seen among animals result from the regenerative capacity of the species involved, cleanliness or contamination of the injury, and the tissue in which repair in occurring.

REGENERATION

Regeneration is an amazing property of lower animals. Wounds heal rapidly and lost parts may be replaced. Hydra and other coelenterates can be cut into small pieces and each will develop into a completely new organism. Earthworms cut in half regenerate new heads and tails. Some of the lower vertebrate forms retain these remarkable capacities. When a newt's leg is amputated, the stump gives rise to pluripotential mesenchymal cells which differentiate to form a new leg including bone and muscle. Growth is not inherent in the stump, for if it is transplanted to the tail region it develops into a new tail. Frog

tadpoles have similar powers of regeneration, but they are largely lost during metamorphosis.

In mammals, few functional regenerative changes occur. Epithelial and connective tissues may regenerate extensively but most tissues have a very limited ability to reduplicate. The process of repair in higher vertebrates is therefore chiefly the revascularization and fibroplasia that occur in the chronic phases of inflammation. The growth of new epithelial cells over the reconstructed wound is a requirement for complete repair in skin and similar surface tissues.

EPITHELIZATION

Basal cells of the surviving epithelium at the periphery of the wound begin to slide across the bare, fibrin-covered wound surface soon after injury. Migrant epithelial cells are characterized by pleomorphism and blunt pseudopods, which project into the fibrin strands. Their surface structures suggest that ameboid movement has taken place (Odlund and Ross 1968). Epithelial cells also cover gaps in epidermis by growing up from skin appendages such as hair follicles (providing these structures remain intact).

Small wounds may be covered by epithelium within 12 hrs. Mitosis begins in the migrant cells and hyperplasia rapidly fills in the gaps in the new epithelial surface. The development of desmosomes between keratinocytes and hemidesmosomes between keratinocyte and basal lamina completes the repair process (Krawczyk and Wilgram 1973).

Epithelial cell proliferation ceases when cells contact one another. *Contact inhibition* is the poorly understood phenomenon involving cell recognition and the establishment of normal intercellular communication (Loewenstein and Penn 1967). Hemidesmosomes form and basement laminae are present. Information causing epithelization to cease is somehow transferred from cell to cell, for cell proliferation does not cease if mechanical barriers are placed in the path of advancing cells.

Scabs form in wounds exposed to the air. Although the dry exudate is a protective cover against skin bacteria, it may also inhibit healing. The advancing epithelial cells do not attach to the scab and must grow beneath or circumvent the necrotic material. This is accomplished more quickly if the wound is kept moist and free of bacteria.

Mucosal epithelial surfaces regenerate more quickly than epidermis. In small experimental wounds of the rat trachea, the injured mucosa is covered by new epithelium in 48 hrs; cilia and goblet cells appear in 14 days (Wilhelm 1953). Similar experimental wounding of the cat duodenum has shown equally rapid growth. Simple epithelium covers the clot-filled defect in a few days and subsequently remodels to form new villi and glands (Florey and Harding 1935).

CONTAMINATION OF WOUNDS

HEALING OF A CLEAN, INCISED WOUND: FIRST INTENTION

Surgical incisions are generally sharp and are free of large numbers of bacteria and tissue debris. Because the vessels have been ligated and the edges approximated, they contain little free blood. Repair is rapid. Fibroblasts have generally bridged the area in 12 hrs. Capillary buds invade, allowing a framework of blood vessels to form and assisting fibroplasia and collagen deposition which impart tensile strength to the wound. Within 4 or 5 days, epithelium has grown over the wound, acute inflammation has ceased, and repair is sufficient to allow movement of the injured area.

HEALING OF AN OPEN WOUND: SECOND INTENTION

Lacerations of tissue that are not sutured must heal by new tissue formation at the base of the wound. They are usually filled with tissue debris, free erythrocytes, and dead bacteria. While bacteria usually do not persist, continual recontamination has the same effect: it prolongs the phase of chronicity. The regularly spaced invasions of capillary buds in this tissue give it, when freed of exudate, a granular appearance, hence the term granulation tissue.

As resolution of the wound occurs and resorption of exudates takes place, capillary ingrowth and fibroplasia dominate. *Organization,* the regular and uniform bridging by connective tissue, begins to form a scar or cicatrix. As collagen production increases, the fibroblasts become less active. The scar grossly appears white and glistening because of the dominance of collagen. Occasionally, in some species such as the horse, granulation tissue has a tendency to become excessive and may restrict function. This *keloid* or "proud flesh" proliferates massively, often resembling tumor formation.

INFLAMMATION AND REPAIR IN SPECIAL ORGANS

BONE

In the simple traumatic fracture of a long bone, the broken ends of the bone are disaligned and adjacent soft tissues are torn. Blood vessels are ruptured; hemorrhage occurs throughout the fracture zone. Coagulation of blood soon forms a clot which fills the spaces of the fracture. Necrosis occurs because of vascular damage. This is particularly seen in bone because the osteocyte, which depends upon nutrient from the canaliculi of the Haversian system, is deprived of its precarious source of nutrition. Periosteum and marrow are better vascularized normally and necrosis is much less evident in these tissues.

The fracture is repaired by the formation of a *callus,* new mesenchymal tissue which bridges the fragments of bone and cements them together. Within 48 hrs after the fracture, the blood clot is invaded by osteogenic cells of the deep layer of the periosteum, the endosteum, and the marrow. These cells proliferate at the margins of the fracture and quickly invade the clot and adjacent necrotic areas (Fig. 4.23).

By one week, proliferating cells have begun to differentiate into chondroblasts and cartilage is laid down. In calcifying cartilage, small (approximately 100 nm) matrix vesicles play a crucial role. In addition to alkaline phosphatase and mechanisms for ATP-dependent calcium transport, these vesicles possess enzymes that can increase the local concentration of orthophosphate and lead to hydroxyapatitie formation (Ali et al. 1971). The matrix material originates

The virulent bacteria are able, in some unknown way, to circumvent the phagocytosis and processing by the synovial cells (Johnson et al. 1970).

Chronic arthritis involves fibrosis and synovial cell hyperplasia of the synovial membrane. These lesions tend to be self-sustaining, for the projection of proliferative lesions into the synovial cavity provokes not only pain but a superimposed subtle inflammatory response. The chronic arthritis commonly seen in the joints of aged animals begins as a degenerative osteoarthropathy which is accompanied by fibrosing changes in the synovial membrane and synovial cell hyperplasia (Huth et al. 1973).

BRAIN

Inflammations of the brain, meninges, and spinal cord are called encephalitis, meningitis, and myelitis, respectively. The earliest events of inflammation, those involved in fluid accumulation, are critical in the central nervous system, for these organs cannot expand beyond the defined limits of the cranium and spinal canal. Even minimal inflammatory lesions in the brain may cause neurologic signs, and if they occur in the highly sensitive autonomic nuclei of the medulla they may result in death.

Fluid accumulation within the brain substance or neuropil is separated classically into *brain swelling*, which is due to accumulation of fluid within glial cells, and *brain edema*, in which fluid accumulates in the extracellular spaces. This distinction is rarely practical, for in most cases of edema of nervous tissue the fluid is present at both sites.

Experimental fluid accumulation in the brain has been studied in injuries produced by cold, craniotomy, injection of intravenous distilled water, alkyl tin compounds, and microbial toxins (Aleu et al. 1963; Aleu and Thomas 1966; Gonatus et al. 1963; Hirano et al. 1965; Torack et al. 1960). Tissue destruction due to pressure of extravascular fluid is characterized by the accumulation of fluid within glial cells, by splitting of myelin sheaths, and by the formation of gaps in the perivascular ring of astrocytic foot processes. Astrocytes are most severely involved, and the marked swelling of the cell and its processes is responsible for secondary changes in adjacent myelin sheaths.

The exudation of cells bears serious consequences in the brain. Purulent encephalitis is nearly always due to bacterial infection. Neutrophils actively pass the capillary wall and accumulate in the neuropil where they tend to form microabscesses. Bacteria most often arrive by way of the bloodstream, usually during pyemia as metastatic emboli.

Acute nonpurulent (or aseptic) encephalitis is usually viral in origin. Most neurotropic viruses replicate in vascular structures prior to spreading to the glia and neurons, but others arrive hematogenously or via nerve sheaths and affect neurons directly. The cellular response to viral infections is lymphoid; that is, the cells that accumulate in the perivascular spaces ("perivascular cuffing") are mixed populations of small lymphocytes, monocytes, and plasmacytes.

In many of these viral encephalitides age is inversely related to susceptibility. In neonates or very young animals, there may be widespread neuronal and glial destruction with little inflammatory response. In contrast, older animals that have developed only mild clinical signs have marked perivascular lymphoid infiltrates and glial proliferation. This is due to the reactions of lymphocytes and antibody-carrying cells, reactions that lead to recovery. There is no solid evidence that other components of the inflammatory response in the brain substantially prevent the development of encephalitis. On the contrary, glial-vascular and lymphoid reactions are implicated as the cause of clinical disease in some infections. Fortunately, the inhibition of viral replication by immunoreactivity surpasses the deleterious effect of inflammation. It has been demonstrated that cells of the plasmacyte series can and do enter the brain and actually pass into the cytoplasm of neurons (Hughes et al. 1968). It is probable that by fusing with infected neurons and glia, plasmacytes can transfer globulins with antibody activity directly into the cytoplasmic matrix of these cells.

Healing in the brain occurs by the proliferation of fibroblasts and glial cells along vascular networks. When the neuropil is punctured by a sterile instrument, the lesion heals by astrocytic gliosis and by becoming filled with a fibrous core derived from the meninges and perivascular adventitia. The glial reaction to injury is rapid. Astrocytes are less vulnerable than nerve cells and, if they are not destroyed during injury, they react progressively to form a dendritic network around the wounded neuropil. Necrotic brain tissue appears to initiate reactive astrocytosis. The *reactive astrocytes* ("fat astrocytes," gemistocytic astrocytes) have very large cell bodies with homogeneous, acidophilic cytoplasm. Ultrastructurally, these cells are filled with free ribosomes, endoplasmic reticulum, and lysosomes. Nuclei are eccentric and there may be several of them. There are invariably increased numbers of dendritic processes (Long et al. 1973). These giant astrocytes are stimulated by foci of edema and ischemia and are characteristic of most slowly progressing and diffusely sclerotic lesions. They occur at the margins of the lesion and their cell processes extend into the affected area. The reactive astrocytes are phagocytic and may contain cell debris and microorganisms within their phagosomes (Raine and Bornstein 1970).

Oligodendrogliocytes undergo acute swelling in injured areas. Their nuclei become pyknotic and the cytoplasmic matrix increasingly lucid and vacuolated. These cells bear the same relation to myelin as do the Schwann cells of peripheral nerves, and they are most reactive in lesions characterized by extensive demyelination. The presence of several oligodendrogliocytes around a nerve cell body is referred to as *satellitosis*.

Microglia are migratory, actively phagocytic cells of the neuropil. They phagocytize lipids, degenerate portions of dendrites, and necrotic neurons. In the process they accumulate large amounts of lipids and are referred to as foam cells ("Gitter cells" or "lipid phagocytes"). *Neuronophagia,* the phagocytosis of nerve cells by microglia, should be distinguished from satellitosis, which is the residence of oligodendrogliocytes around neurons. In the process of reacting to injury in the brain, microglia undergo enlargement, hyperplasia, and autophagy. Nodules of hyperplastic microglial cells, called glial nodules, are characteristic of some of the rickettsial and arboviral encephalitides.

Although microglia are actively phagocytic, it appears that most of the macrophages found in inflammatory lesions in the brain originate from circulating monocytes. By labeling circulating monocytes with H^3-thymidine it has been found that they extravasate at sites of injury and transform into macrophages, and that virtually all of the macrophages at such sites bear the label in autoradiographic preparations (Kitamura et al. 1973).

REFERENCES

Able, M. E., Lee, J. C. and Rosenau, W. Lymphocyte-target cell interaction in vitro. *Am. J. Path.* 60:421, 1970.

Abramson, N. et al. The interaction between human monocytes and red cells. *J. Exp. Med.* 132:1191, 1970.

Adam, W. S. Fine structure of synovial membranes: Phagocytosis of collidal carbon from joint cavity. *Lab. Invest.* 15:680, 1966.

Aleo, J. J., Orbison, J. L. and Hawkins, W. B. Histochemical and biochemical studies of strain L fibroblasts treated with lathyrogen. Increased synthesis of polysaccharides. *Lab. Invest.* 17:425, 1967.

Aleu, F. and Thomas, L. Studies of PPLO infection. III. Electron microscopic study of brain lesions caused by *Mycoplasma neurolyticum* toxin. *J. Exp. Med.* 124:1083, 1966.

Aleu, F. P., Katzman, R. and Terry, R. O. Fine structure and electrolyte analysis of cerebral edema induced by alkyl tin intoxication. *J. Neuropath. Exp. Neurol.* 22: 403, 1963.

Ali, S. Y., Sajdera, S. W. and Anderson, H. C. Isolation and characterization of calcifying matrix vesicles from epiphyseal cartilage. *Proc. Nat. Acad. Sci.* 67:1513, 1971.

Anderson, H. C., Matsuzama, T. and Sajdera, S. Membranous particles in calcifying cartilage matrix. *Trans. N.Y. Acad. Sci.* 32:619, 1970.

Archer, G. T. and Hirsch, J. G. Motion picture studies on the degranulation of horse eosinophils during phagocytosis. *J. Exp. Med.* 118:287, 1963.

Arora, S., Lahiri, P. K. and Sanyal, P. K. The role of prostaglandin E_1 in inflammatory process in the rat. *Int. Arch. Allergy* 39:186, 1970.

Astrup, T. Blood coagulation and fibrinolysis in tissue culture and tissue repair. In *Chemical Biology of Inflammation.* B. K. Forscher, ed., p. 241. Pergamon Press, Oxford, 1968.

Atkins, E. and Heijn, C. Studies on tuberculin fever. *J. Exp. Med.* 132:207, 1965.

Atkins, E. and Huang, W. C. Studies on the pathogenesis of fever with influenzal viruses. *J. Exp. Med.* 107:383, 1958.

Atkins, E., Cronin, M. and Isacson, P. Endogenous pyrogen release from rabbit blood cell incubated in vitro with parainfluenza virus. *Science* 146:1469, 1964.

Bainton, D. F. Sequential degranulation of two types of polymorphonuclear leukocyte granules during phagocytosis of microorganisms. *J. Cell Biol.* 58:249, 1973.

Bainton, D. F. and Farquhar, M. G. Segregation and packaging of granule enzymes in eosinophile leukocytes. *J. Cell Biol.* 45:54, 1970.

Basten, A. and Beeson, P. B. Mechanism of eosinophilia. II. Role of the lymphocyte. *J. Exp. Med.* 131:1288, 1970.

Beeson, P. B. Tolerance to bacterial pyrogens: Role of reticuloendothelial system. *J. Exp. Med.* 86:39, 1947.

Bennett, W. E. and Cohn, Z. A. The isolation and selected properties of blood monocytes. *J. Exp. Med.* 123:145, 1966.

Berlin, R. D. and Wood, W. B. Studies on the pathogenesis of fever. XIII. The effect of phagocytosis on the release of endogenous pyrogen by polymorphonuclear leukocytes. *J. Exp. Med.* 119:715, 1964.

Bhawan, J., Das Tandon, H. and Roy, S. Ultrastructure of synovial membrane in pyogenic arthritis. *Am. J. Path.* 96:155, 1973.

Bhoola, K. D. and Dorey, G. The intracellular localization of kallikrein, trypsin and amylase in dog pancreas. *J. Physiol.* 214:553, 1971.

Bonucci, E. Fine structure and histochemistry of calcifying globules in epiphyseal cartilage. *Zt. Zellf.* 103:192, 1970.

Boyden, S. V. The hemotactic effect of mixtures of antibody and antigen on polymorphonuclear leukocytes. *J. Exp. Med.* 115:453, 1962.

Bullen, J. J., Ward, C. G. and Wallis, S. N. Virulence and the role of iron in *Pseudomonas aeruginosa* infection. *Inf. Immun.* 10:443, 1974.

Cantin, M. and Veilleux, R. Globule leukocytes and mast cells of the urinary tract in magnesium-deficient rats. *Lab. Invest.* 27:495, 1972.

Carr, I. The fine structure of the mammalian lymphoreticular system. *Int. Rev. Cytol.* 27:283, 1970.

Casley-Smith, J. R. An electron microscope study of injured and abnormally permeable lymphatics. *Ann. N.Y. Acad. Sci.* 116:810, 1964.

Chapman, L. F. and Goodell, H. The participation of the nervous system in the inflammatory reaction. *Ann. N.Y. Acad. Sci.* 116:990, 1964.

Cheville, N. F. The gray collie syndrome. *J.A.V.M.A.* 152:620, 1968.

Cheville, N. F. et al. Generalized equine cutaneous mastocytosis. *Vet. Path.* 9:394, 1972.

Chusid, M. J. and Atkins, E. Studies on the mechanisms of penicillin-induced fever. *J. Exp. Med.* 136:227, 1972.

Clark, E. R. and Clark, E. L. Microscopic observations on the growth of blood capillaries in the living mammal. *Am. J. Anat.* 64: 251, 1939.

Clark, J. M. and Higgenbotham, R. D. Significance of the mast cell response to a lysosomal protein. *J. Immun.* 101:488, 1968.

Cliff, W. J. Observations on healing tissue. A combined light and electron microscope investigation. *Phil. Trans. Roy. Soc. B* 246:305, 1963.

Cochrane, C. G. and Aikin, B. S. Polymorphonuclear leukocytes in immunologic reactions. The destruction of the vascular basement membrane in vivo and in vitro. *J. Exp. Med.* 124:733, 1968.

Cochrane, C. G. et al. The first component of the kinin-forming system in human and rabbit plasma. *J. Exp. Med.* 134:986, 1971.

Cohen, S. G. and Ward, P. A. In vitro and in vivo activity of a lymphocyte and immune complex-dependent chemotactic factor for eosinophils. *J. Exp. Med.* 133:133, 1971.

Cohn, Z. A. and Hirsch, J. G. The isolation and properties of the specific cytoplasmic granules of rabbit polymorphonuclear leukocytes. *J. Exp. Med.* 112:983, 1960.

Coleman, E. J. and de Salva, S. J. Mast cell response to cestode infection. *Proc. Soc. Exp. Biol. Med.* 112:432, 1963.

Colley, D. G. Eosinophils and immune mechanisms. *J. Immun.* 110:1417, 1973.

Colten, H. R. et al. Synthesis of the first component of guinea pig complement by columnar epithelial cells of the small intestine. *J. Immun.* 100:788, 1968.

Combs, J. W. Maturation of rat mast cells. An electron microscope study. *J. Cell Biol.* 31:563, 1966.

Comoglio, P. Antigen-dependent mast cell differentiation in vitro. *Exp. Cell Res.* 72: 404, 1972.

Cotran, R. S. Delayed and prolonged vascular leakage in inflammation. III. Immediate and delayed vascular reactions in skeletal muscle. *Exp. Mol. Path.* 6:143, 1967.

Cotran, R. S. and Litt, M. The entry of granule-associated peroxidase into phagocytic vacuoles of eosinophils. *J. Exp. Med.* 129:1291, 1969.

Cotran, R. S. and Majno, G. A light and electron microscopic analysis of vascular injury. *Ann. N.Y. Acad. Sci.* 116:750, 1964.

Crocker, D. J., Murad, T. M. and Geer, J. C. Role of the pericyte in wound healing. An ultrastructural study. *Exp. Mol. Path.* 13:51, 1970.

Cutlip, R. C. and Cheville, N. F. Structure of synovial membrane of sheep. *Am. J. Vet. Res.* 34:45, 1973.

Dale, D. C. and Graw, R. G., Jr. Transplantation of allogenic bone marrow in canine cyclic neutropenia. *Science* 183:83, 1974.

Davis, J. M. G. The ultrastructural changes that occur during transformation of lung macrophages to giant cells and fibroblasts in experimental asbestosis. *Brit. J. Exp. Path.* 44:568, 1963.

Davis, W. C. et al. Ultrastructure of bone marrow granulocytes in normal mink and mink with the homolog of the Chediak-Higashi trait of humans. *Lab. Invest.* 24:303, 1971.

DePetris, S., Karlsbad, G. and Pernis, B. Localization of antibodies in plasma cells by electron microscopy. *J. Exp. Med.* 117:849, 1963.

Devine, C. E. and Simpson, F. O. The fine structure of vascular sympathetic neuromuscular contacts in the rat. *Am. J. Anat.* 121:153, 1967.

Dunphy, K. E. and Udupa, K. N. Chemical and histochemical sequences in the normal healing of wounds. *New Engl. J. Med.* 253:847, 1955.

Dvorak, H. F. and Mihm, M. C. Basophilic leukocytes in allergic contact dermatitis. *J. Exp. Med.* 135:235, 1972.

Dvorak, H. F. et al. Cutaneous basophilic hypersensitivity. *J. Exp. Med.* 132:558, 1970.

Ebert, R. H. and Florey, H. W. Extravascular development of monocytes observed in vivo. *Brit. J. Exp. Path.* 20:342, 1939.

Edwards, L. C. and Dunphy, J. E. Wound healing. I. Injury and normal repair, *New Engl. J. Med.* 259:224, 1958.

Ellman, L. et al. In vivo studies in C4-deficient guinea pigs. *J. Exp. Med.* 134:162, 1971.

Epstein, W. L. Granulomatous hypersensitivity. *Progr. Allergy* 11:36, 1967.

Eschenbach, C. and Seebach, G. Anomalie der Lysosomenmembran von neutrophilen Granulocyten als Ursache der progressiven septischen Granulomatose. *Virch. Arch. B* 7:16, 1971.

Fischer, H. et al. Studies on phagocytic cells of the omentum. In *Mononuclear Phagocytes*. R. Van Furth, ed., p. 528. Davis Co., Philadelphia, 1970.

Florey, H. W. and Harding, H. E. The healing of artificial defects of the duodenal mucosa. *J. Path.* 40:211, 1935.

Florey, H. W., Poole, J. and Meek, G. Endothelial cells and cement lines. *J. Path.* 77: 625, 1959.

Friederici, H. H. R. et al. The fine structure of capillaries in experimental scurvy. *Lab. Invest.* 15:1442, 1966.

Friedman, M. and Byers, S. O. Excess lipid leakage: A property of very young vascular endothelium. *Brit. J. Exp. Path.* 43:363, 1962.

Gabbiani, G. et al. Granulation tissue as a contractile organ: A study of structure and function. *J. Exp. Med.* 135:719, 1972.

Gallin, J. I. et al. Granulocyte function in the Chediak-Higashi syndrome of mice. *Blood* 43:201, 1974.

Gething, M. A. Suspected Ehlers-Danlos syndrome in the dog. *Vet. Rec.* 89:638, 1971.

Gigli, I. and Austen, K. F. Phylogeny and function of the complement system. *Ann. Rev. Micro.* 25:309, 1971.

Ginsburg, H. and Lagunoff, D. The in vitro differentiation of mast cells. *J. Cell Biol.* 35:685, 1967.

Gleich, G. J., Loegering, D. A. and Maldonado, J. E. Identification of a major basic protein in guinea pig eosinophil granules. *J. Exp. Med.* 137:1459, 1973.

Goldberg, B. and Green, H. An analysis of collagen secretion by established cell lines. *J. Cell Biol.* 22:227, 1964.

Goldstein, I. et al. Mechanisms of lysosomal enzyme release from human leukocytes. *J. Nat. Acad. Sci.* 70:2916, 1973.

Gonatus, N. K., Zimmerman, H. M. and Levine, S. Ultrastructure of inflammation with edema in the rat brain. *Am. J. Path.* 42:455, 1963.

Gothlin, G. and Ericsson, J. L. E. Electron microscopic studies on the uptake and storage of thorium dioxide molecules in different cell types of fracture callus. *Acta Path. Micro. Scand. A* 81:523, 1973.

Gowans, J. L. Life-span recirculation and transformation of lymphocytes. *Int. Rev. Exp. Path.* 5:1, 1966.

Hard, G. C. Electron microscopic study of the differentiation of mouse peritoneal macrophages stimulated by *Corynebacterium ovis* infection. *Lab. Invest.* 21:309, 1969.

Hegreberg, G. A. et al. A heritable connective tissue disease of dogs and mink resembling Ehlers-Danlos syndrome of man. *J. Invest. Derm.* 54:377, 1970.

Henson, P. M. The immunologic release of constituents from neutrophil leukocytes. *J. Immun.* 107:1547, 1971.

Hirano, A., Zimmerman, H. M. and Levine, S. The fine structure of cerebral fluid accumulation. *J. Neuropath. Exp. Neurol.* 24:386, 1965.

Hirsch, J. G. Cinemicrophotographic observations on granule lysis in polymorphonuclear leukocytes during phagocytosis. *J. Exp. Med.* 116:827, 1962.

Hirsch, J. G. and Cohn, Z. A. Degranulation of polymorphonuclear leukocytes following phagocytosis of microorganisms. *J. Exp. Med.* 112:1005, 1960.

Horton, E. W. Action of prostaglandin E_1 on tissues which respond to bradykinin. *Nature* 200:892, 1963.

Hughes, D., Raine, C. S. and Field, E. J. Invasion of neurones in vitro by non-immune lymphocytes. An electron microscopic study. *Brit. J. Exp. Path.* 49:356, 1968.

Huth, G. et al. Fine structural changes of the synovial membrane in arthrosis deformans. *Virch. Arch. A* 359:201, 1973.

Jackson, D. S. Some biochemical aspects of fibrogenesis and wound healing. *New Engl. J. Med.* 258:814, 1958.

Jenis, E. H. et al. The May-Hegglin anomaly. *Am. J. Clin. Path.* 55:187, 1971.

Johnson, A. H. et al. Infection of rabbit knee joints after intra-articular injection of *Staphylococcus aureus*. *Am. J. Path.* 60:165, 1970.

Johnson, R. B. et al. The role of superoxide anion generation in phagocytic bactericidal activity. *J. Clin. Invest.* 55:1357, 1975.

Jones, D. B. The morphology of acid mucosubstances in leukocytic sticking to endothelium in acute inflammation. *Lab. Invest.* 23:606, 1970.

Kauder, E. et al. Leukocyte degranulation and vacuole formation in patients with chronic granulomatous disease of childhood. *J. Clin. Invest.* 47:1753, 1968.

Kelenyi, G. et al. Effect of corticosteroids on eosinophil leukocytes in hypereosinophilic syndromes. *Acta Haem.* 49:235, 1973.

Kitamura, T., Hattori, H. and Fujita, S. Autoradiographic studies on histogenesis of brain macrophages in the mouse. *J. Neuropath. Exp. Neurol.* 31:502, 1973.

Kosunen, T. U. et al. Radioautophotographic study of cellular mechanisms in delayed hypersensitivity. *Immunology* 6:276, 1963.

Kramer, J. W. et al. An inherited disorder of Persian cats with intracytoplasmic inclusions in neutrophils. *J.A.V.M.A.* 166:1103, 1975.

Krawczyk, W. S. and Wilgram, G. F. Hemidesmosome and desmosome morphogenesis during epidermal wound healing. *J. Ultr. Res.* 45:93–101, 1973.

Krishan, A. Fine structure of cytochalasin-induced multinucleated cells. *J. Ult. Res.* 36:191, 1971.

Kurtz, S. M. and Feldman, J. D. Experimental stimulation of the formation of the glomerular basement membrane. *J. Ult. Res.* 6:19, 1962.

Lachmann, P. J. et al. Localization of in vivo bound complement in tissue sections. *J. Exp. Med.* 115:63, 1962.

Leak, L. V. and Kato, F. Electron microscopic studies of lymphatic capillaries during inflammation. *Lab. Invest.* 26:572, 1972.

Leduc, E. H., Avrameas, S. and Bouteille, M. Ultrastructural localization of antibody in differentiating plasma cells. *J. Exp. Med.* 127:109, 1968.

Legler, D. W. and Evans, E. E. Comparative immunology: Hemolytic complement in elasmobranches. *Proc. Soc. Exp. Biol. Med.* 124:30, 1967.

Litt, M. Studies in experimental eosinophilia. *Am. J. Path.* 42:529, 1963.

———. Studies in experimental eosinophilia. *J. Reticuloend. Soc.* 103:158, 1973.

Loewenstein, W. R. and Penn, R. D. Intercellular communication and tissue growth. *J. Cell Biol.* 33:235, 1967.

Long, D. M., Maxwell, R. E. and French, L. A. The effects of glucosteroids upon cold-induced brain edema. *J. Neuropath. Exp. Neurol.* 32:245, 1973.

Lund, J. E., Padgett, G. A. and Ott, R. L. Cyclic neutropenia in gray collie dogs. *Blood* 29:453, 1967.

Lust, G., Pronsky, W. and Sherman, D. M. Biochemical and ultrastructural observations in normal and degenerative canine articular cartilage. *Am. J. Vet. Res.* 33:2429, 1972.

Lutzner, M. A., Tierney, J. H. and Benditt, E. P. Giant granules and widespread cytoplasmic inclusions in a genetic syndrome of Aleutian mink. *Lab. Invest.* 14:2063, 1965.

Majno, G. and Palade, G. E. Studies on inflammation. I. The effects of histamine and serotonin on vascular permeability: An electron microscopic study. *J. Biochem. Biophys. Cytol.* 11:571, 1959.

Mandel, G. L., Rubin, W. and Hook, E. W. The effect of an NADH oxidase inhibitor (hydrocortisone) on polymorphonuclear leukocyte bactericidal activity. *J. Clin. Invest.* 49:1381, 1970.

Mann, P. R. An electron microscope study of the relation between mast cells and eosinophil leukocytes. *J. Path.* 98:183, 1969.

Marchesi, V. T. The passage of colloidal carbon through inflamed endothelium. *Proc. Roy. Soc. (Biol.)* 156:550, 1962.

Margolis, J. and Bishop, E. A. Studies on plasma kinins. *Austr. J. Exp. Biol. Med. Sci.* 41:293, 1963.

Matakas, F., Cervós-Navaro, J. and Risch, W. Die Ultrastruktur des Retikulins. *Virch. Arch. B* 10:67, 1972.

McCall, C. E. Lysosomal and ultrastructural changes in human toxic neutrophils during bacterial infection. *J. Exp. Med.* 129:267, 1969.

Movat, H. Z. and Anwar, A. O. The interrelationship between the kinin and the blood clotting system. *Fed. Proc.* 30:451, 1971.

Movat, H. Z. and Fernando, N. V. P. Acute inflammation. The earliest fine structural changes at the blood tissue barrier. *Lab. Invest.* 12:895, 1963.

Movat, H. Z. et al. Demonstration of a kinin-generating enzyme in the lysosomes of human polymorphonuclear leukocytes. *Lab. Invest.* 29:669, 1973.

Nelson, D. S. *Frontiers of Biology: Macrophages and Immunity,* Vol. 11. American Elsevier, New York, 1969.

Nichols, B. A., Bainton, D. F. and Farquhar, M. G. Differentiation of monocytes. *J. Cell Biol.* 50:498, 1971.

Odlund, G. and Ross, R. Human wound repair. I. Epidermal regeneration. *J. Cell Biol.* 39:135, 1968.

O'Hara, P. J. et al. A collagenous tissue dysplasia of calves. *Lab. Invest.* 23:307, 1970.

Olsen, B. R. and Prockop, D. J. Ferritin-conjugated antibodies used for labeling of organelles involved in the cellular synthesis and transport of procollagen. *Proc. Nat. Acad. Sci.* 71:2033, 1974.

Padawer, J. Phagocytosis of particulate substances by mast cells. *Lab. Invest.* 35:320, 1971.

———. The reaction of rat mast cells to polylysine. *J. Cell Biol.* 47:352, 1970.

Page, A. R. and Good, R. A. A clinical and experimental study of the function of neutrophils in the inflammatory response. *Am. J. Path.* 34:645, 1958.

Page, R. C., Davies, P. and Allison, A. C. Pathogenesis of the chronic inflammatory lesion induced by group A streptococcal cell walls. *Lab. Invest.* 30:568, 1974.

Parakkal, P. F. Macrophages: The time course and sequence of their distribution in the post partum uterus. *J. Ult. Res.* 40:284, 1972.

Zeva, H. I. and Spitznagel, J. K. Arginine-rich proteins of polymorphonuclear leukocyte lysosomes. *J. Exp. Med.* 127:927, 1968.

Zucker-Franklin, D. and Hirsch, J. G. Electron microscopic study on the degranulation of rabbit peritoneal leukocytes during phagocytosis. *J. Exp. Med.* 120:569, 1964.

Zucker-Franklin, D., Elsbach, P. and Simon, E. J. The effect of the morphine analog levorphanol on phagocytyzing leukocytes. A morphologic study. *Lab. Invest.* 25:415, 1971.

Zurier, R. B. Prostaglandins, inflammation and asthma. *J.A.M.A.* 133:101, 1974.

Immunopathology

INTRODUCTION

Immunity in its broadest sense is resistance to disease. An animal is considered immune when it is resistant to a known disease process. In this chapter, however, we will consider immunity in its narrowest definition. In essence, *immunology* is concerned with antigens and with those humoral and cellular factors that develop to destroy them. For reactions to qualify as immunologic, two criteria must be fulfilled. (1) they must be specific—reacting antibodies or cells must be specific for the antigens involved, and (2) a memory must be involved, that is, the system must be able to be recalled on second exposure to the antigen. Further encounter thereupon produces a more rapid and stronger immunologic response.

Immunoreactivity in vertebrates is divided into two major mechanistic pathways: humoral and cellular. Each functions by receiving information from foreign proteins called antigens and by giving back subsequently a product that can act upon that antigen. The antigen-acceptance and product-synthesis phases are viewed as afferent and efferent wings of the immune system.

In humoral immunity, antigens contact the cell surfaces of an immunocompetent population of small lymphocytes called B cells. These cells arise from the bone marrow and undergo residence in lymphoid tissues associated with the gut where they acquire their special character. The contact of antigen and B-cell surface transforms this cell into a plasmacyte that secretes globulins (with antiantigen activity) called antibodies. Antibodies are stable and can persist for long periods in serum and extracellular spaces of tissues.

In cellular immunity, the afferent wing involves contact of antigen with T cells, small lymphocytes that are immunocompetent by virtue of residence in the thymus. In the efferent wing, these cells transform to large lymphocytes that secrete soluble substances called lymphokines or lymphotoxins. These humoral factors act in their immediate environment but, unlike antibody, are rapidly destroyed and are not effective when circulating in the bloodstream.

The primary event in the immune response is the direct interaction of antigen and lymphocyte cell surface immunoglobulin receptors. Immunoglobulin molecules synthesized by the small lymphocyte are retained on the cell surface. These are demonstrable only on B lymphocytes. When antigen combines with these surface globulins, the complexes migrate on the plasma membrane to form a polar cap. They are then taken into the cell by pinocytosis (Karnovsky et al. 1972; Perkins et al. 1972; Taylor et al. 1971). This event triggers the lymphocyte into proliferation, differentiation to plasmacyte precursor, and synthesis of the antibody.

How far antigen-induced transformation of small lymphocytes will proceed is determined by the lineage of the lymphocyte involved. The thymic-independent B lymphocytes transform into plasmablasts, and thence into plasmacytes, by the progressive and extensive reduplication of endoplasmic reticulum. The endoplasmic reticulum provides the machinery for the synthesis of globulin (Janossy et al. 1973). As plasmacytes mature, there is also a pro-

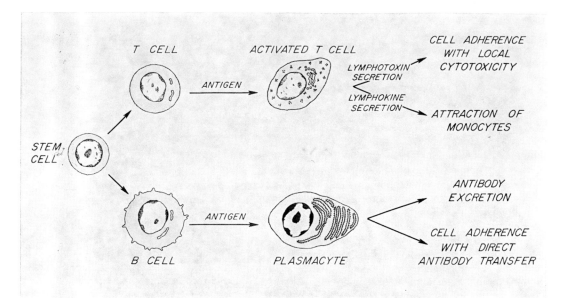

Fig. 5.1. Cells involved in efferent and afferent wings of immune response.

gressive decrease in the numbers of cell-surface immunoglobulin receptors. In contrast, thymus-derived T lymphocytes undergo little ultrastructural change after stimulation to transform. Cells enlarge and develop abundant free ribosomes and aggregates of polyribosomes but remain relatively devoid of endoplasmic reticulum (Fig. 5.1).

In the following consideration of immunopathology, we shall examine the structural alterations in lymphoid and reticuloendothelial tissues resulting from the animal's attempts to protect itself against antigen. This encompasses a wide variety of changes brought about by antigen-antibody reactions and by excesses or deficiencies of globulin synthesis and lymphocyte production. The task before us is to relate the newer knowledge of immunology, which is of necessity acquired in simple in vitro systems, to concepts of the pathogenesis of diseases as they occur in animals.

PHYLOGENY OF THE IMMUNE RESPONSE

The ability of an organism to recognize and eliminate foreign material is necessary for its continuing integrity. The lower animals, in addition to physical and chemical defense barriers (such as skin and gastric juice) and specific internal protective factors (such as lysozyme in body fluids, complement, and polyelectrolytes) depend heavily on the sequence of cell proliferation, phagocytosis, encystment, and digestion for the elimination of foreign antigens. These invertebrates do not form antibody and do not reject foreign cells when they are inserted into tissue.

Vertebrates, however, beginning with the lowest forms (the cyclostomes) possess highly specific immunological mechanisms capable of neutralizing foreign (nonself) antigenic material. The lamprey has small lymphocytes in its blood and these cells show definite signs of organization into tissues, especially in the gut wall. A primitive thymus is present. Its duty, as has been clearly established in mammals and birds, is to confer on undifferentiated stem cells the capacity to interact with antigens; that is, to translate information received on contact with an antigen into an effector mechanism for subsequent destruction of the same antigen. These adaptive (acquired and induced) immunologic mechanisms, which have evolved in concert with the evolution of vertebrates, increase in complexity phylogentically. They parallel increasing complexity in the development of the thymus, spleen, and gut-associated lymphoid tissues.

Although lampreys and other cyclostomes have small lymphocytes that appear to react in cell-mediated pathways, they do not have plasmacytes in their tissues or antibodies in their serum. Sharks and fishes, slightly higher in the evolutionary scale, do (Clawson et al. 1966). The globulin-synthesizing plasmacytes are the principal producers of antibodies, which in the fishes tend to be rudimentary. Undifferentiated small lymphocytes are present in shark and fish intestinal tracts and they are thought to play an instructive role in the capacity of fish to develop plasmacytes (Fichtelius et al. 1968). On stimulation with antigen the small lymphocytes transform into plasmacytes. The undifferentiated small lymphocyte and the plasmacyte represent the beginning and the end of the process of antigen-induced lymphocyte transformation.

Birds possess a unique separation of immunologic systems. Lymphocytes that circulate in the blood, even though they cannot be distinguished microscopically, are the progenitors of two distinct populations of cells. The first population arises early in embryonic life and depends upon the thymus for differentiation. These T lymphocytes (which enter, replicate through several generations, and egress from the thymus) are programed only for interactions with antigens and for limited direct lymphocyte-antigen interaction. The other population, the B lymphocytes, originate in a large central lymphoid organ, the bursa of Fabricius, which is attached to the end of the intestinal tract. These lymphocytes have the capacity to transform into antibody-producing plasmacytes. When the bursa is removed before hatching, the bird does not form antibodies, and plasmacytes cannot be identified in its tissues.

Mammals possess the most complex immunologic apparatus. Small lymphocytes circulate in their blood and transfer to lymph in specialized capillaries in lymph nodes. The circulating small lymphocytes consist of populations of thymus-derived T lymphocytes and thymus-independent, bone marrow–derived B lymphocytes (Table 5.1). These two populations, although they are structural look-alikes, can be differentiated by detecting differences in the antigens within their plasma membranes or the globulin receptors on their surfaces (Muscoplat et al. 1974).

The simplest methods of separating B and T cells involve the application of a specific antiglobulin antibody that is conjugated with a detector substance such as fluorescein or a radioactive label. The antiglobulin antibody will attach to the surface globulins of B cells, but does not complex with T cells, which lack these receptors. It is also reported the fluorescein-labeled antibodies prepared against thymic and bone-marrow lymphocytes will stain their respective T and B cells.

T and B cells have been differentiated by scanning electron microscopy on the basis of cell size and surface configuration. T lymphocytes make up the largest percent in the circulating blood of most mammals, are slightly smaller in size, and have smooth cell surfaces. B lymphocytes are larger and have complex villous surfaces (Polliack et al. 1973).

ANTIGEN

An *antigen* is any substance capable of stimulating an immunologic response. Only macromolecular substances behave as antigens, and in general, proteins are the strongest antigens. The specificity of antigen-antibody reactions, however, is determined by relatively small surface configurations known as determinant groups or

Table 5.1. Theoretical designation of functional states of small lymphocytes

	T cell	B$_1$ cell	B$_2$ cell
Derivation	Thymus	Gut-associated lymphoid tissue	
Function	Cell-mediated immunity	Antibody-mediated immunity	
Immune status	Committed or not	Uncommitted (virgin)	Committed (memory)
Blood-lymph recirculation	+	−	+
Life span	Long	Short	Long
Role in immune response	Primary and secondary	Primary	Secondary
Progeny cell	Large blastic lymphocyte	B$_2$ cell	Plasmacyte

sites that are present on the antigen molecule.

When foreign antigens first gain entrance past epithelial and inflammatory barriers, they drain into regional lymph and circulate in the blood. In mammals, they must pass the elaborate biological filters of the lymph nodes and spleen. Upon entering lymph nodes for the first time, antigens are taken up nonspecifically by macrophages in the medullary sinuses and peripheral lymph channels. In these areas there is a close association of macrophages with plasmacyte precursors which are destined to produce antibodies. Particulate antigens are first localized on cytoplasmic extensions of macrophages and are rapidly processed by these cells (Miller and Nossal 1964).

Macrophages clear antigens by pinocytosis or phagocytosis and sequester them into lysosomes, where they are rapidly processed or degraded. Despite the rapid disappearance of the antigen, macrophages appear to retain immunogenicity (their ability to transmit information to lymphocytes) for long periods. Small amounts of antigen unassociated with lysosomes may remain in the cytoplasmic matrix adjacent to the cell membrane. Recent studies have stressed the role of messenger-RNA of macrophages in the transmission of information from macrophage to lymphoid cell. The reaction of macrophage and antigen yields an immunogenic RNA which, when added experimentally to lymph node cells, elicits antibody.

Whether or not macrophage action is required for immune responses to occur is unresolved. Macrophages may participate nonspecifically, simply as bystanders. It appears however that processing is necessary for and particularly effective with weak antigens. Partial degradation in the lysosomes confers an adjuvant effect upon the antigen (Unanue 1972).

The trapping of antigens by macrophages in the immune animal appears to be more efficient. Upon reexposure, that is, in the presence of specific antibody, antigen is dramatically taken up in specialized sites at the periphery of germinal centers in lymph nodes and spleen (Hanna and Szakal 1968; Nossal et al. 1967). Elaborate extensions of macrophage cell membranes are interpreted as a response of "sensitized" macrophages to antigen (see Fig. 4.21). Antigens are retained extracellularly by a large dendritic web of interlocking cell membranes of specialized reticular cells. They may be held there for several weeks, allowing exceptional access to the lymphoid tissues which are destined to produce antibody-forming lymphoid cells.

MEDIATION OF IMMUNITY: ANTIBODY AND CELLS

For a century, pathologists have recognized lymphoid cells in tissues involved in stages of complete or attempted recovery from infectious diseases. It was known that persistent unresolved infections such as chronic purulent endometritis of dogs had massive infiltrates of plasmacytes and other large basophilic cells. When these lesions healed, the cellular residue was apt to consist of large focal aggregates of small lymphocytes. How these cells acted in bringing about the elimination of microorganisms from tissue and the recovery of the host was not easily resolved.

This section concerns the effector or efferent limb of the immune response—the mediation of immunity. We will see that when information from the processing of antigens is disseminated through the lymphoid system, immunocompetent small lymphocytes are transformed (according to their individual capacities). They may become plasmacytes, secreting antibody that acts directly; they may become large lymphocytes, secreting lymphokines that exert an influence on macrophages, which act as effector cells.

ANTIBODY-MEDIATED IMMUNITY

Near the turn of the century, von Behring discovered antibodies. He observed that serum of animals that had recovered from experimental diphtheria contained a specific substance capable of neutralizing the toxin produced by *Corynebacterium diphtheriae,* the causal bacterium of the disease. It was called "antibody" because it appeared to be directed against the "foreign body" of the disease.

With the discovery of the protective nature of serum antibodies in other diseases, histologists began to suspect that large basophilic blast cells (now called plasmablasts) were in some way associated with antibody production. Experiments in which lymphoid tissues were examined at regular intervals after injection of antigen gave some assurance that this was so. Subsequent use of purified antigens demonstrated that the earliest reaction involved the appearance of these large "pyroninophilic" blast cells in areas where antigens had been sequestered. The clarification of the role of these cells in antibody production awaited basic advances in knowledge of antibodies themselves.

ANTIBODY

An *antibody* may be defined as a protein of the globulin type which is produced following antigenic stimulation and which has combining sites capable of reacting specifically with determinant groups on the antigen that has stimulated its production. The specificity of an antibody is determined by a relatively small part of the molecule that is constructed to combine with a particular determinant site on the antigen.

Antibody molecules are composed of two heavy and two light polypeptide chains that are joined by disulfide bridges. Each chain is divided into constant regions, in which amino acid sequences are similar in all antibody classes, and variable regions, in which the sequence is different. The variable regions provide the specificity that characterizes the antibody.

The antibody-active proteins of serum were narrowed by Tiselius and Kabat in 1938 to the globulin fraction showing the least electrophoretic mobility, the gamma globulins. Electrophoretic migration is determined by the net charge of the protein, and this separates the protein fractions of whole serum. Serum globulins may also be purified by inducing their precipitation in saturated solutions of ammonium sulfate. The precipitate is centrifuged and redissolved in distilled water and provides large amounts of crude antibody.

The net charge of serum globulins is also the basis of ion exchange chromatography. Ion exchange resins (such as DEAE cellulose) absorb serum proteins according to their size and net charge. When serum is poured into a column of DEAE cellulose and the column is eluted successively with buffers of increasing molarity and decreasing pH, it yields successive γ-globulin peaks of increasing net charge.

Ultracentrifugal sedimentation will separate globulin on the basis of molecular size and weight and an appropriate S (for Svedberg constant) number applied according to its sedimentation. Two major globulin sizes are readily distinguished and occur in the 7S and 19S ranges. The slow sedimenting 7S globulin thus is also slow electrophoretically and is the first fraction to come off the ion exchange column.

Ouchterloney developed the agar gel diffusion technique on the basis that globulin (with antibody activity) will, when serum is placed in wells in agar, diffuse and precipitate with similarly diffusing antigen, thus forming observable lines. This technique readily distinguishes the various globulins immunologically when serum is reacted with appropriate antisera. Precipitate lines are often difficult to distinguish however. Immunoelectrophoresis combines this technique with electrophoresis: serum is applied to agar or cellulose acetate and induced to migrate in a charged field; antiserum is then applied, allowed to diffuse, and the resulting precipitate stained for observation.

The term immunoglobulin (Ig) was introduced to describe proteins with known antibody activity, a functional rather than physical description. Immunoglobulins are separated into classes on the basis of molecular structure. The classes of mammalian immunoglobulins now known include several different molecular structures (Table 5.2). The order of appearance of Ig classes in both ontogeny and phylogeny follows the sequences IgM, IgG, IgA.

ANTIBODY CLASSES

The factors that determine which class of Ig results from a particular antigenic stimulus are not completely understood. Different Ig classes may be produced against the same antigen (Table 5.2). In many instances IgM is the first response, but is followed and overtaken by subsequent IgG production. The Ig classes are synthesized by different plasmacytes.

Physicochemical studies have shown that

Table 5.2.   Characteristics of immunoglobulin classes

Class Ig[a]	Sedimentation Constant	Molecular Weight	Electrophoretic Migration	Characteristic
IgG	7s	150,000	γ	2 subclasses in most species
IgM	19s	890,000	β_2	Macroglobulin
IgA	10–12s	180,000	β_2	Secretory antibody
IgE				Reaginic antibody

[a] IgY = 7.1 S Ig of chickens, probably is functionally comparable to mammalian IgG (Leslie 1971); IgT = an equine Ig; IgI = a second poorly characterized equine Ig.

IgG is composed of heavy (55,000 MW) and light (22,000 MW) polypeptide chains united by disulfide bridges (Fig. 5.2). The specific determinants of different classes are a property of their heavy chains; i.e., the notations G, A, M, and D distinguish these globulins according to the properties of their heavy chains. The major common antigen determinants of immunoglobulins lie in their light chains, and only two types of light chains are known (kappa and lambda). While in any one Ig molecule only one type is present, normal sera has light chains of both types. Electron microscopic studies indicate that IgG exists in Y-form (Green 1969).

In most species, IgG has been divided into subclasses such as IgG$_1$ and IgG$_2$. These often have differing biologic activity (measured in terms of complement-fixation, induction of anaphylaxis, fixation to skin, or presence in body secretions). Bovine IgG$_1$, for instance, fixes complement and is the chief IgG in milk and saliva. It is the chief IgG in passive immunization of the calf.

IgM ("macroglobulin") is made up of 5 immunoglobulin units linked by disulfide bonds and theoretically has 10 identical binding sites. This gives IgM a peculiar effectiveness in activating complement to produce lysis of cell membranes: a thousand times more effective per molecule than IgG. This suggests that IgM may have adapted for dealing with larger particulate antigens such as bacteria and cells. Early primary immune responses are often IgM and are gradually replaced by IgG antibody. In bovine anaplasmosis, for instance, 19S IgM is produced 4–5 days prior to the appearance of IgG antibody.

IgA ("secretory antibody") is the predominant immunoglobulin in most external secretions such as saliva, tears, bile, and nasal and intestinal mucus (Tomasi et al. 1965). It does not always predominate; for example, IgG is the major globulin in cow's milk. Secretion of IgA appears to be

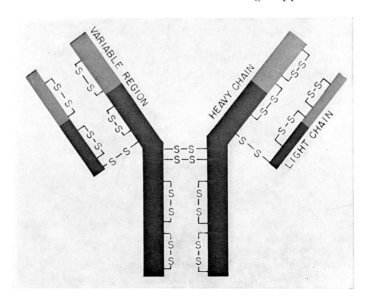

Fig. 5.2.   Diagram of immunoglobulin molecule.

more than mere passive transfer, since its concentration in body fluids may be 20 times that in serum; colostrum of dogs and horses contains IgA in much higher concentration than is present in sera.

IgA in these external secretions has a unique antigenicity conferred upon the molecule by a nonimmunoglobulin component called secretory piece. IgA is synthesized in plasma cells below mucous membranes and the secretory piece is added in its transit through glandular epithelium (Leslie et al. 1971; Poger and Lamm 1974; Schofield and Atkins 1970). In the intestine of the pig, the secretory component has been localized in crypt epithelial cells and associated mucins by immunofluorescent studies; it is not present in submucosal plasmacytes that stain for IgA (Allen and Porter 1973). Synthesis of secretory piece and IgA proceed separately and independently. In vitro, secretory piece is specific for IgA.

The presence of IgA is essential to the antimicrobial activity of the respiratory and intestinal tracts. In mammalian tears, the dominant immunoglobulin appears to be IgA. Disease of the eye is characterized by large accumulations of plasma cells in the lacrimal glands, and most of these contain IgA. Extracellular IgA is demonstrable along basement membranes, between and within the cytoplasm of acinar cells, and in the lumens of lacrimal acini (Franklin et al. 1973). This is evidence of the secretion of IgA through the lacrimal gland epithelium.

The occurrence of pure IgA myeloma proteins (in cancerous animals) and selective secretion of IgA into colostrum allows the IgA class to be identified with assurance in at least some species (Hurvitz et al. 1971; Porter 1972; Vaerman 1971). In the dog, a fast-migrating (electrophoretically) 10S myeloma protein has been described similar to that in colostrum and serum (Rockey and Schwartzman 1967). Ultrastructurally, IgA differs from IgG.

IgE ("reaginic antibody") has the peculiar ability to fix itself firmly to cells. It is implicated only in the production of disease; no known protective function exists. IgE is a homocytotropic antibody because it sensitizes host cells for hypersensitivity reactions such as anaphylaxis, asthma, and atopic dermatologic reactions. Disease induced by antigens combining with IgE in the dog are manifested as dermatitis; rhinitis is more typical of other animals, especially humans. IgE disease was first demonstrated when Prausnitz injected serum from his allergic patient Kustner into his own forearm (inducing passive sensitization). When fish, the allergen, was applied later to the same site, it produced the erythema-wheal reaction.

BIOLOGIC PROPERTIES OF ANTIBODIES

It is not proper to consider antibodies solely on the basis of molecular structure, for their important biologic properties are variable and may be shared by antibodies of more than one class. All classes participate in several types of antigen-antibody reactions in vitro. Adjectives such as agglutinating, neutralizing, complement fixing, and others define this reactivity (Table 5.3). An individual immunoglobulin molecule may react in several of these tests.

Cytophilic antibodies bind to certain cells through binding sites on the antibody molecule which are independent of the sites that react with antigen. Cytophilia is determined both by the antibody molecules and by the character of the cell membrane of the target cell. IgE is known for its strong cytophilic affinity for mast cells and basophils. By attaching, it confers im-

Table 5.3. Definitions of antibodies

Antibodies	Characteristics
Autoantibodies	Those produced in a host which react with the host's own tissue
Cell-associated	Those in or on cells, either on antibody synthesizing cells or cytophilic antibodies on other cells (syn: cell-bound antibodies)
Cytophilic	Those with affinity for cells due to mechanisms unrelated to antigenic binding (syn: cytotropic antibodies)
Isoantibodies	Those produced in one individual which react specifically with an antigen present in another individual of the same species (syn: alloantibodies)
Natural	Those occurring naturally without deliberate antigenic stimulation
Opsonins	Those acting on particulate antigens to induce phagocytosis
Precipitating	Those reacting specifically with soluble antigens to form a precipitate (syn: precipitins)

munologic reactivity to these cells should they encounter the specific antigen again. The result is an immediate hypersensitivity reaction. Subclasses of IgG in some species are also cytophilic for mast cells.

Some antibody molecules are cytophilic for macrophages and this is of great significance in infectious processes. Macrophages armed with specific cytophilic antibodies readily phagocytize antigens. They can also destroy target cells by nonphagocytic contact mechanisms which do not require all components of complement (Tizard 1971). We will again take up this subject under cell-mediated immunity.

IMMUNOLOGIC TAGGING OF ANTIBODY

Antibody molecules can be labeled with specific substances that serve as indicators for the detection of antigens. The fluorescent antibody (FA) test devised by Coons is widely used in diagnostic microbiology and in research in general. Globulins are precipitated from serum of immunized animals and the antibody molecules are conjugated with fluorescein isothiocyanate. Smears, frozen sections of tissue, and infected cell culture monolayers are fixed, stained with the conjugate, and examined under ultraviolet light which induces fluorescein (attached to the antigen sites) to fluoresce.

Important variations in the basic test are used. For electron microscopy, tagging of antibody is done with substances such as dense, iron-containing ferritin molecules which can be visualized ultrastructurally. An indirect FA test utilizes an initial application of unlabeled but specific antibody which attaches to the antigen being sought. This is followed by fluorescein-labeled antiglobulin which binds to the unlabeled specific antibody. The advantage of this procedure is that one labeled antibody preparation can be used for the detection of many different antigens. Tagged antigens can be used in the same way to detect antibody in cells.

PLASMACYTES

Plasmablasts and plasmacytes develop from the activation and transformation of B lymphocytes upon contact with antigen. When antigens combine with immuno-

globulins on the B-cell surface, they initiate polar cap formation and pinocytotic activity. The antigens enter the B lymphocyte and induce transformation from B cell to plasmablast. This progression involves extensive reduplication of rough endoplasmic reticulum, the appearance of globulin with antibody activity in the cisternae, and decrease in the number of cell-surface immunoglobulin molecules (Fig. 5.3).

Plasmacytes release immunoglobulins directly into the tissue environment by merocrine secretion. Antibodies enter the lymphatics and bloodstream and circulating antibodies are particularly effective in combating systemic infections. Plasmacytes also release antibody when directly adjacent to an infected cell and, by the process of empiripolesis, fuse with its plasma membrane and release antibody molecules into its cytoplasm.

The use of Jerne's agar plaque technique to recognize antibody-producing cells has provided intriguing results on how plasmacyte morphology relates to antibody excretion. Cell suspensions of spleen and lymph node from an animal immunized with sheep red cells are mixed with cool melted agar containing sheep red cells. After hardening, antibody diffusing from the plasmacytes reacts with the red cells surrounding them and, when complement is added, causes lysis. These hemolytic plaques provide a quantitative measurement of cellular activity. By cutting out cells in blocks of agar and processing for electron microscopy, experimenters have shown that many of the antibody-producing cells do not have elaborate endoplasmic reticulum, but resemble hemocytoblasts (Gudat et al. 1970; Harris et al. 1966). Plasmacytes synthesizing IgM antibodies, which are more efficient in inducing hemolysis, are detected by this technique.

The immunocytoadherence (rosette) tests are also useful for detecting single antibody-forming cells. Lymphoid cells harvested from an animal immunized against erythrocytes are mixed with a suspension of the same kind of erythrocytes. The suspension is observed for rosette formation: a rosette being a central antibody-carrying cell surrounded by a minimum of four erythrocytes. This highly sensitive test detects IgG or IgM antibodies on synthesiz-

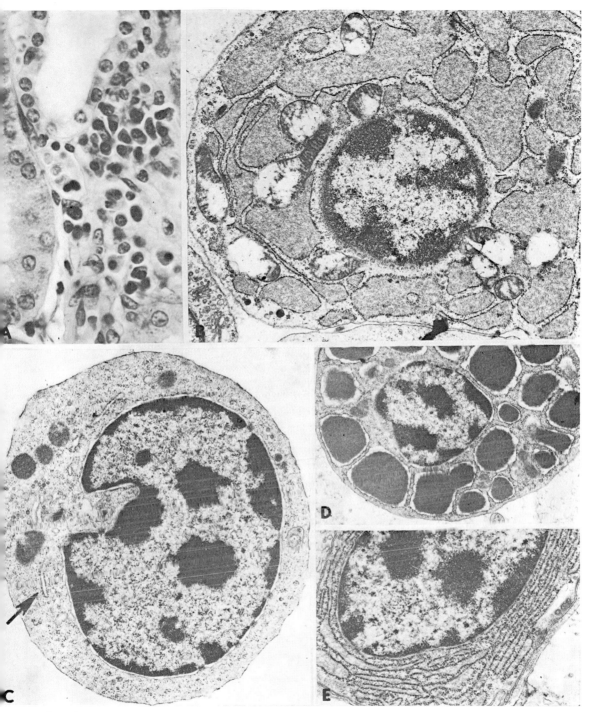

Fig. 5.3. Plasmacytes. A. Histology, interstitium of kidney, pig with leptospirosis. B. Ultrastructure, cisterna of endoplasmic reticulum is distended with globulin precipitates. C. Plasmablast from circulating blood, dog. Small amount of rough endoplasmic reticulum (arrow). Cell classified by light microscopy as large lymphocyte. D. Plasmacyte from circulating blood, dog. E. Plasmacyte in brain, viral encephalitis, chicken.

ing or carrying cells (Pavlovsky et al. 1970). It does not require complement.

ANTIBODY SYNTHESIS

Fluorescent antibody studies of single synthesizing plasmacytes indicate that only one species of immunoglobulin is produced at one time. Light and heavy chains of the antibody molecule are synthesized on separate ribosomes. The polypeptide backbone of the antibody molecule is synthesized in the rough endoplasmic reticulum and transported to the Golgi apparatus where carbohydrate moieties are incorporated (Zagury et al. 1970). There is some evidence that light chains are formed on endoplasmic reticulum, while heavy chain production is associated with polyribosomes (Suzuki et al. 1970).

Plasmacytes may be distinguished on the basis of which Ig class they produce. By purification of the globulin class used to produce fluorescein-labeled antisera, specific IgG, IgM, or IgA is detectable in plasmacyte cytoplasm in immunofluorescent tests (Crabbe et al. 1969). The route by which antigens enter animals is important in the type of plasmacyte response. In animals being immunized subcutaneously, large numbers of IgM-containing plasmacytes appear in peripheral lymphoid tissues, and this is followed by a progressive increase in IgG-containing cells. A few IgA-containing plasmacytes are found in the intestine. In oral immunization, however, IgA antibody-containing cells are abundant throughout the intestine. From this it appears that plasmacytes in the gut are selectively committed to IgA synthesis. Recent studies of IgA in other species have shown similar locations of IgA-containing plasmacytes (Curtain and Anderson 1971; Vaerman and Heremans 1969).

Plasmacytomas (also called myelomas) are tumors composed of malignant plasmacytes. The tumor plasmacytes do not differ markedly in structure from normal plasmacytes. In man and mice these tumors are characterized by massive production of light chains of the antibody molecule and defective assembly with the heavy chain components. Because the malignant plasmacyte produces one specific light chain type, the disease is termed *monoclonal*. Light chains accumulate in the blood and, being of low molecular weight, spill over into the urine as Bence-Jones proteins. Serum from affected individuals provides large amounts of relatively pure immunoglobulin components. A monoclonal macroglobulin (IgM) has also been described in the dog associated with anemia and macroglobulinemia (Hurvitz et al. 1971).

Plasmacytomas that synthesize both heavy and light chains have been reported (Zucker-Franklin and Franklin 1971). Marked vacuolation of the Golgi region was interpreted to indicate that defective assembly occurred and incomplete polypeptide chains were present in that area. There was no distention of endoplasmic reticulum cisternae with excess globulin molecules, as in other plasmacytes.

CELL-MEDIATED IMMUNITY

Cell-mediated immunologic reactions are caused by the reactivity of small T lymphocytes. The events in cell-mediated immunoreactivity include (1) recognition phenomena, which occur on immune (sensitized) T lymphocytes due to specific surface receptors and which trigger (2) activation, the conversion of the resting small (T) lymphocyte to a biosynthetically active cell. The activated T lymphocyte can function as a killer cell directly by secreting lymphotoxins during its attachment to target cells, or it can influence macrophages and other cells to function as effectors by secreting lymphokines (Dumonde et al. 1969). The core of the cellular theory is that specifically sensitized T cells have antigen recognition sites (not present on B cells) and that the reaction is initiated by union of these receptors with specific antigen.

Cell-mediated immunity seems adapted to deal with antigens existing peripherally

Fig. 5.4. Cutaneous tuberculin reaction. A. Perivascular accumulation of small lymphocytes and monocytes, evidence of cell-mediated reactivity. B. Ultrastructure of reaction around postcapillary venules. Most cells are small lymphocytes. C. Small lymphocytes (1) with macrophage (m).

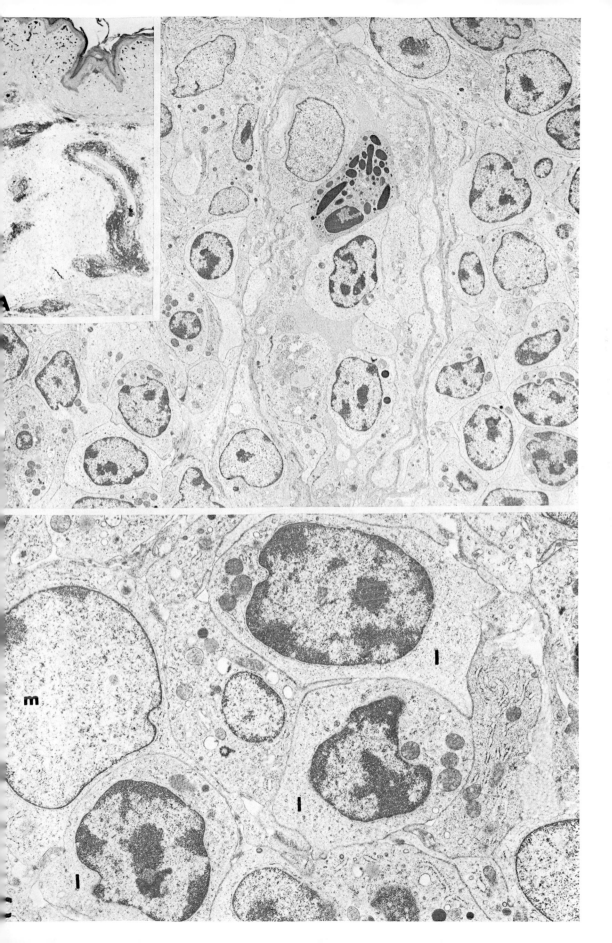

that do not contact lymphoid tissue. It is more readily produced by antigens that are sequestered by macrophages than by antigens that rapidly diffuse. Organisms that can survive and replicate intracellularly are especially prominent in their capacity to induce cell-mediated immunity. Cell-mediated immunoreactivity is the most significant reaction in tuberculosis, brucellosis, salmonellosis, and some of the fungal infections.

To examine the mechanisms involved in cell-mediated immunity we will consider three experimentally induced lesions that have been basic models for study: the tuberculin reaction, contact hypersensitivity, and graft rejection. Characteristics these models share are: (1) the challenge reaction is specific for the sensitizing antigen; (2) passive transfer of the reaction to a normal recipient animal, with cells from one undergoing a cell-mediated reaction, can be done with live cells but not with serum; and (3) the specific cellular reaction in tissue is characterized by perivenous accumulation of monocytes, macrophages, and lymphoid cells (Fig. 5.4). Most effector cells in the tissue lesions are monocytes and macrophages that are attracted by lymphokines excreted by activated T lymphocytes. It must be remembered that circulating antibodies may be present in these reactions, but by definition they are not considered mechanistic.

T-CELL TRANSFORMATION

When immune (sensitized) T cells are antigenically stimulated, they enlarge and become intensely basophilic. Their cytoplasm is filled with enormous numbers of free ribosomes and they contain almost no rough endoplasmic reticulum (Fig. 5.5). How T cells differ on their surfaces is not known, but in theory, surface antigens acquired by development in the thymus are important. Recent descriptions of an antigenic marker (θ antigen) on mouse T cells has allowed the direct study of this phenomenon. T cells carrying the θ antigen are destroyed by anti-θ antibody and complement. This treatment suppresses delayed hypersensitivity, contact sensitivity, the graft rejection, and the in vitro reactivity to certain mitogens.

Mitogens are substances that induce blastogenesis and mitosis in lymphocytes. They are important in the laboratory differentiation of T cells. Some mitogens are specific; others are nonspecific. The specific mitogens are antigens such as tuberculin that stimulate lymphocyte blastogenesis only in specifically immune, tuberculin-sensitized lymphocytes. The blastogenic response to these agents is considered to be due to interaction of the stimulant with immunoglobulin or immunoglobulinlike sites on the surfaces of the responding cell and is a reflection of immunocompetence.

Nonspecific mitogens include the plant mitogens: phytohemagglutin (PHA), pokeweed mitogen (PWM), and conconavalin A. The mechanism of action of these mitogens is not fully understood, but is considered to involve alteration in cell membrane permeability. The plant mitogens are important in B-cell and T-cell differentiation. T cells respond to PHA but not to PWM. B cells respond to PWM and not to PHA. This differential reactivity does not totally discriminate between T and B lymphocytes but is useful in general studies in the laboratory (Greaves et al. 1968; Janossy and Greaves 1972).

LYMPHOTOXINS

Transformed T cells have the capacity to attack cells containing specific antigens in their plasma membranes. They appear to do so through the mediation of some poorly defined soluble protein. *Lymphotoxin* is the name applied to these lymphocyte effector molecules which are synthesized by lymphocytes when they attach to target cells, and which in some unknown way cause cell destruction (Able et al. 1970; Woodruff et al. 1972). Cytolysis appears to be mediated through a depressant action on RNA function; no alterations are detectable in the plasma membrane lecithins or sodium pump (Rosenau et al. 1973). The models for study of this action have been mitogen- or antigen-stimulated lymphocytes. Lymphotoxin appears to bind specifically to the plasma membrane of target cells but cannot damage other, nontarget cells to which it may become adjacent (Hessinger et al. 1973).

The target cells must contain specific receptor molecules because, in experiments in vitro, treatment with trypsin renders

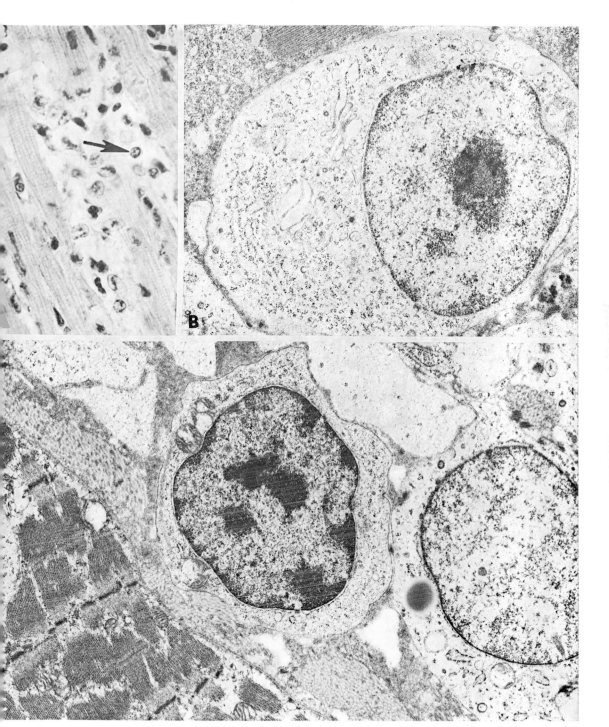

Fig. 5.5. Invasion of muscle cells of bursectomized (nonantibody-forming) chicken infected with Newcastle disease virus. A. Focal histiocytic myocarditis. Few small lymphocytes are present (arrow). B. Small T lymphocyte with well-developed golgi complex but no endoplasmic reticulum. C. Ultrastructure of an immune (sensitized) small lymphocyte which has invaded myocyte. This cell does not form endoplasmic reticulum or synthesize antibody.

them nonsusceptible to lymphotoxin, and they become again fully susceptible when allowed to regenerate these molecular sites on their cell surfaces.

LYMPHOKINES

On contact with specific antigen, immune (sensitized) lymphocytes release soluble factors called *lymphokines* which are attractant to monocytes. By virtue of lymphokine secretion, the transformed T cell induces large numbers of nonspecific effector cells to participate in the cell-mediated reaction.

Lymphokines are a poorly characterized group of humoral factors that modify the behavior of monocytes and, in some cases, eosinophils and basophils. The cacophony of terms used to designate lymphokines results from the diverse methods utilized to establish their existence. Macrophage inhibition factor (MIF) was the first lymphokine described. It inhibits the migration of macrophages on glass surfaces (Dumonde et al. 1969).

The growth of macrophages that are obtained from immune (sensitized) animals and grown in cell cultures is markedly inhibited by the presence of specific antigen. This can be clearly demonstrated by placing peritoneal macrophages from normal and sensitized guinea pigs in capillary tubes and allowing them to migrate from the end of the tube into the culture in the presence of antigen. Macrophages from the normal animal grow in a fan-shaped pattern extending outward from the end of the tube. Those from sensitized animals clump together and are inhibited in growth (David 1966).

When a few peritoneal cells from a sensitized guinea pig are added to cultures of macrophages from a nonsensitized animal, the latter fail to migrate away from the end of the tube. Transfers of pure populations of macrophages do not do this but those containing as few as 1% lymphocytes do. The fact that so few lymphocytes can inhibit migration implicates a soluble factor that mediates inhibition. This factor is found in supernates of incubated small lymphocytes and is called macrophage inhibition factor or MIF.

This evidence indicates that two cells are involved in mediation. Sensitized lymphocytes, which are stimulated to release soluble MIF on contact with antigen, inhibit MIF macrophage migration in vitro and local monocyte mobilization in vivo.

Macrophages cultured in the presence of sensitized lymphocytes and specific antigen behave as if they have lost contact inhibition (semantics become a problem here: the development of macrophage inhibition is associated with loss of contact inhibition). Macrophages clump together and form aggregates of tightly associated cells instead of migrating into loosely arranged monolayers. Macrophage inhibition involves loss of material from the cell membrane. Whereas macrophage migration with normal contact inhibition is a widespread biological phenomenon, its depression may be regarded as an immunologically mediated loss of contact inhibition.

The practicality of MIF tests in the diagnosis of animal diseases has been examined in bacterial and protozoal infections. Although MIF reactivity develops concomitant with infection, the tests are sufficiently cumbersome that they are not accepted as uniform and valid criteria for the routine diagnosis of disease.

Lawrence has successfully transferred tuberculin sensitivity passively by administration of lymphoid cell extracts. His *transfer factor* is a nonantigenic, nonantibody, dialyzable extract of leukocytes which is capable of transferring delayed hypersensitivity. It converts normal lymphocytes in vitro and in vivo to a specific, antigen-responsive state (Lawrence 1969). Therapy with transfer factor in human patients with immunodeficiency disease has had significant effects in warding off systemic fungal infections.

Concerning the lymphokines, it must be emphasized that, by definition. delayed hypersensitivity is a reaction of living animals to antigenic challenge. The validity of soluble factors induced in vitro can only be proven by their demonstration in animals at sites of reactivity.

IMMUNOCOMPETENCE OF FETUS AND NEWBORN

The mammalian fetus, having inherited antigens from its sire, is immunologically incompatible with its mother. Following implantation of the embryo, it becomes, in a sense, a homograft in utero (Lanman and Herod 1965). Cell-mediated rejection of the fetus and placenta by the mother is prevented by several factors. The major barrier involves the curious nonreactivity of the *placental trophoblasts,* which are the cells in direct contact with the maternal tissues. Not only are trophoblasts covered with coats of acidic mucopolysaccharides which tend to mask surface antigens, but also their plasma membranes appear to lack histocompatibility antigens and thereby fail to induce sensitizing of lymphocytes. Other factors of minor importance reinforce the trophoblastic barrier. The lack of vascular interchange between dam and fetus (which varies depending upon the species involved) does not permit large numbers of maternal immunocompetent cells to pass the placenta. The endocrine function of the placenta suppresses the immune system of the pregnant female, probably through adrenal corticosteroid suppression of lymphoid tissues.

ANTIBODY IN THE FETUS

Because its environment is sheltered from antigens, the fetus usually does not make antibodies and is born "virgin." Passive immunity in the developing animal is acquired from the dam (Brambell 1970; Simpson-Morgan and Smeaton 1972). Transmission of immunoglobulins from dam to young may occur before birth, after birth via the colostrum, or, as in most species, by a combination of these pathways (Table 5.4). While the maternal antibodies transmitted are usually protective, they may also inhibit fetal antibody production or cause disease.

If fetal antigens (which are not present in the mother's tissue) enter the maternal circulation, antibodies are formed against them by the dam. When these antibodies are returned to the fetus in the circulation, they may induce disease. The fetal immunogenic substances of most significance are the plasma globulins, erythrocytes, and platelets.

Fetal blood reaches the dam, even in species with tight epitheliochorial placentation (such as the horse and pig), by way of placental trauma and hemorrhage. Anemia may result from the return of antierythrocytic antibodies to the fetus. In primates, where antibodies pass the hemoendothelial placental barrier prenatally, anemia may occur in utero. In horses, mules, and pigs, where antibodies are transmitted in colostrum, hemolytic anemia occurs following suckling.

This situation would be far worse if all immunoglobulins passed the placental barrier. Fortunately, only IgG enters the fetus. The failure of IgA, IgM, and IgE to pass the placenta in significant amounts is important. The major blood group isoantibodies in primates are IgM. The reaginic antibodies associated with hypersensitivity are IgE. If these immunoglobulins reached the fetus, intrauterine disease would be an immense problem.

Prenatally, the fetuses of some species receive maternal antibody via the yolk sac. In others, antibody arrives by direct passage through the placenta. In some species, both the yolk sac and fetal membranes pass immunoglobulins.

In the chicken embryo, antibody transmission occurs through the yolk sac. The

Table 5.4. Transfer of antibody in different species

Species	Route of Transfer	Selective	Time and Duration of Transfer
Chicken	Yolk sac	+	17 days incubation to 2 days after hatching
Rat, Mouse	Yolk sac Placenta Intestine	+	Prenatal and to 18 days after birth
Rabbit	Yolk sac	+	Prenatal from 15 days of gestation
Cat	Intestine		Postnatal (variable)
Dog	Intestine		Birth to 8 days
Pig	Intestine	−	36 hours after birth
Cow, Sheep	Intestine	−	36 hours after birth
Horse	Intestine	−	36 hours after birth
Primate	Placenta	+	Prenatal (late in gestation)

process also continues after hatching, since the yolk sac persists in the newly hatched chick. Even before the ovum is ovulated, antibodies (IgG) are selectively secreted by the ovarian follicular epithelium and are eventually stored in the yolk. The close relation of the oocyte and follicle in the hen's ovary apparently permits this early globulin transmission. Saline extraction of yolk reveals a series of globulins which are probably identical to serum globulins. The yolk sac membrane continues to secrete globulins into the yolk. By injecting I^{131}-labeled chicken γ-globulin into hens (Patterson et al. 1962), the labeled globulin is revealed (by autoradiographs) in the yolk; transmission becomes increasingly rapid during the final growth of the oocyte.

Transmission of maternal antibodies to fetal circulation in rodents is often from uterine lumen into the fetal yolk sac. Yolk sac endoderm is exposed to uterine fluids and absorbs their antibodies. Transmission of immunoglobulins is highly selective. The homologous γ-globulin is transported to far greater extent than other maternal serum proteins. It may be that specific receptors are present on the absorptive cells of the yolk sac endoderm. Absorption of globulins by yolk sac endoderm is by pinocytosis. The absorptive capacity of these cells is indicated by a microvillous border, glycocalyx, many cytoplasmic pinocytotic vesicles, and lysosomes.

Although the developing fetus is immunologically virgin, it becomes immunocompetent with the embryonic development of its lymphoid system. If stimulated antigenically, it will produce plasmacytes and immunoglobulins. Fetuses infected with pathogenic microorganisms have extensive plasmacytosis of affected tissues and develop high serum antibody titers. If a pregnant cow develops leptospirosis, the fetus becomes infected and reacts immunologically against the leptospires (Fennestad and Borg-Petersen 1962).

ANTIBODIES IN THE NEONATE

Nearly all newborn mammals receive antibodies from the colostrum of the mother. The pregnant female develops antibodies against potential pathogens in her immediate environment and therefore can offer, in her milk, passive protection to her newborn. Passive immunity protects the neonatal animal until its own rapidly developing immunologic mechanisms are sufficiently mature for active protection.

MAMMARY GLAND SECRETION OF GLOBULIN IN COLOSTRUM

IgA is the major immunoglobulin in colostrum in many species. In theory, the globulin molecule is produced in plasmacytes within the gland or arrives from the maternal circulation and is stored within the mammary gland acinar cells. These molecules are complexed with a secretory piece and are secreted as IgA. The acinar cell of the mammary gland also functions to transport maternal serum antibodies during colostrum formation. Circulating IgG is concentrated by these cells immediately after birth, but this ability is reduced sharply after initial colostral secretion.

In the cow, the immunoglobulins in colostrum are chiefly IgG from the serum; IgA makes up a smaller proportion of colostral antibody than in most animals. During colostrum secretion, the interstitial fluid of the bovine mammary gland stroma increases markedly (Dixon et al. 1961; Feldman 1961). Immunofluorescent studies reveal globulins as well as albumin and other serum proteins in this fluid. Few plasmacytes are present and it is therefore believed that most globulins arrive from the maternal circulation. The secretory vacuoles of the hypertrophic acinar cells become loaded with globulin (but not albumin) and this is consistent with the function of transporting maternal serum proteins during colostrum formation.

ABSORPTION OF GLOBULIN BY THE INTESTINE

Most colostrums contain trypsin inhibitors that facilitate the passage of globulins undegraded through the stomach. In the intestine of most species, the capacity to absorb globulin molecules intact is transitory, lasting only a few hours. The structure and function of the intestinal absorptive epithelial cell rapidly becomes tight and selective. If colostrum is not fed until 48 hrs after birth, it is then too late for antibodies to be absorbed. They may act within the gut but will be digested and destroyed, for only degraded proteins will reach the circulation.

Colostral proteins are taken into the intestinal epithelial cell nonselectively by pinocytosis. In the apical and basal portions of the active intestinal absorptive cell, there is a dramatic increase in vesicles and vacuoles; globulin can be demonstrated within these structures histochemically. The globulins are not transmitted to the circulation with equal facility in different species (Kraehenbuhl and Campiche 1969). In the pig, whole molecules are transmitted intact. In other animals, selective degradation by epithelial cell lysosomal enzymes transmits fragments of globulin.

The newborn pig has been used as a model for the study of intestinal absorption of colostral globulins. The rapid transmission of globulins from sow to suckling pig is revealed in parallel changes in serum proteins of the piglets. Globulin levels, low at birth, increase rapidly after suckling. By 24 hrs, the piglet has absorbed enough colostral immunoglobulin to give serum concentrations as high as or higher than those of the sow (Jönsson 1973). If pigs are deprived of colostrum, immunoglobulins in their serum are usually too low to be detected. Following injection of antigen into the newborn pig, a true primary immune response results within 48 hrs. The first molecules to appear are IgM and these are followed by synthesis of IgG (Kim et al. 1968).

EMBRYONIC DEVELOPMENT OF IMMUNOCOMPETENCE

The first hematopoietic cells of the avian and mammalian embryo are formed early in the yolk sac. Called *hemocytoblasts* by Maximow, these stem cells have large basophilic cytoplasmic areas that consist of masses of free ribosomes. Hemocytoblasts migrate and seed other sites. Yolk sac suspensions from 4-day chick embryos (when erythroid hemopoiesis is occurring) can repopulate both lymphoid and myeloid organs of irradiated 13-day embryos (Moore and Owen 1967). After seeding begins, hemopoiesis in the yolk sac is gradually replaced by that in the liver and spleen and finally in the bone marrow, where it persists throughout life. The first real evidence of lymphoid development is the appearance of the thymus.

In most species the bone marrow is the source of undifferentiated stem cells, called by some "bone marrow lymphocytes" (Ford et al. 1966; Goldschneider and McGregor 1966; McGregor 1968). When mice are irradiated to destroy immunocompetence, they will recover and produce antibody and lymphocytes near normal levels if bone marrow sites are shielded during radiation. Mice not shielded can be repopulated by injection of normal syngeneic bone marrow cells. However, these cells correct the mouse's immunologic defect only if that mouse has an intact thymus. From this and other data, it is now believed that small lymphocytes of marrow origin are trapped in the thymus and other organs for further differentiation. Specialization at these sites confers upon the lymphoid cell progeny of marrow lymphocytes their special ability to react immunologically.

CENTRAL LYMPHOID ORGANS

The responsibility for conferring immunoreactivity on developing lymphoid cells is associated with the central lymphoid organs: the thymus and gut-associated lymphoid tissues. These organs resemble one another in respect to their endodermal origin, embryonic development, lymphoid content, and postnatal involution. Although immune reactions do not normally occur in these structures, their presence in neonatal life is essential if normal populations of immunologically competent lymphocytes are to develop.

THYMUS

The function of the thymus is to trap marrow-derived lymphocytes, to confer specialization upon them, and to induce them to replicate. Thymic or T lymphocytes can be differentiated from other small lymphocytes by the antigenic makeup of their cell membranes (although this is possible only in mice where purified antigen preparations can be obtained). Their progeny function in cell-mediated immu-

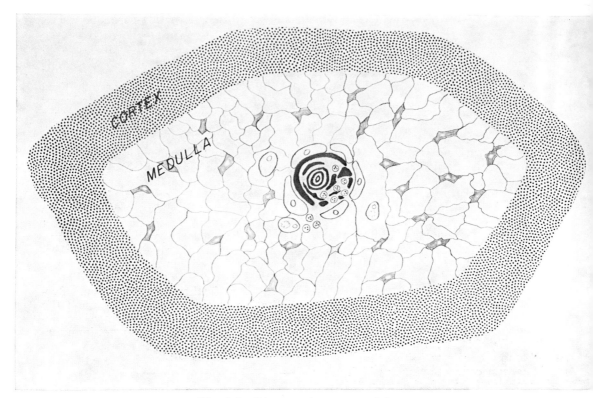

Fig. 5.6.   Diagram of structure of thymus.

nity and as helpers in the afferent limb of antibody production.

The thymus is already a prominent lymphoid organ at birth, when the spleen and lymph nodes are poorly developed. Within the thymus, small lymphocytes multiply, with local death of many and emigration of a few. Lymphocytopoiesis, since it is weighted toward small lymphocyte production, does not fully maintain the thymic lymphocyte population. The marrow-derived lymphocytes are believed to be more efficient as thymic lymphocyte precursors than as thymic lymphocytes themselves.

All animals phylogenetically above the lamprey have a thymus. Even in the lamprey, a primitive prothymus consisting of small foci of lymphocytes within the epi-thelium of the pharyngeal gutter is present. In mammals and birds, the thymic lobule consists of a distinct small lymphocyte-rich cortex and a medulla of epithelial cells in a reticular cell framework.

The thymic cortex is made of a loose network of stellate epithelial-reticular cells filled with heavy populations of small dense lymphocytes. The reticular cells contain tonofibrils and are attached to one another by desmosomes (Fig. 5.6). Necrobiosis of lymphocytes during lymphopoiesis activates the reticular cells, which phagocytize lymphocyte debris and enlarge to immense pale macrophages containing cell debris or "tingable bodies" (Fig. 5.7). The thymic cortex is supplied exclusively by capillaries which have impermeable endothelial junctions (Raviola and Karnovsky

Fig. 5.7.   Thymic atrophy, pig, hog cholera. A. Focal lymphocytolysis and phagocytosis by cortical macrophages (early change). B. Complete atrophy of cortex. C. Atrophic thymic macrophage (m) contains lysosomes and cell debris. It is surrounded by small lymphocytes and is adjacent to the dark cortical reticulum (arrow).

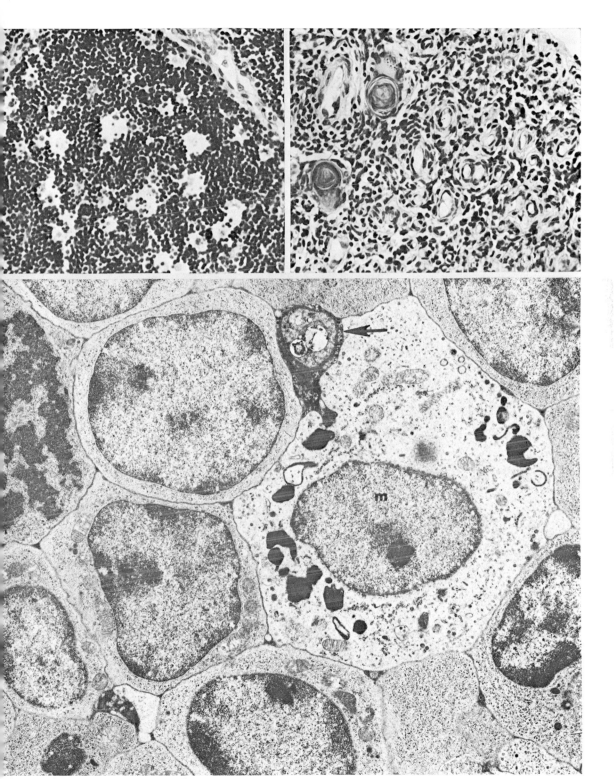

1972). Although small amounts of macro-molecules are transported through the endothelium by pinocytotic vesicles, they are promptly taken up by perivascular macrophages and do not contact the lymphocytes.

In contrast, the blood vessels of the medulla are of the "leaky" variety, arterioles and postcapillary venules. Tracer materials injected intravenously escape readily into medullary areas, and cells in this zone are freely exposed to bloodborne substances. *Thymic corpuscles* (of Hassall) consist of immense epithelial cells (Curtis et al. 1972; Mandel 1968). Ultrastructurally, the various forms of these cells are called: (1) squamous, which are filled with tonofilaments and keratinize in the corpuscles; (2) villous, which line the cleftlike spaces around the corpuscle periphery and contain surface microvilli which stain for acidic mucopolysaccharides; and (3) cystic, which contain dense granules and cytoplasmic canaliculi also with microvilli (Fig. 5.8). These cells concentrate S^{35} and glucosamine and their structure is consistent with a secretory function (Clark 1968). Thymic corpuscles are active structures. They are involved in uptake of plasma globulin, phagocytosis, antigen localization, and the accretion of dead thymic lymphocytes and debris (Blau 1973).

Thymic epithelial cells synthesize polypeptides that promote transformation of T cells. These extracts of thymus include thymic factor (MW 1000), thymosin (MW 12000), and thymopoietin (MW 7000); all induce the in vitro differentiation of bone marrow precursor cells. Thymosin has been used clinically to treat human patients with congenital immunodeficiency disease and is credited with some success (Goldstein 1974).

Pathologic states of the thymus that indicate clinical disease include atrophy and hypoplasia (or aplasia). The thymus is considered a barometer of nutrition and atrophy is a response to many factors: mal-nutrition, cortisone, radiomimetric drugs, toxins, and systemic infectious diseases. The direct effect of some viruses on thymic destruction with clinical sequelae is an intriguing but poorly understood phenomenon. When atrophy occurs, the early stages are characterized by enlargement and proliferation of the epithelial and reticular cells of the medulla (van Haelst 1969). Thymic corpuscles become immense and are filled with necrotic debris and eosinophils. Thymic aplasia is described in human infants with clinical syndromes involving defects in cell-mediated immunity. There is absence of thymic tissue and hypoplasia of regions in peripheral lymphoid tissues (spleen and lymph nodes) that are populated in the neonate by thymic or T lymphocytes.

In the chick embryo, the thymus becomes functional on the seventh day of incubation, the day on which large hemocytoblasts are first visible. Timing of lymphocyte invasion was determined by evaluating the capacity of thymic rudiments (removed from embryos of various ages) to develop lymphocytes in vitro: 6-day thymuses remained epithelial, 7-day thymuses became lymphoid (Moore and Owen 1967).

Experimental studies on thymic function utilize removal of the thymus (thymectomy), a difficult task in some animals and impossible in most. Even if the thymus is totally removed, the animal must be heavily irradiated to remove thymic lymphocytes which are seeded into the peripheral tissues before birth.

Thymectomy in chickens does not markedly inhibit antibody formation, but causes marked inhibition of cellular immune responses (Cooper 1966). This has given rise to the concept of separate immune systems in the chicken. The thymus is responsible for lymphocytes involved in cellular immunity; the bursa (gut-associated lymphoid tissue) is associated with antibody formation. In mammals, separateness

Fig. 5.8. Thymic corpuscle. A. Ultrastructure of young squamous epithelial cell. B. Histology of purulent inflammatory reaction, cow. Corpuscle is filled with neutrophils and surrounded by squamous epithelial cells. C. Ultrastructure of microvilli, villous epithelial cell. D. Histochemical staining of mucopolysaccharides, cystic epithelial cell. E. Cytoplasmic canaliculus, cystic epithelial cell. F. Necrosis of a cystic epithelial cell.

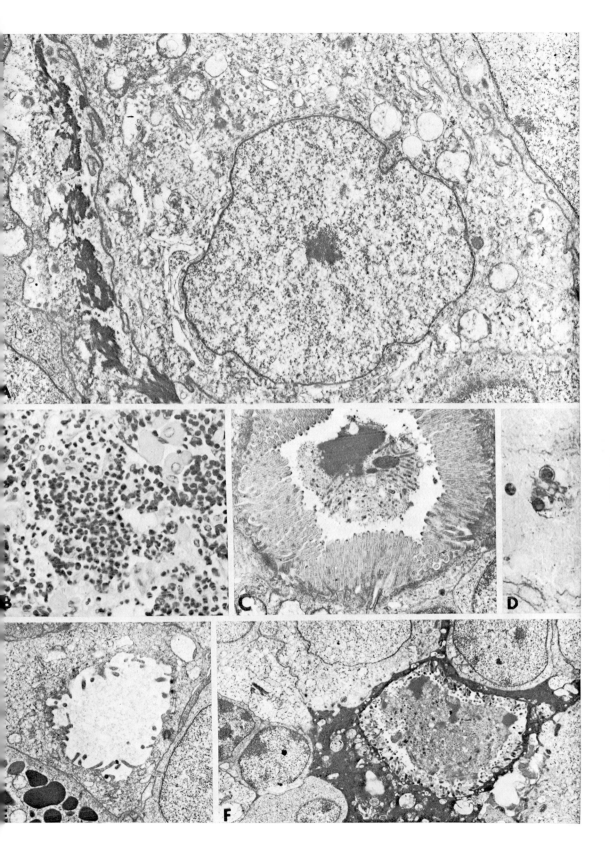

of function is not clearcut, and thymus-derived cells are believed to be required for some humoral responses.

Thymectomy in neonatal mice impairs the immune response, although immunoglobulin levels are not significantly lower. It causes depletion of the recirculating pool of lymphocytes; thymectomized mice develop a wasting syndrome evidenced by emaciation, ruffled fur, and death (Miller 1962). Microscopic examination reveals: (1) lymphoid depletion (lymphopenia and absence of germinal centers in spleen and lymph nodes); (2) impaired immune responses to soluble antigens and skin homografts; and (3) endocrine disturbances (atrophy of anterior pituitary and thyroid L cells). Secondary sex characteristics fail to develop.

GUT-ASSOCIATED LYMPHOID TISSUE

Immunoincompetent bone marrow lymphocytes acquire the capacity to transform into antibody-producing plasmacytes somewhere beyond their bone marrow origin. At present this area is not precisely defined in mammals. Evidence points toward lymphoid tissues within the alimentary canal which function as central lymphoid organs to confer immunocompetence upon thymic-independent, undifferentiated lymphocytes. Epithelium within these structures has the selective capacity to pinocytose and transport antigens and this may be associated with differentiation of lymphocytes (Bockman and Cooper 1973).

THE BURSA OF FABRICIUS IN BIRDS

The bursa has many structural similarities to the thymus (Fig. 5.9). Each lymphoid follicle contains a cortical zone filled with small dense lymphocytes which is separated from a reticular medullary area by a single layer of undifferentiated endodermal epithelial cells. The epithelial cells become prominent during age-related atrophy and may form mucus-secreting glandular epithelium (Fig. 5.10).

The significance of the bursa in establishing the capacity to produce antibodies was clearly demonstrated by Glick's bursectomy experiments. Removal of the bursa at hatching (accompanied by radiation to kill lymphocytes that had seeded periph-

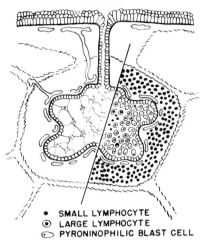

BURSA
LUMEN

• SMALL LYMPHOCYTE
◉ LARGE LYMPHOCYTE
◎ PYRONINOPHILIC BLAST CELL

Fig. 5.9. Diagram of avian bursa.

erally before this time) left the chick without the ability to form plasmacytes and antibodies. Bursal function was most critical around the hatching period; bursectomy after this time had little effect. The functions of the bursal lymphocytes were distinct from those of the thymic-dependent lymphocytes; cell-mediated reactions remained intact unless the thymus was also removed (Cooper 1966; Warner et al. 1962).

Near the end of embryonic development crucial changes occur in the bursa. Stem cells, arriving from the yolk sac, liver, or marrow, are induced to undergo a switch in genetic commitment to become B lymphocytes. IgM is synthesized by these cells and can be found on their surfaces (Cooper et al. 1972). After several generations of these cells have replicated, some of their progeny switch to begin making IgG. It is probable that a subsequent switch to IgA production occurs later. When these cells leave the bursa, contact with antigen drives them to become plasmacytes.

Although the bursa is of unquestionable importance as a central lymphoid organ, it also functions as a peripheral organ that participates in responses to antigens. Microbial antigens enter the bursal duct during passage through the alimentary tract. They also enter via the anus, picked up by

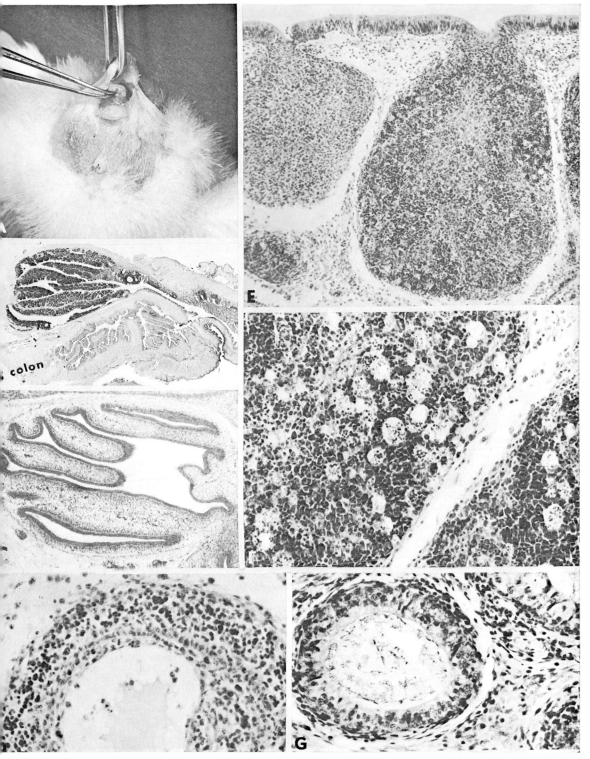

Fig. 5.10. Bursa, chicken. A. Bursectomy. Bursa is at tip of lower forceps. B. Histology, full development. C. In 11-day chick embryo. D. Cystic degeneration of bursal follicle. E. Relation of bursal epithelium to follicle. F. Viral-induced lymphocytolysis in the bursa (Gumboro disease). G. Complete bursal atrophy after viral destruction. Only mucopolysaccharide-producing epithelium remains.

the peristaltic movements of the anal lips. Within the lumen of the bursa, antigens first localize in the epithelial pad overlying the follicle and penetrate the follicle to participate in the instruction of antibody-producing cells.

PEYER'S PATCHES OF MAMMALS

The Peyer's patches are islands of lymph-oid tissue in the submucosa of the mammalian small intestine. Located in the terminal ileum, they are closely associated with the epithelial layer and its microbial flora. The lymphocyte population of the Peyer's patches contains both B and T cells (Kagnoff and Campbell 1974). There is growing evidence that these lymphoid organs and the appendices of the intestine have the same relationship to antibody production in mammals as does the bursa in birds (Heim et al. 1972; Perey and Guttman 1972). Removal of these tissues, although impossible to do completely, appears to negate much of the antibody-producing capacity of the animals. Like the thymus, these organs do not contain antibody but give rise to precursor cells which do (Bienenstock and Dolezel 1971). They should not be confused with tissues of the lamina propria of the intestine which contain large numbers of plasmacytes and are known to respond by the production of antibody. Putting all evidence together, it seems most likely that lymphoid tissues in the gut function both as central and peripheral lymphoid organs. They not only contain the capacity to participate in the normal IgG-producing mechanisms of the host, but also contain most of the IgA-producing plasmacytes of the secretory antibody system.

TONSILS

Tonsils have a highly penetrable epithelium. They receive antigens from the oropharynx and transmit them via efferent lymphatics to cervical lymph nodes (there are no afferent lymphatics). The epithelial cells of the tonsillar crypts are phagocytic and may play important roles in antigen processing (Williams and Rowland 1972).

SEEDING OF PERIPHERAL LYMPHOID TISSUES

Small lymphocytes that have differentiated in the central lymphoid organs are seeded into peripheral tissues at or near birth. They appear to be attracted to specific anatomical sites in the lymph nodes and spleen. The interpretation of abnormal lymphoid tissue in these organs in terms of function is complex. In animals with naturally occurring disease, tissue changes, which encompass different processes occurring simultaneously, are far different from those in animals inoculated experimentally with well-defined antigens.

In lower vertebrates, aggregates of lymphocytes develop at sites of antigen localization throughout the body. True germinal centers develop and persist. Well-defined lymph nodes assume this function in mammals. They are located along lymph vessels for the purpose of trapping and processing particulate material. When antigens occur in lymph, they are thus brought into close contact with the machinery that will provide both the translative and effector (or afferent and efferent) limbs of the immune response.

LYMPH NODE

A thorough knowledge of the anatomy of the mammalian lymph node is essential to an understanding of immunopathology (Fig. 5.11). Antigens, which arrive in the efferent lymphatics, percolate through the loose reticular-cell networks of the subcapsular or cortical sinus and into those of the medullary sinus. They are trapped on the dendritic webs of the reticular cells and phagocytized. During the first immune response the vascular structures of the node expand in association with lymphoid proliferation and the medullary cords become filled with proliferating plasmablasts. In the presence of antibody the uptake of antigens become extremely efficient and plays a significant role in retention of these substances at sites of antibody production (Fig. 5.12).

Germinal centers in the cortex provide the most efficient structures for the continuing formation of immunocompetent B-lymphoid cells. These aggregates are seeded by B lymphocytes and develop through

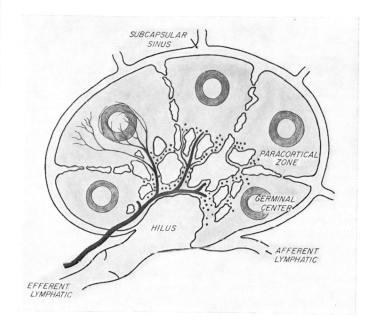

Fig. 5.11. Diagram of structural components of a mammalian lymph node.

stages of cell production which can be artificially divided into: (1) primary centers, small foci of dense lymphocytes in the cortical bed; (2) secondary centers, large active nodules with pale centers and dense outer rims; and (3) tertiary centers, large nodules composed of exhausted reticular cells. The active secondary germinal centers consist of a center zone (TPA, or thinly populated area), a corona of dense small lymphocytes, and a mantle zone. Bone marrow stem cells appear to populate the center zone but differentiated B cells of bursal or gut origin are required for functional mantle zones (Nieuwenhuis and Keuning 1974)

Animals not competent immunologically (by reason of immaturity, exhaustion of old age, disease, or therapy) do not form germinal centers efficiently. When the organs responsible for differentiating bone marrow lymphocytes into immunocompetent antibody-forming cells are removed, germinal centers do not develop. For example, the removal of gut-associated lymphoid tissues from rabbits causes the lymph nodes of these animals to be devoid of germinal centers.

The paracortical areas are theoretically seeded by thymic-dependent T lymphocytes (De Sousa and Parrott 1969; Parrott et al. 1966). In these areas are located the post-capillary venules with high endothelium through which the small lymphocytes of the recirculating pool emigrate. Lymphocytes migrate through endothelial cell junctions (Howard et al. 1971; McGregor 1964; Schoefl 1972). The high endothelium is a special adaptation to allow excessive fluid loss. High endothelium does not develop in response to antigens to the same extent as it is developed in venules of germ-free and conventional animals (Claesson and Jørgensen 1974). Although in experimentally thymectomized rodents paracortical areas are atrophic, it is difficult to assess similar lesions in the pathologic examination of clinical material. In animals responding to cell-mediated reactions such as contact hypersensitivity, the paracortical areas are enlarged and filled with large blastic lymphocytes (Anderson and McKeating 1970; De Sousa et al. 1969).

In one sense, the lymph nodes are chiefly instruments for collecting, reacting with, and transmitting small lymphocytes. They receive large numbers of lymphocytes from blood and discharge them into lymph. In sheep, which have been extensively studied, at least 30 million lymphocytes an hour are discharged in efferent lymph. They enter the lymph nodes from blood, traverse the high endothelium of postcapillary venules in the subcortical re-

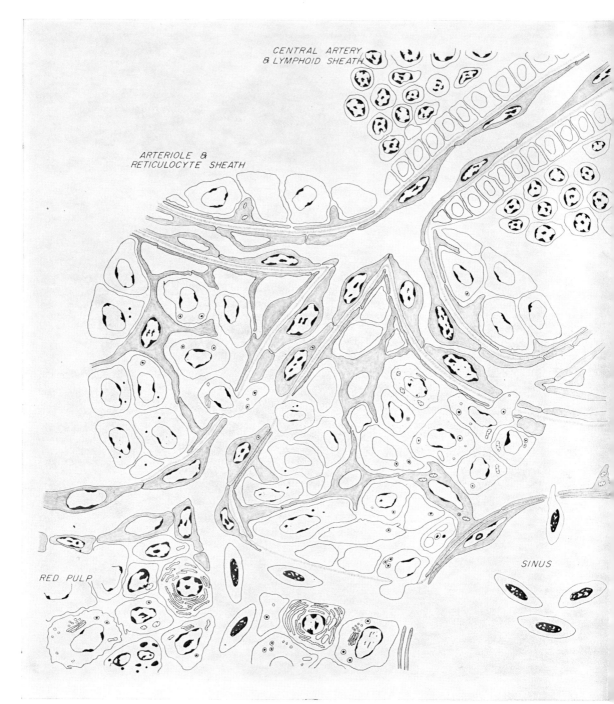

CENTRAL ARTERY
& LYMPHOID SHEATH

ARTERIOLE &
RETICULOCYTE SHEATH

RED PULP

SINUS

Fig. 5.15. Diagram of components of spleen. Periarterial lymphoid
sheath, periarteriolar reticular sheath, red pulp, venous sinus.

Table 5.5. Immunodeficiency syndromes

Primary
  Humoral: agammaglobulinemia (Bruton type,
    man)
  Cellular: thymic aplasia (DiGeorge syndrome,
    man) (Nu-nu mouse; De Sousa 1969)
  Combined: agammaglobulinemia (Swiss type,
    man)
  Specific Ig deficiency: IgA deficiency reported in
    man
  Partial deficiency: Wiskot-Alrich syndrome, man
Secondary
  Postviral immune deficiency: hog cholera, pan-
    leukopenia (cat) bovine viral diarrhea, mea-
    sles, etc.
  Neoplasm-associated: plasmacytoma, thymoma,
    lymphosarcoma
  Aging
  Malnutrition
  Drug-induced

production is depressed but cell-mediated immunity is normal. The commonest and most severe genetic defects are combined immunodeficiencies; both B- and T-cell populations are defective and antibody production and cell-mediated immunity are both depressed (Table 5.5).

COMBINED IMMUNODEFICIENCY OF HORSES

A fatal genetic combined B- and T-lymphocyte immunodeficiency occurs in Arabian foals. The clinical diagnosis is based on lymphopenia (less than 1000/cmm), hypoplasia of the thymus, absence of germinal centers and periarteriolar lymphoid sheaths in the spleen, and absence of one or more serum immunoglobulin classes. IgM is invariably absent and IgA is missing in about 50% of the affected foals (McGuire et al. 1974). Foals with combined immunodeficiency are highly susceptible to respiratory disease and usually die with some form of pneumonia. High mortality occurs from adenoviral infections and from *Pneumocystis carinii* lesions. Neither of these diseases is of clinical importance in normal horses. Combined immunodeficiency in Arabian horses appears to be an autosomal recessive trait. Affected foals do not live to breeding age; they include both males and females; and their sires and dams are not afflicted.

THYMIC APLASIA IN MICE

Nude mice (nu/nu) are a hairless, growth-retarded strain that is affected with thymic dysgenesis (not agenesis). The thymic rudiment does not contain lymphocytes or Hassal's corpuscles, but consists of cysts whose walls are lined with squamous or cubic cells of glandular character. Ciliated and mucous cells are present and plasmacytes and mast cells can be found in the interstitium (Cordier 1974). As a result of this defect, nude mice are deficient in the inductive capacity of normal thymic epithelium. They have bone marrow precursor T cells but lack T lymphocytes. Their circulating lymphocytes all contain surface immunoglobulins indicating that they are B cells. Serum globulin levels are relatively unchanged, although IgA levels may be low and antibody formation is retarded.

Nude mice are totally deficient in cell-mediated immunoreactivity. They will accept skin grafts not only from allogenic mice but from other animal species including birds and reptiles (Rygaard and Povlsen 1974). T-cell function can be restored by grafting a neonatal thymus from a normal mouse (Crewther and Warner 1972; De Sousa et al. 1969). It is also alleged that administration of the thymic polypeptide hormone called thymosin will correct many of the deficits of nude mice.

THYMIC APLASIA OF CATTLE

Several immunodeficiency syndromes have been reported in cattle, but none has been adequately examined immunologically. A lethal syndrome due to an autosomal recessive mode of inheritance occurs in calves of the Black Danish breed. It is characterized by exanthema, hair loss, and parakeratosis. There are severe hypoplasia of the thymus and depletion of peripheral lymphoid tissues (Brummerstedt et al. 1974). Antibody production is depressed, but probably secondary to the primary thymic deficit. Selective deficiency of IgG_2 has also been reported in cattle with increased susceptibility to infection (Nansen 1972).

DYSGAMMAGLOBULINEMIA OF CHICKENS

A dysgammaglobulinemia has been reported in chickens in which thymic and bursal tissues appear normal. The defect was not precisely defined but was believed to be a secretory disturbance in plasma-

Table 5.6. Methods of immunosuppression

Surgical	Bursectomy; removal of gut-associated lymphoid tissue
	Thymectomy
	Thoracic duct cannulation
Biological	Antilymphocyte globulin (ALG)
	Adrenal corticosteroids
	Viruses (lympholytic)
Chemical	Folic acid antagonists (methotrexate)
	Purine analogs (6mp, 5fu)
	Nitrogen mustards
Physical	Radiation
	Burns

cytes characterized by delayed maturation (Lösch and Hoffman-Fezer 1973).

ACQUIRED IMMUNOLOGIC DEFECTS

Transient immunosuppression develops during many systemic viral diseases. This is particularly characteristic of the viruses causing hog cholera, bovine viral diarrhea, canine distemper, and Newcastle disease which replicate in the reticuloendothelial and lymphoid systems. Immunosuppression can be induced therapeutically by many different mechanisms (Table 5.6). These methods are used clinically to prolong the survival of grafts, to suppress immunologic components of acute inflammation, and to kill neoplastic cells. Some agents cause selective destruction of either cellular or humoral mechanisms. For example, antilymphocyte serum preferentially affects cell-mediated immunoreactivity, and there is evidence that radiomimetic drugs have a greater effect on the T-cell population than on B cells (Stockman et al. 1973).

CHEMICAL IMMUNOSUPPRESSION

Alkylating agents produce profound suppressive effects on immune responses by their toxicity to lymphocytes. They alkylate nucleic acids by forming cross-links with nucleoside bases and thereby interfere with DNA biosynthesis. Cyclophosphamide can be used to completely suppress the antibody formation of newly hatched chicks and can be used to suppress the incidence of the B-cell–dependent lymphoid leukosis virus. Purine analogues with substitution of a sulfhydryl group on the sixth position of the purine ring are

effective immunosuppressants. Mercaptopurine, like most, inhibits multiple enzymes involved in purine synthesis and may suppress a number of cellular functions. Methotrexate functions as a powerful inhibitor of dihydrofolate reductase and thereby depresses DNA synthesis due to suppressed thymidylate formation.

Clinically, two major drawbacks exist for chemical immunosuppressants. First, there is rarely a clearly defined correlation between clinical responsiveness to a grafted tissue and the measurement of immunoreactivity. Second, because most immunosuppressive drugs were developed as anticancer agents, a wide variety of distressing side effects occur.

VIRAL IMMUNOSUPPRESSION

Many of the viruses that cause systemic disease are known to produce transient immunosuppression by virtue of replication in the reticuloendothelial and lymphoid systems. Acute hog cholera, avian Newcastle disease, bovine viral diarrhea, and canine distemper all develop because the host's immune system has lost a race with a particularly virulent strain of virus during the incubation period.

Lymphocytic choriomeningitis (LCM) of mice has been studied as a model of viral immunosuppression. The effect of LCM virus is reflected in both altered antibody production and cell-mediated reactivity. Selective destruction of T lymphocytes and necrosis of the thymus and thymic-dependent areas of the lymph nodes and speen are responsible for the term "viral thymectomy" applied to the biologic effect of LCM virus. Why these lympholytic effects do not occur in the persistent infections of newborn mice is not clearly established.

IMMUNOLOGIC TOLERANCE

Historically, the dominant theory of antibody production was that the pattern to fit the determinant groups of a specific antigen was formed upon the antibody molecule during its synthesis by an antigen template. Burnet pointed out that this did not account for: (1) continued antibody production after antigen had disappeared or (2) the lack of antibody formation to "self" proteins. He theorized that when immunocompetent cells encounter antigens in fetal life, they are deflected forever from antibody production against that antigen. Medawar's experiments on skin grafting soon confirmed that if a pure-line mouse was inoculated as a fetus with cells from a donor mouse of a different allogeneic strain, it would subsequently accept a skin homograft from the same donor mouse while skin from a second unrelated donor was rejected. Medawar called this acquired tolerance.[1] By injection of syngeneic sensitized lymphoid cells into "tolerant" graft-bearing mice, rapid rejection of the graft occurred. Tolerance was promptly ended by the activity of the lymphoid cells on the graft.

The first naturally occurring example of immune tolerance was pointed out by Medawar as red blood cell chimerism in nonidentical cattle twins with vascular anastomoses and mixing of the placental circulations. Such dizygotic twins will also accept skin grafts from one another. Similar red blood cell chimerism has been reported in lambs.

Tolerance is thought to be the absence of specific reactive immunocompetent cells. The presence of antigen is required in the thymus where stem cells differentiate to immunocompetent cells. Here the newly differentiated thymic-dependent lymphocytes are sensitive to and are destroyed by antigen. Tolerance wanes as the antigen

1. Experimental induction of tolerance was first shown by prolonged graft survival in chicks. It was not understood and was interpreted as "antigenic adaption."

disappears from the recipient. Antigens that diffuse fully are more apt to induce tolerance than those that concentrate on macrophages, the latter being more immunogenic. Some interpret this as antigen reaching cell surfaces of many lymphocytes and inducing in some unknown way their nonreactivity.

IMMUNOLOGIC DISEASE

Antibody and immune cell production are usually associated with immunity, the absence of clinical disease on exposure to antigen. The extremes of the range in which an animal reacts to antigen, however, include, on the one hand, *tolerance,* where antigen inhibits antibody production, and on the other, *hypersensitivity* (allergy), which is an exaggerated reaction to antigen. The hypersensitivity diseases may be classified into four categories (Table 5.7) based upon the mechanisms responsible for inducing tissue changes. The first three are immediate hypersensitivities, and are examples of how antibody acts in producing disease. Antibody is present in serum; the reaction can be passively transferred to normal recipient animals. The fourth, cell-mediated hypersensitivity, is mediated through interaction of small lymphocytes and macrophages and can only be transferred passively with cells, not serum. The tissue reaction, in contrast to that of immediate hypersensitivity, is delayed in appearance.

It must be emphasized that many naturally occurring diseases are mixtures of

Table 5.7. Categories of hypersensitive disease with experimental models and naturally occurring examples. Groups I, II, and III are mediated by antibody (the immediate hypersensitivities)

Disease	Experimental Model	Natural Disease
I. Anaphylaxis	Passive cutaneous anaphylaxis	Allergic shock Allergic rhinitis
II. Cytotoxic disease	Experimental immune anemia	Hemolytic disease of the newborn Transfusion reaction Autoimmune hemolytic anemia Drug reaction
III. Immune complex disease	Arthus reaction	Serum sickness Glomerulonephritis
IV. Cellular (delayed) hypersensitivity	Tuberculin reaction	Contact hypersensitivity Homograft rejection Extrinsic allergic alveolitis Autoimmune thyroiditis

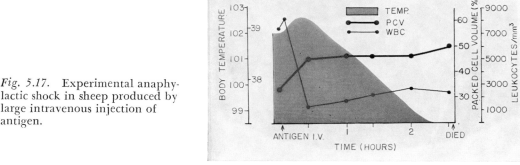

Fig. 5.17. Experimental anaphylactic shock in sheep produced by large intravenous injection of antigen.

ATOPIC ALLERGY

The term *atopic* is used in allergic phenomena to imply a familial association. Reactions of this type are immediate and involve such shock organs as skin (urticaria), upper respiratory tract (rhinitis, or "hay fever"), and bronchioles (as in asthma). Antigens (reagins) can be demonstrated bound to affected tissues, particularly mast cells (Rappaport 1969).

Rhinitis occurs in some species when antigens such as ragweed pollen are inhaled. In dogs, allergic respiratory reactions do occur but the chief response is dermatitis (Arkins et al. 1967; Patterson and Sparks 1962; Walton 1971). The reagins can be demonstrated in serum and react with reaginic antibody (IgE) in the skin. Reaginic antibody will also passively transfer anaphylaxis. Skin reactivity proving atopic allergy can be demonstrated in affected animals by injecting dilute antigen intradermally. An immediate wheal-and-flare reaction due to histamine release differentiates this mechanism from Arthus reactivity and cellular hypersensitivity.

POSTVACCINAL WHEAL AND FLARE REACTIONS

Vaccines prepared in cell cultures and chicken embryos are capable of inducing *wheal and flare* lesions in the skin when used repeatedly. These "anaphylactoid" reactions usually involve several mechanisms, but mast-cell degranulation and localized edema are often dominant. The repeated use of a live foot-and-mouth virus vaccine grown in baby hamster kidney (BHK) cells was responsible for a severe disease in cattle. Eczema and proliferative and nodular dermal lesions with ulceration developed on the udder, perineal skin, and coronary band. Abortion was allegedly part of the syndrome. The reaction was traced to antibodies against proteins of normal BHK cells (Mayr et al. 1969).

Measles vaccines have been implicated in postvaccinal hypersensitivity in humans. Live measles vaccine grown in chicken embryos causes the syndrome when given repeatedly to children with egg protein allergies. Inactivated measles and mumps vaccines induce similar reactions (Harris et al. 1969). It is probable that repeated bee stings and other insect venoms induce transitory postvaccinal-type reactions of edema and swelling.

CYTOTOXIC DISEASE

These diseases are mediated through the lytic reaction of circulating antibody (either IgG or IgM) to antigens that are components of tissues and cells. In most diseases, complement is involved. Most naturally occurring examples are quite complex and many also involve cell-mediated mechanisms of reactivity, the direct action of sensitized lymphocytes on tissue antigens.

TRANSFUSION REACTION

Isoantibodies are those formed against antigenic cell proteins (isoantigens) which differ among individuals of the same species. Generally, isoantibodies are important in relation to cellular antigens such as those on erythrocyte surfaces. In normal baby pig sera, isoantibodies may develop against γ-globulin that has crossed the maternal-fetal barrier.

Landsteiner in 1900 discovered the iso-antigens A and B (and consequently the blood groups A, B, AB, and O) in human red blood cells. These form the strict lim itations of red blood cell transplantation (transfusion) in man. Human blood type is based upon differences in the sugar moiety of the glycoprotein components of the erythrocyte's plasma membrane. Type A contains an enzyme that transfers acetyl-galactosamine to the core protein; type B contains an enzyme that transfers galac-tose. Type O lacks both enzymes.

Similar antigenic differences exist in an-imals. While some of these are termed A, B, etc., they are unrelated serologically to human isoantigens or to each other (Stone and Irwin 1963). The human isoantigens A and B are not confined to red blood cells, but are present on the surfaces of endothelial and epithelial cells of the epi-dermis, thymic corpuscles, and intestine (Sulzman 1960).

Transfusion reactions result when blood with erythrocyte isoantigens of one type is transfused to individuals with isoantibod ies against it; for example, blood with A isoantigen is given to an individual with type B blood (and A isoantibodies). Clump-ing and lysis of the donor erythrocytes in the vascular system of the recipient result in embolization, pulmonary vascular block-ade, and death. The opposite reaction of clumping of recipient erythrocytes by do-nor isoantibodies does not occur because of the rapid dilution of donor antibodies.

HEMOLYTIC DISEASE OF THE NEWBORN

Hemolytic disease is known to occur in newborn horses, mules, calves, and swine (Dennis et al. 1970; Linklater et al. 1973). The fetus, by virtue of inheritance from the sire, develops erythrocyte antigens not present in the mother. When these cells gain access to the mother's bloodstream they induce antibody formation. If these antibodies are returned to the newborn animal via colostrum, severe hemolytic anemia is induced. Whereas absorption of antibodies occurs by way of milk in hors-es and swine, in man, transplacental trans-fer of antibody occurs, resulting in a simi-lar disease called erythroblastosis fetalis.

Thrombocytopenia caused by a similar mechanism also occurs. It has been stud-ied in dogs (Wilkins et al. 1973). Neona-tal thrombocytopenia of piglets of similar mechanism has been reported in Norway (Nordstoga 1965). It was described in 5-day-old piglets with thrombocytopenia and hemorrhages.

IMMUNE COMPLEX DISEASE

Immune complex diseases are due to the damage induced in tissues by antigen-antibody-complement complexes that pro-duce inflammatory responses. They occur when antigens localize in vascular walls and subsequently complex with circulating precipitating antibodies. These complexes attract complement, and the lesions are caused by neutrophils for which the com-plement-containing complexes are chemo-tactic. The development of lesions paral-lels the levels of antibodies in serum. Im-mune complex disease may also result from the direct deposition of circulating antigen-antibody-complement complexes in vascular basement membranes (Hensen 1971).

Circulating immune complexes are nor-mally phagocytized by macrophages. When present in the serum in large amounts or when the reticuloendothelial system is overloaded, they may pass into the vascular walls by simple diffusion. Histamine re lease by platelets at sites of existing vascu-lar injury opens the way for a more active deposition of complexes. In some cases, it appears that a platelet-activating factor is released from IgE-containing basophils when they contact specific antigen. This factor induces platelets to aggregate and release histamine which increases vascular permeability, allowing the large immune complexes ($> 19S$) to pass vessel walls.

ARTHUS REACTION

The classic experimental model of im-mune complex disease is the *Arthus reac-tion*. It is produced in rabbits by two in-tradermal injections of the same antigen at the same site with an interval of greater than 24 hrs. Antibody is produced lo-cally after the sensitizing injection and re-acts with the antigen injected on the sec-ond, challenge dose. Variants of the phe-nomenon are the *local passive Arthus reac-tion,* which results from antibody injected

intradermally followed in 1 hr with antigen injection at the same location, and the
reverse passive Arthus reaction, in which
antigen is injected intravenously and antibody is injected intradermally within 1 hr.

The basic lesion of the Arthus reaction
is an intense vasculitis. It is characterized
by perivascular neutrophil cuffing, vascular
necrosis of the media with neutrophil invasion, and hemorrhage (Cochrane and
Aikin 1966; Venkatachalam and Cotran
1970). These changes result from the complexing of antibody and antigen within the
vascular wall and the subsequent attachment of complement. The complement
complex is strongly chemotactic for neutrophils, which rapidly degrade antigen
and carry it away from the site of localization. Unfortunately, lysis of neutrophil
granules occurs with the disastrous tissue
injury described above. By immunofluorescent studies, antigen, host globulin, and
the third component of complement (C3)
can be detected near the internal elastic
membrane at the beginning of the lesion.

Arthus reactions are common subtle
components of parenteral immunization
procedures. Antigens present in the vaccine localize on the vascular wall, are complexed with antibody (induced by previous
immunization), and combine with complement. Most of these reactions are transient and subclinical, although occasionally
bothersome dermal lesions arise. Although
an Arthus component is probably present
in most vaccine reactions, it must be
pointed out that, mechanistically, these are
more likely to be due to either delayed hypersensitivity reactions or immediate wheal-
and-flare reactions induced by reaginic antibodies and histamine release.

Arthus-type reactions occur in the recovery stages of some infectious diseases.
The ocular lesions following acute infectious canine hepatitis are alleged to be an
example. Partial resolution of the acute
primary viral-induced iridocyclitis may occur with viral antigens persisting in the
anterior uvea. Antibody produced locally
by plasmacytes in the iris and limbus reacts with cell-associated antigen and produces a hypersensivity reaction which is
manifested clinically as corneal opacity or
"blue eye" (Carmichael 1965).

ALLERGIC ALVEOLITIS

An immunologic reaction of the Arthus
type is induced on the alveolar wall of
sensitized animals by large aerosols of extrinsic particulate antigens. *Allergic alveolitis* occurs in cattle and horses exposed to
spores of thermophilic Actinomycetes, such
as *Micropolyspora faeni,* which are common in moist hay. Lesions in the lung include infiltration of the alveolar wall with
plasmacytes, lymphocytes, and macrophages (Pauli et al. 1972; Pirie et al. 1971).
Epithelioid granulomas and obliteration
of bronchioles are seen. The immunologic
mechanism of a respiratory disease is proven
by demonstrating: (1) a latent period between exposure and onset of symptoms,
(2) precipitating antibodies in serum, (3)
Arthus-type skin reactivity to suspect antigens, and (4) complement and immunoglobulins in lesions.

The large number of hypersensitivity
pneumonitides that occur in humans are
named according to the occupational hazard involved: "farmers' lung" (due to *Micropolyspora faeni*), "pigeon breeders' disease," "maple-bark strippers' disease,"
"bagassosis," and so forth. The lesion is
usually a chronic Arthus reaction, for there
are multiple exposures of the lung to antigen. Lung biopsies usually reveal extensive fibrosis, vascular reactions, and perivenular lymphocyte accumulations. This
suggests the participation of cellular hypersensitivity which is often the case in these
complex reactions.

The immunologic reaction of the respiratory system to organic dusts depends on
the host and on the distribution of antigens. Atopic humans and dogs (and presumably most other animals) give bronchial asthmatic reactions, which are mediated by nonprecipitating reaginic antibodies. Nonatopic individuals react to dust
antigens predominantly with precipitating
antibodies which induce alveolitis typical
of an Arthus-type reaction.

SERUM SICKNESS

Serum sickness was a disease of man and
animals in days when large amounts of
horse serum were injected intramuscularly
for passive immunity to infectious diseases.
Serum sickness begins mechanistically by

the deposition of antigen-antibody complexes in kidney, joints, and other organs. It becomes complicated by associated immunologic phenomena and such nonimmunologic factors as coagulation defects. Nonetheless, experimental serum sickness has been used as a convenient model for the study of immune complex diseases (Germuth 1953).

The pathogenesis of acute serum sickness is illustrated by the intramuscular injection of large amounts of bovine serum albumin (BSA) in rabbits. The antigen, BSA, is eliminated in three patterns from the circulation (Fig. 5.18). Clinical and pathological signs of disease accompany the onset of antibody formation 5–6 days after the injection of antigen. Necrotizing vascular lesions are widespread in kidney, heart, lung, and joints. The renal glomerulus is the significant site of injury. There is a rapidly developing proliferative glomerulonephritis with deposits of antigen, antibody, and complement below the capillary endothelium (Arakawa and Kimmelsteil 1970). Ultrastructurally, endothelial cells are swollen severely and separated from their basement membranes. Granular deposits are present below the membrane. In acute glomerulitis there is little emigration of leukocytes. With immunofluorescent techniques, BSA antigens, host globulin, and complement can be detected in the granular deposits along the basement membrane. Regression of lesions follows the disappearance of detectable circulating antigen-antibody complexes.

GLOMERULONEPHRITIS

Immunologic injury to the renal glomerulus can result from cross-reactivity of antibodies and glomerular basement membranes and from immune complex disease (Table 5.8). Under immune complex *glomerulonephritis* are included a group of glomerular diseases wherein antigen-antibody complexes localize in the renal glomerulus. Lesions are characterized by irregular granular hyaline deposits beneath the vascular endothelium (Fig. 5.19). Immunofluorescent staining techniques reveal the localization of antigen, complement, and globulin within the deposits. Ultrastructurally, they are found on either side of the capillary basement membrane and in the mesangium.

Several examples of chronic viral disease associated with glomerulonephritis are known. These occur in Aleutian disease of mink, equine infectious anemia (Banks et al. 1972), chronic hog cholera, lymphocytic choriomeningitis, and lactic dehydrogenase virus infection of mice. Glomerular lesions are based on the peculiar ability of these viruses to induce persistent viremia despite antibody production by the host. In all of these diseases, there occur progressive defectiveness of the immune systems and reticuloendothelial hyperplasia. Glomerulonephritis develops in direct relation to the chronicity of the disease.

Membranous glomerulonephritis is a striking lesion in the late stages of Aleutian

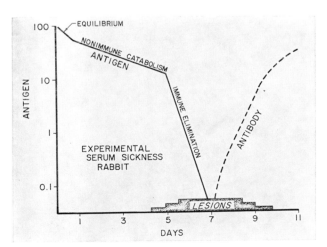

Fig. 5.18. Presence of antibody and antigen in circulating blood in experimental serum sickness, rabbit. Antigen was given at day 0.

Table 5.8. Glomerulonephritis of immune complex and autoimmune origin

Immune complex type. Antibody produced against exogenous antigens and antigen-antibody-complement complexes accumulates in discrete deposits on the outer portion of the glomerular basement membrane.

Clinical:	Viral diseases: Aleutian disease, equine infectious anemia, chronic hog cholera, lymphocytic choriomeningitis, NZB disease
	Lupus erythematosus
	Membranous nephritis of cats (?)
	Streptococcal glomerulonephritis (human)
	Malarial infection (primates)
	Idiopathic globulin deposition (sheep, horse)
Experimental:	Serum sickness (acute and chronic types)
	Nephrotoxic nephritis (kidney tubule antigen)
	Chronic allogeneic disease

Autoimmune type. Antibody produced against glomerular basement membrane antigens. Host antibody reacts with its own tissue producing uniform, linear patterns of antibody and complement along the inner glomerular basement membrane.

Clinical:	Anti-GBM glomerulonephritis (horse)—rare
	Goodpasture syndrome (human)
	Subacute glomerulonephritis (human)—etiology unknown
Experimental:	Masugi nephritis—GBM is antigenic portion of nephrotoxic serum
	Steblay nephritis—anti-GBM nephritis

disease of mink (Henson et al. 1968; Pan et al. 1970). This disease is a slowly progressive systemic plasmacytosis accompanied by persistent viremia and hypergammaglobulinemia. Antigen-antibody complexes accumulate below the vascular endothelium and stain with the periodic acid-Schiff stain and for immunofluorescent techniques for γ-globulin and complement. In the early phase of the glomerular lesions, ultrastructural examination reveals foci of irregular, dense, granular material immediately below the capillary endothelial cells. Globules are often encompassed by basal cytoplasmic folds of the endothelium. Later, dense deposits occur throughout the glomerular filtration barrier: below the endothelium, throughout the basement membrane, and within the epithelial cell foot processes and slit pores. Proliferation of mesangial cells occurs, and dense material accumulates in the cytoplasm of these cells. The final stages of the glomerular lesion are characterized by neutrophil infiltration, fibrin deposition, necrosis, and effacement of glomerular architecture.

Chronic membranous glomerulonephritis is a common finding in malignant lymphoma in cats, mice, and humans (Anderson and Jarrett 1971; Branca et al. 1971; Sutherland and Mardiney 1973). The granular material which is deposited along the capillary basement membrane represents antibodies against leukemia viruses, deposited either directly as preformed antigen-antibody complexes or as the attachment of circulating antibodies to antigens localized in the glomerulus. In mice, virions have been demonstrated within the glomerular basement membrane and the antigen involved appears to be a glycoprotein of the viral envelope (Batzing and Hanna 1973; Pascal et al. 1973; Yoshiki et al. 1974).

In addition to immune complex-induced glomerulopathy, renal glomerular lesions

Fig. 5.19. Glomerulonephritis, chronic hog cholera. A. Histology. Hypertrophy and hyperplasia of mesangial cells (arrow). B. Glomerular mesangium (right) and capsule (left). Capsular parietal epithelium is necrotic and basement membrane is thickened. Monocyte (M) is present in the capillary at center and a neutrophil (N) in vessel at lower right. C. Mesangium (top), urinary space (with debris at center), and capillary with neutrophil (bottom). Mesangial cell filled with dense residual bodies and surrounded by electron-dense mantle. Epithelial foot processes are coalesced (arrow) and contain dense material, particularly at the mesangial surface. D. Subendothelial accumulations of dense granular material (arrow).

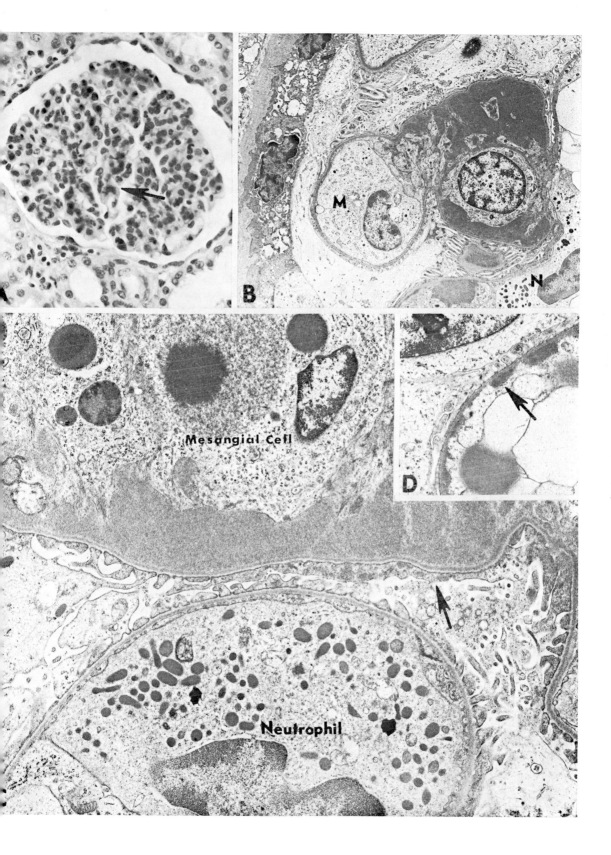

have been described in humans and horses due to trapping of antibodies against glomerular basement membrane antigens. In contrast to the irregular deposits of immune complex disease, these deposits occur in smooth linear fashion along the capillary basement membrane. Anti-GBM–induced glomerulopathy occurs spontaneously in horses although such lesions have not been established as the cause of renal disease (Banks et al. 1972).

ANTIBODY-MEDIATED RESPIRATORY
SYNCYTIAL VIRUS DISEASE

Respiratory syncytial (RS) viruses are recognized as common, widespread, and recurring etiologic agents of respiratory disease in humans. RS virus in normal adult humans causes respiratory disease of limited severity. Lung parenchyma is affected by bronchiolitis and patchy areas of interstitial pneumonitis, and disease is followed by detectable, neutralizing antibodies in both serum and nasal secretions. Most RS infections are secondary and adults are protected by IgA antibodies in the secretions of the respiratory tract. Experimental clinical trials have revealed that humans with little or no antibody in nasal secretions will, upon being infected, shed large amounts of virus and develop serum and nasal-secretory antibodies. In contrast, patients with large amounts of antibodies in their respiratory tract secretions will shed very little virus and do not develop serum antibodies (Chanock et al. 1970).

IMMUNOLOGIC-MEDIATED RS DISEASE

Newborn infants develop far more serious disease during infection than do older children or adults. Although there is an age-related resistance basis for this peculiar epidemiologic pattern of infection in infancy, there is also a defined immunologic component that may dominate the disease. The presence of neutralizing antibodies in serum without the presence of protective IgA secretory antibodies in the respiratory tract is responsible for the immune reaction. During infection of the lower respiratory tract, edema of the bronchiolar mucosa and alveolar wall occurs. This allows the nonspecific leakage of globulins through the vascular wall

and the specific antibodies complex with viral antigens in the tissues to produce an immune complex (or type 3) allergic reaction.

The pattern of severe disease in children occurs in primary infections during the first few months of life and the timing correlates with the retention of passive serum antibodies (acquired maternally). This suggests that anti-RS virus antibodies, which are widespread in the general population, do protect the infant. The immunologic phenomenon has been confirmed in vaccine trials using parenteral inoculation of a killed cell cuture vaccine that induced only serum neutralizing antibodies. In one nursery, a naturally occurring RS outbreak took place 9 months after vaccination and revealed that the frequency of viral isolation did not differ from vaccines and controls and that 60% of vaccinated children developed bronchiolitis or pneumonia as compared with 8% of the nonvaccinated control children.

In summary, the conditions required for immunologic disease to occur are: (1) virus must produce specific antigen at cell surfaces and/or excess soluble antigens in the respiratory tract epithelium; (2) specific IgA antibodies must be absent in respiratory secretions; (3) serum antibodies must be present (either maternally or vaccine-induced); and (4) there must be a high rate of infection in early life. Influenza fails in this regard because of the different antigenic makeup of viruses involved in successive epidemics. Parainfluenza does not induce similar lesions since the disease is not severe in neonates.

CELL-MEDIATED IMMUNOLOGIC DISEASE

Cell-mediated immunologic diseases are those caused by the recognition of antigens by small lymphocytes (T cells) and their secretion of lymphokines and lymphotoxins. These substances cause necrosis and infiltration of monocytes and macrophages at sites of antigen localization. Lesions tend to be large and proliferative and contain large numbers of macrophages, lymphoid cells, and other leukocytes. The experimental models studied previously include the tuberculin reaction, graft rejection, and contact hypersensitivity.

Severe skin diseases involving cell-mediated reactivity have arisen after immunization with some viral agents, notably foot-and-mouth disease in cattle and measles in humans (Harris et al. 1969). The foot-and-mouth vaccine prepared in vitro in hamster kidney cells contains a protein antigen that induces large nodular lesions in the skin, characteristic of delayed hypersensitivity (Mayr et al. 1969).

CONTACT HYPERSENSITIVITY

These immune responses produce common allergic disease in animals and man. Dermatitis due to poison ivy, cosmetics, or drugs is often seen. In humans, one of the most frequent contact hypersensitivities is "cement eczema" caused by allergy to hexavalent chromium salts present in cement. The contact hypersensitivities have been useful for investigating cell-mediated immunoreactivity because percutaneous tests do not elicit masking antibody-induced Arthus reactions.

When a large vesiculant dose of picryl chloride is applied to skin it induces sensitivity, so that subsequent small dose application will cause a highly specific contact reaction. Intercellular edema and lymphoid cell migration disrupt the upper dermis and epidermis (Flax and Caulfield 1963). Intact sensitized lymphocytes must arrive at the challenge site for the reaction to develop. Very small numbers are required and they appear to arrive at the site randomly, not selectively. Thus, following union of antigen and sensitized lymphocytes, lymphokines are released and attract monocytes. The final inflammatory reaction is therefore comprised of immunologically nonspecific cells (McCluskey et al. 1963).

The term "delayed hypersensitivity" was coined in 1942, when Landsteiner and Chase discovered that picryl chloride contact hypersensitivity could be passively transmitted by viable cells, but not by serum. They recognized the resemblance to the long known bacterial hypersensitivities. The specific histologic reactions identifying cell-mediated changes are often referred to as "delayed-hypersensitivity type" reactions.

Testing is generally by patch; a 1 cm piece of filter paper soaked in dilute sensitizer is placed on the skin and covered with adhesive tape for 24 hrs. After a lag of 12 hrs, erythema and swelling appear and reach a peak at 24–48 hrs. Hydrophobic solutions penetrate and react readily; higher concentrations of hydrophilic solutions such as tuberculin and penicillin are required.

THE TUBERCULIN REACTION

Following his discovery that tubercle bacilli placed intradermally into tuberculous guinea pigs produced severe necrotic reactions in 1–2 days (instead of 10–14 as in normal animals), Koch established that crude extracts of infected growth medium would act similarly. This dermal *tuberculin reaction* now produced with purified protein derivatives (PPD), has been the prototype in the study of cell-mediated immunity.

PPD tuberculin is a relatively nonantigenic extract of soluble mycobacterial proteins. When injected intradermally into a tuberculous (or artificially sensitized) animal, it incites an inflammatory reaction characterized by increased vascular permeability to fluid and neutrophils and perivascular accumulation of lymphocytes and macrophages. Even though PPD does not appear to be retained locally any longer than in nonsensitized animals (Oort and Turk 1963), it most likely has an increased avidity for the cell membrane of sensitized macrophages (Eisen 1969); it is taken up by macrophages, lymphocytes, and neutrophils. The questions to be resolved are: how is information transferred to sensitized, memory-containing small lymphocytes; and how do these in turn induce other cells to produce the reaction?

Early in this century, Zinsser had perceptively differentiated tuberculin hypersensitivities from the immediate antibody reactions such as the Arthus reaction. While the tuberculin reaction was specific for tuberculoprotein-sensitized animals, many early pathologists were unable to histologically differentiate it from nonspecific inflammatory responses. Dienes and Mallory in 1932, however, suggested that it was predominantly a mononuclear cell infiltration in contrast to the neutrophil exudate of the more immediate antibody reactions. These views predominate among immunologists (if not pathologists), and it is now accepted that the delayed, peri-

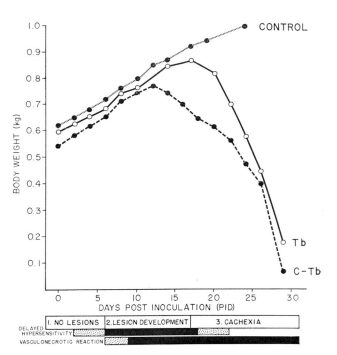

Fig. 5.20. Development of lesions, delayed hypersensitivity, and vasculonecrotic (Arthus) reactivity in experimental avian tuberculosis. Body weights of three groups of birds are plotted: control, infected (Tb), and cortisone treated-infected (C-Tb).

vascular accumulation of lymphocytes and monocytes represents the specific cell-mediated phase of the tuberculin reaction. Ultrastructurally, it is clearly seen that the initial lesions consist of small lymphocytes accumulating around venules. By 24 hrs, monocytes and macrophages dominate the tuberculin reaction (Weiner et al. 1969).

The character of the lesion is determined by the purity of the tuberculin and the severity of tuberculosis. Crude tuberculin is apt to provoke exudative reactions with many neutrophils. Although in the early stages of tuberculosis vigorous tuberculin reactions develop, in the terminal stages anergy occurs. Anergic animals do not respond to tuberculin, probably because of extensive dissemination of bacillary antigens throughout the host (Fig. 5.20).

Generally, when the tuberculin reaction is evoked in clinical medicine the specific cell-mediated component is accompanied by other phenomena. Studies of vascular permeability involving extravasation of

I^{126}-albumin emphasize the complexity of the reaction (Baumgarten and Wilhelm 1969). Three peaks of exudation were described (Table 5.9). The intermediate peak, present only when killed bacilli were used for immunization, is an Arthus reaction to tuberculoproteins. In the presence of high antibody titers, this exudation may mask the specific phase of the tuberculin reaction.

The production of the tuberculin reaction passively by transference of lymphoid cells from sensitized donors to normal recipients has been a profitable model for study. H^3-labeled lymphocytes are obtained from lymph node suspensions (or better, thoracic duct) of sensitized host animals. When injected into a recipient animal that is challenged with PPD, the transferred cells appear to localize specifically at the reaction site (Najarian and Feldman 1961). Most of the cells in the reaction are not labeled, however, and experiments using other antigens dispute

Table 5.9. Vascular permeablity and exudation in the tuberculin reaction

Phase	Begins	Subsides	Mediation by
Primary	Immediately	20 min	Histamine (anaphylactic antibody) blocked by antihistimine
Intermediate	½ hr	2 hrs	Arthus reaction to protein
Secondary (delayed)	3 hrs	48 hrs	Cell-mediated mechanism: the specific phase

this specificity (McCluskey et al. 1963). The kinetics of the in vivo reaction make this controversy difficult to resolve.

It is known that, on contact with specific antigens, immune lymphocytes release soluble lymphokines which attract monocytes. How these factors function is not certain.

CUTANEOUS BASOPHILIC HYPERSENSITIVITY

Cutaneous basophilic hypersensitivity is a poorly understood expression of cellular immunity. It occurs transiently, early in the course of immunization with soluble antigens, and as part of reactions involving contact hypersensitivity and graft rejection. Antigenic requirements and histopathology differentiate it from classic delayed hypersensitivity (Dvorak et al. 1970).

The lesion is characterized by massive perivascular accumulations of basophils and monocytes. It is initiated by a primary interaction between sensitized (thymus-derived) small lymphocytes and antigen. Basophils, originating in the bone marrow, are attracted to the sites of reaction by lymphokines released by the lymphocyte. The reaction can be initiated by passively transferred lymphocytes but not by serum. It is inhibited by anti-lymphocyte serum. The local lesion is associated with enlargement of thymic-dependent areas of the draining lymph nodes.

Sites at which positive tuberculin skin tests have been elicited exhibit an accelerated reaction on later reinjection of tuberculin. This *retest phenomenon* may persist for several months. The edematous erythematous papule reaches its peak in 6–8 hrs, and its distinguishing feature is the massive accumulation of eosinophils (Arnason and Waksman 1963). It is not affected by antineutrophil sera, being thus distinguished from the Arthus and Shwartzman reactions.

GRAFT REJECTION

Skin transplants between syngeneic[2] animals vascularize and are accepted. Those between allogeneic animals become ne-

crotic and slough in 10–14 days. Rejection of grafted skin is characterized by massive intravascular and perivenous accumulations of small lymphocytes and monocytes, which invade the grafted epithelium and its blood vessels (Waksman 1963; Weiss and Smyth 1970; Wiener et al. 1969). Vascular damage induces ischemia, which in turn causes death of the graft.

Medawar, in his classic experiments on skin transplantation in mice, noticed that the rejection of grafts closely resembled delayed hypersensitivity on the basis of histologic appearance, timing, and independence of antibody. Although grafts did elicit antibodies, they did not appear to play a major role in rejection. A second skin transfer and graft from the same donor resulted in a more rapid rejection by the recipient. This rapid "second set" reaction was specific for the original donor skin and had other characteristics of immunologic reactivity. Rejection was inhibited by immunosuppressant drugs; tolerance could be induced; and rejection could be transferred with lymph node cells but not with serum (Medawar 1958).

The immunologic basis of rejection of grafted tissue is a direct expression of genetic difference between donor and recipient. Rejection occurs against histocompatibility antigens located on the cell membrane of grafted cells. The complex histocompatibility antigens have not been defined in most mammals and experiments are confined to highly inbred syngeneic mice or chickens. Syngeneic animals accept grafts; allogeneic animals do not. Among highly inbred animals one exception occurs. The hybrid offspring of two inbred strains contain antigens present in both parents. They are unique; they will accept tissues from each other and from either parent. Their tissue, however, will not be accepted by either parent.

Assuming that the technical aspects of grafting are correct (proper surgical alignment, absence of infection, etc.), the survival of a graft depends on suppression of the host's immunity. Xenografts[3] are rejected immediately, probably on the basis

2. Syngeneic = genetically identical; lack of tissue incompatibility (isogenic). Allogenic = not identical but same species. Xenogeneic = genetically dissimilar, between species (heterogenic).

3. Syngraft = between syngeneic animals (syngeneic graft, isograft). Allograft = between outbred individuals of the same species (allogeneic graft, homograft). Xenograft = between different species (xenogeneic graft, heterograft).

of antibody formation. Allografts are rejected by several mechanisms.

Clinical research on human organ transplantation has revealed the complex nature of rejection. For example, kidney allografts may be rejected at three different time periods after grafting, and each represents different dominant mechanisms: (1) Peracute rejection begins immediately and appears to be mediated through cytotoxic antibody; neutrophils are dominant in the lesions and accumulate in glomerular and peritubular capillaries (Milgrom et al. 1971). (2) Acute rejection begins in a few days and is due to the cellular immunological processes described by Medawar; small lymphocytes accumulate around intertubular capillaries in the graft and destroy it. (3) Chronic rejection may occur after many months and is related to vascular degeneration.

The majority of grafted organs in nonimmunosuppressed recipients are rejected within 4 wks by mechanisms of cell-mediated immunity. Contact between sensitized lymphocyte and foreign cell destroys the latter. How the small lymphocyte mediates graft rejection is not precisely known. It is theorized that sensitized cell-antigen interaction releases a factor involving nonsensitized monocytes. The latter dominate in the graft, and release of lysosomal enzymes is responsible for tissue damage.

Macrophages from immune animals also destroy target cells carrying the antigen used for immunization. This in vitro reaction again occurs at contact, not by phagocytosis. If animals are immunized with sheep erythrocytes and rosette tests performed (immune animal spleen cells mixed with sheep red cells), less than 10% of lymphocytes attach to sheep erythrocytes, yet macrophages adhere readily. Such discrepancy is due in large part to the presence of cytophilic antibody firmly adhered to the macrophage surface.

Graft rejection reactions were extended to tumor research by the demonstration that (in mice) lymphosarcoma rejection was accelerated on second or challenge grafting, and that lymphocytes could cause this reaction when transferred from a sensitized to a syngeneic nonsensitized host. The development of specific tumor antigens which are distinct from host antigens is currently an intense area of research.

Tumor immunity is best illustrated in laboratory animals. A primary chemically induced tumor is excised, minced, and pieces of tumor are grafted onto the original host and onto several syngeneic animals. Tumor growth occurs in the latter but is suppressed in the original tumor-bearing host. If tumor cells are cultured, their growth is inhibited by the addition of lymph node cells of the host animal.

Clinical use of anticancer therapy based on immune rejection has been done in human medicine. Insurmountable difficulties are encountered and no effective regimen has been established.

GRAFT-VERSUS-HOST REACTION

The *graft-versus-host* reaction (GVH) is an immunologic response in which transplanted lymphocytes react against histocompatibility antigens of the host. The recipient of immunologically active lymphocytes is destroyed by the attack of these cells on its tissues (Walker et al. 1972).

It was demonstrated by Billingham in Medawar's laboratory that animals sensitized to skin by homograft reacted against intradermal injection of lymphocytes from the skin donor. Reinforcing the concept that this was cellular-immune reactivity due to injection of a dose of transplantation antigen present in lymphocytes was the production of similar reaction with killed cells and cell-free extracts. Conversely, lymphocytes from a sensitized recipient when injected intradermally into the graft donor produced the same type of phenomenon.

Subsequent experiments with two highly inbred strains of mice revealed startling results. Injection of immunologically competent lymphoid cells from an adult of one strain into newborn recipients of another inbred strain (having different strong histocompatibility genes/antigens) produced a fatal runting syndrome. It was shown that, if donor lymphocytes come from allogeneic strains lacking tissue antigens present in the host, they react against the host itself, initiating a graft-versus-host reaction. While the host could not destroy the grafted lymphocytes, they (the grafted lymphocytes) proliferated and destroyed the host.

Requirements for this reaction are: (1) Recipient must be incapable of an efficient immune response to reject the graft (therefore neonatal animals are best). (2) Donor cells must be immunocompetent. (Adult lymphocytes are best and the reaction is accelerated with cells from a pre-immunized donor. Grafts such as epithelium cannot mount an immune response and are incapable of initiating this reaction.) (3) The donor and recipient must differ at strong histocompatibility genes (Fig. 5.21).

Clinical signs associated with runt disease are growth failure, diarrhea, emaciation, hepatosplenomegaly, and lymphoid exhaustion (Hildemann et al. 1964). Progressive lymphocyte depletion occurs in the peripheral and central lymphoid organs, with conversion to histiocytes. There are also lesions with macrophage accumulations in the myocardium, intestinal mucosa, synovia, and liver. While infant recipients of parental lymphocytes are usually killed by the graft-versus-host reaction, adult recipients, if they develop disease, show lesions of anemia, glomerulonephritis (Lewis et al. 1968), and increased incidence of lymphoma. Graft-versus-host disease can activate C-type RNA leukemia viruses in mice (Hirsch et al. 1970), and it is possible that similar reactions occur naturally in animals that live to old age.

LYMPHOCYTIC CHORIOMENINGITIS

Lymphocytic choriomeningitis (LCM) is an acute disease of young field and laboratory mice characterized by wasting and CNS signs. LCM virus, in susceptible mice, is known to cause two distinct syndromes: acute disease and asymptomatic persistent infection.

Immunolymphocyte-mediated CNS disease, an acute systemic disease, runs a course which ends in death or recovery with immunity. Viral antigens (as revealed by immunofluorescence) are present in lymphocytes, macrophages, platelets, mega-karyocytes, and epithelial cells at various sites. Virus in the brain appears to be limited to the meninges and choroid plexus.

Development of immunity is associated with circulating antibody and clearance of virus from tissues. Coincident with the drop in infectious virus, cytotoxic lymphocytes appear in the meninges and virus-antibody-complement complexes occur in the circulation. CNS disease is caused by the mouse's antiviral immune-lymphocyte response, and immunosuppression will prevent fatal disease. The effectiveness of thymectomy, antilymphocyte serum, cortisone, and irradiation to suppress disease indicates that lesions are caused by a graft rejection-type process involving immune lymphocytes acting against infected tissue. Experimentally, mice are permanently protected against lethal intracerebral challenge with LCM virus if given an immunosuppressive dose of cyclophosphamide up to the third day after infection. The protected mice develop a persistent lifelong infection. If they receive donor lymphocytes from syngeneic, LCM-immunized mice, an acute fatal CNS disease will result.

Neonatal infection with persistent viremia, the second type of LCM infection, occurs in mice exposed in utero or during or shortly after birth. These mice survive with high titers of circulating virus which often persist for the life of the mouse (carrier state). This was previously thought to represent tolerance to viral infection but mice are now known to produce both humoral and cellular immune responses. The absence of circulating antibody is due to the combination of circulating virus with newly formed antibody molecules. Persistently infected mice may develop a chronic wasting disease with trapping of antigen-antibody complexes in the renal

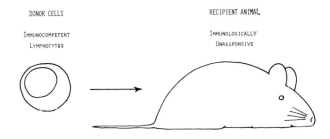

DONOR CELLS

IMMUNOCOMPETENT LYMPHOCYTES

RECIPIENT ANIMAL

IMMUNOLOGICALLY UNRESPONSIVE

Fig. 5.21. Requirements for the graft-versus-host reaction.

glomerulus and chronic glomerulonephritis (Cole 1971).

One concept of LCM disease hypothesizes that LCM virus modifies the infected cell by forming new antigens on the host cell plasma membrane. An immune response is initiated by thymic-dependent lymphocytes against LCM antigens and these lymphocytes are capable of lysing infected cells. Cytolysis can be demonstrated in vitro by adding immune mouse lymphocytes to infected cell cultures. This constitutes a graft rejection by the host of its own viral-infected cells. Subsequent liberation of intracellular antigens stimulates a more powerful antibody response by plasmacytosis and antibody formation (Hotchin 1971).

The final result of the rejection process determines the status of the animal: death, if too extensive; immunity, if successful; and tolerance, if the attack is incomplete. Failure of the immune response may be complete (as with congenital carrier infections) or partial, resulting in "split tolerance," chronic, persistent, and slow wasting disease with glomerulonephritis.

AUTOALLERGIC DISEASE

In *autoallergic* (autoimmune) *disease,* the animal's own tissue acts as an endogenous antigen with subsequent production of humoral antibody or sensitized lymphocytes. The state of tolerance is broken. By the clonal selection theory, it is necessary to postulate that only the lymphoid mutants potentially capable of producing immune responses against autoantigens are suppressed and destroyed by encounter before birth with the corresponding autoantigen. It can, therefore, be viewed that the development of autoimmune disease results from: (1) failure of the autoantigen to encounter the corresponding lymphoid mutant during fetal life with failure to induce tolerance or (2) breakdown of the tolerant state with production of autoantibodies and lymphocytes following circulation of autoantigenic material.

Autoimmune disease is broadly grouped into (1) organ-specific disease and (2) non-organ systemic disease. The first is characterized by chronic inflammatory changes in the tissue and circulating autoantibodies directed specifically against antigens in the disease organ. Examples are autoimmune thyroiditis, polymyositis, and ulcerative colitis. Lymphocytes and/or antibodies are detectable against the host's thyroglobulin, muscle, and colonic mucosa respectively. An example of non-organ systemic disease is lupus erythematosus.

Naturally occurring autoimmune diseases usually embody several patterns of disease. Autoimmune hemolytic anemia of dogs develops due to autoantibody production against erythrocytes, but affected animals are apt to show a wide variety of tissue changes. The clinical disease may be considerably clouded by nonhematologic signs.

AUTOIMMUNE HEMOLYTIC ANEMIA OF DOGS

This syndrome is characterized by severe hemolytic anemia, thrombocytopenia, and reticulocytosis (Lewis et al. 1963). Clinical tests corroborating the diagnosis include a positive direct antiglobulin (Coombs) test (Fig. 5.22) and low hemoglobin with observed spherocytosis. Erythrocytes have antibodies attached to their cell membranes which induce hemolysis and anemia. The

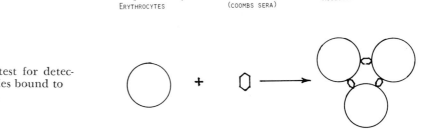

Fig. 5.22 Coombs test for detection of autoantibodies bound to surface erythrocytes.

spleen becomes filled with degenerate and dead erythrocytes. In Lewis's report of 19 cases, 14 had thrombocytopenia (6 of these with purpura). Other cases of thrombocytopenic purpura have been described, but the nature of the autoimmune phenomena was not investigated (Wayne 1960). Glomerulonephritis with "wire-loop" type lesions is seen in some of the cases. These phenomena must be differentiated from lupus erythematosus.

IMMUNE THYROIDITIS OF CHICKENS

Thyroiditis was discovered in a strain of white Leghorn chickens with excess body fat, small skeletal structure, silky feathers, poor laying record, and sensitivity to low environmental temperature. All these are changes associated with hypothyroidism. The disease was recognized by 8 wks of age and was accompanied by atrophy and lymphoid infiltration of the thyroid (Kite et al. 1969). The pituitary was not affected. By selective breeding, the incidence was raised from 10% to over 80% and the strain designated OS (obese strain). Large lymphoid cells and germinal centers are present in the thyroid by 2 wks and reach peak incidence at 4–5 wks. Plasmacytes migrate through the follicular epithelium, causing breakdown and rupture of intercellular connections (Wick and Graf 1972). Bursectomy causes a significant decrease in incidence and severity, indicating that antibody-forming cells are essential to the disease (Wick et al. 1970). Circulating autoantibodies to thyroglobulin are present in a large percent of affected chickens.

Autoimmune thyroiditis (Hashimoto's disease) occurs in man but, like experimental autoimmune thyroiditis, it appears to involve small lymphocytes and cell-mediated mechanism rather than autoantibodies (Harris 1969; Jankovic et al. 1963).

LUPUS ERYTHEMATOSUS (LE)

LE is a rare disease of dog and man characterized by arthritis, anemia, lymphadenopathy, and nephritis. Widespread vascular lesions are induced by a circulating antibody against host tissue DNA. Anti-DNA antibodies are the basis of the LE test, wherein suspect serum is added to leukocyte suspensions. Nuclei of susceptible cells undergo dissolution with release of nuclear chromatin which is then phagocytized by other leukocytes. These appear as large cells with hematoxylin-staining inclusions, called LE cells. Immunologic glomerulonephritis, an immune complex reaction, is an integral part of the disease.

Canine LE is a complex disorder characterized by progressive development of hemolytic anemia, thrombocytopenic purpura, proteinuria, and polyarthritis (Lewis 1965; Lewis et al. 1965). Renal failure is a frequent cause of death and is due to irregular, spotty, chronic membranous glomerulonephritis with focal accumulations of plasmacytes. Thymic lesions include the development of lymphoid follicles and germinal centers in medullary areas.

In canine LE, anemia occurs as acute severe hemolytic crises, during which there is a strong direct positive antiglobulin (Coombs) test. Eluates from affected erythrocytes will sensitize normal canine erythrocytes to an indirect antiglobulin test (confirming that autoantibodies are responsible for the hemolysis). The LE cell test is highly specific for canine systemic LE (Lewis et al. 1963). The most significant serologic abnormalities include autoantibodies against IgG, nucleoprotein, DNA, RNA, thyroglobulin, and erythrocyte membrane antigens.

Thrombocytopenic purpura episodes occur due to platelet destruction and are manifested as hematuria, epistaxis, and petechiae or ecchymoses in the skin and mucous membranes. Autoantibodies to platelets have not been demonstrated, and it may be that circulating antigen-antibody complexes (unrelated to platelets) exert a cytotoxic effect.

Genetic analysis of affected dogs does not support the hereditary nature of the disease as postulated for human LE (Lewis and Schwartz 1971). Recent studies implicate a viral agent, and cell-free filtrates have been shown to induce immunologic abnormalities in mice.

NZB DISEASE OF MICE

A unique spontaneous progressive hemolytic anemia distinguished by reticulosis and autoantibody directed against erythrocytes occurs in the New Zealand Black

(NZB) strain of mice (Comerford et al. 1968; East 1970). NZB disease has been studied extensively as a model for autoimmune diseases. Clinically, mice begin to develop splenomegaly and lymphadenopathy by 10 months and die by 18 months. Other changes typical of NZB disease are hemosiderosis, extramedullary hematopoiesis, and hyalin changes in the splenic arteries. Lymphoid hyperplasia occurs in the early stages, but later lymphoid atrophy and reticuloendothelial hyperplasia are present.

Erythrocytic autoantibodies (7S, IgG) coat the plasma membranes of affected erythrocytes, the basis of the positive Coombs test. Erythrocytes from healthy, Coombs-negative donors are rapidly destroyed in the spleen of older Coombs-positive recipients (but not vice versa) indicating that these cells also become coated with antibody. Splenectomy delays autoantibody formation and removes the organ of erythrocyte destruction; clinically, the anemia is thereupon improved. Sera of affected mice also contain large amounts of IgM. The macroglobulinemia is apparent even in germfree NZB mice. Humoral responses are "enthusiastic" but not aberrant.

Membranous glomerulonephritis develops as mice age and is characterized by irregular thickening of the capillary basement membrane and cresentric epithelial proliferation of the capsule. Ultrastructurally, there are proliferation of the mesangium, endothelial cell proliferation, fibrinoid thrombi, and the development of sclerosis. Electron-dense deposits are due to trapping of specific antigen-antibody complexes. Deposits are composed of IgG and components of complement but, after effacement of glomerular architecture, albumin and fibrinogen can also be identified (Lambert and Dixon 1968). Lymphocytes and plasmacytes cluster around the arteries in the kidney, some of which show sclerosis (Hicks 1966). There is no correlation between the renal and blood diseases.

Thymectomy (which should restrict immune reactivity) does not affect Coombs reactivity. Germinal centers are detected in the thymus of NZB mice, but are not unique and are not related to Coombs positivity (Siegler 1965). The disappearance of thymic epithelial cells may be important (Vries and Hijmans 1966).

POSTVACCINAL ENCEPHALOMYELITIS

Postvaccinal allergic encephalomyelitis is a rare complication of immunization using rabies virus grown in central nervous system tissues. It occurs in dogs, humans, and other mammals which have been repeatedly immunized against rabies after being bitten by a rabid animal. The clinical signs of paralysis and disorientation are a result of lymphocytic cuffing and demyelination that occur in the white matter of the brain and spinal cord.

Experimental allergic encephalomyelitis (EAE) is produced by injecting an animal with brain tissue extracts and is a widely studied model of immunologic CNS disease. The encephalitogenic antigen has been identified as a positively charged protein present in myelin. The lesion is mediated by the T-lymphocyte system and is characterized by foci of demyelination surrounded by perivascular lymphocytic infiltration and inflammation. The disease is transferable from donor to recipient by immune lymphocytes, but not by serum. Antibodies are not mechanistic and are, in fact, protective; by binding to the basic protein they inhibit its access to autoreactive T lymphocytes.

IDIOPATHIC POLYNEURITIS (GUILLAIN-BARRÉ SYNDROME)

Idiopathic polyneuritis is a postinfectious paralytic disease of humans which is usually transient and follows upper respiratory infections. An autoimmune mechanism has been proposed to explain the segmental demyelinating lesions in the spinal nerve roots and peripheral nerves which are responsible for the clinical signs.

Idiopathic polyneuritis of dogs (Coonhound paralysis) is a similar condition (Cummings and Haas 1972). Progressive paralysis begins 7–14 days after the dog has been bitten or scratched by a raccoon. Affected dogs are afebrile and alert; signs of disease vary from weakness to flaccid symmetric quadriplegia. The ventral nerve roots of the spinal cord and some peripheral nerves have lesions characterized by segmental demyelination and perivenular lymphoid infiltrates. Unfortunately, the lesions and pathogenesis of the disease are not clearly understood.

PEMPHIGUS

Pemphigus refers to a group of diseases of man characterized by bullous lesions of the skin and mucous membranes. Canine pemphigus arising as an autoallergic disease has been described in dogs. Bullae develop due to loss of coherence of epithelial cells with subsequent acantholysis. The autoantibodies present in serum appear to be directed against glycoproteins of the epithelium (Hurvitz et al. 1975).

AMYLOIDOSIS

Amyloidosis is the disease resulting from the deposition of amyloid in tissue. Early observations of its association with chronic antigenic stimulation and abnormal plasmacytosis implicated the immune system in the etiology.

Amyloid is a fibrous protein produced by aberrant reticuloendothelial cells and deposited in tissues in association with polysaccharides. Discovered by Rokitansky and clarified by Virchow as an iodine-staining starchy substance, it has been defined by generations of light microscopists as an homogeneous extracellular glycoprotein, distinguished from other hyaline material by staining, specific sites of deposition, and its association with specific disease states. Amyloid fibrils and their polysaccharide matrices constitute pure amyloid (Pras et al. 1971). In most lesions, however, the fibrils represent a spongelike scaffold upon which other substances have been absorbed.

Amyloid in tissue is confirmed by: (1) ultrastructural demonstration of amyloid fibrils 10–15 nm wide and of indeterminant length since they crisscross into and out of the plane of section (Shirahama and Cohen 1967) and (2) histochemical staining with Congo red. Amyloid fibrils have a high affinity for Congo red, which induces birefringence under polarized light due to the peculiar alignment of stain on the parallel fibrils (Puchtler et al. 1962). Fibrils have a characteristic x-ray diffraction pattern indicating a β-pleated sheat configuration.

Violet dyes (crystal violet) and fluorochromes (thioflavin T) are also useful, but staining is too variable and nonspecific for proof. Histochemical techniques such as the PAS reaction and specific procedures for fibrin, collagen, complement, globulin, and acid mucopolysaccharides may also give positive results, chiefly because amyloid, depending on its stage of deposition, is contaminated with varying amounts of these substances. Plasma globulins can usually be demonstrated in amyloid, and current research indicates that human primary amyloids represent the deposition of immunoglobulin fragments in tissue (Glenner et al. 1972).

Amyloid in tissue is commonly found at necropsy, incident to diseases involving chronic infections, sepsis, or tissue-destructive processes. In these cases, amyloid is usually present in the spleen and the clinical sequelae are masked by the severity of the causal septic disease. It occasionally exists as a disease in its own right, and the clinical manifestations depend upon the organ affected (Trautwein 1965).

The spleen is the chief site of amyloid deposition in most animals. Amyloid is formed in three sites: (1) at the periphery of the periarteriolar sheath, (2) between the adventitia and smooth muscle cells of the central artery, and (3) in cells in the red pulp. The greatest amount is deposited at the marginal zone at the periphery of the periarteriolar lymphoid sheath and results in the term "perifollicular amyloid." Amyloid accumulates in large masses surrounded by reticular cells, and in the early stages of deposition is generally free of contaminating collagen, fibrin, and other proteins. The relation of amyloid in this location to the reticular sheaths around the penicillar arterioles is not known. Amyloid is also commonly seen infiltrating the central arteriole. Here it is closely associated with abnormal smooth muscle cells and is generally interspersed with collagen, probably due to a close association with adventitial cells. Amyloid may also be seen associated with degenerating plasma cells in the sinuses of the red pulp, where it forms at the periphery of the cell (Figs. 5.23 and 5.24).

Renal amyloidosis produces the most serious consequences. It is common in old

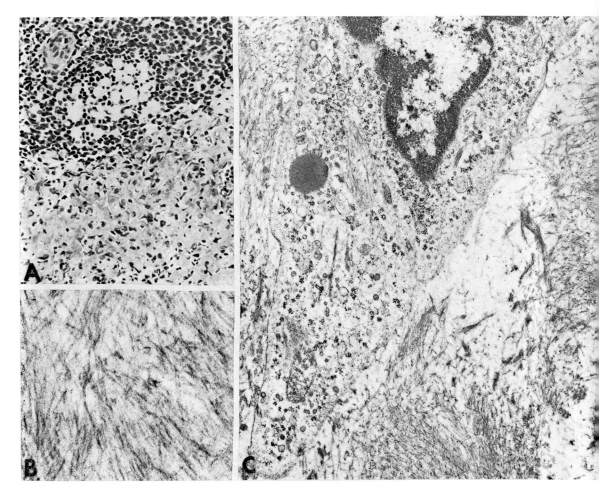

Fig. 5.23. Amyloidosis. Spleen, dog with cyclic neutropenia. A. Perifollicular accumulation of dense amyloid (bottom) in the spleen. Large globules of new amyloid within the lymphoid sheath. Central artery (top left) is also affected. B. Amyloid fibrils at high power. C. Amyloid-producing cell. Cytoplasm filled with polyribosomes. Amyloid fibrils present extracellularly.

dogs and the glomerulus is severely affected (Fig. 5.25). Death results from uremia. The liver is the chief site of deposition in some species and is the usual site in birds. Amyloid is deposited adjacent to hyperplastic Kupffer cells and within blood vessels. In rare instances, death may be due to massive liver deposits and hepatic rupture. In even less common situations, pancreatic islet cell destruction may lead to diabetes mellitus, or deposition in the adrenal zona glomerulosa may influence salt and water metabolism.

Amyloidosis is progressive, and amyloid is inefficiently removed by the reticuloendothelial system. Amyloid fibrils are curiously resistant to phagocytosis and proteolysis; they are not remarkably immunogenic. These characteristics probably result from the large size of the amyloid molecules. When amyloid is incubated with neutrophils and monocytes experimentally, very little is phagocytized (Franklin and Zucker-Franklin 1972). However, if the molecules are slightly altered or distorted by the addition of heterologous antibody,

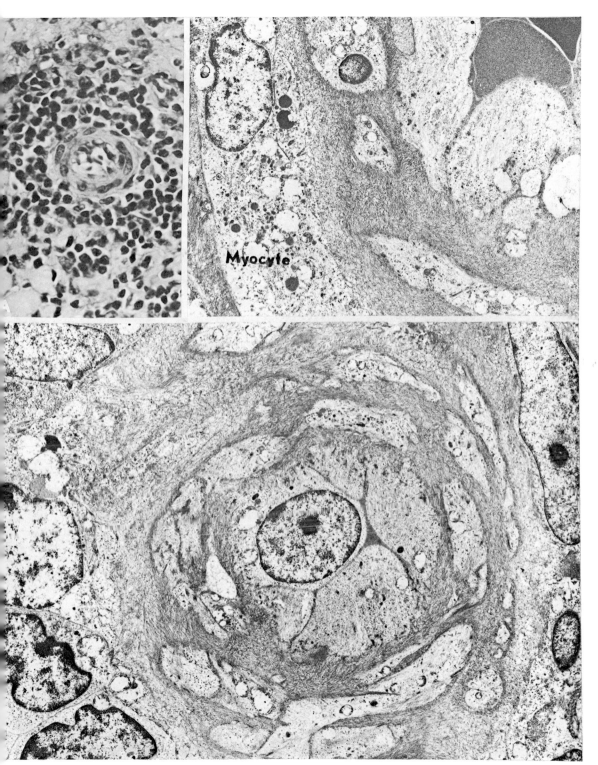

Myocyte

Fig. 5.24. Amyloid in muscular artery. A. Histology. Splenic central
artery. B. Ultrastructure. Infiltration of vascular wall with fibrils.
C. Degeneration of vascular myocyte.

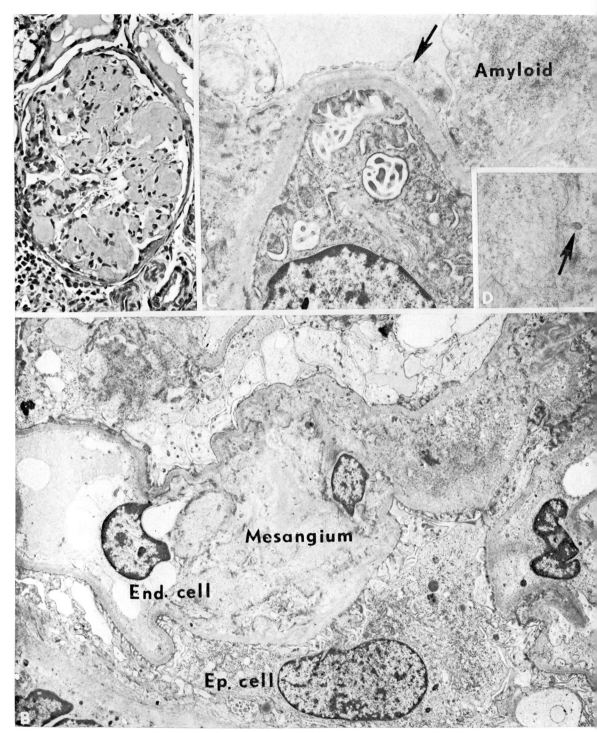

Fig. 5.25. Renal amyloidosis in a dog. A. Histology. B. Amyloid fibrils in the mesangium. Marked degenerative changes occur in the endothelial and epithelial cells. C. Amyloid fibrils beneath the fenestrated endothelium (arrow). D. Streaming of fibrils from a transport vesicle, endothelial cell.

Table 5.10.   Amyloidosis

Primary (idiopathic)
  Plasmacytoma-associated (amyloid produced by
    tumor cells)
  Aging-associated (vascular amyloid is dominant)
  Local amyloidosis (seen in pancreatic islet cells,
    nasal mucosa of horses, thyroid interstitium,
    and mammary gland)
  Systemic amyloidosis (widespread accumulation
    in mesenchymal tissues, especially heart,
    tongue, and intestine)
Secondary to chronic disease
  Chronic bacterial infection (tuberculosis, osteo-
    myelitis, and deficiencies of immune and in-
    flammatory mechanisms)
  Hyperimmunization (especially in horses used
    for antitoxin production)
  Extensive tissue destruction of any cause

phagocytosis readily occurs. Even though some phagocytosis and elimination occur in vivo, the persistence of the underlying defect usually causes amyloid production to dominate its resorption. If the cause of the disease is removed, amyloid disappears from organs with active macrophages such as spleen, but may not do so from the renal glomerulus.

Traditionally, amyloidosis is classified into primary and secondary types (Table 5.10). While there may be pathogenetic differences between them, it is more likely that they represent variations that depend upon the cell type involved in production and the manner of tissue deposition (Jakob 1971). In humans, primary amyloid is composed of Ig light chains; secondary amyloid is a non Ig protein.

PATHOGENESIS

Amyloid is a fibrous protein, and one assumes that in amyloidosis there is an underlying abnormal proliferation of protein-synthesizing cells. There are indeed atypical reticular cells present in lesions (Figs. 5.24 and 5.25). It is reasonable to call them "amyloid cells," for they appear to be irrevocably directed toward abnormal protein synthesis. Amyloidosis is associated with dysfunction of the immune systems and is frequently accompanied or preceded by proliferation of lymphoid cells and increases in globulin production. In those rare lesions we classify as primary amyloidosis, it is conceivable that other protein-synthesizing cells, such as thyroid or pancreatic islet cells, may participate in amyloid formation.

The *two-phase cellular theory* of local amyloid secretion (Teilum 1964) is based upon amyloid formation in situ by fixed reticuloendothelial (RE) cells due to secretion of insoluble polysaccharide-containing globulins. An initial pyroninophilic phase is characterized by proliferation of reticuloendothelial cells and a rise in serum gamma globulin. The second or amyloid phase is characterized by development of PAS-staining cells (with abnormal glycoprotein) and decrease in gamma globulin levels. The transition from the initial phase to the amyloid phase is dependent upon suppression of proliferating RE cells, either by exhaustion of the immune mechanism following protracted antigenic stimulation or by immunorepressive drugs. The breakdown of immunoglobulin production results in formation of amyloid in situ as glycoprotein products of plasmacytic cells.

The pathogenesis of naturally occurring amyloidosis in animals has not been adequately studied. To illustrate the progression of the disease, we show serum proteins and spleen biopsies of a gray Collie which had cyclic neutropenia (Fig. 5.26). The dog

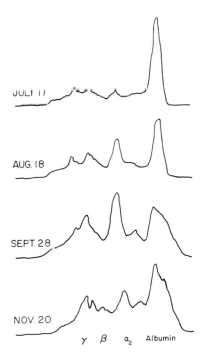

Fig. 5.26. Plasma proteins in dog with progressive amyloidosis.

suffered periodic episodes of gingivitis, rhinitis, and enteritis (beginning at 2 months of age) which were initiated by the cyclic depression of its neutrophils. Gradually, elevations in alpha$_2$ globulin were seen, and progressive increases in all plasma globulins characterized late disease. A splenic biopsy taken at 3 months had no amyloid but contained small lymphocyte sheaths with no germinal centers. At 4 months there were wide cuffs of large pyroninophilic lymphoblasts in the sheaths but no amyloid. At necropsy at 6 months of age marked splenic amyloidosis was present.

Experimental amyloidosis can be produced by repeated injections of highly antigenic material. Casein given to mice or rabbits is most commonly used (Christensen and Rask-Nielsen 1962; Heefner and Sorenson 1962). The process is hastened by use of cortisone or x-radiation. If spleen cells (from mice in the preinduction phase of casein treatment) are harvested and transferred to normal syngeneic recipient mice, the latter will rapidly develop splenic amyloid if suppressed immunologically (Werdelin and Ranlov 1966). The spleen cells that form amyloid are large PAS-staining reticular cells.

It has been demonstrated unequivocally that these cells secrete amyloid (Bari et al. 1969). Spleen cells from amyloidotic mice were maintained in cell culture for 6 months. Only dark stellate reticular cells survived in old cultures and these produced increasing amounts of amyloid. The fibrils accumulated at the cell surface and in some cases were present in cell membrane invaginations.

IMMUNOLOGIC ASPECTS OF AMYLOIDOSIS

Amyloid has been examined immunologically by attempts to produce antibodies against amyloid components and by the search for immunoglobulins within tissue amyloid. Antibodies against purified fibrils or degraded subunits induced in a heterologous host can be produced; these antibodies have value in the preparation of fluorescein-conjugated stains for the immunofluorescent detection of amyloid in tissue. Antibodies against purified human amyloid fibrils (produced in rabbits) react in agar gel diffusion tests with alpha$_2$ globulin; the reaction implicates this protein in the pathogenesis of amyloid (Cathcart et al. 1965).

The concept that primary amyloid results from aberrant immunoglobulin production finds substantiation in the analysis of concentrated amyloid fibrils produced by purification of amyloid from human tissue. Amino acid sequences are similar to plasmacytoma (Bence-Jones) proteins and it is asserted that the major protein component of the amyloid fibril is derived from light polypeptide chains (Glenner et al. 1972). Evidence has been presented that amyloid fibrils can be synthesized in vitro from Ig light chains. By proteolytic digestion of Bence-Jones proteins from human patients with amyloidosis, a precipitate results that has the characteristics of the amyloid fibril. This suggests that amyloid fibers may be formed by intralysosomal proteolytic digestion of circulating light Ig chains. The variable region of the light chain appears to play an essential role. Each amyloid protein appears homogeneous and this indicates an origin from a single aberrant clone of cells.

It has been proposed that the genesis of casein-induced amyloid involves a B-cell population. Mice with T-cell defects form amyloid as readily as normal mice.

If amyloid represents the abnormal synthesis of immunoglobulin polypeptide fragments, amyloidosis should be repressed by factors that negate plasmacytosis and antibody formation. This does not appear to be the case. Bursectomized chickens treated with casein are devoid of plasmacytes and do not form antibody. They do develop amyloid at the same rate as intact chickens (Druet and Janigan 1966).

Attention has been focused on the relation of amyloid formation and impaired cellular immunity. Factors such as thymectomy, splenectomy, irradiation, and cortisone therapy, which promote depletion of small lymphocytes, all accelerate amyloid formation. Specific cellular unresponsiveness to casein (used to induce amyloidosis) has been shown to develop during amyloid formation in guinea pigs, even though cellular immunity to other antigens remained intact. It was suggested that tolerance to specific immunogens may therefore play a role in amyloid production, and that amyloid is the end product of a specific clone of inactivated lymphocytes (Cathcart et al. 1970; Letterer and Kretschmer 1966).

REFERENCES

Able, M. E., Lee, J. C. and Rosenau, W. Lymphocyte-target cell interaction in vitro. *Am. J. Path.* 60:421, 1970.

Aitkin, M. M. and Sanford, J. Experimental anaphylaxis in cattle. *J. Comp. Path.* 79:131, 1969.

Allen, W. D. and Porter, P. Localization of immunofluorescence of secretory component and IgA in the intestinal mucosa of the young pig. *Immunology* 24:365, 1973.

Anderson, L. J. and Jarrett, W. F. H. Membranous glomerulonephritis associated with leukemia in cats. *Res. Vet. Sci.* 12:179, 1971.

Anderson, L. J. and McKeating, F. J. Immunological response in lymph nodes of the cat. *Immunology* 19:935, 1970.

Arakawa, M. and Kimmelsteil, P. The glomerulonephritis of acute serum sickness. *Am. J. Clin. Path.* 54:60, 1970.

Arkins, J. A. et al. The characterization of skin-sensitizing antibody induced in non-sensitized dogs. *J. Allergy* 40:50, 1967.

Arnason, B. G. and Waksman, B. H. The retest reaction in delayed hypersensitivity. *Lab. Invest.* 12:737, 1963.

Banks, K. L., Henson, J. B. and McGuire, T. L. Immunologically mediated glomerulonephritis of horses. *Lab. Invest.* 26:701, 708, 1972.

Bari, W. A., Pettengill, O. S. and Sorenson, G. D. Electron microscopy and electron microscopic autoradiography of splenic cell cultures from mice with amyloidosis. *Lab. Invest.* 20:234, 1969.

Batzing, B. L. and Hanna, M. G., Jr. Localization of endogenous C type virus in the glomerular basement membrane of aged AKR mice. *J. Immun.* 110:1189, 1973.

Baumgarten, A. and Wilhelm, C. L. Vascular permeability responses in hypersensitivity. *Pathology* 1:305, 1969.

Bienenstock, J. and Dolezel, J. Peyers patches: Lack of specific antibody-containing cells after oral and parenteral immunization. *J. Immun.* 106:938, 1971.

Blau, J. N. Hassall's corpuscles—a site of thymocyte death. *Brit. J. Exp. Path.* 54:634, 1973.

Bockman, D. E. and Cooper, M. D. Pinocytosis by epithelium associated with lymphoid follicles in the bursa of Fabricius, appendix, and Peyer's patches. An electron microscopic study. *Am. J. Anat.* 136:455, 1973.

Booth, B. H., Patterson, R. and Talbot, C. H. Immediate-type hypersensitivity in dogs: Cutaneous anaphylactic and respiratory responses to Ascaris. *J. Lab. Clin. Med.* 76:190, 1970.

Brambell, F. W. R. *Frontiers of Biology: The Transmission of Passive Immunity from Mother to Young,* Vol. 18. American Elsevier, New York, 1970.

Branca, M. et al. Immune complex disease. I. Pathological changes in the kidneys of BALB/c mice neonatally infected with Moloney leukemogenic and murine sarcoma viruses. *Clin. Exp. Immun.* 9.853, 1971.

Brummerstedt, E. et al. Lethal trait A46 in cattle. *Nord. Vetmed.* 26:279, 1974.

Carmichael, L. E. The pathogenesis of ocular lesions of infectious canine hepatitis. *Vet. Path.* 2:344, 1965.

Cathcart, E. S., Comerford, F. R. and Cohen, A. S. Immunologic studies on a protein extracted from human secondary amyloid. *New Engl. J. Med.* 273:143, 1965.

Cathcart, E. S., Mullarkey, M. and Cohen, A. S. Amyloidosis: An expression of immunologic tolerance. *Lancet* 2:639, 1970.

Chanock, R. M. et al. Influence of immunologic factors in respiratory syncytial virus disease. *Arch. Envir. Hlth.* 21:3471, 1970.

Christensen, H. E. and Rask-Nielsen, R. Comparative morphologic histochemical and serologic studies on the pathogenesis of casein-induced and reticulosarcoma-induced amyloidosis in mice. *J. Nat. Cancer Inst.* 28:1, 1962.

Claesson, M. H. and Jørgensen, D. Comparative studies of the paracortical post-capillary venules of normal and nude mice. *Acta Path. Micro. Scand. B* 82:249, 1974.

Clark, S. L. Incorporation of sulfate by the mouse thymus. *J. Exp. Med.* 128:927, 1968.

Clawson, C. C., Finstad, J. and Good, R. A. Evolution of the immune response. V. Electron microscopy of plasma cells and lymphoid tissue of the paddle fish. *Lab. Invest.* 15:1830, 1966.

Cochrane, C. G. and Aikin, B. S. Polymorphonuclear leukocytes in immunologic reactions. The destruction of vascular basement membrane in vivo and in vitro. *J. Exp. Med.* 124:733, 1966.

Jönsson, Å. Transfer of immunoglobulins from mother to offspring. *Acta Vet. Scand. Suppl.* 43:1, 1973.

Kagnoff, M. F. and Campbell, S. Functional characteristics of Peyers patch lymphoid cells. *J. Exp. Med.* 139:398, 1974.

Karnovsky, M. J., Unanue, E. R. and Leventhal, M. Ligand-induced movement of lymphocyte membrane macromolecules. II. Mapping of surface moieties. *J. Exp. Med.* 136:907, 1972.

Kim, Y. B., Bradley, S. G. and Watson, D. W. Ontogeny of the immune response. *J. Immun.* 101:224, 1968.

Kite, J. H. et al. Spontaneous thyroiditis in an obese strain of chickens. *J. Immun.* 103: 1331, 1969.

Kraehenbuhl, J. P. and Campiche, M. A. Early stages of intestinal absorption of specific antibodies in the newborn. *J. Cell Biol.* 42:345, 1969.

Lambert, P. H. and Dixon, F. J. Pathogenesis of the glomerulonephritis of NZB/W mice. *J. Exp. Med.* 127:507, 1968.

Langevoort, H. L. The histophysiology of the antibody response. *Lab. Invest.* 12:106, 1963.

Lanman, J. T. and Herod, L. Homograft immunity in pregnancy. *J. Exp. Med.* 122:579, 1965.

Lawrence, H. S. Transfer factor. *Adv. Immun.* 11:195, 1969.

Leslie, C. A., Crandall, R. B. and Crandall, C. A. Studies on the secretory immunological system of fowl. II. Immunoglobulin producing cells associated with mucous membranes. *Immunology* 21:983, 1971.

Letterer, E. and Kretschmer, R. Experimental amyloidosis and tolerance. *Nature* 210: 390, 1966.

Lewis, R. M. An evaluation of the clinical usefulness of the LE cell phenomenon in dogs. *J.A.V.M.A.* 147:939, 1965.

Lewis, R. M. and Schwartz, R. S. Canine systemic lupus erythematosus. Genetic analysis of an established breeding colony. *J. Exp. Med.* 134:417, 1971.

Lewis, R. M., Schwartz, R. S. and Henry, W. B. Canine systemic lupus erythematosus. *Blood* 25:143, 1965.

Lewis, R. M. et al. Canine systemic lupus erythematosus. Transmission of serologic abnormalities by cell-free filtrates. *J. Clin. Invest.* 52:1893, 1973.

Lewis, R. M. et al. Chronic allogeneic disease. I. Development of glomerulonephritis. *J. Exp. Med.* 128:653, 1968.

Lewis, R. M. et al. A syndrome of autoimmune hemolytic anemia and thrombocytopenia. *Proc. Am. Vet. Med. Ass.*, p. 140, 1963.

Linklater, K. A., McTaggart, H. S. and Imlah, P. Hemolytic disease of the newborn. *Brit. Vet. J.* 129:36, 1973.

Lösch, U. and Hoffmann-Fezer, G. Vergleichende histologische und immunologische Untersuchungen an immunologisch defekten Huhnern. *Zentr. Vetmed. A* 20:596, 1973.

Mandel, T. Ultrastructure of epithelial cells in the medulla of the guinea pig thymus. *Austr. J. Exp. Biol. Med. Sci.* 46:755, 1968.

Mayr, A. et al. Untersuchungen über Art, Umfang und Uraschen von Impfschäden nach der Maul- und Klauenseuche-Schutzimpfung in Bayern in den Jahren 1967/68. *Zentr. Vetmed. B* 16:488, 1969.

McCluskey, R. T., Benacerraf, B. and McCluskey, M. W. Studies on the specificity of the cellular infiltrate in delayed hypersensitivity reactions. *J. Immun.* 90:466, 1963.

McGregor, D. D. Bone marrow origin of immunologically competent lymphocytes in rat. *J. Exp. Med.* 127:953, 1968.

———. Studies by thoracic duct drainage of the function and potentialities of the lymphocyte. *Fed. Proc.* 25:1713, 1964.

McGuire, T. L., Poppie, M. J. and Banks, K. C. Combined (B- and T-lymphocyte) immunodeficiency: A fatal genetic disease in Arabian foals. *J.A.V.M.A.* 164:70, 1974.

McMaster, P. D. and Franzl, R. E. The primary immune response in mice. *J. Exp. Med.* 127:1109, 1968.

Medawar, P. B. The homograft reaction. *Proc. Royal Soc. B* 149:145, 1958.

Milgrom, F., Klassen, J. and Fuji, H. Immunologic injury to homografts. *J. Exp. Med.* 134:193s, 1971.

Miller, J. F. A. P. Role of the thymus in transplantation immunity. *Ann. N.Y. Acad. Sci.* 99:340, 1962.

Miller, J. J. Studies of the phylogeny and ontogeny of the specialized lymphatic venules. *Lab. Invest.* 21:484, 1969.

Miller, J. J. and Nossal, G. Antigens in immunity. VI. The phagocytic reticulum of lymph node follicles. *J. Exp. Med.* 120:1075, 1964.

Mitchell, J. and Abbot, A. Antigens in immunity. XVI. Light and electron microscopic study of antigen localization of the rat spleen. *Immunology* 21:207, 1971.

Moore, M. A. S. and Owen, J. J. T. Experimental studies on the development of the thymus. *J. Exp. Med.* 126:715, 1967a.

———. Studies in the irradiated chick embryo. *Nature* 215:1081, 1967b.

Muscoplat, C. C. et al. Lymphocyte surface immunoglobulin: Frequency in normal and lymphocytotic cattle. *Am. J. Vet. Res.* 35:593, 1974.

Nagy, Z. A., Horvath, E. and Urbán. Z. Antigen capture in spleen and relationship to phagocytic activity in chickens. *Nature NB* 242:241, 1973.

Najarian, J. S. and Feldman, J. D. Passive transfer of tuberculin sensitivity by tritiated thymidine-labeled lymphoid cells. *J. Exp. Med.* 114:779, 1961.

Nansen, P. Selective immunoglobulin-deficiency in cattle and susceptibility to infection. *Acta Path. Micro. Scand.* 80:49, 1972.

Nieuwenhuis, P. and Keuning, F. J. Germinal centers and the origin of the B-cell system. *Immunology* 26:509, 1974.

Nordstoga, K. Thrombocytopenic purpura in baby piglets caused by maternal isoimmunization. *Vet. Path.* 2:601, 1965.

Nossal, G. et al. Antigens in immunity. XV. Ultrastructural features of antigen capture in primary and secondary lymphoid follicles. *J. Exp. Med.* 127:277, 1967.

Oort, J. and Turk, J. L. The fate of I131-labeled antigens in the skin of normal guinea pigs and those with delayed-type hypersensitivity. *Immunology* 6:148, 1963.

Pan, I. C. et al. Glomerulonephritis in Aleutian disease of mink: Ultrastructural studies. *J. Path.* 102:33, 1970.

Parrott, D., De Sousa, A. B. and East, J. Thymus dependent areas in the lymphoid organs of neonatally thymectomized mice. *J. Exp. Med.* 123:191, 1966.

Pascal, R. R., Koss, M. N. and Kassel, R. L. Glomerulonephritis associated with immune complex deposits and viral particles in spontaneous murine leukemia. *Lab. Invest.* 29:159, 1973.

Patterson, R. and Sparks, D. B. The passive transfer to normal dogs of skin reactivity asthma and anaphylaxis from a dog with spontaneous ragweed pollen sensitivity. *J. Immun.* 88:262, 1962.

Patterson, R. et al. The metabolism of serum proteins in the hen and chick and secretion of serum proteins by the ovary of the hen. *J. Gen. Physiol.* 45:501, 1962.

Pauli, B., Gerber, H. and Schatzmann, U. "Farmers lung" beim Pferd. *Path. Micro.* 38:200, 1972.

Pavlovsky, S. et al. Etude de la réponse immunologique au niveau cellulaire. I. Identification des cellules formatrices de rosettes en microscopie optique et électronique. *Ann. Inst. Pasteur* 119:63, 1970.

Perey, D. Y. E. and Guttman, R. D. Peyer's patch cells. Absence of graft-versus-host reactivity in mice and rats. *Lab. Invest.* 27:427, 1972.

Perkins, W. D., Karnovsky, M. J. and Unanue, E. R. An ultrastructural study of lymphocytes with surface-bound immunoglobulins. *J. Exp. Med.* 135:267, 1972.

Pirie, H. M. et al. A bovine disease similar to farmer's lung: Extrinsic allergic alveolitis. *Vet. Rec.* 88:346, 1971.

Poger, M. E. and Lamm, M. E. Localization of free and bound secretory component in human intestinal epithelial cells. *J. Exp. Med.* 139:629, 1974.

Polliack, A. et al. Identification of human B and T lymphocytes by scanning electron microscopy. *J. Exp. Med.* 138:607, 1973.

Porter, P. Immunoglobulin in bovine mammary secretion. *Immunology* 23:225, 1972.

Pras, M. et al. The significance of mucopolysaccharides in amyloid. *J. Histochem. Cytochem.* 19:443, 1971.

Puchtler, H., Sweat, F. and Levine, M. On the binding of Congo red by amyloid. *J. Histochem. Cytochem.* 10:355, 1962.

Raviola, E. and Karnovsky, M. J. Evidence for a blood-thymus barrier using electron-opaque tracers. *J. Exp. Med.* 136:466, 1972.

Rockey, J. H. and Schwartzman, R. M. Skin sensitizing antibodies: A comparative study of canine and human PK and PCA antibody and a canine myeloma protein. *J. Immun.* 98:1143, 1967.

Rosenau, W., Goldberg, M. L. and Burke, G. C. Early biochemical alterations induced by lymphotoxin in target cells. *J. Immun.* 111:1128, 1973.

Rygaard, J. and Povlsen, C. O. Effects of homozygosity of the nude (Nu) gene in three inbred strains of mice. *Acta Path. Micro. Scand.* 82:48, 1974.

Santos-Buch, C. A. and Treadwell, D. E. Disruption of Kupffer cells during systemic anaphylaxis in the mouse. *Am. J. Path.* 51:505, 1968.

Schoefl, G. The migration of lymphocytes across the vascular endothelium in lymphoid tissue. *J. Exp. Med.* 136:568, 1972.

Schofield, G. C. and Atkins, A. M. Secretory immunoglobulin in columnar epithelial cells of the large intestine. *J. Anat.* 107:491, 1970.

Shirahama, T. and Cohen, A. S. High-resolution electron microscopic analysis of the amyloid fibril. *J. Cell Biol.* 33:679, 1967.

Siegler, R. Pathogenesis of thymic changes in NZB mice with hemolytic anemia. *J. Exp. Med.* 122:929, 1965.

Simpson-Morgan, M. W. and Smeaton, T. C. The transfer of antibodies by neonates and adults. *Adv. Vet. Sci.* 16:355, 1972.

Söderström, N. and Stenström, A. Outflow paths of cells from the lymph node parenchyma to the efferent lymphatics. *Scand. J. Haem.* 6:186, 1961.

Stockman, G. D. et al. Differential effects of cyclophosphamide on the B and T cell compartments of adult mice. *J. Immun.* 110:277, 1973.

Stone, W. H. and Irwin, M. R. Blood groups in animals other than man. *Adv. Immun.* 3:315, 1963.

Sulzman, A. E. The histological distribution of blood group substances in man as determined by immunofluorescence. *J. Exp. Med.* 111:789, 1960.

Sutherland, J. C. and Mardiney, M. R., Jr. Immune complex disease in the kidneys of lymphoma-leukemia patients: The presence of an oncornavirus-related antigen. *J. Nat. Cancer Inst.* 50:633, 1973.

Suzuki, I. et al. Intracellular distribution of immunoglobulin heavy and light chains within tissue cultured cells of human lymphoid origin detected by electron microscopy. *J. Immun.* 104:907, 1970.

Taylor, R. B. et al. Redistribution and pinocytosis of lymphocyte surface immunoglobulin molecules induced by antiimmunoglobulin antibody. *Nature New Biol.* 233:225, 1971.

Teilum, G. Pathogenesis of amyloidosis. *Acta Path. Micro. Scand.* 61:21, 1964.

Thomlinson, J. R. and Buxton, A. Anaphylaxis in pigs and its relation to the pathology of oedema disease and gastroenteritis associated with *Escherichia coli. Immunology* 6:126, 1963.

Tizard, I. R. Macrophage cytophilic antibodies and the function of macrophage-bound immunoglobulins. *Bact. Rev.* 35:365, 1971.

Tomasi, T. B. et al. Characteristics of an immune system common to certain external secretions. *J. Exp. Med.* 121:101, 1965.

Trautwein, G. Vergleichende Untersuchungen über das Amyloid und Paramyloid verschiedener Tierarten. *Vet Path.* 2:493, 1965.

Unanue, E. R. The regulatory role of macrophages in antigenic stimulation. *Adv. Immun.* 15:95, 1972.

Vaerman, J. P. Studies on the IgA system of the horse. *Immunology* 21:443, 1971.

Vaerman, J. and Heremans, J. F. Distribution of various immunoglobulin containing cells in canine lymphoid tissue. *Immunology* 17:627, 1969.

van Haelst, J. J. G. Light and electron microscopic study of the normal and pathological thymus of the rat. *Zt. Zellf.* 99:198, 1969.

van Rooijen, N. Antigens in spleen. *Immunology* 22:757, 1972.

Venkatachalam, M. A. and Cotran, R. S. Ultrastructure of the local Arthus phenomenon using horseradish peroxidase as antigen. *Lab. Invest.* 23:29, 1970.

Waksman, B. H. The pattern of rejection in rat skin homografts and its relation to the vascular network. *Lab. Invest.* 12:46, 1963.

Walker, K. Z., Schoefl, G. I. and Lafferty, K. T. The pathogenesis of the graft-versus-host reaction in chicken embryos. *Austr. J. Exp. Biol. Med. Sci.* 50:675, 1972.

Walton, G. S. Allergic responses involving the skin of domestic animals. *Adv. Vet. Sci.* 17:201, 1971.

Warner, N. L., Szenburg, A. and Burnet, F. M. The immunological role of different lymphoid organs in the chicken. *Austr. J. Exp. Biol. Med. Sci.* 40:373, 1962.

Wayne, J. W. Idiopathic thrombocytopenic purpura in a dog. *Can. Vet. J.* 1:569, 1960.

Webb, R. A. The mechanism of anaphylactic leucopenia in dogs. *J. Path. Bact.* 27:79, 1924.

Weiss, L. and Smyth, P. Primary rejection of homologous intraperitoneal fibroblasts: An electron microscopic study. *J. Immun.* 105:1375, 1970.

Werdelin, O. and Ranlov, P. Amyloidosis in mice produced by transfer of spleen cells from casein treated mice. *Acta Path. Micro. Scand.* 68:1, 1966.

White, R. G. and Gordon, J. Macrophage reception and recognition mechanisms in the chicken spleen. In *Mononuclear Phagocytes.* R. van Furth, ed., p. 510. Davis, Philadelphia, 1970.

Wick, G. and Graf, J. Electron microscopic studies in chickens of the obese strain with spontaneous hereditary autoimmune thyroiditis. *Lab. Invest.* 27:400, 1972.

Wick, G., Kite, J. H. and Witebsky, E. Spontaneous thyroiditis in obese strain of chickens. IV. The effect of thymectomy and thymobursectomy on the development of the disease. *J. Immun.* 104:54, 1970.

Wiener, J., Lattes, R. G. and Pearl, J. S. Vascular permeability and leukocyte emigration in allograft rejection. *Am. J. Path.* 55:295, 1969.

Wilkins, R. J., Hurvitz, A. I. and Dodds-Laffin, W. J. Immunologically mediated thrombocytopenia in the dog. *J.A.V.M.A.* 163:277, 1973.

Williams, D. M. and Rowland, A. C. The palatine tonsils of the pig—an afferent route to the lymphoid tissue. *J. Anat.* 113:131, 1972.

Woodruff, J. M., Burcher, W. I. and Hellerstein, L. J. Early secondary disease in the Rhesus monkey. *Lab. Invest.* 27:85, 1972.

Wray, C. and Thomlinson, J. R. Anaphylaxis in calves and the development of gastrointestinal lesions. *J. Path.* 98: 61, 1969.

Yoshiki, T. et al. The viral envelope glycoprotein of murine leukemia virus and the pathogenesis of immune complex glomerulonephritis of New Zealand mice. *J. Exp. Med.* 140:1011, 1974.

Zagury, D. et al. Immunoglobulin synthesis and secretion. *J. Cell Biol.* 46:52, 1970.

Zucker-Franklin, D. and Franklin, E. C. Ultrastructural and immunofluorescent studies of cells associated with u-chain disease. *Blood* 37:257, 1971.

CHAPTER SIX

Neoplasia

Neoplasia involves an intrinsic heritable abnormality in cells which gives rise to autonomous growth. Neoplastic cells do not behave as integrated, interdependent populations, which we expect in metazoan animal tissue. The regulatory mechanisms of cell contact inhibition, differentiation, and mitosis are defective, and the cells grow in rapidly expanding masses that ultimately compromise host structure and function.

To understand the neoplastic cell, one must reconsider hyperplasia and metaplasia (Chapter 1). The capacity to undergo mitosis is inherent in all cells. Throughout life, mitotic activity is repressed or controlled in some way. Neoplastic cells lack this repression, and must be considered cells which are unresponsive to the controlling mechanism or in which the mechanism itself is imperfect.

Cancer is a chronic disease and extends backward for many months from the time clinical signs first appear. The clinical phases of the disease represent only a fraction of the pathogenetic process. Some epithelial lesions are termed *precancerous,* for they are known to smoulder silently for months or even years before malignant foci of cells can be readily demonstrated.

Neoplastic cell transformation in many cases probably involves the development of a series of discrete cell populations. That is, the progressive development of a tumor is characterized by the evolution of successive clones of cells, each coming one step closer to the overt cancer cell type which proliferates to stop only with the death of the host.

The methods and provisions for the study of animal neoplasms are dependent largely upon human medicine because of the enormous importance of cancer in man. There are therefore important differences in the statistical evidence available and the limitations of clinical treatment, which should be emphasized. Tumors do occur in invertebrates but the characteristic biologic behaviors, as they are manifested in mammals, do not. The phylogenetic development of neoplasms and of the immune system appear to have evolved in consort with vertebrate speciation. The implication that these two biologic systems are interdependent, however, has yet to be established (Wellings 1968).

Studies on the incidence of neoplasms in many species of animals cannot be relied upon. With the exception of pets, animals have short life spans: wild species because of predation, and domestic food-producing animals because they are slaughtered during young adulthood. If these animals do develop neoplasms, the lesion itself is often responsible for killing the individual before the tumor has been fully manifested.

The spectra of neoplasms for the cat and dog are well documented and those of some domesticated species reasonably so. For wild mammals many isolated reports exist, but few systematic collections of tumors have been made. Series of neoplasms in the lower vertebrate species including fish and reptiles exist (Lucké and Schlumberger 1949; Mawdesley-Thomas 1971; Wadsworth 1960).

GENERAL CONSIDERATIONS

TERMINOLOGY

Neoplasms that are well differentiated, grow slowly by expansion, and do not invade below basement membranes are called *benign*. A neoplasm is benign when its cellular characteristics are considered innocent, and this implies that the tumor will remain localized and is removable by simple excision. Benign tumors are often encapsulated (but lack of capsule does not imply malignancy). It must be added that benign tumors can be the cause of serious disease by exerting pressure on ducts, arteries, or the nervous system. Parathyroid adenomas may be tiny, yet can generate disease that is lethal to the animal.

Benign tumors are classified according to their histology. They are designated by adding the suffix *-oma* to the cell type of origin. A benign tumor of fibrocytes is therefore a *fibroma*. *Adenoma* is applied to benign epithelial tumors that produce glandular patterns (Table 6.1) (Fig. 6.1).

At the other extreme of tumor behavior are the *malignant* tumors whose cells are anaplastic and which metastasize and invade. The aggressive neoplastic cells invade and, in some cases, destroy normal tissues (Fig. 6.2). Malignancy is a clinical concept and its determining character must relate to the growth of the neoplasm within the animal. A "cancer" is a malignant neoplasm. Those of ectodermal derivation are called *carcinomas* and those of mesodermal origin are termed *sarcomas*.

Special terms are sometimes applied to malformations and tumors derived therefrom. A *hamartia* is a tissue defect of cells normally found in a particular area; a *hamartoma* is a tumor of these components, that is, an excessive, focal overgrowth of mature cells in an organ of identical cellular elements. A *choristia* is a tissue defect of structure not found normally in the area; a *choristoma* is a tumor of the same.

DEFINITION

Virchow is quoted as having said that no man even under torture can say what a tumor really is. A century later, definitions are little better, for they break down at one or more points. The definition of a neoplasm is made vague by the all-inclusive-

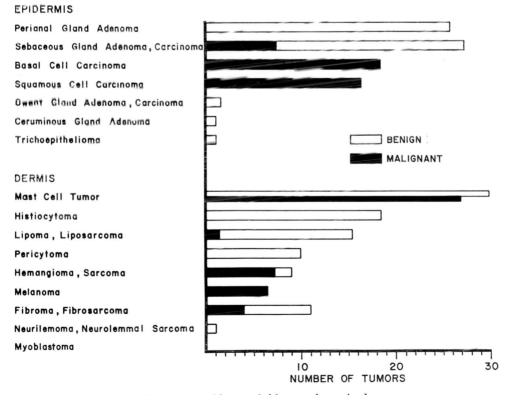

Fig. 6.1. Incidence of skin neoplasms in dogs.

Table 6.1. Classification of some neoplasms

Organ of Origin	Cell of Origin	Benign Tumor	Malignant Tumor
Epidermis	Squamous cell Basal cell	Acanthoma (Borland and Webber 1966)	Squamous cell carcinoma Basal cell carcinoma
Adnexae	Hair follicle Sweat gland Sebaceous gland Perianal gland	Trichoepithelioma Adenoma of Adenoma of Adenoma of (Kuhn 1968)	Adenocarcinoma of Adenocarcinoma of Adenocarcinoma of Adenocarcinoma of
Other glands	Salivary gland	Adenoma (Koestner and Buerger 1965)	Mixed tumor Adenocarcinoma
	Mammary gland	Adenoma (Bomhard 1973)	Adenocarcinoma Mixed tumor Duct tumor
Neurectoderm	Melanoblast	Melanoma	Malignant melanoma (Mishima 1967)
Connective tissue	Fibrocyte Adipose cell Undifferentiated cell	Fibroma Lipoma Histiocytoma Myxoma	Fibrosarcoma (Todd et al. 1973) Liposarcoma (Kalderon and Fethiere 1973) Reticulum cell sarcoma Myxosarcoma (Merkow et al. 1969)
	Mast cell Schwann cells Nerve sheath cell	Mastocytoma Neurilemmoma (Schwannoma) Neurofibroma (Duncan and Harkin 1969)	Mast cell sarcoma Malignant neurilemmoma Neurofibrosarcoma
Vascular tissue	Endothelium	Hemangioma Hemangioendothelioma (Ramsey 1966) Hemangiopericytoma (Battifora 1973) Vascular leiomyoma	Angiosarcoma Hemangioendotheliosarcoma Malignant hemangiopericytoma
Muscle tissue	Skeletal muscle Smooth muscle	Rhabdomyoma Leiomyoma	Rhabdomyosarcoma (Peter and Kluge 1970) Leiomyosarcoma (Ferenczy et al. 1971)
Skeletal tissue	Cartilage Bone	Chondroma Osteoma	Chondrosarcoma (Wellman 1969) Osteosarcoma (Franks et al. 1973; Perk and Hod 1973)
Other	Synovium Mesothelium Meninges	Synovioma Mesothelioma Meningioma	Synovial sarcoma (Gabbiani et al. 1971) Mesothelial sarcoma Meningioma, malignant

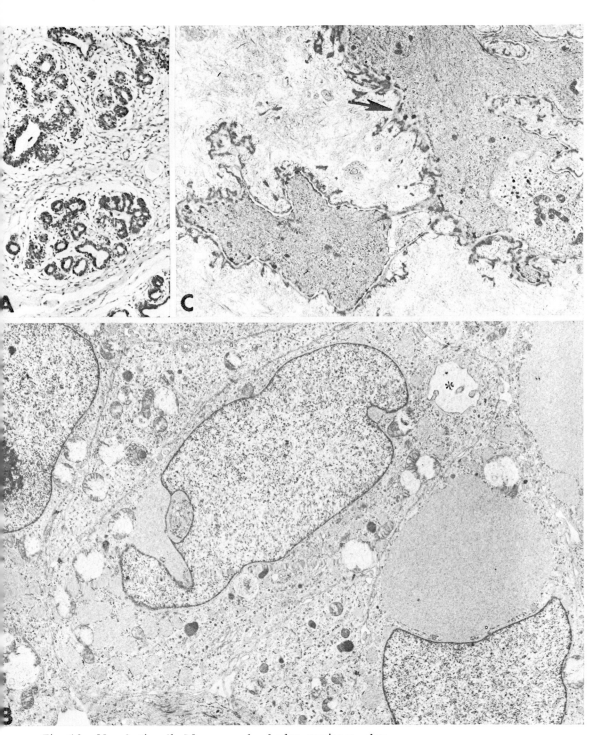

Fig. 6.2. Neoplastic cell. Mammary gland adenocarcinoma, dog.
A. Histology. Neoplastic cells lack normal organization and relation
to ducts and vascular tissues. B. Nuclei are irregular and contain
indentations and invaginations. Cytoplasm is filled with accumulation
of light granular secretory material and aberrant canaliculi (asterisk).
C. Markedly irregular basal plasma membrane of invasive neoplastic
cell with reduplication of dense basement membrane material (arrow).

ness of this group of diseases. Like infectious diseases, the term includes lesions of varying causes and pathobiologic behavior. Furthermore, the current intense research effort in oncology renders a static definition suspect almost immediately. It is not proper to make the term neoplasm appear oversimple and we therefore retrace some definitions as given by distinguished pathologists over the last century.

NEOPLASMS ARE ". . . CIRCUMSCRIBED
ATYPICAL PRODUCTIONS OF TISSUE FROM A
MATRIX OF SUPERABUNDANT OR ERRATIC
DEPOSITS OF EMBRYONIC ELEMENTS. . . ."
(Cohnheim, 1872)

This definition, one of the first, indicates that all neoplasms arose from embryonic tissue that remained latent. The development of the light microscope in the years preceding it initiated the scientific evaluation of tumor tissue. Virchow and his contemporaries believed that tumors grew by accretion of cells from surrounding tissues which were stimulated by a primary tumor nodule. The great contribution of this era was the demonstration by Muller that tumors were actually composed of cells and that they grew independently or, as put by Ribbert, "aus sich heraus." With the application of the microscope to the study of human neoplasms, lesions from all organs were documented and classified. Classification schemes were developed, based upon the correlation of histologic appearance and clinical behavior. The value in prognosis was outstanding. The histogenesis, or tissue-origin of tumors was established as a necessary clinicopathologic tool.

In those years, neoplasms of animals were rarely found, looked for, or reported. To an enlightened few it became obvious that the domestic animals suffered the same neoplastic diseases as did humans, and Leblanc, a French veterinarian, published a report on the cellularity of animal tumors in 1858.

The amazing success of microbiologists in transmitting infectious diseases in the latter half of the nineteenth century prompted similar attempts to transmit tumors. Scattered reports of transmission occurred, but evidence pointed to accidental or fallacious interpretation, and the consensus was that these attempts had consistently failed. The singular success was that of the Russian veterinarian Novinsky who in 1876 established the transplantability of the canine venereal tumor, a "discovery" made by medical pathologists no less than four times since. In the early 1900s, Jensen in Denmark passed tissue suspensions of a mouse mammary carcinoma through several generations. By careful histologic examination, his efforts established that transmission was effected by transplantation and not by inciting host cells to transform. The reasons why transplanted neoplastic cells so often failed to graft awaited the basic immunologic discoveries of Medawar in the 1940s.

"A TUMOR IS A NEW FORMATION OF CELLS
WHICH PROLIFERATES CONTINUOUSLY AND
WITHOUT CONTROL. . . ."
(F.B. Mallory, 1914)

Mallory's definition went on to state that tumor cells tended to differentiate toward their cell of origin, lacked an orderly structural arrangement, and served no useful function. This definition emphasized the lack of host control over tumor cell growth. It summed up a half century of histologic examination and classification of neoplasms and provided a sound basis for the differentiation of the neoplasms from other space-occupying lesions. Its failure relates to its ignorance of the study of causes of neoplasms which was beginning to emerge at this time.

At the beginning of the twentieth century, studies on animal tumors were still largely ignored, both as significant by veterinary clinicians and as models of human disease by medical scientists. Long-term exposures to x-radiation and coal tar were established as carcinogenic in animals, but these models related to only a few rare instances of naturally occurring neoplasms. These years represent an era of shame in medical research, for two highly significant discoveries were made at this time. First, lymphoid neoplasms of the chicken were shown to be transmissible by cell-free filtrates in Denmark by Ellerman and Bang. Second, a sarcoma of the chicken was readily transmitted in a similar way by Rous at the Rockefeller Institute and produced a rapidly expanding sarcoma in the recipient bird. Rous persisted for some years with his chicken sarcoma and belatedly received the Nobel prize in 1967. The results of these experiments should have implied not only that viruses were causal in cancer, but that the neoplastic process required a fundamental change in the cell. Unfortunately, medical scientists ignored these studies. The fact that the neoplasms were transmissible was even used as evidence against their being tumors. James Ewing, in his book *Neoplastic Diseases,* spoke for the age: ". . . it was impossible to regard as a valid hypothesis the conception of a specific group of parasites living in symbiosis with the cancer cell and stimulating its growth."

"A TUMOR IS AN ABNORMAL MASS OF TISSUE, THE GROWTH OF WHICH EXCEEDS AND IS UNCOORDINATED WITH THAT OF NORMAL TISSUE AND PERSISTS IN THE SAME EXCESSIVE MANNER AFTER CESSATION OF THE STIMULI WHICH EVOKED THE CHANGE. . . ,"

(Willis, 1948)

This definition is still a practical one. It correctly stresses the lack of coordinated growth of the tumor cells with other tissue cells of the organism. Previous definitions had asserted that neoplasms grew autonomously or without control, and this is not so. Tumor cells are dependent upon vascular architecture and host blood and lymph for survival. Despite their loss of autoregulatory mechanisms that normally control mitotic activity, they still are susceptible to some biologic regulation.

In the 1930s, experimental oncology gained momentum (Table 6.2). It was soon obvious that many bona fide animal tumors were transplantable, and that some were transmissible by cell-free filtrates. An agent transmissible in milk was shown to induce mammary tumors in mice. Most important, however, was the discovery that a virus was responsible for lymphosarcoma in mice. This initiated the reinvestigation of avian and mammalian models of cancer, and mobilized the discipline of virology to play its role in cancer research.

A great deal of work was done on viral-induced hyperplasias, such as the Shope rabbit papilloma that regressed when the

Table 6.2. Milestones in experimental oncology

1838	Möller (Germany) demonstrates the cellular nature of neoplasm by examining tumor tissue with the light microscope.
1858	Leblanc (France) establishes that animal tumor has a similar cellular composition.
1876	Novinsky (Russia) demonstrates transplantability of the canine venereal tumor.
1903	Jensen (Denmark) inoculates suspension of mouse mammary gland tumor into mice, reproduces tumors, and passes them serially.
1908	Ellerman and Bang (Denmark) discover transmissibility of avian lymphoid tumors.
1910	Rous transmits a sarcoma of a chicken by cell-free suspensions.
1910	Clunet (France) produces tumors experimentally by X radiation.
1912	Murphy shows that rat tumors will grow on the chicken chorioallantoic membrane.
1914	Yamamoto (Japan) proves carcinogenicity of coal tar by long-term application to skin of rabbits.
1924	Little and Strong develop inbred strains of mice for genetic analysis of tumors.
1932	Shope demonstrates viral nature of rabbit papilloma.
1936	Lücke discovers viral-induced renal carcinoma of the frog.
1936	Bittner discovers a viral agent in milk causing mammary gland carcinoma of mice.
1951	Gross isolates virus causing naturally occurring lymphoma in mice.
1956	Billingham shows survival of skin grafts in recipient mice.

virus was destroyed. Although these lesions, by definition, represented hyperplasia rather than neoplasia, the information obtained by study of the cells provided an important basis for future oncologic research.

The above definition emphasizes that one of the most distinctive characteristics of the neoplastic cell is the persistence of its excessive mitotic capacity in the absence of the stimulus that initiated mitosis. The current relevant questions of oncologic research are related to the mechanisms whereby cells are transformed to malignancy.

"NEOPLASIA RESULTS FROM CELL VARIATION WHICH REPRESENTS SOMATIC MUTATION AND/OR ABERRANT DIFFERENTIATION. . . ."

(Prehn, 1971)

It has become obvious in the last few decades that there is no such thing as the "cancer cell." This would have implied that all malignant neoplastic cells possessed, in common, some distinctive definable abnormality. No abnormal gene structure or abnormality of the total genome has ever been documented in a specific neoplasm. Cancer is not a mutation in the customary sense of that word. Those chromosomal abnormalities which have been reported are consequences of the neoplastic process and not involved in its causation. The search for a common basis for neoplastic cell behavior has directed attention toward two basic changes: somatic mutation and defects in the regulatory system of cells.

Since mitotic activity is generated by and largely occurs in the nucleus, it is most obvious to view this structure as responsible for neoplastic replication. The genetic information or genome of the cell is encoded in molecules of DNA and is written in a four-letter alphabet, the "letters" being four different chemical bases. In normal cells, the genetic information is transcribed from DNA to a closely related single strand of RNA and, in turn, translated from that strand into a protein constructed of amino acids. It seems that if the DNA molecules of the cell were altered, either by chemical oncogens or by insertion of viral material into the chromosome, this most readily would explain the abnormalities of growth which characterize the neoplasm.

In some cancers the DNA strand is certainly broken. Drugs such as dimethylnitrosamine break single strands of DNA, and the acetylaminofluorine compounds cause disruption of double-stranded molecules. Oncogenicity seems to be inversely related to the rapidity of strand repair in experiments in vivo.

It has been suggested that the major biologic characteristic of a neoplasm is an alteration in the control of cell metabolism. According to this view, an alteration of the regulator genes may be responsible, but there may also be disruption through the regulatory circuits of the Jacob-Monod type[1] that promote the continued repli-

1. The *Jacob-Monod theory* implies that the total genome in the cell is functionally discontinuous. It is segmented into "units of transcription"— the operons. Transcription of operons is regulated by cytoplasmic factors linking regulator genes to operons. Control is negative and effected by repressors produced by regulatory genes. The system comprises two genetic sites on the chromosome and incorporates a negative feedback control of transcription.

Table 6.3. Biological characteristics of malignant neoplastic cell

Metastasize—transfer to other tissues by blood and lymph.
Invade—cells not contained by barriers of connective tissue and basement membrane.
Anaplastic—large nuclei and nucleoli; fewer mitochondria and other organelles; are concerned with replication and not with normal cell metabolism.
Mitotic—mitotic activity is greater.
Nondifferentiated—growth pattern is haphazard and does not resemble normal tissues.
Nonencapsulated.

cation of neoplastic cells. The *deletion hypothesis,* which is based upon work with transplantable hepatomas, is that neoplasms result from the deletion of specific proteins (involved in growth control) by oncogens. This gives rise to altered mechanisms for regulating DNA synthesis and cell replication. While increased cell replication is not an absolute criterion for this concept, it remains the basis for naturally occurring neoplasms.

THE NEOPLASTIC CELL

There are certain features that separate malignant tumors from their benign counterparts (Table 6.3). These are not requisites of malignancy but are general characteristics of malignant tumors. *Differentiation* refers to the extent to which cells resemble the cells of their tissue of origin (in embryology, differentiation is used to indicate a change from a lower to a higher state of specialization). *Undifferentiation* is synonymous with *anaplasia* and refers to the loss of specialization and organization, with anarchic changes in cell organelles.

Cellular differentiation, the derivation of specialized cells from less specialized ones, is an expression of specific genetic activity. This is initiated by derepression of sections of the genome and results in synthesis of specific proteins (enzymatic or structural) that characterize a particular tumor cell type. Epigenetic mechanisms operate at two levels: (1) transcription of genetic information and (2) translation of transcribed information. Neoplastic transformation appears to be a pathologic counterpart of normal differentiation and arises from a misprograming of gene activity by

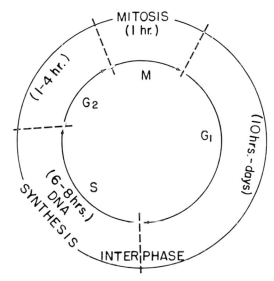

MITOSIS
(1 hr.)

M

(1-4 hr.)

G2

G1

(10 hrs.-days)

S

(6-8hrs.)
DNA
SYNTHESIS

INTERPHASE

Fig. 6.3.   Phases of the cell mitotic cycle.

these epigenetic mechanisms (Sherbet 1974).

Histologic examination provides the basis for the histogenetic classification of neoplastic tissues. Although specific organelles, inclusions, and other structures can often be identified histochemically and by fluorescent antibody procedures, ultrastructural studies clearly establish the definitive cell type of the tumor.

MITOSIS

The *cell cycle* is that period which extends from one mitosis to the next (Fig. 6.3). During each cycle, the structural components of the cell cytoplasm and nucleus undergo doubling. All the activities, how-ever, are geared to the nuclear cycle of chromosome replication and segregation which define the four periods: G1, S, G2, and M. Control, regulation, and inhibition of cell reproduction are achieved by interruption of the nuclear cycle. The three major chromosomal events in cell division, i.e., reproduction, movement, and cleavage, all occur with strict continuity in the cycle. If one is blocked, the others do not occur (Table 6.4).

G1 is the resting phase, and RNA and protein synthesis are necessary for cells to progress through it. The *S* phase is initiated by a new protein, which stimulates the reaction of DNA and DNA duplicase, which in turn initiate DNA synthesis. Subsequent progress through the cycle is governed by a temporal sequence of genetic transcriptions that are held in sequence by the dependency of one upon the next.

The growth rate of a tumor depends upon several kinetic factors: (1) the length of the cell cycle, that is, the interval between mitosis and completion of subsequent mitoses in the daughter cells; (2) the fraction of cells that participate in the growth process; and (3) the number of cells lost by death, exfoliation, and metastasis. The length of the tumor cell cycle is usually (but not always) shorter than that of its normal cellular counterpart.

NEOPLASTIC CELL STRUCTURE

The ultrastructure of the neoplastic cell provides many clues to its degree of differentiation. The leiomyoma, a common tumor in dogs, is a well-differentiated neoplasm whose cells closely resemble the par-

Table 6.4.   Indices of mitotic activity

Term	Definition	Comment
Mitotic index	% of cells in a population in mitosis at a given time	Low mitotic index may indicate few cells are dividing rapidly or all cells are dividing slowly
Mitotic time	Time from prophase to telophase	
Generation time	Prophase to prophase (mitotic time + interphase time)	
Turnover time	Time required for the production of a number of cells equal to the number already present	Does not equal cell cycle time unless all cells are dividing
Labeling index	Number of cells taking up thymidine-H[3] (in DNA synthesis) over total number of cells	Analogous to mitotic index but greater since DNA synthesis duration is greater than mitotic time.

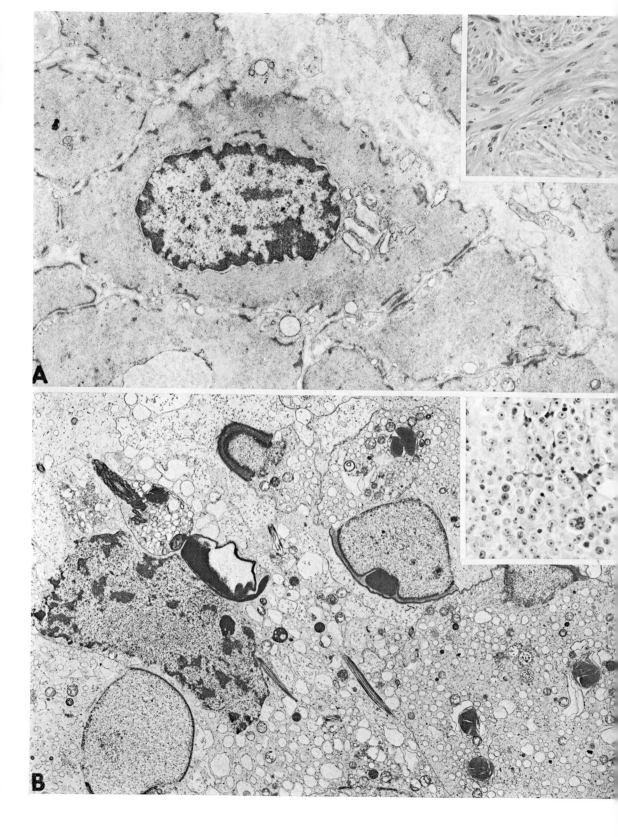

ent smooth muscle cells. They cannot be differentiated with assurance from normal smooth muscle by electron microscopy (Fig. 6.4). In contrast, the leiomyosarcoma may show little histologic resemblance to smooth muscle. By use of the electron microscope, however, characteristic myofilaments can be demonstrated that establish the diagnosis. The mammary gland adenocarcinoma of dogs contains groups or acini of tumor cells that vary considerably in their differentiation. Cells that are less anaplastic usually contain secretory granules near the luminal surface; secretions may be present in the lumen (Fig. 6.5). The well-differentiated seminoma, a neoplasm of the germ cells of the testicle, may reproduce spermatozoa and may contain abnormal forms of all cell types found in spermatogenesis: spermatogonia, spermatocytes, and spermatids (Fig. 6.4). In contrast, the far more common poorly differentiated seminoma has few distinguishing features. Similarly, interstitial cell tumors of the testicle may closely resemble steroid-secreting cells or, if more malignant, have few indices of normal cell type (Fig. 6.6).

Cellular anaplasia and invasion of tissue are the two most reliable hallmarks of malignancy (if the tumor has metastasized, there is no doubt). The characteristics of *anaplasia* are: (1) pleomorphism (differences in cell size and shape), (2) large hyperchromatic nuclei with irregularities of the nuclear membrane, (3) increase in size and number of nucleoli, and (4) decrease in numbers of normal cytoplasmic organelles with the presence of many aberrant forms. Pseudopodia, microfilaments, and clumps of membranous sacs and tubules are commonly found. There is usually a deficiency of endoplasmic reticulum, mitochondria, and other cell work-associated organelles. The nuclear membrane is often convoluted, irregular, and doubled over upon itself. In summary, the cells appear to function in reproduction and not in metabolic activity of other kinds.

Mitoses are numerous and are often abnormal. Malignant cells are usually aneuploid and have a variety of chromosomal defects. Athough most have pathologic karyotypes (including chromosomal deletions, translocations, and other changes), few have specific abnormalities that are faithfully reproduced in the tumor. (One is the "Philadelphia chromosome" associated with chronic granulocytic leukemia of humans.)

Mitosis is more rapid in malignant tumors than in most normal tissue. The mitotic process itself resembles that in normal cells. The replication and migration of centrioles, the appearance and disappearance of spindle tubules and kinetochores, and the movement and replication of chromosomes can rarely be distinguished from normal (Chang and Gibley 1968). Nucleoli and some cytoplasmic organelles tend to persist during mitosis of neoplasms, which they do not do in normal cell cycles (Bernhard and Granboulan 1963).

One of the most important characteristics of malignant cells is their tendency to lose cohesiveness with neighboring cells. This decreased adhesiveness represents a change in the plasma membrane and is manifested as the capacity of malignant tumors to spread by invasion of tissue, by implantation on new surfaces, or by metastasizing to new sites in lymphatics or blood vessels. Some of the changes observed in plasma membranes of tumor cells have been a more negative surface charge, decrease in calcium content, the presence of new "tumor" antigens, and the elaboration of humoral substances which enhance invasiveness. High negative charges on the cell surface tend to repel cells from one another. These charges may reflect the production of abnormal amounts of sialomucopeptide at the plasma membrane or the uncovering of previously masked components. In epithelial tumors the desmosomes, which form strong attachment sites, are sometimes abnormal (Martinez Palomo 1970). Base-

Fig. 6.4. Well-differentiated neoplasms. A. Leiomyoma from the intestine of a dog. Cells resemble normal smooth muscle cells but the tissue organization is haphazard. *Inset:* Histology. B. Seminoma, testicle, dog. Neoplasm contains abnormal forms of cells seen in spermatogenesis: spermatogonia, spermatocytes, and spermatids. Cells are large and polyhedral and have large, round nuclei. *Inset:* Histology.

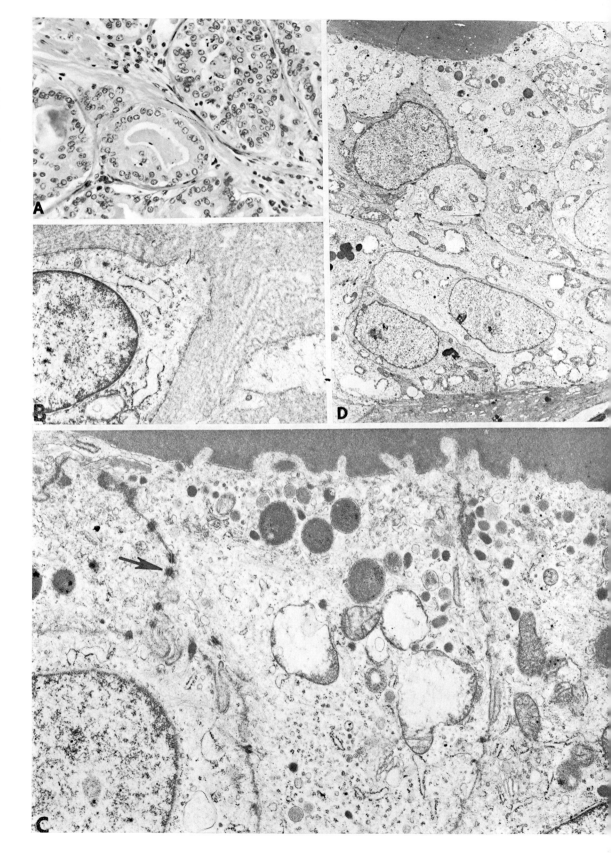

ment membranes are usually lacking at the basal surfaces of malignant epithelial tumors.

Neoplastic cells lack "contact inhibition." When normal cells grow in vivo and in culture, there is inhibition of movement and mitosis when they contact each other. It is presumed that contact allows the exchange in some way of information and the establishment of organelles such as desmosomes for maintaining contact. When tumor pieces are placed in culture, cells migrate away from the explant more quickly than do cells from normal tissue. They do not grow in organized radial strands but in random, haphazard patterns.

Changes in the surface topography of tumor cells in regard to loss of contact inhibition and decreased surface adhesiveness have been examined in vitro by treating transformed cells with plant lectins such as conconavalin A. The plant lectins are multivalent ligands that bind to sugar residues (glucosides, galactosides, etc.) which extend outward from the plasma membrane. The lectin-binding sites (or "receptors") are aggregated into small clusters on most tumor cells whereas in normal cells they are distributed in random fashion. Clustering of sites is actually induced by the lectin molecules. The transforming event that leads to increased lectin-binding–site mobility on tumor cells appears to be related to alterations in the metabolism of cyclic AMP and to the consequent disruption of the interaction between microtubules and plasma membrane that brings about changes in surface topography.

TUMOR CELL FUNCTION

The biochemical characteristics of neoplastic cells tend to converge into a common pattern in the most malignant tumors. Warburg established in the 1920s that malignant cells have a high degree of glycolytic activity (both anaerobic and aerobic

glycolysis). These neoplasms produce large amounts of lactic acid from glucose, and this pathway is not markedly reduced in the presence of oxygen, as it is in normal tissue. From this it was theorized that malignancy correlated with increased fermentation and decreased respiration. Currently, this metabolic defect is viewed as characteristic of tumor cells but is not thought to be significant in the definition of cause (Knox 1967; Potter 1964).

In some tumors, the activity of a particular enzyme is more invariable in the tumor than in its normal tissue counterpart. That is, normal cells adapt their enzymes to changing conditions; tumor cells do not. It is now believed that the normal regulatory flexibility of programed mRNA translation is lost (Pitot 1968).

The function of tumor cells plays an important role in the death of animals by cachexia (providing the tumor does not kill early by the obliteration of some vital organ). Neoplastic cells may, by virtue of tumor cell enzymes, act as an amino acid trap which irreversibly drains the host of essential amino acids.

In summary, cancer cells differ functionally from their normal counterparts and the magnitude of change correlates with the extent of anaplasia. To date, the biochemical alterations described have been a reflection of rapidly dividing cells and not of a crucial change in the development of cancer. Exciting and hopeful results are expected from the discovery of biochemic differences in cancer cells. Cells of some human lymphatic leukemia patients have low levels of the enzyme asparagine synthetase. Because they require asparagine, treatment with L-asparaginase is effective; it deprives the cell of its necessary asparagine.

VASCULARITY

The growth of a neoplasm is dependent upon concomitant growth of a supporting

Fig. 6.5. Adenocarcinoma of the mammary gland, dog. A. Histology. Some differentiated neoplastic cells have formed acini which are filled with secretions; more anaplastic-appearing cells occur in solid cords. B. Mesenchymal cell associated with tumor has produced large amounts of basement membrane material. C. Luminal surface of a differentiated cell from a tumor acinus. Note secretion granules and intact desmosomes (arrow). D. Ultrastructure of portion of tumor acinus.

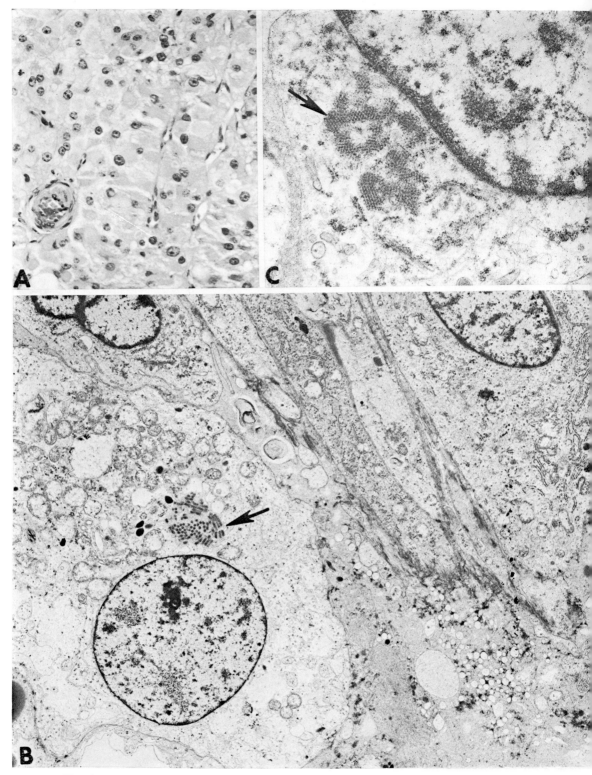

Fig. 6.6. Interstitial cell tumor, testicle, aged dog. A. Histology. Neoplastic cells arranged on cords of connective tissue. Large areas of dense cytoplasm and eccentric nuclei. B. Ultrastructure. Organelles of steroid synthesis are disoriented. Dense granules are pleomorphic. Large arrays of annulate lamellae present (arrow). C. Small dense particles in crystalline patterns (arrow) within cisternae of endoplasmic reticulum.

vascular system. The probability of a neoplastic cell entering mitosis decreases with increasing distance of the cell from its nearest capillary. In the mouse mammary tumor, for example, the turnover time of endothelial cell populations lags behind that of the tumor cells. As the tumor expands, neoplastic cell proliferation is diminished and this is reflected in slowed growth in tumor size (Tannock 1968, 1970). When tumor cells are implanted into susceptible hosts experimentally, they grow to a diameter of a few mm and then lie dormant unless vascularization takes place.

New capillary growth within neoplasms is often more vigorous than capillary bud formation as seen in the repair phase of inflammation (Algire and Chalkley 1945; Toth 1973; Warren and Shubik 1966). Endothelial cells are kinky, enlarged, and have extensive contortions and surface projections of the luminal plasma membrane (Fig. 6.7). Tumor blood vessels are often more permeable than normal vessels (Underwood and Carr 1972). The hypertrophic characteristic of the endothelial cells is particularly common in malignant animal tumors. In most cases, the vessels are not considered neoplastic, but as a host response that is induced in some way by the tumor itself. Tumor vascular systems are never normal, however, and the supply of oxygen, glucose, and other nutrients to the tumor is usually less efficient than in normal tissue. The vascular pattern reflects tumor histology, not the tissue of origin (Milne et al. 1967). The vascular pattern of a neoplasm can be revealed by perfusion with radiopaque substances and radiographic examination or by perfusion with latex and erosion of tumor tissue. By these methods, tumor blood vessels are revealed as haphazard networks with a predisposition to form capillaries from arterial vessels of all sizes.

It is now appreciated that in many cases the populations of neoplastic cells and of host endothelial cells constitute an integrated system; the mitotic indices of one population depend upon the other. Tumor cells stimulate endothelial cell proliferation, and vascularization has an indirect effect on tumor growth (Folkman et al. 1971).

It appears that some diffusable soluble substance is released from tumor cells and acts upon adjacent host endothelium. New capillary buds are induced even when the tumor implants are enclosed in filter chambers (Ehrmann and Knoth 1968). Induction of DNA synthesis in resting endothelial cells of capillaries and venules can be demonstrated within a few mm of an implanted tumor.

A soluble factor which is mitogenic for capillary endothelium has been extracted from animal neoplasms (Cavallo et al. 1972, 1973; Folkman et al. 1971). Called *tumor angiogenesis factor*, it is assayed in artificial subcutaneous air sacs in rats. It is proposed that growth of solid tumors can be deliberately arrested by blockade of angiogenesis factor and prevention of vascularization (Gimbrone et al. 1972).

When growth of tumor cells extends beyond that of the supporting vasculature, necrosis results. This is a characteristic of highly malignant tumors in which ischemic necrosis and hemorrhage are often striking (Fig. 6.7). Necrosis may be accompanied by some decrease in tumor size, but the rapidly dividing malignant cells soon make up the loss.

SPREAD OF NEOPLASMS

There are four basic mechanisms by which neoplastic cells spread within an animal. These are: (1) continuity through tissue planes (invasiveness); (2) implantation on new surfaces, particularly serosal surfaces; (3) dissemination through the vascular system by eroding veins or, in rare cases, arteries; and (4) dissemination through lymphatic vessels and lymph nodes.

INVASIVENESS

The capacity to invade host tissue is largely an intrinsic property of the neoplastic cell. The extension of pseudopodia below basement membranes and between connective tissue planes involves changes in the plasma membrane (Fig. 6.8). Some of these relate to increased negative charges and decreased calcium content. Whether these cause or result from cell transformation is not known.

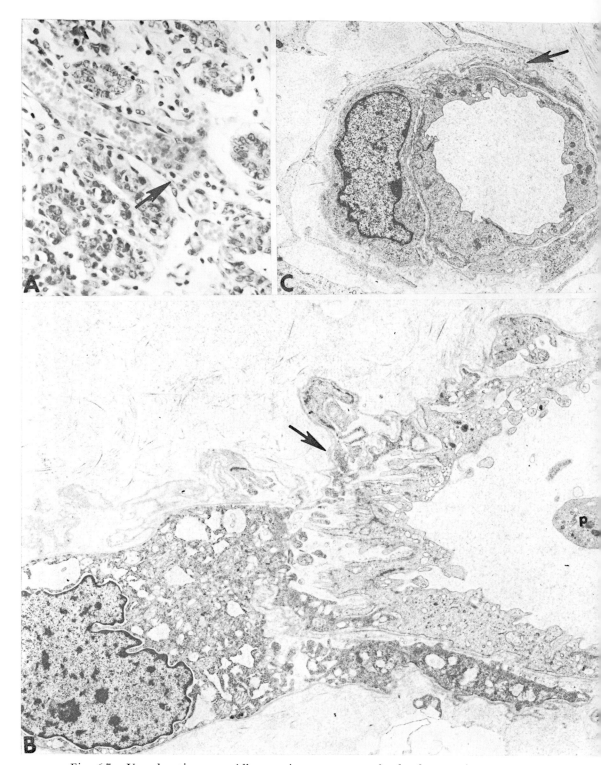

Fig. 6.7. Vascular tissue, rapidly growing mammary gland adeno-carcinoma, dog. A. Histology. Large, thin-walled blood vessels ramify between acini of neoplastic cells. Mesenchymal cells attached to vascular wall (arrow) are source of new vascular tissue. B. Ultrastructure of a thin-walled blood vessel and its perivascular cell. Cell swelling and vacuolation. Note pseudopodia on the luminal surfaces of endothelial cells, irregular basement membranes (arrow), intravascular platelet (p), and collagen fibers and granule precipitates in the interstitium. C. Ultrastructure of small arteriole. Basement membrane is thickened and irregular (arrow).

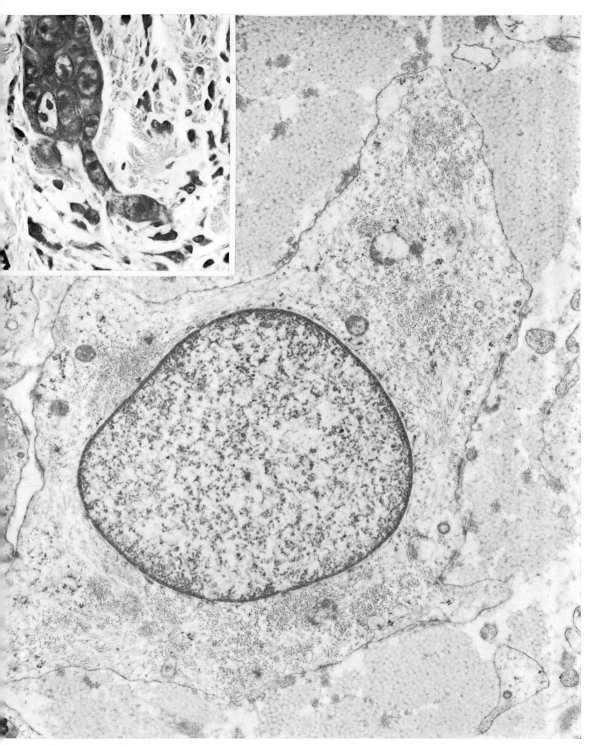

Fig. 6.8. Invasion of neoplastic cells of squamous cell carcinoma into the subcutaneous connective tissue. A. Histology. B. Ultrastructure.

Carcinomas are known to elaborate enzymes that degrade connective tissues. For example, some basal cell epitheliomas are collagenolytic, that is, they produce collagenase which degrades dermal collagen. This can be demonstrated ultrastructurally adjacent to the neoplastic cells (Hashimoto et al. 1972). Most tumors, however, invade without releasing proteolytic enzymes. Contact of tumor cell with normal cell may re-sult in lysis of the former with liberation of cytoplasmic enzymes. This, in turn, may be responsible for injury to normal tissues (Brandes et al. 1967).

METASTASIS

Metastasis is the hallmark of malignant neoplasms (Fig. 6.9). All neoplasms that metastasize are malignant, although not all

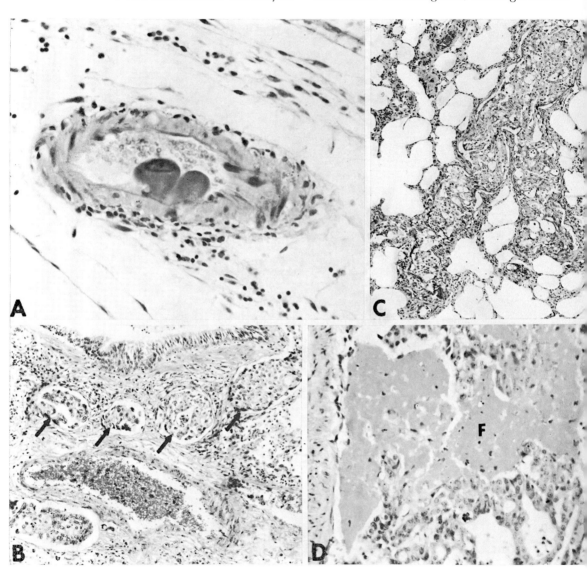

Fig. 6.9. Metastases. A. Metastatic carcinoma cells attached to arterial wall. B. Large collections in peribronchial lymphatics, lung (arrows), canine mammary gland adenocarcinoma. C. Infiltration and growth of tumor cells in the pulmonary artery. D. Collections of carcinoma cells in a pulmonary artery enmeshed in fibrin (F).

malignant neoplasms metastasize. Highly malignant tumor cells have relatively little tendency to adhere to one another (McNutt et al. 1971) and may be washed by lymph from the tissue spaces and enter the thoracic duct. Neoplastic cells may also directly erode vascular walls. Most cancer cells that enter the bloodstream die without initiating new metastatic foci (Zeidman 1965). Factors which influence whether tumor cells initiate new growths at sites distant from the primary tumor include: (1) the way in which metastasis occurs—whether from single cells or from tumor emboli; (2) the intrinsic capacity of the malignant cell to lodge in and attach to host endothelial cells; and (3) the existence and efficiency of a host immune response (see Chapter 5, cell-mediated immunity) (Greene and Harvey 1964; Wood 1958). Tumor cells at metastatic sites usually resemble the cells of the primary tumor, although this is not always true. The remarkable variation one occasionally sees may be due to formation of new clones of cells. The absence of surface glycocalyx is responsible for the metastasis of some tumor cells (Kim 1975).

In animals, most malignant tumors metastasize to the lung. In Misdorp's collection of 56 canine mammary gland carcinomas, the metastatic foci were: 86% to lymph nodes, 72% to lungs, and 10–12% each to adrenal, kidney, liver, and bone. Lung metastases occur because of the immense flow of blood through this organ and its large network of capillaries through which circulation is slowed. The pulmonary capillary bed serves as a filter for aggregates of tumor cells. Tumor cells lodge in the pulmonary vascular tree, insert pseudopodia between endothelial cells, and emigrate into the lung parenchyma (Ludatscher et al. 1967).

LYMPHATIC SPREAD

Lymphatic drainage provides a common pathway of metastatic spread of many carcinomas. This involves drainage to regional lymph nodes (Fisher et al. 1973). Thus, adenocarcinoma metastases of the posterior mammary gland tend to be found in the inguinal lymph nodes; tumors in the anterior mammary gland drain anteriorly. Spread via lymphatics should not be equalled with vascular metastasis, for its bearing to the animal is not the same.

IMPLANTATION

Because of their lack of cohesiveness, tumor cells growing on epithelial surfaces are prone to be shed into the surrounding spaces. Exfoliation of cells into fluids of the body cavities and respiratory and urogenital tracts is the basis for the cytologic examination of these fluids for cancer cells. Unfortunately, it is also the basis for massive implantation of cells and the development of immense numbers of tumors on serosal surfaces.

This pattern of growth is characteristic of some glandular tumors. For example, pancreatic adenocarcinomas may seed through the peritoneal cavity; these lesions are referred to as *peritoneal carcinomatosis*. When the cavity is opened, massive growth of neoplastic cells may present the misleading appearance of an acute fibrinous peritonitis (Fig 6.10). Tumor cell localization on the peritoneal membranes is enhanced when serosal surfaces are injured. Tumor cells adhere on exposed collagen fibrils and grow more rapidly (Buck 1973).

Transplantation of neoplastic cells from contaminated surgical instruments and gloves is a significant potential hazard during cancer surgery. Although rarely reported in animal neoplasms, this is a well-documented sequel to cancer surgery in man.

RESTRAINT OF NEOPLASMS

The natural course of malignant neoplasms differs. In some, the tumor can be seen to grow from day to day with death of the animal occurring in a few weeks. Conversely, some animals with cancer may survive several years. These instances represent extremes and both are rare. It is usual for an animal with a malignant neoplasm to survive from six months to a year after the lesion becomes manifest.

There are multiple factors that restrain cancer. In addition to intrinsic properties of the tumor (genotype, its vascular arrangement, etc.) there are factors which can be altered in the host such as nutrition, endocrinologic status, and immunoreactivity.

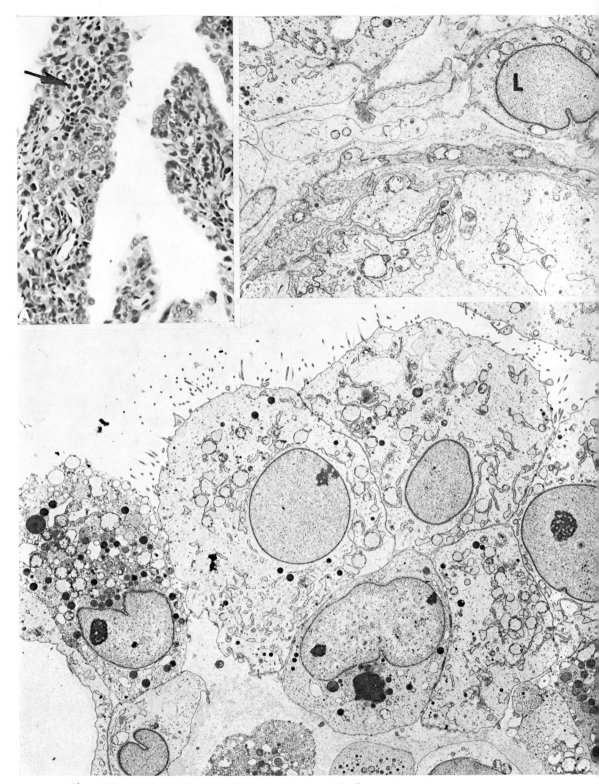

Fig. 6.10. Implantation of malignant cells (aortic body carcinoma) onto serosal surface, mediastinum (carcinomatosis). A. Histology. Fronds of tumor composed of vascular and connective tissue supports on which tumor cells proliferate. Infiltration of lymphoid cells has occurred (arrow). B. Ultrastructure. Note surface microvilli, difference in cell structure, and lack of granules. C. Ultrastructure of tumor capillary (lower), lymphocyte (L), and interstitium.

ENDOCRINE-DEPENDENT NEOPLASMS

Neoplasms of the human prostate and mammary gland are, to varying degrees, endocrine-dependent. Growth is enhanced by the sex hormone appropriate to the host and is inhibited by its absence or therapy with opposing endocrine secretions. For example, prostatic carcinoma develops under the influence of testosterone. Orchiectomy inhibits growth, as does treatment with estrogens. Several endocrine-dependent tumors of laboratory animals are known, but there are few among the naturally occurring neoplasms of mammals. Carcinoma of the prostate is one example. Human carcinomas of the prostate are enhanced and inhibited by testosterone and estrogen respectively (Huggins 1967). The canine prostatic carcinoma is not as androgen-dependent as its human counterpart. Neoplastic cells are more refractory to castration due to an apparent shift to an androgen-independent state, from a reductive to an oxidative pathway of steroid metabolism (Leav et al. 1974).

NUTRITION AND CANCER

It appears that the nutritive status of an animal may play some role in susceptibility to neoplasia. The evidence favoring that premise is spotty and it is difficult to apply statistics to incidence in naturally occurring tumors. In general, animals on very high calorie diets have a slightly increased incidence of tumors. Most of this information relates to large colonies of rats and mice. It has been reported that when two groups of cattle were placed on high and low calorie diets and exposed to sunlight, there was a higher incidence of squamous cell carcinoma in the well-fed animals (Anderson et al. 1970). In laboratory animals, it even appears that transient caloric restrictions for periods during development (even when followed by standard dietary regimes) has an inhibitory effect on tumor development (Ross and Bras 1971).

After the appearance of tumors, high calorie diets also appear to enhance neoplastic growth. Experimentally, fasting and starvation greatly prolong the G_2 period of Ehrlich ascites tumor cells growing in the mouse peritoneal cavity.

CHEMOTHERAPY

Chemotherapy as a method of treatment is largely restricted to human neoplasms, where it has seen most widespread use in tumors of the lymphoreticular system. The drugs used include corticosteroids, antimetabolites, radiomimetic drugs, and selective toxins (Table 6.5). Tumor cells affected by cyclophosphamide, a common chemotherapeutic drug, exhibit nonspecific features of degeneration. These are dominated by autophagy, and there is widespread development of lysosomes and organelle-containing residual bodies (Anton and Brandes 1968). The canine venereal tumor treated with cyclophosphamide regresses rapidly. Its cells vacuolate, mitotic activity is depressed, and acid phosphatase levels (found in lysosomes) increase markedly in tumor tissue. Experiments show that tumors disappear more slowly in females than in males, allegedly because of the lysosomal stabilizing effect of estrogens (Hernandez-Jauregui et al. 1973).

In some types of tumors of humans, chemotherapeutic drugs have been curative. For example, a single dose of cyclophosphamide produces complete disappearance of Burkitt's lymphoma in about 60% of the children treated. Extraordinary success has also been obtained with chemotherapy in humans with embryonal nephroma, retinoblastoma, and Ewing's sarcoma of bone. The first neoplastic disease in which cure was demonstrated was the trophoblastic tumor choriocarcinoma, in which methotrexate was highly effective.

The chemotherapeutic sensitivity of an individual tumor depends on active growth by that tumor. Tumor growth rate is related largely to the growth fraction, that is, the number of cells in mitosis at any one time. It is also contingent upon the number of cells dying or becoming differentiated. Drug-sensitive tumors are those in which most cells are in an active mitotic cycle (Skipper 1971; Zubrod 1972).

Chemotherapy depends on a well-developed vascular system within the tumor, for the drugs must reach the neoplastic cell in concentrations sufficient to exert an effect. Within the tumor, it appears that mitotic and labeling indices decrease with increasing distance of the tumor cell from

Table 6.5. Chemotherapeutic agents against neoplasms

Drug	Type	Action
Bleomycin	Antibiotic from *Streptomyces verticillatus*	Inhibits DNA synthesis
Cyclophosphamide (nitrogen mustard)	Alkylating agent	Cross-linkage of DNA
Cytosine arabinoside	Pyrimidine analog	Inhibition of DNA synthesis
Daunorubicin	Antibiotic from *Streptomyces peucetius*	Inhibition of DNA synthesis
5-fluorouracil (5FU)	Pyrimidine analog	Inhibition of DNA synthesis
L-asparaginase	Enzyme catalyzing hydrolysis of L-asparagine	Depletion of L-asparagine required by tumor cells
6-mercaptopurine (6MP)	Purine analog	Inhibition of DNA synthesis
Methotrexate	Folic acid antagonist	Inhibition of dihydrofolate reductase required by DNA synthesis
Prednisone	Synthetic adrenocorticosteroid	Lysis of lymphocytes; inhibition of DNA-directed RNA synthesis
Vincristine	Alkaloid from periwinkle plant	Inhibits DNA synthesis

a viable blood vessel. Therefore, there will tend to be a decreased chemosensitivity with an increase in mass of the tumor.

TUMOR IMMUNOLOGY

One of the most intriguing aspects of the cancer cell is that, in transition to the neoplastic state, it may undergo a biochemical change that distinguishes it from normal cells of the host. It is now certain that at least some naturally occurring tumors may develop measurable tumor antigens located on the plasma membrane, that these tumor antigens can evoke both antitumor antibodies and lymphocytes, and the tumor will be thereby inhibited in growth by specific immunologic mechanisms. Despite these exciting facts, the hopes of effective tumor immunosuppression are clouded by the capricious and elusive nature of the immune mechanisms and the difficulty in making them operable in the living animal. Nowhere is the diversity of "cancer" more pointed than in the differences of individual tumors in their immunoreactivity.

One of the most important facts at present is that naturally occurring animal tumors possess measurable specific antigens on their cell surfaces. Other than the viral-induced lymphomas, there is very little real evidence of the antigenicity of tumors. Two important points emerge from the demonstration of tumor antigens: (1) immunologic detection of specific tumors should be feasible, and (2) specific immunologic attachment should be practical in the treatment of neoplasms.

Specific tumor antigens are capable of inducing a selective cell-mediated reaction that destroys malignant cells. This type of immunity can be transferred experimentally with leukocytes but not with serum. Many tumors contain lymphocytes in their connective tissue stroma, and tumors with lymphocytes appear to have a better prognosis (Stewart 1969). Lymphocytes harvested from tumor-bearing laboratory animals will attack identical tumor cells when grown in culture and will inhibit tumor growth in syngeneic animals. If blood lymphocytes from animals with tumors are combined in vitro with those tumor cells, they will inhibit tumor cell growth (Hellström et al. 1971; Perlmann et al. 1973). Ultrastructurally, sensitized lymphocytes attach to tumor cells, which then appear to lyse. Sensitized macrophages in culture may phagocytize tumor cells, which become enclosed within giant phagosomes. These fuse with lysosomes which initiate intracellular digestion (Chambers and Weiser 1973). Quantitation appears highly important, for the level of immunity may be sufficient to reject small numbers of tumor cells while larger inoculae result in tumor acceptance.

Humoral antibodies are also important in some tumors. For example, in lymphosarcoma of cats (which is caused by a virus), a clear correlation has been established between humoral antibodies to virus-associated plasma-membrane antigens and the failure of cats to develop progressive malignant tumors (Essex et al. 1971). How antibodies prevent tumor initiation or growth in vivo is not clear. In some instances, antibodies may enhance rather than inhibit tumor growth, and this has led to the suggestion that antibodies and cell-mediated immunity have opposing effects on tumor growth.

One consequence of tumor-associated cell-surface antigens and specific immune response by the host to them is the current use in humans of immunostimulation. BCG vaccine, a potent immunizing agent against human tuberculosis, is used as a nonspecific adjuvant to stimulate the reticuloendothelial system. Macrophages so stimulated aggressively attack and cause degeneration of the target tumor cells (Snodgrass and Hanna 1973). Having been demonstrated to be effective in animal model systems, BCG vaccine is now being used in the leukemias and melanomas of humans and is credited with some success.

The technology now available does little to explain why immunotherapy is not more effective. Why doesn't tumor immunotherapy work? First, the immunoreactivity induced by the tumor is probably insufficient quantitatively to inhibit an already rapidly growing tumor. By continual antigen shedding, very large tumors could provide sufficient tumor antigens that would combine with immune cells or antibody to prevent them from reacting with neoplastic cells. Second, there is a close relation between oncogenesis and immunosuppression, and it may be that tumors develop in an already immunodefective host. The establishment of a graft-versus-host reaction is a potent activator of leukemia in mice (Hirsch et al. 1973), and many of the chemical oncogens are also strong immunosuppressive agents. Third, humoral antibodies may even enhance tumor growth. It is proposed that they combine on the tumor cell surface and block the effect of more potent immunotoxic mechanisms (Hellström et al. 1969). Antigens on the cell surface may also

be blocked by sialomucins (Curie and Bagshave 1968). Last, prolonged exposure to tumor antigens may induce a partial or split state of tolerance in the host where immunoreactivity is ineffective.

IMMUNOLOGIC ENHANCEMENT

The concept of immunologic enhancement originated in the field of experimental tumor immunology. During the early enthusiastic attempts to demonstrate the immunologic repression of tumors it was found, unexpectedly, that the opposite results occurred. That is, there developed an enhanced susceptibility of the host to the tumor graft. This was manifested as increased numbers of tumor "takes," increased size of tumors, and greater numbers of metastases.

It is now hypothesized that immunologic enhancement involves the prevention of antigens from inducing immune rejection by antibody or immune cells. It is believed that immune complexes are formed between antibodies (with enhancing capacity) and antigens. The latter are hidden from recognition at certain levels of the immune cycle. The specific inhibition of the immune response to antigens by passive antibody has been a principle of immunology since its demonstration by Theobald Smith in 1909. Enhancement appears to be the result of complex interaction of several mechanisms (Kaliss and Bryant 1958; Voisin 1971).

CAUSES OF NEOPLASMS

The simpleminded statement that the cause of cancer is not known is an intellectual cop-out. First, because the causes of some cancers are known and, second, because an enormous amount of evidence exists about many neoplasms to justify presumptive statements as to their cause. This discussion will consider some of the agents known to be oncogenic and theories of the mechanisms involved in oncogenicity (Table 6.6).

One must keep distinct the wide range of oncogens proven in laboratory rodents from those agents actually shown to cause naturally occurring cancer in animals.

Table 6.6. Causes of naturally occurring neoplasms

Organ	Tumor	Species	Agent Associated	Exposure
Liver	Hepatoma	Trout	Aflatoxin B_1	Contaminated feed
	Carcinoma	Rat	*Taenia taeniaformis*	Parasitic infection, liver
	Angiosarcoma	Man	Vinyl chloride gas	Aerosol, plastic industry
Kidney	Carcinoma	Frog	Herpesvirus	Infected water (via urine)
Bladder	Carcinoma	Cow	Bracken fern toxin	Feeding
	Carcinoma	Man	Azo dye (naphthaline)	Dye manufacture
Lung	Mesothelioma	Man	Asbestos	Asbestos industry
	Carcinoma	Man	Cigarette smoke	Smoking
Mammary gland	Adenocarcinoma	Mouse	Oncornavirus	Nursing (milk)
Esophagus	Sarcoma	Dog	*Spirocirca lupi*	Parasite localization
Rumen	Carcinoma	Cow	Plant toxin (?)	Feeding
Thyroid	Carcinoma	Man	Radiation (X rays)	Therapeutic radiation
Eye	Carcinoma	Cow	Radiation (solar)	Exposure to sun (UV)
Tongue	Carcinoma	Man	Radiation (radium)	Licking contaminated brushes (watch making)
Scrotum	Carcinoma	Man	Soot (benzpyrene)	Chimney sweeping

Furthermore, as in toxicology, dosage is critical. Enormous amounts of many chemicals are oncogenic. The massive doses required render their study highly artificial and such models should be viewed with suspicion. Even among the reliable models of oncogenicity, there are very few instances where the direct cause of cancer is determined and its mechanism reasonably explained. In these, it is often suspected that the agent involved merely unmasks a viral oncogen which thereupon exerts the primary oncogenic effect.

ONCOGENESIS BY PHYSICAL AGENTS

SOLAR RADIATION

Cancer of the skin develops in nonpigmented animals exposed to intense sunlight for long periods. Heavily pigmented animals are practically resistant to this type of lesion. A great deal of epidemiologic evidence in humans incriminates solar radiation. Skin cancer is more prevalent in: (1) geographical areas where sunlight is most intense, (2) light-skinned (than in dark-skinned) races, and (3) the exposed (than unexposed) areas of the body. The relation between solar radiation and carcinoma induction has been proven experimentally and the carcinogenic effect shown to be in the ultraviolet spectrum between rays of 2800 and 3200 Å (Blum 1954).

One of the outstanding examples of solar radiation–induced cancer is the squamous cell carcinoma of the eye which develops in white-faced Hereford cattle in the southern United States (Anderson and Skinner 1961; Russell et al. 1956). The incidence of these tumors in Angus cattle in similar localities is much less. The squamous cell carcinomas develop at the corneal periphery in the medial and lateral aspects of the eyeball which are not covered by the eyelid when the eyes are open.

X-RADIATION

Since the early days of the use of X rays, it has been known that these physical forces can induce cancer. An enormous amount of evidence exists for radiation-induced cancer in humans. The pioneers in radiology were often affected by carcinomas of the skin overlying the hands and arms, which were most exposed to radiation. The oncogenic changes of whole body radiation have been recently dramatically illustrated in the studies on the survivors of Hiroshima and Nagasaki. Not only was leukemia commoner in these populations, but the incidence of solid tumors increased as well. Fallout of I^{131}, as one example, has caused adenomatous change in the thyroid of exposed individuals. Similarly, young children who were irradiated in infancy for "enlarged thymus" returned several years later with adenocarcinoma of the thyroid. Radiation-induced bone cancer occurs in adults irradiated for arthritis of the spine.

The primary event in radiation-induced oncogenesis is the production of specific genetic alteration, that is, a somatic mutation (Cole and Nowell 1965). The dose-rate and quality of radiation influence the frequency of mutation. It appears the mutation may occur by direct damage to the mitotic apparatus, by damage to epigenetic sites with secondary damage to chromosomes, or by activation of latent oncogenic viruses. None of these theories adequately explains the long period between exposure to radiation and tumor formation.

When dogs or other large mammals are given whole-body radiation by exposure to cobalt or ingestion of Sr^{90}, a spectrum of neoplasms results which includes lymphosarcoma, reticulum cell sarcoma, and myeloid leukemia (Upton and Cosgrove 1968). The mechanism of tumor induction in these animals has not been explained. Experimental radiation-induced lymphosarcoma in mice is a commonly studied model. It is thought that radiation immunosuppresses the mice and in some unknown way activates latent viruses which are the direct cause of lymphocyte transformation (Siegler et al. 1966).

CHEMICAL ONCOGENESIS

One of the earliest reports on the cause of cancer was the finding by Sir Percival Potts that English chimney sweeps suffered a high incidence of carcinoma of the scrotum because of continual exposure to substances in soot. Although it was soon obvious that an oncogenic factor involved in scrotal cancer was present in soot, the substance was not identified for nearly 150 years. In 1915, Yamagawa, by the patient painting of rabbits' ears with coal tar, reproduced a squamous cell carcinoma similar to that which developed in chimney sweeps. The precise chemical oncogen, dibenzanthracene, a polycyclic aromatic hydrocarbon, was identified in 1930, the first known chemical carcinogen.

The polycyclic hydrocarbons are the most powerful chemical oncogens known and are present in tobacco smoke and in the urban atmosphere. Of several of these potent chemicals which are available for the experimental oncologist, the most widely used are dibenzanthracene (DBA), 3-methylcholanthrene (MC), and 7:12-dimethylbenzanthracene (DMBA) (Becker 1971; Homberger 1969). By painting these substances on the skin, it is possible to produce epidermal carcinomas regularly in most laboratory animals. The same agents act directly when injected subcutaneously to induce sarcomas and when taken orally to induce intestinal carcinomas.

The clearest picture of chemical oncogenesis comes from studies involving the chronic application of oncogens to skin. When polycyclic hydrocarbons are painted on the skin of laboratory animals, they accumulate in hair follicles and sebaceous glands and produce a necrotizing effect. Following death of random cells, a transient hyperplastic reaction develops. Cells immediately above the germinal layer are enlarged and have large nuclei and nucleoli (Raick 1973). Hyperplastic foci disappear within several days unless the oncogen is repeatedly applied. With each successive application the epidermal cells show an increasing resistance to the toxic effect of the chemical, but hyperplasia becomes more intense. In time, anaplastic cells appear and the tumor progresses to malignancy even if the oncogen is removed from the skin. Ultrastructurally, the malignant cells are little different from cells in naturally occurring epidermal carcinomas (Clarke 1969; Kakefuda et al. 1970; Parry and Ghadially 1965).

MECHANISMS OF CHEMICAL CARCINOGENESIS

The concept that different mechanisms may be involved in the chemical induction of cancer has given rise to a two-stage theory of carcinogenesis. Although the carcinogen induces an irreversible transformation in some of the epidermal cells, their neoplastic characteristics may remain unexpressed for the life span of the animal. The subsequent presence of a promoter will determine whether the neoplastic character is expressed.

If mouse skin is painted with a subcarcinogenic dose of methylcholanthracene, papillomas result from subsequent painting with croton oil (the reverse order does not elicit a tumor). The methylcholanthracene is considered the initiator and the croton oil the promoter. The initiator converts normal skin cells to latent tumor cells, which persist until activated by the promoter (Berenblum and Shubik 1947).

The assay of oncogenic chemicals is largely limited to the use of laboratory animals. In vitro techniques have been devised but generally prove ineffective for assay. A new method utilizes cell culture–animal combinations. Suspected substances are injected into pregnant hamsters, where they act transplacentally upon the fetus. Fetal tissues are then cultured in series and, where carcinogens were used, develop colony and cell changes which show their presence. These changes represent oncogenesis and when cells are injected back into the living hamster they produce tumors.

Chemical oncogens may induce cancer by genetic or by epigenetic (nongenomic or nonmutational) mechanisms. The polycyclic hydrocarbons bind to nuclear DNA, chiefly in the heterochromatin (Harris et al. 1973), and somatic mutation may thereby occur. A correlation usually exists between nucleic acid binding and oncogenic potency. The somatic mutation appears to result from the direct injury to the nucleic acid molecule and the long time period required for the molecule to reform.

Other chemical oncogens have an epigenetic mode of action. The alteration of metabolic pathways and inactivation of repressors may secondarily affect gene expression. This *deletion hypothesis* of tumor induction implies the deletion of some regulatory metabolic circuit within the cell (Pitot and Heidelberger 1963). Reconciliation of the above theories is offered by allowing that nongenomic changes in metabolic circuitry in some way pave the way for mutation.

Neoplastic cells always exhibit some loss of differentiation and control. Both may depend upon acquired defectiveness in mRNA template stability. That is, the capacity of mRNA templates to faithfully express cell differentiation is altered. A new, altered set of mRNA templates is manifested as anaplasia and may be measurable chemically as a loss in control of enzyme synthesis.

Many chemicals that are not oncogenic directly induce tumors by virtue of oncogenic metabolites. Some of the azo dyes are potent oncogens of this type. N-methyl-e-aminoazobenzene (MAB, butter yellow) has been widely fed to rats as a model for the study of liver carcinoma. This chemical requires the conversion, during detoxification in the liver, to the oncogenic metabolite N-hydroxy-MAB. The metabolite induces foci of hyperplasia in the liver that progressively change to adenoma and, in turn, to adenocarcinoma.

The so-called "industrial cancers" of the bladder of humans are caused by the storage of urine containing oncogenic chemicals or their oncogenic metabolites. These tumors occur in workers in the dye industry and are caused by three primary aromatic amines: 2-naphthylamine, benzidine, and 4-aminodiphenyl. Not only are the chemicals causally related to human transitional cell carcinomas, but they reproduce the equivalent tumors experimentally in dogs.

Some aromatic amines such as dimethylnitrosamine are widely used as experimental oncogens (Hard and Butler 1971). They allegedly break single strands of DNA. A single intraperitoneal injection will induce fibroblastic tumors of the kidney. Sheep have been intoxicated with dimethylnitrosamine-contaminated herring meal but the lesions involved were hepatotoxic.

CARCINOGENS IN FOOD

Food supplies are a major route of exposure of animals to chemical oncogens. A great many chemicals are intentionally added to foods during processing. Antioxidants, preservatives, and flavoring agents are potential oncogens. Other examples include dyes added to fruits and those used for labeling meats. Oncogens may be present in food grains as unrecognized plant contaminants (senecio, crotolaria, etc.) or as spoilage molds on feed (aflatoxin). These known oncogenic substances must be recognized as such and eliminated from the food source.

Food grains are often contaminated during growth and processing by chemicals (Kraybill and Shimkin 1964). In general, these include the oncogenic agricultural chemicals, pesticides, and mycotoxins. Contamination may be direct, or may involve residues in plants and water supplies. In the past, concern has been projected into regulatory action when chemicals in use already have been found, upon testing in laboratory rodents, to produce neoplasms. Thioacetamide and thiourea, which are used as fungicides on fruit, produce hepatomas in rats. Aramite, for the control of mites on fruit trees, induces hepatomas in several species. The herbicide aminotriazole, used to control weeds in cranberry bogs, produces thyroid adenomas in rats. Release of this latter item to the press at the height of the holiday sales season produced disastrous results in the marketing of cranberries. The political furor that inevitably results from events of this kind can in turn adversely affect appropriate decisions concerning the danger of oncogens which are based on real scientific evidence. It is difficult to place the true danger of these chemicals in perspective between valid scientific evidence and careless exploitation by the journalist. Considering our ignorance of those diseases induced by longterm exposure, it is often impossible to provide an accurate prediction of oncogenicity.

AFLATOXIN AND HEPATIC CARCINOMA

Hepatomas were found to be widespread in fish farms and hatcheries in 1960. The cause was commercially pelleted cottonseed meal fish feed which contained the aflatoxins of *Aspergillus flavus*. Experiments promptly established that aflatoxin B_1 was the cause. Most species of trout were susceptible to aflatoxin-induced hepatoma, but tumors developed more rapidly in fish reared commercially in waters of higher temperature. Dietary aflatoxin B_1 at 1–20 ppb induced hepatoma in trout in 3–6 months. If aflatoxin levels were high (1–15 mg/kg), fish died of acute hepatic necrosis and hemorrhage.

The trout hepatomas are well differentiated and grow by expansion. Metastases are rare, although they do occur (Ashley and Halver 1963). Most tumors become fibrotic, cystic, and regressive. The tumor cells faithfully reproduce the structure of normal hepatocytes (Unuma et al. 1967; Wood and

Larson 1961). Aflatoxin-induced liver carcinomas have also been produced in rats (Unuma et al. 1967) and monkeys (Adamson et al. 1973). Marmosets on chronic low levels of aflatoxin develop cirrhosis and tumorous changes (Lin et al. 1974). In contrast, rats have tumor nodules in noncirrhotic livers.

Naturally occurring hepatomas have been reported in turkeys fed on feed contaminated with aflatoxin, and circumstantial evidence has incriminated the aflatoxins in other species. As contaminants of peanuts and other feed grains, the aflatoxins have enormous public health significance. Chronic aflatoxicosis has been suggested as one factor in the high incidence of human hepatocellular carcinoma in Africa and Asia.

BRACKEN FERN AND BOVINE BLADDER TUMORS

Bovine enzootic hematuria is a disease of grazing cattle largely confined to woods and areas containing bracken fern (*Pteris aquilina*). Hematuria has been shown to be caused by carcinomas of the bladder in Turkish cattle and water buffalo. Experimentally, bladder carcinomas were induced in cattle from nonenzootic geographical areas by feeding bracken fern. Tumors developed in all animals that survived over three years on the feeding program, and were indistinguishable from the naturally occurring lesions (Pamukcau et al. 1967). Bracken fern feeding also produces intestinal and urinary tumors in rats, aplastic anemia in cattle, and leukemia and pulmonary tumors in mice (Pamukcau et al. 1972). The chemical carcinogen present in the fern is not completely characterized, but is believed to be a metabolic breakdown product of a fern toxin.

CYCASIN NUTS AND LIVER TUMORS

Nuts of the plant *Cycas circinalis* contain a carcinogenic glycoside termed cycasin. When flour from these nuts is fed to rodents, they develop renal, small intestinal, and hepatic carcinomas. Methylazoxymethanol, an aglycone moiety of cycasin, is cleaved away by intestinal flora that possess a β-glucosidase and is the active carcinogen. Experimentally, methylazoxy-

genic herpesvirus genome with the lymphoid target cell is responsible for the proliferative lymphosarcomas that develop in the animal. It appears to be due to the action of the viral genome within the lymphoid cell and not merely to a lymphoid hyperplastic reaction to some extrinsic event. The uniclonality of the Burkitt's lymphosarcoma is a strong argument for this statement.

The status of viral DNA in the neoplastic cell, and whether it is linked with the host cell genome (or merely carried along in a nonintegrated state), is not known. Provided a ligating enzyme is present, the theoretical reasons for the usurping of host cell DNA synthesis by a herpesviral DNA template are logical. It is probable that, in the tumors, herpesviral DNA combines with cell DNA, mRNA is transcribed, and proteins are produced that migrate to the cell surface and are involved in transformation of the cell.

Large multilobular metastasizing renal adenocarcinomas occur in 2–5% of many frog populations in some parts of North America. The finding of large intranuclear inclusion bodies in the kidney tumor cells prompted successful transmission studies (Lucké 1938). The inclusions within the tumor cell nuclei are filled with large numbers of herpes virions and the herpesvirus was shown to be the cause of the tumor (Lunger 1965; Zambernard et al. 1966). Tumors could be induced in susceptible frogs by injection of suspensions of tumor, and successive transplantations were maintained in frogs for many generations.

The renal adenocarcinoma herpesvirus infects frog eggs when they are developing in the water in spring; carcinomas appear in the third or fourth summer of the frog's life. These "summer tumors" do not produce virus but do contain viral genetic material. During the summer months the tumor grows and may expand sufficiently to kill the frog. If it does not, tumor growth ceases at hibernation in the autumn. As the tumor cells cease their growth cycles, they become virogenic. That is, they produce infectious virions which lyse the tumor cell. Virus is excreted into the urine and, with the end of hibernation, is expelled into the pond water where it infects the eggs and tadpoles during the spring season (Skinner and Mizell 1972).

The growth of the frog herpesvirus is temperature-dependent, and this intriguing temperature-dependent tumor growth phenomenon has been demonstrated in the laboratory. Tumor cells can be converted from a virus-free summer state (in which the viral genome is present but unexpressed) to a virus-containing state by merely lowering the environmental temperature of the host frog.

The Epstein-Barr (EB) virus is the cause of human infectious mononucleosis and will probably be proven to be the cause of some lymphomas. It was discovered during electron microscopy of cell cultures derived from a case of the intriguing lymphosarcoma of African children known as Burkitt's lymphoma. This lymphosarcoma is characterized by multifocal solid tumors of the viscera and occurs in an epidemiologic pattern reminiscent of an infectious disease. Chemotherapy has a dramatic cure rate in affected children (Achong and Epstein 1966; Zur Hausen et al. 1967).

EB virus has not been definitely established as a cause of human lymphosarcoma but the epidemiologic implications are impressive. The virus will transform lymphocytes in vitro into permanently growing cells resembling lymphoma cells. It induces lymphoproliferative disease in nonhuman primates (Epstein et al. 1973). It leaves fingerprints in the form of membrane antigens and nucleic acid remnants within tumor tissue of affected children. Patients with Burkitt's lymphoma have levels of antibodies to EB virus that are greater than those found in unaffected children. Lymphosarcomas nearly identical with Burkitt's lymphoma occur in other primates and it may be that this virus is responsible (Di Giacomo 1967).

RNA VIRUSES

Members of the RNA *oncornavirus group* cause cancer in three orders of vertebrates: mammals, birds, and reptiles. Naturally occurring diseases where this has been established include the malignant lymphomas of cats, mice, and chickens. These viruses are also implicated in the lymphomas of cattle, dogs, and other mammals. The expression of oncogenicity of these viruses relates both to the character of the virus (how closely homologous its RNA is to host cell DNA) and age of the host. The relatively rapid mitotic activity and the immaturity of the immune systems are important factors in the susceptibility of the young animal.

In previous years, the most perplexing problem of oncogenesis by RNA viruses related to how the viral RNA molecule could influence the synthesis of cellular DNA. One of the central dogmas of molecular biology had been that information was transferred from DNA to RNA and from RNA to protein; it could not be transferred from protein to protein or from protein to nucleic acid. A major discovery in viral oncogenesis was therefore the finding of an RNA-directed DNA polymerase (reverse transcriptase) in viral-infected tumor cells and thereafter in the core of the RNA virions. This established the concept of a "reverse" flow of genetic information from RNA to DNA (Baltimore 1970; Temin 1972). The genetic information of the RNA-oncornaviruses, which is coded in RNA, transfers information by synthesizing a new DNA from the viral RNA template. The reverse transcriptase of one oncornavirus may even influence cellular reactivity of another, for Spiegelman et al. have shown that purified polymerase from avian leukosis virus can transcribe the RNA of other oncornaviruses to specific DNA production.

A provirus hypothesis was proposed by Temin to explain the replication of oncornaviruses through DNA intermediates and why such long periods exist between infection and cellular transformation. Reverse transcriptase uses the viral RNA genome to produce a DNA copy called the provirus. The provirus then serves as a template for virion production or is integrated into the host cell genome. An enzyme related to DNA replication, polynucleotide ligase, has been found in purified preparations of oncornaviruses. This enzyme repairs breaks in DNA molecules; it has been hypothesized that it functions to join viral DNA to cellular DNA on the chromosome, thus integrating the two.

Viral genetic material would be replicated with that of the host cell and passed to new daughter cells. The virions would disappear for months or even years and would reappear later due to some form of activation.

The viral oncogene hypothesis of Huebner proposes that most animals contain genetic information (in unexpressed form) for producing RNA-tumor viruses within their somatic cells. This information is transmitted from parent to offspring and has been a part of the genetic makeup of vertebrates since their early evolution. The genetic information for making the RNA viral material and causing the virion to assemble is repressed in all cells but is potentially inducible by oncogenic and mutagenic agents (Todaro and Huebner 1972).

Genetic information is located in hypothetical oncogenes that are segments of a larger virogene area of the chromosome. An oncogene, the DNA of which is complimentary to viral RNA, is integrated into the host cell genome and is inherited like a gene. The gene may be wholly or partially expressed, leading to (1) virion production, (2) viral-coded protein synthesis, or (3) cell transformation. This hypothesis resembles the provirus hypothesis of Temin but differs in implying that viral genetic material is an intrinsic part of the cell and was not received during recent infecting events. In either case, the virogene oncogene hypothesis stipulates that a complete copy of the information required for virus production and malignant transformation is transmitted from parent to offspring and is present in the DNA of all animals prone to cancer. The endogenous virogenes have evolved like the other cellular genes in a manner consistent with phylogenetic development.

After an oncornavirus enters the cell, it sheds its protein coat and initiates, by virtue of its reverse transcriptase, the production of a DNA copy of the viral genome. The intermediate copy, called the provirus, is integrated into the host cell's genome to produce a virogene, a gene that is the template for the production of virions. The type C virion contains all the enzymes necessary for cleaving cellular DNA, inserting the provirus, and mending the break in DNA. Proliferation of the infected cell results in transmission of the virogene to daughter cells without the appearance of viral proteins or virions. Integration also provides a way for the provirus to avoid the host's immune system. In the new host, if the virogene is activated, (1) the host cell becomes virogenic and begins to make new virions and/or (2) the host cell transforms into a tumor cell.

Endogenous type C virogenes are detectable in the DNA of chickens, mice, cats, and primates by the determination of nucleic acid sequences (comparable to those in the virion) and by detection of RNA in normal tissue that is expressed by these virogenes. Thus, even though infectious type C viruses cannot be isolated, the transcription of their virogene information can be identified. For example: nucleic acid sequences of type C viruses isolated from baboons have been found in DNA of normal baboon tissue, indicating that they are endogenous, vertically transmitted viruses of baboons. In contrast, the nucleic acid sequences of two type C viruses isolated from tumors of woolly monkeys and gibbon apes cannot be detected in their corresponding normal primate tissue but are found instead in DNA of normal mice. This is an indication that these viruses originated from viruses endogenous (or xenotropic) to mice.

SOME COMMON NEOPLASMS OF ANIMALS

Confrontation with enormous lists of neoplasms during a discussion of tumor classification is usually overwhelming to the beginning student of pathology. Separation into carcinoma and sarcoma or into adenoma and adenocarcinoma seems simple enough, but this is complicated by the capricious use of terms such as "mixed mammary gland tumor" or "transmissible venereal tumor" which have been established by precedent for neoplasms that do not fit comfortably within a rigid classification scheme. Even worse, the discipline of pathology is saddled with some confusing (and often humorous) eponyms such as "Wilm's tumor" (embryonal nephroma) or "Sticker tumor" (canine venereal tumor).

Compared with medical pathology, veterinary pathology is largely free of such nonsense and every effort should be made to avoid these meaningless names.

Classification is the means by which the pathologist communicates with the clinician who must provide a prognosis for the patient. With the advent of studies using clinical material, tumor classification gradually begins to make some practical sense. To present some indication of the incidence of tumors, we now examine the biological behavior of some of the commoner neoplasms encountered in the animal kingdom. Emphasis is placed on the behavior of these abnormal cells in their host animal and upon current research in experimental oncology.

MALIGNANT LYMPHOMA

Malignant lymphoma (lymphosarcoma) is one of the most common malignant neoplasms in the animal kingdom. It involves the malignant transformation of lymphocytes that become disseminated throughout the affected animal. The disease is important because it kills large numbers of animals and humans. In human medicine, the terms used are acute leukemia of children and chronic lymphatic leukemia of adults. Malignant lymphoma has been a cause of enormous economic loss to the poultry industry; in cattle, the viruses involved are viewed as significant potential contaminants of meat and milk.

Malignant lymphomas appear as solid, fleshy, white masses that destroy the architecture of lymphoid tissue and develop in the parenchyma of visceral organs. The malignant cells vary from normal-appearing small lymphocytelike cells to large blastic cells (Fujimoto et al. 1969; Laird et al. 1968a) (Fig. 6.12). When the malignant cells are disseminated through the bloodstream, the disease may be called lymphoid leukemia. The white blood cell counts done on leukemic animals may exceed 100,000 WBC per cmm.

Some lymphosarcomas are leukemic even though space-occupying lesions are not found. In contrast, some animals with extensive involvement by large tumor masses never become leukemic. The pathogenetic factors responsible for release or peripher-

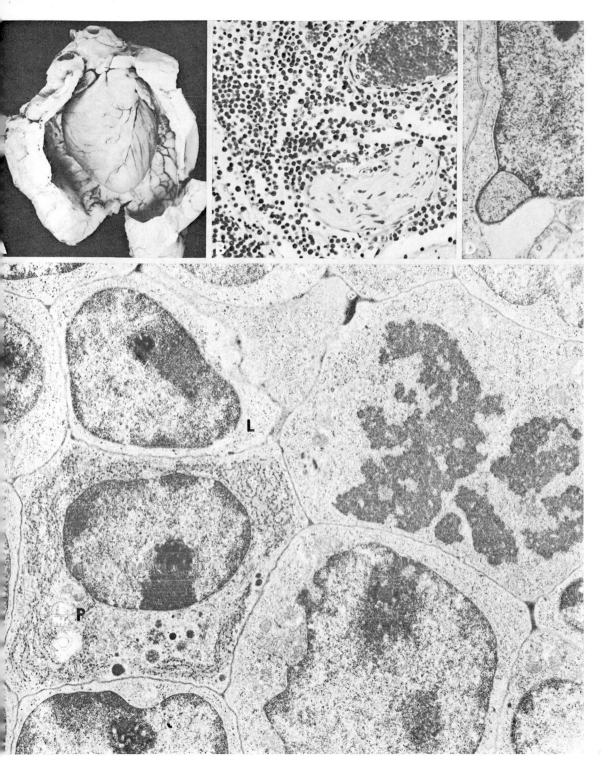

Fig. 6.12. A. Lymphosarcoma with massive involvement of the mediastinum and pericardium, cat. Tumor encircles heart and surrounds great vessels. B. Histology. Malignant lymphoblastic cells have infiltrated throughout connective tissues of mediastinum. C. Ultrastructure. Tumor cells resemble those of lymphoid tissue including small lymphocytes (L) and plasmacytes (P). One mitotic cell is fixed in metaphase (right). D. Nuclear pockets in neoplastic lymphocyte.

Table 6.7. Lymphosarcoma in animals

Species	Transmissible	Viral Etiology Established	Virus
Fish			
Cod	?	—	—
Herring			
Amphibians			
Toad	+	—	? (Balls and Ruben 1967)
Reptiles			
Viper	+	—	
Birds			
Chicken	+	+	Herpesvirus (Marek's disease)
		+	Oncornavirus (leukosis)
Mammals			
Mouse	+	+	Oncornavirus (Gross virus)
Cat	+	+	Oncornavirus
Monkey	+	+	*Herpesvirus saimiri*
Dog	+	—	? (Kakuk et al. 1968)
Cow	+	—	? (Miller et al. 1969)

alization of tumor cells is not known. The best theories of why malignant lymphoma cells remain restricted to solid lumps in spite of their demonstrated ability to spread freely throughout the body relate to the restricting influence of the host's immune response.

Lymphosarcoma is a tumor of virtually every vertebrate species and has been reported in the more primitive vertebrates and fish (Balls and Ruben 1967; Dunbar 1969; Hadji-Azimi and Fischberg 1972; Wolke and Wyand 1969) (Table 6.7). Phylogenetically, it appears to have arisen coincidentally with the development of the immune system. Because of the intense research endeavor in the field of leukemia of humans, many of these models have been widely investigated concerning their transmissibility and identification of causal viral agents. Oncornaviruses are established as etiologic agents in chickens, mice, and cats and are suspect in guinea pigs (Opler 1967), rabbits (Fox et al. 1970), and cattle (Miller et al. 1969; Olson et al. 1972; Wittmann and Urbaneck 1969). Transplantation of malignant cells as grafts to immunosuppressed recipients has been done with lymphosarcomas of dogs (Cohen et al. 1970; Kakuk et al. 1968; Owen 1971) and swine (Case and Simon 1968), but the oncornaviruses implicated have not been shown to be causal.

AVIAN LYMPHOSARCOMA

Malignant lymphoid neoplasms of the chicken are induced by two viruses. The leukosis viruses, which are RNA oncornaviruses, induce a variety of hematopoietic and mesenchymal tumors of which lymphoid leukosis is by far the most common. Host response is determined by both viral genome and host cell. The Marek's disease viruses are DNA herpesviruses. With both these viral agents, the incidence of infection is high, but the incidence of tumor development is low (Table 6.8). Lymphoid leukosis is a neoplastic disorder involving B cells; Marek's disease is one of T cells.

LYMPHOID LEUKOSIS OF CHICKENS AND THE LYMPHOID LEUKOSIS VIRUS (LLV)

LLV-induced lymphosarcoma is characterized by foci of whitish, solid tumors in the bursa, liver, and spleen. Other organs may be affected and the clinical appearance is related to muscle wasting, anemia, and hepatosplenomegaly. Neoplastic lymphoid cells are large stem cells with large nucleoli and few cytoplasmic organelles. Endoplasmic reticulum is sparse and does not appear to be an efficient source for globulin production, even though large amounts of IgM may be produced. Virions may be found budding from the cell surface but are not readily detectable in naturally occurring tumors. LLV exerts its oncogenic effect by interrupting the switch from IgM to IgG that occurs in the normal bursa (Cooper et al. 1974).

When newly hatched chicks of a susceptible strain are inoculated with an oncogenic isolate of LLV, transformation of

Table 6.8. Avian lymphosarcoma

	Lymphoid Leukosis	Marek's Disease
Etiology	Leukosis virus (Oncornavirus)	MD virus (Herpesvirus)
Incidence		
Earliest appearance	16 wks	6 wks
Peak mortality	24–40 wks	10–20 wks
Cytology	B cell	T cell
Manifest	Originate in bursa, nodular/diffuse Viscera, affects liver, spleen, kidney, gonad, heart, bone marrow	PNS lesion (neural lymphosarcoma) Gray infiltration of iris (gray eye) Nodular skin lesions Bursa-atrophy/interfollicular infiltration
Natural transmission	Vertical (mother-daughter, via egg)	Horizontal (bird to bird)

lymphoid cells in the bursa occurs at about 6–8 wks of age. By 10–16 wks transformed follicles are visible in nearly all birds and metastasis from the bursa to viscera occurs around the time of sexual maturity at 20 wks. Lymphoid leukosis represents neoplastic B-cell transformation and requires the bursa for development (Peterson et al. 1964). The initial change in bursal follicles involves the uncontrolled replication of ribosome-filled B cells that form isolated gigantic follicles. These compress and distort adjacent follicles and eventually spread to involve the entire bursa. The process is confined to the bursa for a period of 2–4 wks but then disseminates throughout the chicken.

Obliteration of the bursa prior to transformation (by bursectomy, chemotherapy, or lytic viral infection) destroys the capacity of the virus to induce tumors. Thymectomy has no effect on the course of disease. Even after the tumor has localized in the bursa, the removal of this organ will suppress the dissemination of the tumor's cells and the incidence of lymphosarcoma. Put another way, bursectomy at 12 wks of age will prevent the occurrence of lymphosarcomas in the liver and spleen even though the neoplastic process has already been initiated within the bursa.

In naturally occurring leukosis virus infections, a small percent of tumors arises that involves tissue other than the lymphoid system. The neoplasm that results appears to depend upon both the availability of certain target cells at the time of infection and the degee to which the oncornaviral RNA of a particular virion is homologous to the long deoxynucleotide sequence of the host cells. The mode of transmission influences the availability of

target cells. In vertical transmission (dam to offspring) viral DNA is uniformly distributed among most tissues of the neonate. Horizontal infection after hatching results in increased viral DNA only in dividing target cells. The expression of oncogenicity may therefore involve: (1) myeloblasts and their precursors that give rise to acute myeloblastic leukemia, (2) erythroblasts which account for acute anemia and occasionally erythroid leukemia, (3) embryonic kidney cells that give rise to embryonal nephromas, and (4) osteoblasts that develop into bone destruction and osteopetrosis (Mladenov et al. 1967).

In natural conditions, leukosis virus is transmitted from hen to chick via the egg. In the hen, virions are demonstrable in the ovary and oviduct (Di Stefano and Dougherty 1966). They bud from the plasma membrane of cells in direct contact with the oogonia and germinal epithelium. Large numbers of virions are also present in the albumin-secreting glands of the magnum of the oviduct. They bud from the surface of microvilli into the lumen and the zygote is exposed to high concentrations of virus in the magnum while it is still a single cell.

When the chicken embryo is infected, the chick appears immunologically tolerant to leukosis virus and does not develop antibodies. At hatching, most chicks are viremic although a variable percentage will not have virus. Virions are demonstrable in most tissues, especially the liver and kidney (Dougherty and Di Stefano 1967; Heine et al. 1962; Simpson 1969). In infected flocks, maternal antibody is present in newly hatched chicks, but gradually disappears and is gone in 4–6 wks. These chicks may become infected by carrier birds, but the incidence of tumors is suppressed by humoral antibodies and by some unknown factor associated with aging of the chick.

In summary, the salient facts of naturally occurring lymphoid leukosis are: (1) virus replicates in the female reproductive tract and transmission to offspring occurs vertically; (2) large numbers of chicks may be infected but few develop tumors; (3) neoplastic transformation begins in the bursa and bursectomy prevents the dissemination of neoplastic cells; and (4) neoplastic B cells produce large amounts of IgM.

MAREK'S DISEASE (MD)

In 1907, Marek described a disease of chickens in which the peripheral and central nervous systems were infiltrated by lymphocytes. He designated the disease polyneuritis and believed the basic lesion to be infiltration and focal accumulation of a mixed population of lymphoid cells. Although lymphoid lesions were seen in viscera in some cases, observations on the epidemiology and pathology of the disease suggested that it was distinct from lymphoid leukosis. During the succeeding decades, this herpesvirus-induced neoplastic disease became widespread and is now a major cause of mortality in the domestic chicken. Two forms of the disease are recognized: subacute or classic MD, in which nerves are the chief site of lymphocyte proliferation; and acute MD, in which tumors of the viscera are common.

Successful transmission experiments were followed by isolation of the causal herpesvirus in 1968. MD virus is a highly cell-associated virus. It replicates in the epithelium of the feather follicles and is transmitted from bird to bird by skin flakes in dust aerosols. The morphology of the virion is typical of the herpesvirus group (Epstein et al. 1968). Virions are easily found in cell cultures prepared from tumors but are located with difficulty in tumors themselves.

The first changes seen in lymphoid tissues of chicks inoculated experimentally are lymphocyte destruction and lymphoid atrophy, with subsequent infiltration of pale large reticulum cells. Naked virions are seen mostly in reticulum cells, occa-

sionally in lymphocytes, and rarely in epithelial cells (Frazier 1974). When the disease becomes manifest, virions can readily be found in epithelial cells of the feather follicles with lesions. Affected epithelial cells are hyperplastic and swollen and contain intranuclear inclusion bodies. They contain both naked and enveloped virions, usually in nucleus and cytoplasm respectively, and epithelium is the source of cell-free infectious virus. In contrast, tumor tissue, infected nerves, and viscera contain viral antigens, but only naked virions are demonstrable and viral assays reveal that infectivity is cell-associated (Calnek et al. 1970; Ubertini and Calnek 1970).

In summary, three different host-virus relationships appear possible in MD: (1) both virions and viral antigens are present and extracellular infectious virus can be isolated, as in feather follicle epithelium; (2) viral antigens are present but enveloped virions are not, as occurs in nerve and visceral tumors; and (3) neither virions nor viral antigens are present. In the latter case, the disease is transmissible by intact cells, so the viral genome must be present. It is suggested that there is integration of the viral DNA with host cell chromosomes. Cells not producing virions have been shown to contain viral-specific nucleic acid and can be chemically induced in vitro to produce virus.

The transformation of lymphoid cells in MD is associated with a functional thymus. Thymectomy is rarely successful in chickens but the thymic-dependency of the tumor has been demonstrated by staining tumors cells with fluorescent antibody preparations against thymic antigen (Hudson and Payne 1973). Bursectomy, which so effectively obliterates oncornavirus-induced lymphomas in the chicken, has no effect on the course of MD-induced neoplasia (Payne and Rennie 1970).

Chickens inoculated with blood or other infective material containing Marek's disease herpesvirus may develop acute disease characterized by massive infiltration of peripheral nerves, particularly the sciatic nerve, by proliferating lymphoid cells. These include blast cells, small and medial lymphocytes, and dark-staining "MD" cells. Lesions in the peripheral nervous system enlarge progressively and are associated with death of the bird. Lymphoid tumors develop in other organs such as the liver, gonads, spleen, heart, and lung. Atrophy of the thymus and bursa is prominent. Multifocal lesions develop in the skin in some birds (Lapen et al. 1970).

Some infected chickens develop minimal lesions in the nervous system. These do not progress but regress into an inflammatory-like condition dominated by edema with plasmacytes scattered throughout the spongy nerve tissue (Payne and Biggs 1967). It has been noticed that some of these lesions resemble allergic neuritis, and an immune mechanism has been postulated. It is suggested that the perivascular infiltrates of lymphocytes and primary demyelination represent a herpesvirus-induced autoimmune demyelinating disease, in which there is a cell-mediated immune response to normal myelin.

FELINE LYMPHOSARCOMA AND
FELINE LEUKEMIA VIRUS (FeLV)

Lymphosarcoma, the most common neoplasm of the cat, can be induced with cell-free preparations of FeLV. The disease is progressive and appears as massive enlargement of lymphoid organs. Secondary effects are anemia, emaciation, and glomerulonephritis. Feline lymphosarcoma occurs in four variants, each with distinct sites of cell multiplication and routes of migration through the lymphoid tissues: (1) alimentary, in which the Peyer's patches and lymph node germinal centers are initially involved; (2) multicentric, which begins in the paracortical (thymic-dependent) areas of the lymph nodes; (3) thymic, which also affects the paracortical areas of the lymph nodes; and (4) leukemic, which chiefly affects the bone marrow and the red pulp of the spleen and the medullary areas of the peripheral lymph nodes (Mackey and Jarrett 1972) (Table 6.9).

The cell types that are seen in feline lymphosarcoma allegedly represent both B and T cells which have been transformed. In individual cats, the malignant cells may be predominantly lymphoblastic, prolymphocytic, histiocytic, or lymphohistiocytic. There is little correlation between the cell type and the clinical course of the disease.

Lymphosarcoma of cats is caused by an

Table 6.9. Types of feline lymphosarcoma

Form	Primary Involvement	Occurrence
Alimentary	Mesenteric lymph nodes	Most common
Multicentric	Generalized Lymph node, para-cortical areas	Common
Leukemia	Bone marrow Splenic red pulp	Uncommon
Thymic	Thymus Anterior mediastinum Lymph node, para-cortical areas	Least common

oncornavirus, FeLV. The initial successful transmission experiments by Jarrett in Glasgow were repeated in several laboratories. The virions were identified in tumor tissue (Jarrett et al. 1964; Laird et al. 1968a; Rickard et al. 1969; Theilen et al. 1970). They were seen extracellularly, within cytoplasmic vacuoles, and budding from the plasma membrane. They were most prevalent in bone marrow, thymus, lymph node, and spleen. In cells of the circulating blood, virions are best sought within and budding from the surface of platelets (Laird et al. 1968b).

Megakaryocytes appear to be of major significance in FeLV mediated lymphosarcoma. They may serve as a reservoir of virus or viral oncogens. When young kittens are first infected, it is probable that thrombocytopenia occurs as a direct effect of the virus and may provide an early clue to the preleukemic states.

The induction of lymphosarcoma in cats is related both to the presence of FeLV and to immunologic abnormalities. Experimentally, when kittens are inoculated with FeLV, radiation increases the percent of animals that develop lymphosarcoma. The predisposing factors involved in naturally occurring lymphosarcoma are unknown although it appears that immunosuppressant diseases that occur in kittenhood may play some role. Cats that have recovered from severe anemia induced by *Hemobartonella felis* have a much higher incidence of malignant lymphoma than do nonanemic cats (Priester and Hayes 1973). In the preneoplastic phases of experimental disease, significant depression of cell-mediated immunoreactivity occurs and thymic atrophy is prominent (Perryman et al. 1972). It may be that the immunosuppressive effect of FeLV is a critical factor in the development of neoplastic disease.

It is accepted that, like other oncornaviruses, FeLV can be passed genetically from parent to offspring. It also appears that one cat can infect another with this virus. This discovery was triggered by the observation that feline lymphosarcoma tends to occur in "clusters."

When one cat in a household of several cats develops the disease, unrelated associates are apt to come down with the disease. By examining platelets for the presence of FeLV it was found that of almost 1500 healthy cats from disease-free households, only 2 carried FeLV. In contrast, 177 of 543 cats from households with lymphosarcoma carried FeLV and many of these subsequently developed the disease. These infected cats were followed for several months and it was found that 24% died with feline lymphosarcoma within the next 6 months (Hardy et al. 1973). FeLV is present in blood, saliva, and urine and it appears that cats spread the virus during fighting and mating (which involves biting and scratching). Grooming with the tongue and multiple use of litter boxes may also be involved in spread of the virus.

MYELOPROLIFERATIVE DISEASE OF CATS

Poorly characterized neoplastic syndromes occur in cats involving proliferation of bone marrow cells. The commonest of the feline myeloproliferative diseases is *granulocytic* (myelogenous) *leukemia*. The proliferating marrow seeds the body with immature-appearing, malignant granulocytes. These large cells contain small dense granules typical of progranulocytes. The less differentiated cells are often associated with virions typical of the oncornavirus group (Fig. 6.13). In the spleen, cells infiltrate the pulp cords, sparing the germinal centers until late in the disease (Fraser et al. 1974). This is in contrast to lymphoid leukemia, which involves the germinal centers first. In the liver, periportal areas are first infiltrated with subsequent replacement of parenchymal cells. Ultrastructurally, virions are best sought in bone marrow cells (Herz et al. 1970).

The other myeloproliferative diseases are *erythremic myelosis* (malignant transformation of the RBC series) and *erythroleukemia* (a mixture of neoplastic granulocytes and erythrocytes). Like granulocytic leukemia, they are associated with severe refractory anemia, undifferentiated cells in the circulation, and infiltration of cells into tissues. Ultrastructurally, the malignant cells may be too undifferentiated to characterize the involved types (Hurvitz 1970).

The etiology of the myeloproliferative diseases is not established. Although FeLV may be causally related, other feline oncornaviruses have been isolated. The feline sarcoma virus (FSV), which shares antigens with FeLV, is associated with solid tumors in cats. It probably bears the same relationship to feline neoplastic disease that Rous sarcoma virus bears to lymphoid leukosis in chickens. A third feline C-type virus, "feline endogenous virus" (RD114), has been isolated that, as yet, has not been proven to be involved in oncogenicity.

FELINE FIBROSARCOMA

Fibrosarcomas in cats have been shown to be transmissible. C-type virions similar to FeLV are demonstrable in both naturally occurring and experimental tumors. After inoculation of virus into kittens, tumors arise in over three-fourths of the animals. Rapidly growing masses tend to have loose, myxomatous patterns of stellate cells with vacuolation and pleomorphic nuclei. The more slowly growing tumors are compact and have fusiform-shaped cells with elongate nuclei. Virions of 115 nm diameter bud from the plasma membrane and can also be seen extracellularly and within cytoplasmic vacuoles (Snyder et al. 1970).

LYMPHOSARCOMA IN PRIMATES

Lymphosarcoma is rarely reported in monkeys, chimpanzees, and other nonhuman primates. An exciting laboratory model of a stem cell tumor induced by a simian herpesvirus has emerged, however. *Herpesvirus saimuri* is indigenous and noncytopathic in squirrel monkeys *(Saimiri sciureus)* but can produce rapidly fatal neoplastic disease in some other nonhuman primates (Melendez et al. 1969, 1970, 1971). The virus originally grew out of degenerat-

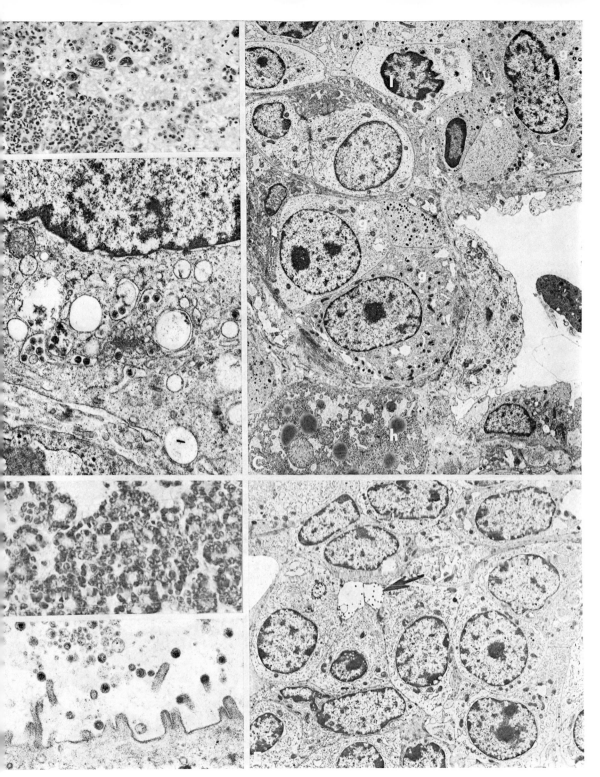

Fig. 6.13. A.–C. Myeloproliferative disease, cat. A. Histology. B. Feline oncornaviruses within the cisternae of the ER in a virogenic reticulum cell. C. Ultrastructure. Lymphoid cells (l), neutrophils (n), and immature granulocytes (g) surround the hepatocytes (h). D.–F. Mouse mammary gland tumor. D. Histology, note acini. E. Ultrastructure. Virions bud from the acinar surfaces (arrow). F. Virions associated with cell surface. Micrographs E and F, R. Cutlip.

ing primary kidney cells cultured from a healthy squirrel monkey. When injected into squirrel monkeys, no disease or lesion developed. However, a rapidly progressive malignant lymphoma of the reticulum cell type developed in owl *(Aotus* sp.) and marmoset *(Saguinus* sp.) monkeys after inoculation. Spider monkeys are similarly affected (Hunt et al. 1972). The disease has a very rapid course of 13–28 days and can be induced with cell-free inoculae.

The neoplasm produces extensive invasion of many organs. The lungs, liver, kidney, adrenal, and lymphoid organs are all affected. The fundamental change is proliferation and invasion of the tissue by neoplastic reticulum cells. The cell response is both necrotizing and proliferative, however. Ultrastructural examination of tumor tissue reveals the cells to be mixtures of lymphoblasts and undifferentiated reticulum cells (King and Melendez 1972). In some animals, lymphoblasts are the dominant cell type. Herpesviruses cannot be demonstrated in tumor tissue, but do appear when cells are removed from the tumor and grown in culture (Morgan et al. 1973).

MURINE LYMPHOSARCOMA

A naturally occurring lymphosarcoma of mice characterized by thymic enlargement is caused by an oncornavirus, the Gross murine leukemia virus (MLV). Gross, in 1951, reported that cell-free preparations of hematopoietic organs of AK mice that had developed lymphosarcoma would induce the same disease in a specific strain of mouse when inoculated soon after birth.

Pathogenesis studies have revealed that the "Gross virus"-induced lymphosarcoma of AKR mice, a "high incidence" strain, is a malignancy of T cells that evolves in an orderly and precise manner (Metcalf 1966; Siegler and Rich 1965). The process begins unilaterally in one of the two thymic lobes. The first change seen histologically is lymphocytolysis, which leads to narrowing of the cortex and loss of small lymphocytes. Subsequently, there is an expansion of the medullary areas due to histiocytosis and follicular aggregation of small lymphocytes. Phagocytic reticulum cells, which become activated and hyperplastic, are an impor-

tant factor in the degradation of dying neoplastic lymphocytes (Izard and De Harven 1968).

Virions are widely distributed throughout the thymus of preleukemic mice, where they occur both in lymphocytes and thymic epithelial cells (De Harven 1964). In very young mice, it appears that virions are most obvious in hematopoietic tissues, from which they appear to seed other lymphoid organs. Later, they are particularly prominent in the germinal centers of the spleen and lymph nodes, where they reside in close approximation to the dendritic webs of the reticulum cells (Hanna et al. 1970; Swartzendruber et al. 1967). The immunosuppressive effect accompanying MLV infection may be mediated by alterations in the lymphoid tissue, possibly as a consequence of competition between virion and the antigen in question for a particular precursor immunocompetent cell.

By electron microscopy, virions are seen free in the cytoplasm and budding from the plasma membrane of the cell. Budding appears to occur at sites on the plasma membrane that are free of the G (Gross) cell-surface antigen and of the major (H-2) histocompatibility antigen of mice (Aoki et al. 1970).

Natural transmission of murine lymphosarcoma is through the embryo. The disease is not prevented by rearing mice derived via hysterectomy or by foster nursing. Virions have been photographed in the ovaries of females, budded from cells of the follicular theca and corpus luteum. They also occur throughout the female genital tract and in the spermatozoa and ductal system of the male genital tract (Feldman and Gross 1967). In utero infection induces tolerance against at least some of the antigens in the virion, and high levels of virus are present in the mouse throughout its life span. Tolerance is partial, for some anti-MLV antibodies are produced and allegedly are responsible for membranous glomerulopathy which develops in aged infected mice (Oldstone et al. 1972).

The naturally occurring lymphosarcomas in mice have been overshadowed by the enormous amount of research done on artificial model systems induced by MLV strains. Thus there is available today a large family of ML viruses named after investigators such as Moloney, Rauscher, Friend, et al. They not only induce lymphosarcoma but reticulum cell sarcomas and myeloid neoplasms as well.

In some colonies of mice with a high incidence of lymphosarcoma a paralytic syndrome occurs wherein affected mice drag their hind limbs about. Examination of these animals has revealed degenerate neurons in the anterior horn of the lower spinal cord which are filled with virions resembling the oncornaviruses (Andrews and Gardner 1974). Whether or not these virions are the Gross virus has not been proven but a possible neurotropism of this agent is intriguing.

MALIGNANT MELANOMA

The production of melanin is phylogenetically an ancient mechanism (see Chapter 2). Malignant melanomas, the neoplasms of melanin-synthesizing cells, are equally distributed throughout the phyla of the animal kingdom (Ghelelovitch 1968). The word melanoma in its common usage denotes malignancy, and the words carcinoma and sarcoma are generally avoided because of the uncertainty concerning the derivation of these tumor cells. Melanomas vary in their behavior, but the malignant variety are vicious neoplasms and this fact imparts a fearsome aspect to the diagnosis of melanoma. Among individual melanomas, the rate of growth is inversely related to the extent of differentiation (melanogenesis) (Gray and Pierce 1964). Melanosis is used to denote nonneoplastic pigmentation caused by melanin pigments. It is commonly seen in the meninges, lungs, and skin; swine and sheep tissues are often affected.

Malignant melanomas arise from melanoblasts anywhere in the body and have been reported in amphibians, reptiles, fish, and birds. They are common in dogs, where they occur in the oral cavity, skin, and the ciliary body and choroid of the eye. Pigmented breeds are especially affected, and there is an increased incidence in the black Cocker Spaniel, Airedale, and Boston and Scottish terriers. Curiously, the spotted Dalmation is not known to develop these tumors.

In horses, depigmented gray individuals are affected. Melanomas are particularly common in the black Percheron which turns gray and white with age (the skin remains black although the hair is gray) (Hadwen 1931). Melanomas are rare in horses of other pigmentations. About 80% of aged gray horses develop malignant melanomas. The commonest location is in the perianal regions. It has been theorized that there is failure of melanin synthesis and the progressive loss of pigmentation stimulates melanoblastic activity which is associated with neoplastic transformation (M'Fadyean 1933).

Malignant melanoma cells are most often large and polyhedral and contain varying amounts of golden-brown to black pigment granules (Fig. 6.14). Cells of individual tumors show considerable variance in shape and pigmentation. Some are composed of elongate, stellate-shaped cells. Some contain only blastic cells which produce little pigment. These "amelanotic melanomas" are detected histochemically by the content of tyrosinase that is present in the endoplasmic reticulum. It oxidizes dihydrophenylalanine (dopa), which is added as part of the histochemical test (called the dopa reaction), to black granular foci in the tumor tissue.

Ultrastructurally, malignant melanoma cells contain melanosomes of various sizes. These bodies are disoriented and more pleomorphic than in normal melanocytes (Crowell et al. 1973; Epstein and Fukuyama 1973; Michima 1967, Toshima et al. 1968). Compound melanosomes, which are membrane-bound lysosomes packed with degenerate primary melanosomes, occur. They arise within melanoma cells by autophagy (Novikoff et al. 1968). In the amelanotic melanomas, few melanosomes are present but the Golgi complex is quite large and contains associated premelanosomes. Melanomas usually contain many large, pigment-filled macrophages.

EXPERIMENTAL ONCOLOGY

Immunotherapy against malignant melanoma holds some promise. Antigens prepared from tumor tissue evoke antibodies that suppress tumor growth in human patients. It is also hypothesized that sera of individuals of the black races, who rarely

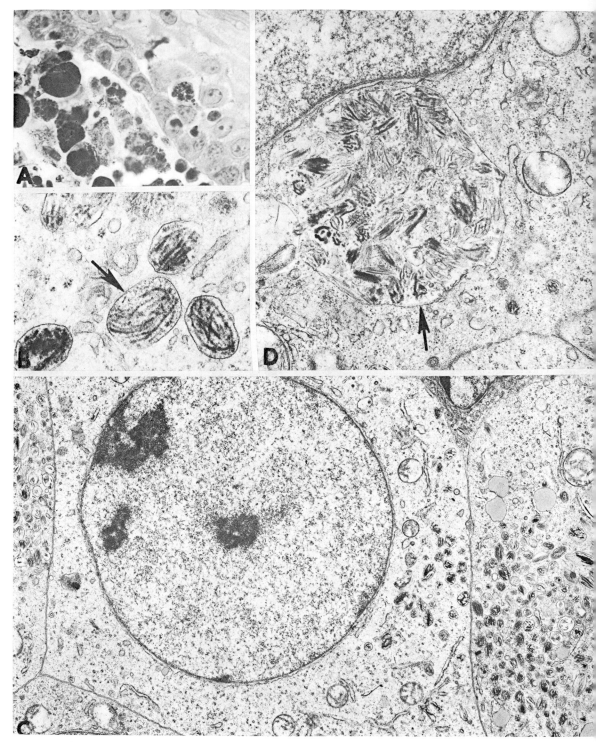

Fig. 6.14. Malignant melanoma. A. Histology. Skin tumor of dog.
B. Melanosomes (arrow). C. Ultrastructure. Transplantable melanoma
S91, mouse. D. Ultrastructure of tumor cell phagosome (arrow) with
melanin.

suffer malignant melanoma, may contain a humoral factor that represses malignant transformation of the melanocyte. Feeding patients on low tyrosine and phenylalanine diets has been tried, with uncertain results. Tyrosine, into which phenylalanine is transformed, is the basic amino acid in melanin production. It is proposed that by depriving the enzyme tyrosinase of its substrate the tumor cell would be inhibited (Jensen et al. 1973).

Two transplantable murine melanomas have been widely studied. The Cloudman melanoma S91 arose from the tail of a DBA mouse at the Jackson laboratory. It is strain-specific, and has been passed through several hundred generations. Subcutaneous implants kill the host within 12 weeks, after metastasizing to the lungs and other viscera. The Cloudman melanoma produces large amounts of melanin via the tyrosinase–dopa oxidase enzyme complex and tumor cells contain large pleomorphic melanosomes (Demopoulos 1965). An amelanotic variety arises when the tumor is transplanted to albino mice. Cells of this neoplasm do not produce tyrosine or dopa oxidase and have few pigment granules (Hirsch and Zelickson 1964). The Harding-Passey melanoma originated on the ear of a stock brown mouse and is not strain-specific. Its cells are more stellate than those of the Cloudman tumor and contain lesser amounts of pigment. This tumor rarely metastasizes.

Melanoma of the swordtail platyfish has been a widely studied model for malignant melanoma. Wild platyfish (*Xiphophorus* spp.) are of several different color patterns, each due to distribution of macromelanophores in the skin. Melanomas develop in hybrids (crosses between species) and the genetics of these tumors have been extensively explored (Anders 1967). A large number of environmental factors can act on the genome of the hybrids to lower the age of appearance of the melanomas.

Normal fish carry a macromelanophore gene S_d which is responsible for melanophore differentiation. The fish's pigment cells differentiate from melanoblasts to melanocytes to melanophores. In tumors, differentiation is blocked by abnormal genes. By combining certain hereditary factors, melanotic or amelanotic tumors can be produced. Those unpigmented fish that develop "albino" or amelanotic melanomas are killed by their rapidly growing tumors more quickly. The albino tumor cells are less differentiated. Ultrastructurally, in contrast to the heavily pigmented melanotic tumors, they contain premelanosomes but few mature pigment bodies (Vielkind et al. 1971). The albino gene is thought to act by inhibiting tyrosinase activity.

MAST CELL TUMOR

The mast cell tumor (mast cell sarcoma, mastocytoma) makes up nearly 20% of all skin tumors in the dog. These circumscribed neoplasms are prone to develop about the genitals and hind limbs, and they occur more often in the Boston Terrier and Boxer breeds. Mast cell tumors have been documented in other species, but the lower incidence and the inadequacy of the reports involved make a valid study of their behavior impossible (Ward and Hurvitz 1972).

CANINE MASTOCYTOMA

Canine mastocytomas begin as delimited foci of mast cells. They are progressive and potentially malignant. Approximately 30% of mastocytomas recur locally or in disseminated form after surgical excision. Local recurrences are apt to be more loosely distributed throughout the connective tissues than are the original tumors. The more malignant neoplasms metastasize widely to regional lymph nodes and also to the spleen, liver, and kidney.

In dogs with localized skin mastocytomas, there is often a subtle generalized mastocytosis. Accumulations of mast cells are present in the regional lymph nodes, spleen, liver, bone marrow, and kidneys. Many dogs with these tumors also have a diffuse plasmacytosis and membranous glomerulonephritis (Hottendorf and Nielsen 1968). The biological and clinical significances of these changes are elusive.

Histaminemia may be present in dogs with large disseminated mastocytomas. Rapid release of histamine produced experimentally by mast cell degranulators may cause hypotension. The production of histamine may also lead to gastric ulceration. In one series of tumor-bearing dogs, 20 of 24 had ulcers; most were in the stomach, but some occurred in the duodenum (Howard et al. 1969). In 3 individuals, the ulceration was sufficiently severe to cause death. Gastric ulcers are also associated with mast cell tumors in the cat, ox, and human.

Cytologically, the neoplastic mast cells are polyhedral or round, and they have round, central nuclei with several nucleoli. Their Giemsa-staining granules vary in size and structure. In old, well-differentiated cells, they are large and tend to be high in histamine and heparin. In poorly differentiated neoplasms, granules may be dustlike or undetectable in routine stains. Because of this absence of metachromatic granules, these tumors may be mistaken for reticulum cell sarcomas. Electron microscopy, however, invariably reveals the presence of at least a few mast cell granules (Bowles et al. 1972; Weiss et al. 1968). Mitotic figures are rare, even in malignant tumor cells. The intercellular spaces of the tumor are characteristically filled with foci of necrotic collagen, aggregates of eosinophils, and fibrinoid necrosis of the arterioles within the tumor.

EXPERIMENTAL STUDY

Transmission studies of the canine mast cell sarcoma indicate that some transmissible agent may be involved (Bloom et al. 1958; Bowles et al. 1972; Lombard et al. 1963; Peters 1969). In the initial transmission studies by Lombard et al., pooled tumor suspensions from an aged Doberman Pinscher with skin mastocytoma, metastatic lesions, and mast cell leukemia were inoculated into newborn Beagle pups. One of 7 developed a mast cell tumor within 30 days. Its tumors were passed into new pups. By the fifth passage generation, the tumor incidence was 11 dogs with tumors out of 14 that had been inoculated. Electron microscopic examination of tumor cells has revealed the presence of virions resembling the murine oncogenic viruses (Lombard et al. 1963; Rudolph and Weiss 1969). Transmissible mastocytomas have also been reported in mice (Dunn and Potter 1957; Rask-Nielsen and Christensen 1963).

TRANSMISSIBLE VENEREAL TUMOR OF DOGS

The canine transmissible venereal tumor is an undifferentiated stem-cell neoplasm of the genitals of dogs, which is usually acquired during mating and which is transferable by living cells. Cells are transferred as a graft to the new host and tumors grow progressively by expansion. Although malignant forms and metastases have been reported, they are rare. The tumors grow rapidly at first, but decreased mitotic activity develops with advancing age in most tumors and is alleged to be due to an increase in the rate of cell loss as a result of an immune reaction (Cohen 1972).

Venereal transmission was established by a Russian veterinarian in 1876, making this the oldest transmissible neoplasm known. Naturally occurring transmission is exemplified by the following excerpt from a report on English dogs by Smith in 1898: "From January to June 1894 a dog, A, served twelve bitches, eleven of whom became infected. About a month after pupping, there was noticed in each case a growth in the vaginal wall, somewhat resembling a raspberry. The growth gradually increased in size and extent until in some cases the whole of the vagina was filled with a mass as large as an orange. An examination of dog A revealed the presence of a similar growth situated on the penis behind the corona . . ."

More recent transmission studies revealed that of 601 dogs inoculated with tumor cells, 68% developed tumors (Karlson and Mann 1952). They first appeared 15 days after inoculation. By 30 days, 37% had developed and by 60 days, 89%. At 80 days most tumors had regressed and only 5 dogs had metastatic lesions. In irradiated dogs, the tumor exhibits the biologic behavior of a malignant neoplasm (Cohen 1973). Tumors have also been transmitted to foxes and to mice and hamsters with immunosuppression.

Cytologically, individual tumor cells are uniform, polygonal, and have large amounts of basophilic cytoplasm. Mitoses and foci of necrosis are common even in small tumors. Connective tissue stroma is present only in small amounts. Ultrastructurally, the cytoplasm contains scattered vacuoles and small mitochondria in a cytosol filled with free ribosomes. The cell surface contains many microvilli, which are in close apposition and cause definite demarcation of cells from each other (Drommer and Schulz 1969; Shubin and Ponomarkov 1971).

Tumor cells have been maintained in cell culture for long periods, and virions have been seen in some cultures (Adams et al. 1968; Sapp and Adams 1970). The virus does not appear to cause tumor growth. Although viral etiologies have been proposed in the past for the venereal tumor, general failure of transmissibility of the neoplasm with cell-free filtrates mitigates against this proposal. Cells in culture have an adherence phenomenon and readily form rosettes (Cohen et al. 1971).

The chromosome number of the transmissible venereal tumor cells (59) differs from that of normal dog cells (78). Even after long-term cell culture, the chromosome number and distribution resemble that of the naturally occurring tumor (Adams et al. 1968). Chromosomes are decreased in number, but are increased in volume. The total number of chromosomes is decreased inversely with an increase in metacentric forms (Barski and Cornefert-Jensen 1966; Makino 1963; Oshimura et al. 1973; Weber et al. 1965). Tumor cells from widely different geographical areas have a similar chromosome number (59 chromosomes with 17 biarmed and 42 acrocentric), and from this karyotypic uniformity it is inferred that this is a transplantable tumor of common origin. The chromosome number and structure represent a distinct pattern necessary for propagation of the tumor cell. Polyploidization through endomitotic division appears to play a fundamental role in the evolution of the tumor cell. A transmissible venereal tumor with a variant chromosomal number has been reported (Sellyei et al. 1970).

Dogs whose tumors have regressed are immune from further experimental inoculation and antibodies appear to play a significant role. Passive immunity, due to treatment with serum from recovered dogs, will cause regression of actively growing tumors and will prevent initiation of tumors when cells are inoculated experimentally. Active immunization induced with multiple injections of tumor extract acts similarly (Powers 1968). There appears to be no evidence relating to the effect of cell-mediated immunity.

CUTANEOUS HISTIOCYTOMA OF DOGS

This tumor, from which the transmissible venereal tumor must be differentiated, has erroneously been called an "extra-genital" transmissible venereal tumor. It is composed of large histiocytes, which probably originate from and bear the pleomorphism of the monocyte-macrophage series of cells (Drommer and Schulz 1969; Kelly 1970). Its biological behavior is different (Taylor et al. 1969) and it does not have the microvillous surface and the frequent mitoses of the venereal tumor.

BASAL AND SQUAMOUS CELL CARCINOMAS

These two carcinomas are among the more common malignant skin tumors of most animal species. The histologic diagnosis depends upon the faithful reproduction of their respective components of the epidermis. Cells of the basal cell carcinoma do not differentiate, whereas those of the squamous cell carcinoma form keratin and the tumors contain circumscribed aggregates of keratinized cells called "squamous pearls."

Benign neoplasms of the epidermal spinous cells are often called papillomas. Since this term is also used for nonneoplastic skin lesions, *acanthoma* is preferable. Epithelioma is sometimes used. The lack of concern for appropriate terminology reflects the scant importance of these tumors to the host. They are usually small pedunculated lesions, bothersome only because of their physical presence.

A major problem in the diagnosis of skin neoplasms is to sort out inflammatory and hyperplastic lesions from the true neoplasms. Many times inflammation is superimposed upon skin tumors to the extent that diagnosis becomes difficult. Secondary infection because of exposure to the trauma of the environment leads to purulent inflammation, ulceration, and necrosis. Treatment of skin lesions may cause allergic sensitivity, chemical irritation, and foreign body reactions. Heat rash during the summer months and the itch-scratch syndrome are complicating factors in nervous breeds of dogs.

Some of the lesions of the epidermis and dermis that must be differentiated histologically from neoplasms are: (1) *Pseudo-epitheliomatous hyperplasia* (see Chapter 4) is a condition in which thick pegs of epithelium are formed around chronic inflammatory processes and may superficially resemble the squamous cell carcinoma. (2) Cutaneous calcification, which is inflammatory in nature, may be confused with tumors (such as trichoepitheliomas) which tend to calcify. (3) Epidermoid, dermoid, follicular inclusion, and pilonidal cysts are common and should be differentiated from true neoplasms. In some cases squamous cell carcinoma has been known to arise within the epithelium of an epidermoid cyst. (4) Viral papillomas are not true neoplasms. They regress when they are rid of the viral agent inducing them.

BASAL CELL CARCINOMA

Basal cell carcinomas are common, slowly growing, invasive (but rarely metastatic) lesions that occur in several species, notably cats, dogs, and humans. The neoplasm consists of invading clusters of neoplastic basal cells, which form clumps of undifferentiated cells in the subcutis. Cells do not differentiate into keratin-producing cells. Neoplastic cells resemble but are different from normal basal cells. They invariably contain hemidesmosomes but the cytoplasmic ultrastructure varies with individual tumors (Brody 1970; Drommer 1968). Some tumors contain scattered sebaceous cells.

An examination of the reproductive cycle of the germinative cell population of human basal cell carcinomas indicates relatively intense cell proliferation despite slow growth (Weinstein and Frost 1970). From this it must be assumed that cell death within the tumor occurs almost as rapidly as cell division.

It is the stratum germinativum or basal cell layer which is the proliferative compartment of normal epidermis. From each dividing basal cell one remains in the basal layer and the other moves upward and differentiates into a keratin-producing cell. Movement in most mammals can be shown to require 12–14 days; that is, if tritiated thymidine is injected into an ani-

Table 6.10. Cell proliferation kinetics in human epidermis and basal cell carcinoma

Cell Cycle	Normal Skin	Basal Cell Carcinoma
S	16 hr.	20 hr.
G2	7	7
M	1	1.5
G1	284	188
Germinative Cell Cycle	308	217
Labeling Index	5.2	9.2

Source: (Weinstein 1970). Use of thymidine-H^3 as DNA marker with autoradiographic analysis.

mal, it is incorporated into the cells during DNA synthesis (S phase). By taking serial biopsies of skin with processing for histology and autoradiography, an upward progression of labeled cells can be determined. They reach the top of the viable epidermis in 12 days in the mouse, and this is considered the transit time through the epidermis. In basal cell carcinomas, the labeling index is markedly increased but the germinative cell cycle is diminished (Table 6.10).

"Basal cell" is often used confusingly and loosely to designate undifferentiated epithelial cells that have a small nucleus and scanty cytoplasm. These cells occur not only in tumors of the epidermis, but also in hair follicles and sebaceous gland neoplasms. The basal cell carcinoma, as viewed by some, encompasses a group of tumors characterized by the presence of cells resembling the stratum germinativum of normal epidermis.

The presence of basal cells does not set aside a distinct kind of tumor. It does not distinguish, for example, basal from squamous cell carcinoma. The basal cell carcinoma is based upon the predominant differentiation of the basal cells to initiate adnexal structures. In other tumors the predominant tendency is to also form keratinocytes and the squamous cell carcinoma results.

SQUAMOUS CELL CARCINOMA

Squamous cell carcinomas are among the commonest tumors of many species of mammals (Priester 1973). They may be derived from either ectoderm (skin, prepuce, etc.) or from endoderm (oral mucosa, esophagus, stomach). Whichever the source, the tumors tend to be so similar that the tissue of origin can rarely be identified with certainty. Despite our knowledge of solar radiation and chemical oncogens as causes of squamous cell carcinomas, the inducing factor for most naturally occurring tumors is not obvious.

Histologically, the tumors are characterized by irregular masses of epithelial cells. At the periphery of the masses are polar, undifferentiated cells resembling the germinal basal cells of normal squamous epithelium. In the central areas are keratinized cells which are often formed into whorls or "pearls" of keratin.

Ultrastructurally, the keratinizing cells of well-differentiated squamous cell carcinomas have large cytoplasmic areas filled with bundles of tonofilaments (Stoebner et al. 1967). Individual cells may be connected by desmosomes, but these intercellular junctions tend to be haphazard. Anaplastic tumors have fewer tonofilaments and desmosomes and show marked irregularities of the nuclear and plasma membranes. If the tumor is ischemic or the patient treated with antimetabolic drugs, the disorganization of cells is exaggerated. In most squamous cell carcinomas, villous projections of the advancing border of the tumor can be seen perforating the basement membrane containing the neoplasm. These invading cells have been shown to contain collagenases which probably play an important role in this activity (Hashimoto et al. 1973).

Growth of the squamous cell carcinoma is dependent upon continued proliferation of the undifferentiated cells. The progeny of these replicating tumor cells may resemble the parent cell or be a differentiated benign cell which keratinizes and which is incapable of replication to form further tumor cells (Pierce and Wallace 1970). In the treatment of human squamous cell carcinomas with bleomycin (an antimetabolite), there is selective destruction of replicating undifferentiated cells. Cells of the treated tumors show increased differentiation and have increased cytoplasmic tonofibrils, desmosomes, and glycogen (Michaels et al. 1973).

MAMMARY GLAND TUMORS

Neoplasms of the mammary gland show distinct species preferences. They are among the commonest tumors of dogs and mice and are relatively common in cats (Weijer et al. 1972). They are among the rarest tumors of cattle, which are subject to intense activity, both normal and pathologic, of the gland. Those rare tumors which have been reported in the bovine mammary gland have been stromal or invasive from surface epidermis (Povey and Osborne 1969).

Investigations on the etiology of mammary tumors have dealt chiefly with pathologic ovarian hormone production and with the potential role of oncogenic viruses. The remarkable story of the Bittner agent and mouse mammary cancer has led to similar approaches in other species. Although virions have been reported in mammary tumors of monkeys (Chopra and Mason 1970), cats (Feldman and Gross 1971), lemmings, and rats (Chopra and Taylor 1970), their causal role remains elusive; these agents may be only passenger viruses. The monkey virus contains an RNA-directed DNA-polymerase and this agent may represent the first primate oncornavirus.

MOUSE MAMMARY GLAND TUMORS

Naturally occurring mammary gland tumors are commonly encountered in older females in colonies of mice. Most are adenocarcinomas, but tumors of the milk-duct system also occur. The adenocarcinomas are usually well-differentiated neoplasms composed of masses of disoriented glandular acini. The epithelial cells exhibit secretory activity, and the lumen of the glands may contain proteinaceous material. The Golgi complex of tumor cells is large but has defects in protein production (Fiske 1967). When cells of naturally occurring adenocarcinomas are examined ultrastructurally, virions are readily found (Fig. 6.13).

The more malignant tumors metastasize chiefly to the lungs. Nodules of adenocarcinoma provoke granular pneumocyte hyperplasia and a basement membrane and connective tissue capsule (Brooks 1970).

The mammary gland tumors of mice can be induced by exogenous agents. Oncogenic viruses act on the glandular parenchyma. Hormones and urethane induce neoplasms of the milk-duct system (Van Ebbenhorst Tengbergen 1970).

The *Bittner mammary tumor virus* (MTV) is the oncornavirus responsible for neoplasms of the glandular parenchyma. The original discovery was made by the staff of the Jackson Memorial Laboratory in Bar Harbor in 1933. They observed that something transmitted extrachromosomally and maternally caused female offspring to develop mammary cancer. Bittner in 1936 demonstrated that an agent was transmitted in the mother's milk: mice of low mammary tumor strains nursed by mothers of high cancer strains developed a high incidence of mammary tumors; conversely, mice of high cancer strains suckled by foster mothers of low cancer strains developed only a few mammary tumors. Biological evidence was soon provided that the agent was a virus.

With the development of the thin-sectioning technique in electron microscopy, virions were photographed in many laboratories (see Bernhard 1960; Calafat 1968; Dmochowski et al. 1968; Feldman 1963; Imai et al. 1966; Pitelka et al. 1964). The virions have been classified as types A (50–70 nm, cytoplasmic) and B (110–120 nm, extracellular). The mature B virions have an eccentric, electron-dense nucleoid; the immature B virions have an electron-lucent nucleoid and four distinct shells. The mature B virions are believed to be the active, mature MTV. The specific antigenicity related to MTV, as measured by immunodiffusion tests, is carried by the B particle. B virions are tagged by specific, ferritin-labeled antibody (Tanaka and Moore 1967). The A virion is the intracellular precursor of the B virion (Smith 1967).

When the virus is ingested, it is disseminated hematogenously and there is ample viral activity in blood samples from infected mice (Moore et al. 1970). Virions infect the immature mammary gland and have been demonstrated in normal acinar cells. The factor which initiates transformation to neoplastic growth has not been identified.

Table 6.11. **Classification and incidence of mammary gland tumors in dogs**

Tumor Type	Percent	Variants
Adenoma	5.1	Papillary, papillary-cystic
Myoepithelioma	1.1	
Mixed tumor, benign	45.1	
Mixed tumor, malignant	8.5	
Carcinoma	39.7	Lobular, papillary, solid
Sarcoma	0.5	Osteosarcoma, chondrosarcoma

Source: (Moulton 1970), 1,366 tumors.

MAMMARY GLAND TUMORS OF DOGS

These are the commonest tumors seen in aged, intact, female dogs. In general terms, 30% are malignant and there is a distinct tendency to metastasize to regional lymph nodes and to lungs (Anderson 1965; Moulton et al. 1970). The classification of canine mammary tumors is one of the bugbears of veterinary pathology (Table 6.11). The best classification should be based on histogenesis, but the origin of the more malignant carcinomas is not always obvious. If it is not, these tumors tend to be prefaced by terms referring to their stromal reaction (fibrosing or scirrhous) or compactness (solid, lobular, papillary).

About 50% of canine mammary neoplasms are *mixed tumors*. That is, they contain neoplastic cells of both glandular and stromal origin. These hard, multilobular tumors contain remarkable foci of myxomatous tissue and cartilage. The myxoid portions represent malignant myoepithelial cells which produce basement membrane material and cartilage (see Fig. 6.5). Ultrastructurally, they are recognized by their stellate shape and abundant fibrils and endoplasmic reticulum (Pulley 1973). The Golgi complex of these cells is large and they contain ample glycogen (Bomhard and Sandersleben 1973).

Adenocarcinomas are lobulated tumors which vary from hard scirrhous lesions to soft fungiform masses. Despite scirrhous, papillary, and solid types, the common denominator is the presence of neoplastic epithelial cells forming acini. Unlike its counterpart in mice and cats, the ultrastructural examination of these tumor cells has not revealed the presence of virions (Feldman and Gross 1967).

Ductal papillomas are papillary growths in the teat canal or the largest lactiferous ducts. Histologically, they are neoplastic epithelial growths containing dilated and cystic ducts which are supported by vasculomesenchymal tissues.

The canine mammary tumors are related to endocrine status of the individual. Ovariohysterectomy has a negative effect on tumor formation and bitches neutered before their first estrus have 0.5% of the mammary cancer risk of intact females. There appears to be lesser incidence in bitches that whelp regularly compared with those that do not. Although mammary tumors are often reported to be associated with irregular or pathologic ovarian function, the only adequate study which has been done did not reveal a significant difference between mammary tumor-bearing and normal dogs in ovarian pathology (Brodey et al. 1966).

LUNG TUMORS

Carcinoma of the lung is a disease of old animals. Primary tumors are rarely reported, except in the dog, and they are uncommon in this species (Brodey and Craig 1965). Carcinomas are best classified according to their pattern of growth and the terms "bronchogenic" and "bronchiogenic" should be avoided. In the dog, adenocarcinomas constitute about 60% of lung tumors. These neoplasms originate at the periphery of the lung and consist of compressed but singular rows of cuboidal cells. Ultrastructurally, the cells are large and have characteristics of neoplastic cells in general (Fig. 6.15). Nuclei are irregular and surface microvilli are present. The many dense cells which are found in these tumors indicate that degeneration and death of neoplastic cells occur as the lesion continues to expand. Squamous cell carcinomas are far less common in dogs. Cytologically, these tumor cells contain tonofilaments and desmosomes and can readily be distinguished on the basis of ultrastructure (Obiditsch-Mayer and Breitfellner 1968). The ultrastructure of most human lung neoplasms has been reported but, like their animal counterparts, little effort has been made to correlate cell structure with growth potential and the electron microscopic examination of lung tumors does not enhance the prognostic ability of the pathologist. The few examples examined have not provided clues to a more sophisticated classification scheme (Giddens and Dillingham 1971; Kuhn 1972; Obiditsch-Mayer and Breitfellner 1968).

Metastatic tumors are commoner in the lungs of most animals than are primary tumors. Most arrive in the lung hematogenously, and when a focus of neoplastic growth begins it provokes connective tissue proliferation and the reduplication of basement membrane material (the beginning of encapsulation) (Brooks 1970).

The cause of primary lung tumors in animals is not known although, as in humans, it is assumed that prolonged low level inhalation of chemical oncogens is significant. The incidence of lung tumors in dogs is allegedly increasing in densely populated urban areas and the increase is believed to be due to airborne automobile emissions and industrial pollutants. Tumors have been experimentally induced in the lung with chemical carcinogens (Mostofi and Larsen 1951; Skoryna et al. 1951; Staub et al. 1965) and radiation (Hahn et al. 1973), but their relation to naturally occurring disease is equivocal. Ultrastructurally, the induced tumors of laboratory animals tend to be mixtures of undifferentiated cells and hyperplastic granular pneumocytes (Straks and Feron 1973).

RENAL TUMORS

Neoplasms of the kidney in animals are rare, and there are no valid statistics on prevalence, histogenesis, or growth patterns. Adenomas may arise in the cortex. They closely resemble renal parenchyma; tubules, cystic areas, and papillary growths are common. These tumors are usually encapsulated and are not known to progress to carcinoma.

RENAL CARCINOMA

Carcinomas of the kidney arise from tubular epithelium. They are most com-

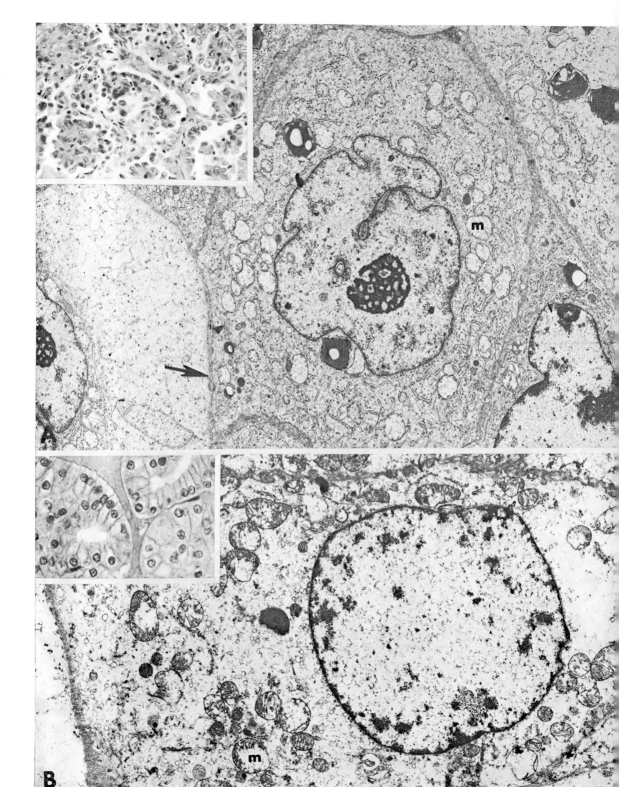

monly found in aged dogs (Sandison and Anderson 1968). Tumor tissue may form tubule structures but papillary growth patterns are rare. Cells are large, cuboidal, and have large amounts of pale, eosinophilic cytoplasm (Fig. 6.15). Nuclei are dark and eccentric and mitotic figures are common. Ultrastructurally, tumor cells contain endoplasmic reticulum and mitochondria typical of dedifferentiating cells of the renal tubular epithelium. Large rarified spaces are present in the cytoplasm.

Renal carcinomas are relatively fast in growth and are prone to invade the renal veins and lymphatics. Growth within the renal pelvis may cause hydronephrosis. Metastases are common and are found in the regional lymph nodes and the lungs. Other viscera are less commonly affected.

Carcinomas of the kidney with renin-secreting activity have been reported in man (Conn et al. 1972), but not in animals. They are associated with elevated plasma renin and increased blood pressure. The tumors resemble hemangiopericytomas, but have high concentrations of renin. Granules are present in the tumor cells which resemble and stain specifically for juxtaglomerular granules.

Renal carcinomas can be induced experimentally by viral and chemical agents (Hard and Butter 1971). Tumors associated with intranuclear inclusion body formation commonly occur in the kidneys of hibernating frogs. They are caused by an oncogenic herpesvirus which can be identified in the inclusions (Rafferty 1964). Renal carcinoma is induced in chickens by nephroblastogenic strains of avian lymphoid leukosis virus. Virions are seen in high numbers in the distal convoluted tubules (Weiler et al. 1971) and provoke a tumor with adenomatous structures resembling this component of the normal nephron. The tumors are mixtures of tissue and also contain cartilage and osteoid cells (Heine et al. 1962). Models of transplantable renal cell carcinoma exist in mice, hamsters, and rats; most

are endocrine-dependent (Murphy and Hrushesky 1973).

EMBRYONAL NEPHROMA

The embryonal nephroma (Wilm's tumor) allegedly arises from the metanephros, and this is attested to by its content of tubule and glomeruluslike structures. These tumors are composed of undifferentiated vestigial renal tissue with primitive characteristics. Epithelial and connective tissue components may dominate in a particular tumor, and foci of muscle, cartilage, and bone may be present. Cytologically, the epithelial tumor cells appear as undifferentiated cells filled with ribosomes and large Golgi areas (Balsaver 1968). They are much smaller than cells of the renal carcinoma. Glomeruluslike structures do not contain capillaries or endothelial cells.

Embryonal nephromas are large, encapsulated, lobular tumors. They grow by expansion and are rarely metastatic or invasive. Except for the pig (Sullivan and Anderson 1959) and chicken, they are reported in only a few species (Elkham 1963; Flir 1954; Magnusson 1970). Transplantable embryonal nephromas have been described in rabbits (Greene 1943) and rats (Olcott 1950). Recently a protein-polysaccharide complex has been obtained from human embryonal nephromas which promotes cell growth in culture (Beierle et al. 1971).

SECONDARY TUMORS

Metastases to the kidney are common among disseminating malignant tumors primary at other sites. Lesions usually develop in the cortex and are sufficiently different cytologically from renal carcinomas that they are readily differentiated. Malignant lymphoma often involves the renal parenchyma in dogs and cats. Malignant lymphocytes infiltrate the interstitium and may form large nodules of neoplastic cells.

Fig. 6.15. A. Bronchiogenic carcinoma, aged dog. Large tumor cells line the alveolar walls and form aggregates that obliterate the alveoli (inset). Tumor cell is cuboidal and contains surface microvilli (arrow). Mitochondria (m) and well-developed endoplasmic reticulum. Nucleus is large, distorted, and contains indentations in nuclear membrane. B. Renal cell carcinoma, aged dog. Cells are large, pale, and clear (inset). Cytoplasm filled with vacuoles and mitochondria (m).

LIVER NEOPLASMS

HEPATOCELLULAR CARCINOMA

Multiple foci of nodular regeneration are common in aged individuals of some species, but true hepatomas are rare. Ultrastructural studies have been reported on hepatocellular carcinomas of swine (Ito et al. 1972), chicken (Beard et al. 1975), and man (Garancis et al. 1969; Horvath et al. 1972). The tumor cells closely resemble hepatocytes from which they are derived. (See Fig. 6.16.)

Hepatocellular carcinomas are significant in terms of long-term sequelae of some hepatotoxins. In fact, assays for the induction of liver lesions are standard procedures in the examination of food additives, drugs, and other chemicals. The hepatocyte is also susceptible to many naturally occurring oncogens. Most of these are not oncogenic themselves, but are metabolically converted to highly reactive derivatives that react with cellular DNA, RNA, and protein. The enzymes for conversion are present on the endoplasmic reticulum. The oncogens trigger a sequence of events that may, if sustained, lead to the development of an overt carcinoma.

The experimentalist views liver carcinogenesis as developing in three stages: (1) initiation, a relatively short term interaction between a chemical oncogen and target organelles; (2) promotion, a longer period wherein initiated cells are influenced to proliferate; and (3) transformation, the selective overgrowth of new neoplastic cell populations.

During initiation, DNA is the common target molecule for most oncogens. The initial damage induced is subject to repair, but if cellular proliferation occurs coincident with injury the DNA defect may be permanent. In an affected liver only a few cells may emerge from injury as potential neoplastic progenitors. This number can be markedly increased by prior partial hepatectomy, a process that stimulates mitotic activity in the liver.

The cytotoxic effect of any oncogen, if it persists, presents a continual suppressant on normal hepatocytes. However, new regenerating cells that survive may not be so inhibited; a new hepatocyte population develops that is resistant to the toxic property of the oncogen and is free to proliferate. Whether or not a neoplasm results appears to depend upon what happens to these nodules of new cells. Subsequent development of new third and fourth cell populations increases the risk of true neoplastic dedifferentiation.

One of the most bothersome problems of liver oncology has been that of how to detect neoplastic transformation. The approach has been to search for new cellular antigens, isoenzymes, or hormones that are present in the neoplastic cell. One of these markers that newly transformed hepatocytes often have is the new antigen α-fetoprotein. This protein is present on embryonic livers and, in human hepatocellular carcinoma, also is present on tumor cells. It has been used as a diagnostic test for hepatocellular carcinoma (Abelev 1971). Other new antigens ("preneoplastic antigen," etc.) have also been found in cells of oncogen-induced liver nodules.

SOME UNIQUE ANIMAL TUMORS

Some tumors and tumorlike conditions of animals which have intriguing aspects in their biologic behavior should be mentioned. In some, there is a clear-cut association with an agent; in others, the growth characteristics merely lead one to believe that they are caused by some exogenous agent. Transmission experiments of many of these have succeeded, but the results have failed to pinpoint the specific mechanism by which the tumor is induced.

Fig. 6.16. A.–C. Hepatocellular carcinoma, liver, aged dog. Large pale tumor mass (arrow) is surrounded by smaller nodules of tumor. Dark nodes of hepatic regeneration (r) are present. B. Histology. Tumor cells are large, pleomorphic, and degenerate. Some are multinucleate. C. Ultrastructure. D.–H. Thyroid carcinoma, dog. D. Tumor in atrophic thyroid (T). Parathyroid gland (P). E. Histology. F. Ultrastructure of carcinoma cell. Large cytoplasmic rodlets (arrow). G. Enlargement of rodlets. H. Rodlets in cross section.

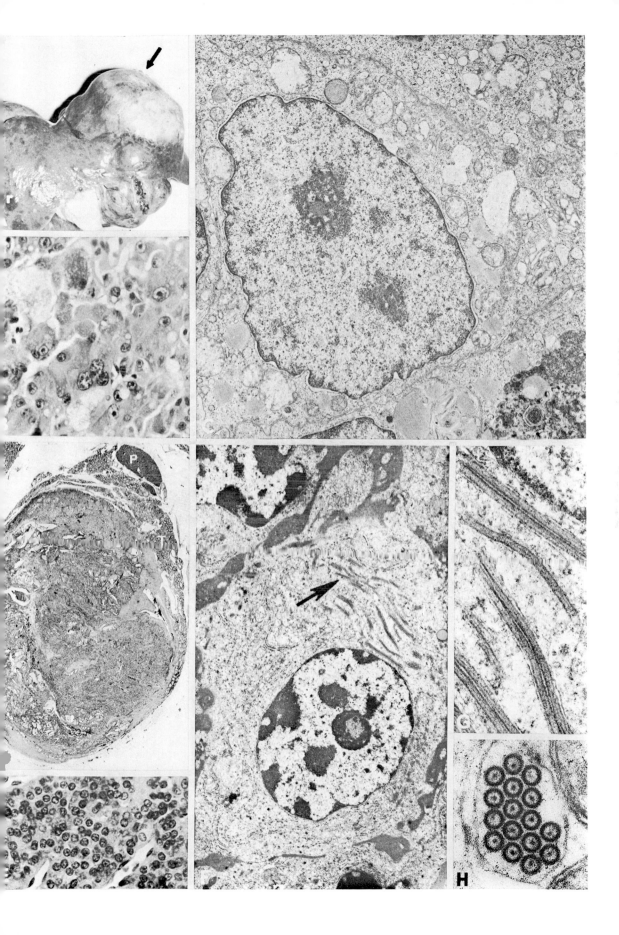

NASAL ADENOPAPILLOMA OF SHEEP

Adenopapillomas (or adenocarcinomas) of the nasal cavity of sheep have been reported as epizootics in various countries (Cohrs 1953; Duncan et al. 1967; Magnusson 1916; Tokarnia et al. 1972). They are composed of well-differentiated epithelial acini and villous projections. The tumors grow into the nasal cavity, the frontal sinus, and the pharynx. Extension to the cranial cavity has occurred due to pressure atrophy of bone. Metastases are not evident. The neoplasm has been transmitted by cell-free filtrates, but the nature of the inciting agent has not been determined (Cohrs 1952).

CANINE ESOPHAGEAL SARCOMA AND SPIROCERCA LUPI

A correlation between the presence of sarcoma of the esophagus and infection with *Spirocerca lupi* has been established in certain geographical areas (Ribelin and Bailey 1958; Seibold et al. 1955). This peculiar parasite encysts and causes granulomas in or near the esophagus. Highly destructive lesions may be responsible for aortic aneurysms and ossifying spondylitis. In a small percentage of cases, a sarcoma develops. The tumors are malignant and are often disseminated; metastatic foci occur in lymph nodes and lung. The mechanism of tumor induction is not known, but experimental work has been done on a similar model in rats (liver sarcomas caused by infection with the larvae of *Taenia taeniaformis*). Secretions of this cestode cause fibroblastic hyperplasia and appear to be oncogenic (Dunning and Curtiss 1953).

EQUINE SARCOID

The equine sarcoid is a naturally occurring locally aggressive fibroblastic tumor of the dermis. It has a tendency to recur after surgical incision and classically was considered to spread from horse to horse on harnesses. The peculiar whorling arrangement of the fibroblasts leads inexperienced pathologists to the diagnosis of nerve sheath tumors. The equine sarcoid has been transplanted from one site to another on individual horses (Olson 1948) but not

between horses. The epidemiology of the disease suggests an infectious nature. Intracytoplasmic virions resembling the oncornaviruses have been seen in cell cultures derived from an equine sarcoid, but not in cells of the lesion in horses (England et al. 1973). Bovine papilloma virus inoculated experimentally into horse skin induces fibroblastic formation remarkably similar to the sarcoid (Olson and Cook 1951; Ragland et al. 1965). While the virus may be responsible for the naturally occurring tumor, this fact has not been established.

PULMONARY ADENOMATOSIS OF SHEEP

Pulmonary adenomatosis (Jaagsiekte) is a transmissible disease of sheep characterized by the slowly progressive development of foci of proliferating epithelial cells. Affected sheep show respiratory distress and emaciation, but there is no loss of appetite or orientation. Lesions are classified as neoplastic on the basis of their structural resemblance to adenomas, because they expand progressively to kill the host, and because similar lesions (presumably metastatic) are occasionally found in the bronchial and mediastinal lymph nodes. Metastatic lesions, some with a fibrous component, have also been seen in skeletal muscle, kidney, and peritoneum.

Lungs of diseased sheep are large, mottled, and frothy and are often complicated by secondary bacterial lesions. Solid foci may be scattered over the surface as in typical lung carcinoma. Histologically, the lesions of pulmonary adenomatosis consist of dense, disorganized collections of epithelial cells which distort the normal lung parenchyma and grow into and along the alveolar walls. Ultrastructural examination indicates that the proliferating adenoma cells are derived from type-II or granular pneumocytes (Nisbet et al. 1971). No organisms connected with the etiology have been seen in adenoma cells (Wandera and Krauss 1971).

Transmission of pulmonary adenomatosis has been accomplished in several laboratories, but the etiologic agent has not been firmly established. A herpesvirus has been isolated from cultures of macrophages from affected lungs in which intranuclear inclusion bodies developed (Mackay 1969;

Smith and Mackay 1969). The virus was transmitted to normal alveolar macrophage cultures, and ultrastructural examination revealed the progressive intranuclear development typical of the herpes group. This herpesvirus is now believed to be the cause of pulmonary adenomatosis and has been isolated in other laboratories (Malm-quist et al. 1972). C-type viruses typical of the leukovirus group have been seen in lung adenoma lesions (Perk et al. 1971) and in cell cultures derived from affected lungs (Malmquist et al. 1972). These viruses may be associated with a second chronic lung disease (maedi) which may exist as a superinfection.

REFERENCES

Abelev, G. I. Alpha-fetoprotein in ontogenesis and its association with malignant tumors. *Adv. Cancer Res.* 14:295, 1971.

Achong, B. G. and Epstein, M. A. Fine structure of the Burkitt tumor. *J. Nat. Cancer Inst.* 36:877, 1966.

Adams, E. W., Carter, L. P. and Sapp, W. J. Growth and maintenance of the canine venereal tumor in continuous culture. *Cancer Res.* 28:753, 1968.

Adamson, R. H., Correa, P. and Dalgard, D. N. Occurrence of a primary liver carcinoma in a rhesus monkey fed aflatoxin B_1. *J. Nat. Cancer Inst.* 50:549, 1973.

Algire, G. H. and Chalkley, H. W. Vascular reactions of normal and malignant tissues in vivo. *J. Nat. Cancer Inst.* 6:73, 1945.

Anders, F. Tumour formation in platyfish-swordtail hybrids as a problem of gene regulation. *Experientia* 23:1, 1967.

Anderson, A. C. Parameters of mammary gland tumors in aging beagles. *J.A.V.M.A.* 147:1653, 1965.

Anderson, D. E. and Skinner, P. E. Studies on bovine ocular squamous cell carcinoma (cancer eye). *J. An. Sci.* 20:474, 1961.

Anderson, D. E., Pope, L. S. and Stephens, D. Nutrition and eye cancer in cattle. *J. Nat. Cancer Inst.* 45:697, 1970.

Andrews, J. M. and Gardner, M. B. Lower motor neuron degeneration associated with type C RNA virus infection in mice. *J. Neuropath. Exp. Neurol.* 33:285, 1974.

Anton, E. and Brandes, D. Lysosomes in mice mammary tumors treated with cyclophosphamide. *Cancer* 21:483, 1968.

Aoki, T. et al. G (Gross) and H-2 cell-surface antigens. Location on Gross leukemia cells by electron microscopy with visually labeled antibody. *Proc. Nat. Acad. Sci.* 65:569, 1970.

Ashley, L. M. and Halver, J. E. Multiple metastases of rainbow trout hepatoma. *Trans. Am. Fish. Soc.* 92:365, 1963.

Balls, M. and Ruben, L. N. The transmission of lymphosarcoma in *Xenopus laevis*, the South African clawed toad. *Cancer Res.* 27:654, 1967.

Balsaver, A. M. et al. Ultrastructural studies in Wilm's tumor. *Cancer* 22:417, 1968.

Baltimore, D. RNA-dependent DNA polymerase in virions of RNA tumour viruses. *Nature* 226:1209, 1970.

Barski, G. and Cornefert-Jensen, F. Cytogenetic study of Sticker venereal sarcoma in European dogs. *J. Nat. Cancer Inst.* 37:787, 1966.

Battifora, H. Hemangiopericytoma. *Cancer* 31:1418, 1973.

Beard, J. W. et al. Neoplastic response of the avian liver to host infection with strain MC29 leukosis virus. *Cancer Res.* 35:1603, 1975.

Becker, F. F. Cell function: Its importance in chemical carcinogenesis. *Fed. Proc.* 30:1736, 1971.

Beierle, J. W. et al. Growth promotion by extracts from Wilm's tumor in vitro. *Experientia* 27:435, 1971.

Berenblum, I. and Shubik, P. A new quantitative approach to the study of stages of chemical carcinogenesis in mouse's skin. *Brit. J. Cancer* 1:383, 1947.

Bernhard, W. The detection and study of tumor viruses. A review. *Cancer Res.* 20:712, 1960.

Bernhard, W. and Granboulan, N. The fine structure of the cancer cell nucleus. *Exp. Cell Res.* 9:19, 1963.

Bloom, G., Larrson, B. and Aberg, B. Canine mastocytoma. *Zentr. Vetmed.* 5:443, 1958.

Blum, H. P. *Carcinogenesis by Ultraviolet Light,* pp. 285–305. Princeton Univ. Press, 1954.

Bomhard, D. V. and Sandersleben, J. V. Über die Feinstruktur von Mammamischtumoren der Hündin. *Virch. Arch. A* 359:87, 1973.

Borland, R. and Webber, A. J. An electron microscope study of squamous cell carcinoma in merino sheep associated with keratin-filled cysts of the skin. *Cancer Res.* 26:172, 1966.

Bowles, C. T. et al. Characterization of a transplantable canine immature mast cell tumor. *Cancer Res.* 32:1434, 1972.

Brandes, D., Anton, E. and Schofield, B. Invasion of skeletal and smooth muscle by L1210 leukemia. *Cancer Res.* 27:2159, 1967.

Brodey, R. S. and Craig, P. H. Primary pulmonary neoplasms in the dog. *J.A.V.M.A.* 147:1628, 1965.

Brodey, R. S., Fidler, I. J. and Howson, A. E. The relationship of estrous irregularity, pseudo-pregnancy and pregnancy to the development of canine mammary neoplasms. *J.A.V.M.A.* 149:1047, 1966.

Brody, I. Contributions to the histogenesis of basal cell carcinoma. *J. Ult. Res.* 33:60, 1970.

Brooks, R. E. Mouse mammary tumor metastases in lung: An electron microscopic study. *Cancer Res.* 30:2156, 1970.

Buck, R. C. Walker 256 tumor implantation in normal and injured peritoneum studied by electron microscopy, scanning electron microscopy and autoradiography. *Cancer Res.* 33:3181, 1973.

Calafat, J. Virus particles of the B and C types associated with mouse mammary tumours. *J. Microsc.* 7:841, 1968.

Calnek, B. W., Obertini, T. and Adldinger, H. K. Viral antigen, virus particles and infectivity of tissues from chickens with Marek's disease. *J. Nat. Cancer Inst.* 45:341, 1970.

Case, M. T. and Simon, J. Transmission studies of swine lymphosarcoma. *Am. J. Vet. Res.* 29:263, 1968.

Cavallo, T. et al. Tumor angiogenesis: Rapid induction of endothelial mitosis demonstrated by autoradiography and electron microscopy. *Cell Biol.* 54:408, 1972.

Cavallo, T. et al. Ultrastructural autoradiographic studies of the early vasoproliferative response in tumor angiogenesis. *Am. J. Path.* 70:345, 1973.

Chambers, V. C. and Weiser, R. S. An electron microscope study of the cytophagocytosis of sarcoma I cells by alloimmune macrophages in vitro. *J. Nat. Cancer Inst.* 51:1369, 1973.

Chang, J. P. and Gibley, C. W., Jr. Ultrastructure of tumor cells during mitosis. *Cancer Res.* 28:521, 1968.

Chopra, H. and Taylor, D. J. Virus particles in rat mammary tumors of varying origin. *J. Nat. Cancer Inst.* 44:1141, 1967, 1970.

Chopra, H. C. and Mason, M. M. A new virus in a spontaneous mammary tumor of a Rhesus monkey. *Cancer Res.* 30:2081, 1970.

Clarke, M. A. The fine structure of methylcholanthrene-induced tumors in mice. *Cancer* 24:147, 1969.

Cohen, D. The biological behavior of the transmissible venereal tumour in immunosuppressed dogs. *Europ. J. Cancer* 9:253, 1973.

――. Detection of humoral antibody to the transmissible venereal tumour of the dog. *Int. J. Cancer* 10:207, 1972.

Cohen, D., Gurner, B. W. and Coombs, R. R. A. A phenomenon resembling opsonic adherence shown by disaggregated cells of the transmissible venereal tumour of the dog. *Brit. J. Exp. Path.* 52:447, 1971.

Cohen, H. et al. Cellular transmission of canine lymphoma and leukemia in beagles. *J. Nat. Cancer Inst.* 45:1013, 1970.

Cohrs, P. Infektiöse Adenopapillome der Riechschleimhaut beim Schaf. *Berl. Muench. Tieraerztl. Wosch.* 66:225, 1953.

――. Übertragbare Adenome der Riechschleimhaut beim Schaf. *Zt. Krebsforsch.* 58: 682, 1952.

Cole, L. J. and Nowell, P. C. Radiation carcinogenesis: The sequence of events. *Science* 150:1782, 1965.

Conn, J. W. et al. Primary renism. *Arch. Int. Med.* 130:682, 1972.

Cooper, M. D. et al. Studies on the nature of the abnormality of B cell differentiation in avian leukosis: Production of heterogeneous IgM by tumor cells. *J. Immunol.* 113:1210, 1974.

Crowell, W. A., Chandler, F. W. and Williams, D. J. Melanoma in cattle: Fine structure and a report of two cases. *Am. J. Vet. Res.* 34:1591, 1973.

Currie, G. A. and Bagshave, K. D. The effect of neuraminidase on the immunogenicity of the Landschutz ascites tumour. *Brit. J. Cancer* 22:588, 1968.

De Harven, E. Virus particles in the thymus of conventional and germ-free mice. *J. Exp. Med.* 120:857, 1964.

Demopoulos, H. B. et al. Comparison of ultrastructure of B-16 and S-91 mouse melanomas and correlation with growth pattern. *Lab. Invest.* 14:108, 1965.

Di Giacomo, R. F. Burkitt's lymphoma in a white-handed gibbon *(Hyalobates lar)*. *Cancer Res.* 27:1178, 1967.

Di Stefano, H. S. and Dougherty, R. M. Mechanisms for congenital transmission of avian leukosis virus. *J. Nat. Cancer Inst.* 37:869, 1966.

Dmochowski, L. et al. Electron microscopic and bioassay studies of milk from mice of high and low mammary-cancer and high and low leukemia strains. *J. Nat. Cancer Inst.* 40:1339, 1968.

Dougherty, R. M. and Di Stefano, H. S. Sites of avian leukosis virus multiplication in congenitally infected chickens. *Cancer Res.* 27:322, 1967.

Drommer, W. Submikroskopische Untersuchungen an Basaliom des Hundes. *Vet. Path.* 5:174, 1968.

Drommer, W. and Schulz, L.-Cl. Vergleichende licht- und elektronenmikroskopische Untersuchungen an übertragbaren venerischen Sarkom und Histiozytom des Hundes. *Vet. Path.* 6:273, 1969.

Dunbar, C. E. Lymphosarcoma of possible thymic origin in Salmonid fishes. *Nat. Cancer Inst. Monogr.* 31:167, 1969.

Duncan, J. R. et al. Enzootic nasal adenocarcinoma in sheep. *J.A.V.M.A.* 151:732, 1967.

Duncan, T. E. and Harkin, J. C. Electron microscopic studies of goldfish tumors previously termed neurofibriomas and Schwannomas. *Am. J. Path.* 55:191, 1969.

Dunn, T. B. and Potter, N. A transplantable mast cell neoplasm in the mouse. *J. Nat. Cancer Inst.* 18:587, 1957.

Dunning, W. F. and Curtiss, M. R. Attempts to isolate the active agent in *Cysticercus fasciolaris. Cancer Res.* 13:838, 1953.

Ehrmann, R. L. and Knoth, M. Choriocarcinoma: Transfilter stimulation of vasoproliferation in the hamster cheek pouch studied by light and electron microscopy. *J. Nat. Cancer Inst.* 41:1929, 1968.

Elkam, E. Three different types of tumors in Salientia. *Cancer Res.* 23:1641, 1963.

England, J. J., Watson, R. E. and Larson, K. A. Virus-like particles in an equine sarcoid cell line. *Am. J. Vet. Res.* 34:1601, 1973.

Epstein, M. A. and Achong, B. G. Observations on the nature of the herpes-type EB virus in cultured Burkitt lymphoblasts using a specific immunofluorescence test. *J. Nat. Cancer Inst.* 40:609, 1967.

Epstein, M. A., Hunt, R. D. and Rabin, H. Pilot experiments with EB virus in owl monkeys *(Aotus trivirgatus)*. *Int. J. Cancer* 12:309, 319, 1973.

Epstein, M. A. et al. Structure and development of the herpes-type virus of Marek's disease. *J. Nat. Cancer Inst.* 41:805, 1968.

Epstein, W. L. and Fukuyama, K. In vitro culture of cloned hamster melanoma cells containing R-type virus. *Cancer Res.* 33:825, 1973.

Essex, M. et al. Correlation between humoral antibody and regression of tumours induced by feline sarcoma virus. *Nature* 233:195, 1971.

Feldman, D. G. Origin and distribution of virus-like particles associated with mammary gland tissue. *J. Nat. Cancer Inst.* 30:477, 1963.

Feldman, D. G. and Gross, L. Electron microscopic study of the distribution of the mouse leukemia virus (Gross) in genital organs of virus-injected C3Hf mice and of AK mice. *Cancer Res.* 27:1513, 1967.

———. Electron microscopic study of spontaneous mammary carcinomas in cats and dogs: Virus-like particles in cat mammary carcinomas. *Cancer Res.* 31:1261, 1971.

Ferenczy, A., Richart, R. M. and Okagaki, T. A. comparative ultrastructural study of leimyosarcoma, cellular leiomyoma, and leiomyoma of the uterus. *Cancer* 28:1004, 1971.

Fisher, E. R., Reidbord, H. E. and Fisher, B. Studies concerning the regional lymph node in cancer. *Lab. Invest.* 28:136, 1973.

Fiske, S. W. C., Courtecuisse, V. and Haguenau, F. High resolution autoradiographic study of normal lactating mammary gland and mammary tumors of the mouse. *J. Nat. Cancer Inst.* 39:209, 1967.

Flir, K. Zur Vergleichenden Pathologie der Nierengeschwulste. *Deut. Tieraerztl. Wosch.* 61:147, 1954.

Folkman, J. et al. Isolation of a tumor factor responsible for angiogenesis. *J. Exp. Med.* 133:275, 1971.

Fox, R. R. et al. Lymphosarcoma in the rabbit: Genetics and pathology. *J. Nat. Cancer Inst.* 45:719, 1970.

Franks, L. M., Rowlatt, C. and Chesterman, F. C. Naturally occurring bone tumors in C57BL/1crf mice. *J. Nat. Cancer Inst.* 50:431, 1973.

Fraser, C. J. et al. Acute granulocytic leukemia in cats. *J.A.V.M.A.* 165:355, 1974.

Frazier, J. A. Ultrastructure of lymphoid tissue from chicks infected with Marek's disease virus. *J. Nat. Cancer Inst.* 52:829, 1974.

Fujimoto, Y., Miller, J. and Olson, C. The fine structure of lymphosarcoma in cattle. *Vet. Path.* 6:15, 1969.

Gabbiani, G. et al. Synovial sarcoma. *Cancer* 28:1031, 1971.

Garancis, J. C. et al. Hepatic adenoma. *Cancer* 24:560, 1969.

Ghelelovitch, S. Melanotic tumors in *Drosophila melanogaster*. *Nat. Cancer Inst. Monogr.* 31:263, 1968.

Giddens, W. E. and Dillingham, L. A. Primary tumors of the lung of nonhuman primates. *Vet. Path.* 8:467, 1971.

Gimbrone, M. A., Jr. et al. Tumor dormancy in vivo by prevention of neovascularization. *J. Exp. Med.* 136:261, 1972.

Good, R. A. Relations between immunity and malignancy. *Proc. Nat. Acad. Sci.* 69:1026, 1972.

Gray, J. M. and Pierce, G. B. Relationship between growth rate and differentiation of melanoma in vivo. *J. Nat. Cancer Inst.* 32:1201, 1964.

Greene, H. S. N. Occurrence and transplantation of embryonal nephromas in rabbits. *Cancer Res.* 3:434, 1943.

Greene, H. S. and Harvey, E. K. The relationship between the dissemination of tumor cells and the distribution of metastases. *Cancer Res.* 24:799, 1964.

Hadji-Azimi, I. and Fischberg, M. Some pathological aspects of the spontaneous lymphoid tumor in *Xenopus laevis*. *Path. Micro.* 38:118, 1972.

Hadwen, S. The melanomata of grey and white horses. *Can. Med. Ass. J.* 25:519, 1931.

Hahn, F. F. et al. Primary pulmonary neoplasms in beagle dogs exposed to aerosols of [144]Ce in fused-clay particles. *J. Nat. Cancer Inst.* 50:675, 1973.

Hanna, M. G., Jr., Szakal, A. K. and Tyndall, R. L. Histoproliferative effect of Rauscher leukemia virus on lymphatic tissue. *Cancer Res.* 30:1748, 1970.

Hard, G. C. and Butler, W. H. Ultrastructural analysis of renal mesenchymal tumor induced in the rat by dimethylnitrosamine. *Cancer Res.* 31:348, 1971a.

——. Ultrastructural aspect of renal adenocarcinoma induced in the rat by dimethylnitrosamine. *Cancer Res.* 31:366, 1971b.

Hardy, W. D., Jr. et al. Horizontal transmission of feline leukemia virus. *Nature* 244:266, 1973.

Harris, C. C. et al. Localization of benzo(a)pyrene-^{3}H and alterations in nuclear chromatin caused by benzo(a)pyrene-ferric oxide in the hamster respiratory epithelium. *Cancer Res.* 33:2842, 1973.

Hashimoto, K., Yamanishi, Y. and Dabbous, M. K. Electron microscopic observations of collagenolytic activity of basal cell epithelioma of the skin in vivo and in vitro. *Cancer Res.* 32:2561, 1972.

Hashimoto, K. et al. Collagenolytic activities of squamous cell carcinoma of the skin. *Cancer Res.* 33:2790, 1973.

Heine, U. et al. Morphologic aspects of Rous sarcoma virus elaboration. *J. Nat. Cancer Inst.* 29:211, 1962a.

Heine, U. et al. Multiplicity of cell response to the BAL strain A (myeloblastosis) avian tumor virus. *J. Nat. Cancer Inst.* 29:41, 1962b.

Hellström, I. et al. Demonstration of cell-mediated immunity to human neoplasms of various histological types. *Int. J. Cancer* 7:1, 1971.

Hellström, I. et al. Serum-mediated protection of neoplastic cells from inhibition by lymphocytes immune to their tumor-specific antigens. *Proc. Nat. Acad. Sci.* 62:362, 1969.

Hernandez-Jauregui, P., Gonzalez-Angulo, A. and de la Vega, G. Ultrastructural and histochemical patterns of regressing canine venereal lymphoma after cyclophosphamide treatment. *J. Nat. Cancer Inst.* 51:1187, 1973.

Herz, A. et al. C-type virus in bone marrow cells of cats with myeloproliferative disease. *J. Nat. Cancer Inst.* 44:339, 1970.

Hinze, H. C. and Chipman, P. J. Role of herpesvirus in malignant lymphoma in rabbits. *Fed. Proc.* 31:1639, 1972.

Hirsch, H. M. and Zelickson, A. S. An enzymatic and electron microscopic characterization of a variant of the Cloudman S-91 melanoma. *Cancer Res.* 24:1137, 1964.

Hirsch, M. S. et al. Leukemia virus activation during homograft rejection. *Science* 180:500, 1973.

Homberger, F. Chemical carcinogenesis in the Syrian golden hamster. A review. *Cancer* 23:313, 1969.

Horvath, E., Kovacs, K. and Ross, R. C. Ultrastructural findings in a well-differentiated hepatoma. *Digestion* 7:74, 1972.

Hottendorf, G. H. and Nielsen, S. W. Pathologic report of 29 necropsies on dogs with mastocytoma. *Vet. Path.* 5:102, 1968.

Howard, E. B. et al. Mastocytoma and gastric ulceration. *Vet. Path.* 6:146, 1969.

Hudson, L. and Payne, L. N. An analysis of the T and B cells of Marek's disease lymphomas of the chicken. *Nature* 241:52, 1973.

Huggins, C. Endocrine-induced regression of cancers. *Cancer Res.* 27:1925, 1967.

Hunt, R. D. et al. *Herpesvirus saimiri* malignant lymphoma in spider monkeys—a new susceptible host. *J. Med. Primatol.* 1:114, 1972.

Hurvitz, A. I. Fine structure of cells from a cat with myeloproliferative disease. *Am. J. Vet. Res.* 31:747, 1970.

Imai, T. et al. The mode of virus elaboration in C3H mouse mammary carcinoma as observed by electron microscopy in serial thin sections. *Cancer Res.* 26:443, 1966.

Ito, T. et al. Fine structure of hepatocellular carcinoma in swine. *Jap. J. Vet. Sci.* 34:33, 1972.

Izard, J. and De Harven, E. Increased numbers of a characteristic type of reticular cell in the thymus and lymph nodes of leukemic mice: An electron microscopic study. *Cancer Res.* 28:421, 1968.

Jarrett, W. F. H. et al. Leukaemia in the cat. *Nature* 202:566, 1964.

Jensen, O. A., Egeberg, J and Edmund, J. The effects of phenylalanine and tyrosine low diet on the growth and morphology of transplantable malignant melanomas of the Syrian golden hamster *(Mesocricetus aurates)*. *Acta Path. Micro. Scand. A* 81:559, 1973.

Kakefuda, T., Roberts, E. and Suntzeff, V. Electron microscopic study of methylcholanthrene-induced epidermal carcinogenesis in mice. *Cancer Res.* 30:1011, 1970.

Kakuk, T. J. et al. Experimental transmission of canine malignant lymphoma to the beagle neonate. *Cancer Res.* 28:716, 1968.

Kalderon, A. E. and Fethiere, W. Fine structure of two liposarcomas. *Lab. Invest.* 28:60, 1973.

Kaliss, N. and Bryant, B. F. Factors determining homograft destruction and immunogenical enhancement in mice receiving successive tumor inocula. *J. Nat. Cancer Inst.* 20:691, 1958.

Karlson, A. G. and Mann, F. C. The transmissible venereal tumor of dogs. *Ann. N.Y. Acad. Sci.* 54:1197, 1952.

Kelly, D. F. Canine cutaneous histiocytoma. A light and electron microscopic study. *Vet. Path.* 7:12, 1970.

Kim, U. et al. Immunological escape mechanism in spontaneously metastasizing mammary tumors. *Proc. Nat. Acad. Sci.* 72:1012, 1975.

Peter, C. P. and Kluge, J. P. An ultrastructural study of a canine rhabdomyosarcoma. *Cancer* 26:1280, 1970.

Peters, J. A. Canine mastocytoma: Excess risk as related to ancestry. *J. Nat. Cancer Inst.* 42:435, 1969.

Peterson, R. D. A. et al. Effect of bursectomy and thymectomy on the development of visceral lymphomatosis in the chicken. *J. Nat. Cancer Inst.* 32:1343, 1964.

Pierce, G. B. and Wallace, C. Differentiation of malignant to benign cells. *Cancer Res.* 31:127, 1970.

Pitelka, D. R. et al. On the significance of virus-like particles in mammary tissues of C3Hf mice. *J. Nat. Cancer Inst.* 33:867, 1964.

Pitot, H. C. Some aspects of the developmental biology of neoplasia. *Cancer Res.* 28: 1880, 1968.

Pitot, H. and Heidelberger, C. Metabolic regulatory circuits and carcinogenesis. *Cancer Res.* 23:1694, 1963.

Plowright, W., Linsell, C. A. and Peers, F. G. A focus of ruminal cancer in Kenyan cattle. *Brit. J. Cancer* 25:10, 1971.

Potter, V. R. Biochemical perspectives in cancer research. *Cancer Res.* 24:1085, 1964.

Povey, R. C. and Osborne, A. D. Mammary gland neoplasia in the cow. *Vet. Path.* 6: 502, 1969.

Powers, R. D. Immunologic properties of the canine transmissible venereal sarcoma. *Am. J. Vet. Res.* 29:1637, 1968.

Priester, W. A. Skin tumors in domestic animals. *J. Nat. Cancer Inst.* 50:457, 1973.

Priester, W. A. and Hayes, H. M. Feline leukemia after feline infectious anemia. *J. Nat. Cancer Inst.* 51:289, 1973.

Pulley, L. T. Ultrastructural and histochemical demonstration of myoepithelium in mixed tumors of the canine mammary gland. *Am. J. Vet. Res.* 34:1513, 1973.

Rafferty, K. A., Jr. Kidney tumors of the leopard frog. A review. *Cancer Res.* 24:169, 1964.

Ragland, S., Spencer, G. R. and McLaughlin, C. A. Experimental viral fibromatosis of equine dermis. *Lab. Invest.* 14:598, 1965 (Abstr.).

Raick, A. N. Late ultrastructural changes induced by 12-0-tetradecanoylphorbol-13-acetate in mouse epidermis and their reversal. *Cancer Res.* 33:1096, 1973.

Ramsey, H. J. Fine structure of hemangiopericytoma and hemangio-endothelioma. *Cancer* 19:2005, 1966.

Rask-Nielsen, R. and Christensen, H. E. Studies on a transplantable mastocytoma in mice. *J. Nat. Cancer Inst.* 30:743, 1963.

Ribelin, W. E. and Bailey, W. S. Esophageal sarcomas associated with *Spirocerca lupi* infection in the dog. *Cancer* 11:1242, 1958.

Rickard, C. G. et al. Transmissible virus-induced lymphocytic leukemia of the cat. *J. Nat. Cancer Inst.* 42:987, 1969.

Ross, M. H. and Bras, G. Lasting influence of early caloric restriction on prevalence of neoplasms in the rat. *J. Nat. Cancer Inst.* 47:1095, 1971.

Rudolph, R. and Weiss, E. Intracytoplasmatische Glykogenablagerungen, lamelläre Strukturen und virus-ähnliche Einschlüsse in Mastzellentumoren des Hundes. Eine elektronenmikroskopische Untersuchung. *Zt. Krebsforsch.* 72:343, 1969.

Russell, W. D., Wynee, E. S. and Loquvam, G. S. Studies on ocular squamous carcinomas (cancer eye). I. Pathological anatomy and historical review. *Cancer* 9:1, 1956.

Sandison, A. T. and Anderson, L. J. Tumors of the kidney in cattle, sheep and pig. *Cancer* 21:727, 1968.

Sapp, W. J. and Adams, E. W. C-type viral particles in canine venereal tumor cell cultures. *Am. J. Vet. Res.* 31:1321, 1970.

Seibold, H. R. et al. Observations on the possible relation of malignant esophageal tumors and *Spirocerca lupi* lesions in the dog. *Am. J. Vet. Res.* 16:5, 1955.

Sellyei, M., Tury, E. and Fellner, F. A new chromosomal variant of the Sticker venereal tumor. *Zt. Krebsforsch.* 74:7, 1970.

Sherbet, G. V. Epigenetic mechanisms and paraneoplastic phenomena. *Ann. N.Y. Acad. Sci.* 230:516, 1974.

Shubin, A. S. and Ponomarkov, V. I. Ultrastructure of transmissible sarcoma in dogs. *Arkh. Patol.* 33:38, 1971 *(Vet. Bull.* 41:6470).

Siegler, R. and Rich, M. A. Pathogenesis of murine leukemia. *Nat. Cancer Inst. Monogr.* 22:525, 1965.

Siegler, R., Harrell, W. and Rich, M. A. Pathogenesis of radiation-induced thymic lymphoma in mice. *J. Nat. Cancer Inst.* 37:105, 1966.

Simpson, C. F. Electron microscopy of the irises of chickens with spontaneous ocular leukosis. *Cancer Res.* 29:33, 1969.

Skinner, M. S. and Mizell, M. The effect of different temperatures on herpesvirus induction and replication in Lucké tumor explants. *Lab. Invest.* 26:671, 1972.

Skipper, H. E. Cancer chemotherapy is many things. *Cancer Res.* 31:1173, 1971.

Skoryna, S. C., Rudis, A. and Webster, D. R. Pathogenesis of feline lung tumors produced by 2-acetylaminofluorine. *Cancer Res.* 11:280, 1951.

Smith, G. H. Cytochemical studies on the mouse mammary tumor virus. *Cancer Res.* 27:2179, 1967.

Smith, W. and Mackay, J. M. K. Morphological observations on a virus associated with sheep pulmonary adenomatosis (Jaagsiekte). *J. Comp. Path.* 79:421, 1969.

Snodgrass, M. J. and Hanna, M. G., Jr. Ultrastructural studies of histiocyte-tumor cell interactions during tumor regression after intralesional injection of *Mycobacterium bovis*. *Cancer Res.* 33:701, 1973.

Snyder, S. P., Theilen, G. H. and Richards, W. P. C. Morphological studies on transmissible feline fibrosarcoma. *Cancer Res.* 30:1658, 1970.

Staub, E. W. et al. Bronchiogenic carcinoma produced experimentally in the normal dog. *J. Thor. Cardiovasc. Surg.* 49:364, 1965.

Stewart, T. The presence of delayed hypersensitivity reactions in patients toward cellular extracts of their malignant tumors. *Cancer Res.* 23:1380, 1969.

Stoebner, P. et al. Ultrastructure of anaplastic bronchial carcinoma. *Cancer* 20:286, 1967.

Straks, W. and Feron, V. J. Ultrastructure of pulmonary adenomas induced by intratracheal instillation of diethylnitrosamine in Syrian golden hamsters. *Europ. J. Cancer* 9:359, 1973.

Sullivan, D. N. and Anderson, W. A. Embryonal nephroma in swine. *Am. J. Vet. Res.* 20:324, 1959.

Swartzendruber, D. C., Ma, B. I. and Murphy, W. H. Localization of C type virus particles in lymphoid germinal centers of C58 mice. *Proc. Soc. Exp. Biol. Med.* 126:731, 1967.

Tanaka, H. and Moore, D. H. Electron microscopic localization of viral antigens in mouse mammary tumor by ferritin-labeled antibody. *Virology* 33:197, 1967.

Tannock, I. F. Population kinetics of carcinoma cells, capillary endothelial cells, and fibroblasts in a transplanted mouse mammary tumor. *Cancer Res.* 30:2470, 1970.

———. The relation between cell proliferation and the vascular system in a transplanted mouse mammary tumor. *Brit. J. Cancer* 22:258, 1968.

Taylor, D. O. N., Dorn, C. R. and Luis, O. H. Morphologic and biologic characteristics of the canine cutaneous histiocytoma. *Cancer Res.* 29:83, 1969.

Temin, H. M. The RNA tumor viruses—background and foreground. *Proc. Nat. Acad. Sci.* 69:1016, 1972.

Theilen, G. H. et al. Experimental induction of lymphosarcoma in the cat with "C"-type virus. *Cancer. Res.* 30:401, 1970.

Todaro, G. J. and Huebner, R. J. The viral oncogene hypothesis: New evidence. *Proc. Nat. Acad. Sci.* 69:1009, 1972.

Todd, G. C., Griffing, W. J. and Koenig, G. R. Fibrosarcoma with metastasis in a rhesus monkey. *Vet. Path.* 10:342, 1973.

Tokarnia, C. H., Dobereiner, J. and Canella, C. F. C. Tumor etmoidal enzootica em bovinos no estado de Rio de Janeiro. *Pesq. Agr. Bras. Ser. Vet.* 7:41, 1972.

Toshima, S., Moore, G. E. and Sandberg, A. A. Ultrastructure of human melanoma in cell culture. *Cancer* 21:202, 1968.

Toth, B. 1,1-dimethylhydrozine (unsymmetrical) carcinogenesis in mice. Light microscopic and ultrastructural study on neoplastic blood vessels. *J. Nat. Cancer Inst.* 50:181, 1973.

Ubertini, T. and Calnek, B. S. Marek's disease herpesvirus in peripheral nerve lesions. *J. Nat. Cancer Inst.* 45:507, 1970.

Underwood, J. C. E. and Carr, I. The ultrastructure and permeability characteristics of the blood vessels of a transplantable rat sarcoma. *J. Path.* 107:157, 1972.

Unuma, T., Morris, H. P. and Rusch, H. Comparative studies of the nucleoli of Morris hepatoma, embryonic liver, and aflatoxin B_1-treated liver of rats. *Cancer Res.* 27: 2221, 1967.

Upton, A. C. and Cosgrove, G. E. Radiation-induced leukemia. In *Experimental Leukemia*. M. A. Rich, ed. Appleton-Century-Croft, 1968.

van Ebbenhorst Tengbergen, W. J. P. R. Morphological classification of mammary tumours in the mouse. *Path. Europ.* 5:260, 1970.

Vielkind, J., Vielkind, V. and Anders, F. Melanotic and amelanotic melanomas in Xiphophorin fish. *Cancer Res.* 31:868, 1971.

Voisin, G. A. Immunological facilitation: A broadening of the concept of the enhancement phenomenon. *Progr. Allergy* 15:328, 1971.

Wadsworth, J. R. Tumors and tumor-like lesions of snakes. *J.A.V.M.A.* 137:419, 1960.

Wandera, J. G. and Krauss, H. The ultrastructure of sheep pulmonary adenomatosis. *Zentr. Vetmed.* A 18:325, 1971.

Ward, J. M. and Hurvitz, A. I. Ultrastructure of normal and neoplastic mast cells of the cat. *Vet. Path.* 9:202, 1972.

Warren, B. A. and Shubik, P. The growth of the blood supply to melanoma transplants in the hamster cheek pouch. *Lab. Invest.* 15:464, 1966.

Weber, W. T., Nowell, P. C. and Hare, W. C. D. Chromosome studies of a transplanted and a primary canine venereal tumor. *J. Nat. Cancer Inst.* 35:537, 1965.

Weijer, K. et al. Feline malignant mammary tumors. *J. Nat. Cancer Inst.* 49:1697, 1972.

Weiler, O., Delain, E. and Lacour, F. Studies on a viral nephroblastic nephroblastoma of the chicken: An electron microscopic comparison of the sequence of development of the virions in different organs. *Europ. J. Cancer* 7:491, 1971.

Weinstein, G. O. and Frost, P. Cell proliferation in human basal cell carcinomas. *Cancer Res.* 30:724, 1970.

Weiss, E., Rudolph, R. and Deutschländer, N. Untersuchungen zur Ultrastruktur und Ätiologie der Mastzellentumoren des Hundes. *Vet. Path.* 5:199, 1968.

Wellings, S. R. Neoplasia and primitive vertebrate phylogeny: Echinoderms, prevertebrates and fishes. *Nat. Cancer Inst. Monogr.* 31:59, 1968.

Wellmann, K. F. Chondroblastoma of the scapula. *Cancer* 24:408, 1969.

Wittmann, W. and Urbaneck, D. Untersuchungen zur Ätiologie der Rinderleukose. *Arch. Exp. Vetmed.* 23:709, 1969.

Wolke, R. E. and Wyand, D. S. Ocular lymphosarcoma of an Atlantic cod. *Bull. Wildlife Dis. Ass.* 5:401, 1969.

Wood, E. M. and Larson, C. P. Hepatic carcinoma in rainbow trout. *Arch. Path.* 77:17, 1961.

Wood, S., Jr. Pathogenesis of metastasis formation observed in vivo in the rabbit ear chamber. *Arch. Path.* 66:550, 1958.

Zambernard, J., Vatter, A. E. and McKinnell, R. G. The fine structure of nuclear and cytoplasmic inclusions in primary renal tumors of mutant leopard frogs. *Cancer Res.* 26:1688, 1966.

Zedeck, M. S. et al. Biochemical and pathological effects of methylazoxymethanol acetate, a potent carcinogen. *Cancer Res.* 30:801, 1970.

Zeidman, I. Fate of circulating tumor cells. *Cancer Res.* 25:324, 1965.

Zubrod, C. G. Chemical control of cancer. *Proc. Nat. Acad. Sci.* 69:1042, 1972.

Zur Hausen et al. Comparative study of cultured Burkitt tumor cells by immunofluorescence autoradiography and electron microscopy. *J. Virol.* 1:830, 1967.

Respiratory System

DEFENSE MECHANISMS IN THE BRONCHIOLES

The lungs receive constant insults of dust, smoke, and toxic gases. The oxygen-exchanging membranous pneumocyte of the alveolar wall is protected from much of this by the mucociliary system of the bronchioles. Ciliated columnar epithelium of the respiratory tract is designed to purify air from the polluted environment for its presentation to the respiratory lobule of the lung. Warmed and humidified by passage through the upper respiratory tract, air is cleansed in the bronchioles by the continuous secretion of mucus, which physically traps and chemically inactivates foreign substances.

Beating in concert, the bed of cilia moves particulate material by wavelike propulsive action through the layer of nonviscous material that exists between the cilia and the mucous layer which is superficial and more viscous. Cilia are quite sensitive to injury and disruption of movement considerably depresses their effectiveness in removal of contaminants of the upper respiratory tract (Fig. 7.1). Sulfur dioxide, a significant air pollutant in industrial areas, causes loss of cilia on short-term experimental exposure at 100 ppm (the concentration in severe London smog is 1.35 ppm). Cilia are also susceptible to low levels of ozone and nitrogen dioxide (Stephens et al. 1973). Ultrastructurally, they are blunted, broken, and their anchors in the basal bodies are disorganized.

In diseases such as influenza and mycoplasmosis, invading organisms attach to cilia, causing them to be rapidly removed from the bronchiolar epithelium (Bang and Bang 1969; Livingston et al. 1972).

The acute inflammatory response (bronchiolitis) is characterized by destruction of cilia, marked intercellular edema, dilatation of subepithelial capillaries, and the exudation of neutrophils through the epithelium into the lumen. Cilia break off and disappear, leaving disoriented and degenerate basal bodies (Dahlgren and Dalen 1972; Frasca 1968; Giddens and Fairchild 1972). If bronchiolar disease persists, the ciliated columnar epithelium undergoes metaplasia. Basal cell hyperplasia causes stratified squamous epithelium to develop (Asmundsson et al. 1973).

One of the first events in inflammation of the lung is the exudation of fluid through the bronchiolar epithelium and into the air passages. These serous exudates contain relatively large amounts of plasma proteins, which can be demonstrated by comparing nasal washings from normal and inflamed nasal cavities. The importance of the respiratory tract as a portal of entry for infectious organisms led to the early observations that respiratory secretions were antimicrobial. One of the most significant studies was the demonstration of the important role of antibody in resistance to influenza. Immunization by the nasal route against aerosolized challenge was far superior to any other method of immunization. Protection correlated better with antibody in bronchial washings than with antibody present in serum.

During microbe-induced inflammation of the respiratory tract, the protein content of respiratory washings markedly increases. This is a nonspecific effect due to increased vascular permeability and, in primary infections, the proteins exuding are albumin and globulins. Unless the an-

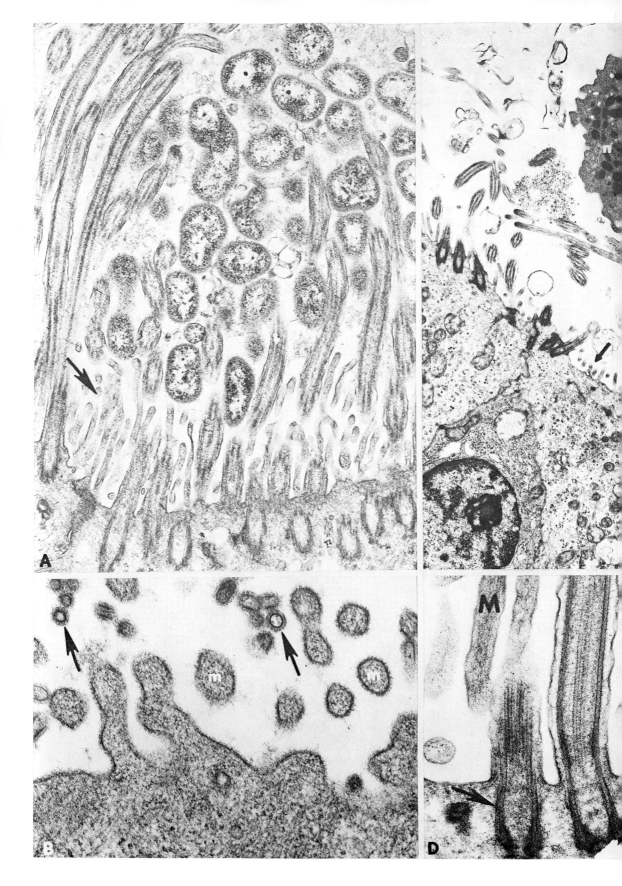

imal has previously experienced the disease, specific antibody activity is not seen in this initial outpouring of globulin. Later, specific antibody activity does develop and can be measured in the secretions (Lüthgen 1972; Potter et al. 1972).

Recent discoveries have illustrated that respiratory secretions contain a higher concentration of antibody than can be accounted for by passive transudation from plasma. Most antibody activity is associated with immunoglobulin A or IgA (Curtain et al. 1971; Lieberman et al. 1971). IgA is synthesized by plasmablasts and plasmacytes, which are located in the lamina propria of the bronchioles and is shed through the epithelium into the lumen. When nasal or lung washings are measured for antibody activity and IgA content, it is seen that these two factors are closely associated (Fig. 7.2). The peribronchiolar lymphoid aggregates have an intimate association with the overlying epithelium (Bienenstock et al. 1973).

Mucous cell hyperplasia of respiratory epithelium (Fig. 7.3) accompanies acute and chronic inflammation. Mucus, which is formed in epithelial goblet cells and subepithelial mucous glands, floods the damaged epithelial surface. It protects and provides the surface with the tenacious material that, when expectorated, removes much of the debris and irritant. Intrapulmonic bronchioles produce mucus of greater acidity than that in the upper respiratory tract (Spicer et al. 1971). The distinctive sulfated mucosubstance which bathes the base of the cilia is probably a glycocalyx produced by the ciliated epithelial cell.

The presence of excess mucus has an irritant effect on sensory nerve endings, and they induce the cough reflex, which is highly important in removing debris. Bronchiolar epithelium, like the exocrine glands, receives autonomic innervation (parasympathetic nerves come via the vagus; sympathetic via the second to fourth thoracic ganglia) through close apposition of membranes of the nerve, which lie in grooves on the surface of the epithelial cell. Synaptic vesicles of the synapse contain acetylcholine which, when released, causes bronchiolar constriction (via action on smooth muscle) and mucus secretion. These mechanisms may be manipulated by the clinician very effectively in treatment of respiratory disease.

Failure of bronchioles to remove irritants and cell debris allows these substances to reach the primary respiratory lobule. The diameter of the terminal bronchioles (estimated as 20μ), the last structure which can effectively trap particulate material, determines what particles enter the alveolus. The bronchioles cannot stop small particles and microorganisms which air turbulence during inspiration does not force against the mucociliary layer of the terminal bronchiole (Asmundsson and Kilburn 1970).

ALVEOLAR WALL

The alveolar wall is a connective tissue interstitium through which capillaries ramify, which is bounded by flattened epithelial cells called membranous pneumocytes. Masked by the tortuosity of the vascular bed is the pattern of connective tissue fibers that lie in a central plane and give tensile strength to the lung parenchyma. The width of the *blood-air barrier* (capillary endothelium, basement membrane, and membranous pneumocyte) is altered in lung disease. These pathologic changes, as determined by electron microscopy, are an indication of the capacity of the alveolar wall for gaseous interchange.

The movement of oxygen and carbon dioxide across the blood-air barrier is con-

Fig. 7.1. Bronchiolar epithelium. A. Mycoplasmal pneumonia, pig. Organisms are enmeshed within cilia producing little damage except distortion and increased length of microvilli (arrow) (Micrograph, W. Wegmann). B. Influenza pneumonia, pig. Virions (arrows) bud from bronchiolar cell surface and distort microvilli (m) and destroy cilia. C. Bronchiolitis, chronic Bordetella pneumonia, pig. Destruction of cilia, increased numbers of surface microvilli (arrow), and neutrophil (n) in lumen. D. Cilia. Note rigid peripheral microtubules (arrow) which are attached to the basal body within the epithelial cells. Long microvillus (M) contains a central core of tiny microfilaments.

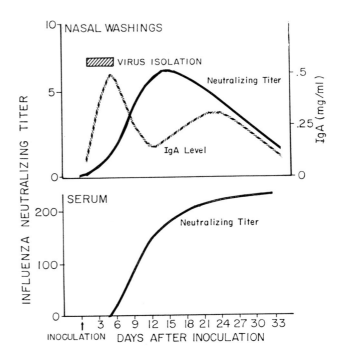

Fig. 7.2. Levels of IgA and antiinfluenza-neutralizing activity in nasal washings and serum. First peak of IgA exudation is nonspecific and is not associated with antibody activity.

sidered to be a process of passive diffusion although the liberation of CO_2 from carbonic acid is greatly accelerated by the enzyme carbonic anhydrase. When gaseous transfer is compromised by injury to the alveolar wall, the capillaries dilate (active hyperemia) and protrude into the alveolus. The exposed surface for interchange is thereby considerably enlarged.

ENDOTHELIUM

The endothelial cell is usually the first component of the alveolar wall to show alteration in injury to the lungs. Cell swelling with rarefaction of the cytoplasm is an early manifestation of damage. In severe injury there is blebbing of the cytoplasm into the lumen of the capillary. If edema of the alveolar wall interstitium is extensive, fluid accumulation may cause focal herniation of the endothelial cell cytoplasm through the basement membrane into the pericapillary spaces. Intercellular junctions are rarely seen open even in severe injury, although dense deposits, presumably acidic mucopolysaccharides, are commonly found in the intercellular spaces. The permeability of alveolar capillary endothelium, especially at intercellular

junctions, depends in part on intravascular volume (Schneeberger 1970). Normal capillary endothelial cells have no fenestrae, but in pathologic conditions such as pulmonary fibrosis fenestrae may develop.

Significant changes occur in systemic deficits of oxygen. Hypoxia is usually accompanied by increases in pinocytotic vesicles, vacuole formation, and degeneration of mitochondria in endothelial cells. Pulmonary capillaries have remarkable capacity to dilate, which they do in response to hypoxia, to increased demand for oxygen, and to many vasoactive drugs.

MEMBRANOUS PNEUMOCYTE

The thin flattened cytoplasm of the membranous pneumocyte (type I cell, respiratory epithelial cell) covers the surface of the alveolar wall. Its nucleus, rarely seen ultrastructurally, is small and elongate. The membranous pneumocyte obtains oxygen directly from the alveolus and is highly susceptible to hypoxia. In hypoxic states, degenerate mitochondria are commonly seen bulging into the alveolus. Cell swelling occurs, and fluid distends perinuclear cisternae and the few cisternae within the cell cytoplasm. The

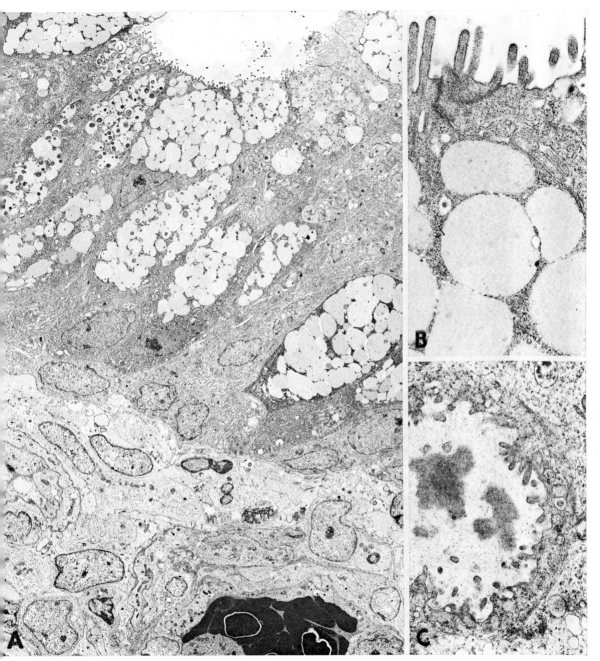

Fig. 7.3. Mucous hyperplasia (cartarrh) following influenza, chicken.
A. Epithelium consists of masses of goblet cells. Capillaries and venules
below the epithelium are swollen and surrounded by macrophages and
lymphocytes. B. Enlargement. Note mucus granules and microvilli.
C. Intracellular canaliculus in a mucin-producing cell. Granular
material in the lumen is composed of mucopolysaccharides.

plasma membrane is associated with large numbers of pinocytotic vesicles, which reflect its function of transferring fluid from capillary to alveolus. In some toxic reactions, membranous pneumocytes, like other components of the alveolar wall, become filled with lysosomes and myeloid bodies (Lüllman et al. 1973). The regenerative capacity of membranous pneumocytes following injury is not known. Even in severe injury to the alveolar wall, hyperplasia or hypertrophy of these cells is rarely seen.

GRANULAR PNEUMOCYTE

The granular pneumocyte (type II cell) is a second type of pneumocyte lining the alveolar walls. It differs from the membranous pneumocyte in being larger, cuboidal, and having dense osmiophilic inclusions and surface microvilli. The dense lamellar inclusions are expelled into the alveolus by merocrine secretion and are the source of *pulmonary surfactant*. Surfactant lines the alveolar wall, stabilizing it by lowering surface tension (Buckingham et al. 1966).

Surfactant has been characterized chemically. Phospholipids are the active component, but are demonstrable only by special techniques (Colacicco and Scarpelli 1970). Granular pneumocytes are selectively labeled with choline-H^3, a specific precursor of phosphatidyl choline, the main phospholipid of surfactant. Labeled choline is first seen in the endoplasmic reticulum, later in the Golgi complex, and finally in the dense lamellar inclusions (Chevalier and Collet 1972).

A mucopolysaccharide layer lining the cell membrane of the granular pneumocyte is demonstrable with colloidal iron stains. It was originally believed to be a component of surfactant (Askin and Kuhn 1971; Bernstein et al. 1969). It is firmly bound to the cell membrane, is not removed by repeated washing of the lungs (as is phospholipid), and is specifically digested by neuraminidase. For these reasons, it appears to be an integral part of the cell membrane and not of surfactant. Mucopolysaccharides have also been demonstrated on the cell membrane of membranous pneumocytes.

Granular pneumocytes are absent in the early fetal lung, but are seen with increasing frequency as birth nears (Kikkawa et al. 1968). This correlates with increasing amounts of measurable surfactant in the fetal lung. During birth, as hypoxia develops and the first breathing begins, there is rapid degranulation of granular pneumocytes with massive release of surfactant. Surfactant not only stabilizes the lung, but also aids in removal of amniotic fluid and cells that lodge in the alveoli prior to birth.

When surfactant is absent or inactivated in newborn animals, the resulting high surface tension at the end of expiration necessarily forces more air out of the lungs, and atelectasis (incomplete expansion of the lungs) results. Lambs born prematurely, for example (Kikkawa et al. 1968), have a respiratory distress syndrome associated with decreased surfactant and this, like hyalin membrane disease of foals (Mahaffey and Rossdale 1959) and premature human infants, may be responsible for the fibrin and mucous membranes that cover the alveoli, preventing adequate gaseous exchange. Peroxisomes also increase in granular pneumocytes as birth approaches but their significance is not known (Schneeberger 1972).

Steroid treatment of pregnant animals accelerates both surfactant and granular pneumocyte inclusions in the lung of the fetus (Wang et al. 1971). In some animals, these hormones are used to induce parturition, and the secondary effects on granular pneumocytes may mimic the natural birth process in the lung.

Granular pneumocyte hyperplasia and release of surfactant are early responses of the alveolar wall to injury (Breeze et al. 1975). Secretion is stimulated by pilocarpine. It also appears that release of surfactant is partially under neural control. Degeneration of granular pneumocytes is seen when the vagus nerves are sectioned bilaterally. There is progressive decrease in osmophilia of the cytoplasmic granules. The edema and atelectasis that follow vagotomy are allegedly due to absence of surfactant, which follows a secondary atrophic reaction in membranous pneumocytes (Goldenberg et al. 1969).

The granular pneumocytes appear to be

the progenitors of the membranous pneumocytes due to their proliferation and repair of the damaged alveolar wall, and their presence and mitotic activity in the early fetal lung (Adamson and Bowden 1975).

Granular pneumocytes show degenerative changes, including fatty degeneration, in intoxications of various causes (Gould and Smuckler 1971). It can readily be seen that suppression of surfactant production has important effects on secondary changes in lung tissue.

ALVEOLAR MACROPHAGES

Foreign substances entering the alveolus are removed by alveolar macrophages. These cells lie free in the alveolus and phagocytize and digest particulate and macromolecular materials. They become engorged and in some diseases have diagnostic significance, for example, the iron-filled "heart failure cells" in chronic heart failure and the lipid-filled "foam cells" found in some toxic lesions (Flodh and Magnusson 1973). Pneumocytes play very little role in clearance of these substances. The clearance of low levels of inert exogenous material (such as carbon, dust, and nonpathogenic microbes) and of endogenous cell debris, surfactant, and fibrin is constant. The engorged, degenerate macrophages are expelled up the tracheobronchial pathways.

Alveolar macrophages originate from blood monocytes. Early studies revealed that carbon-labeled monocytes, when injected into guinea pigs, were concentrated in the lungs (Ungar and Wilson 1935). Recent immunologic studies clearly show that lung alveolar macrophages of irradiated mice originate from blood monocytes (from a donor mouse) inoculated intravenously (Godleski and Brain 1972). The donor cells were from a different mouse strain and contained an identifiable antigenic marker. Macrophages probably also arise from liver Kupffer cells and from activated spleen macrophages (Bowden et al. 1969; McCarthy et al. 1964; Schneeberger and Keeley 1970).

Alveolar macrophages can be harvested and studied in vitro by washing them free through tracheobronchial insufflation with saline. Like other macrophages, they stick rapidly to glass and phagocytize particulate material actively. They differ in being more dependent upon aerobic metabolism, and are in a more activated state than are macrophages obtained from serosal cavities. The intracellular degradation of material in lysosomes can be systematically studied in this manner.

NEURAL CONTROL OF THE ALVEOLAR WALL

Vertebrate lungs are innervated by parasympathetic fibers via the vagus and by sympathetic nerves from the second through the fourth thoracic ganglia. The nerves ramify along the bronchiolar system and the unmyelinated axons extend into the alveolar walls, where they may be seen ultrastructurally between the pneumocytes and underlying capillaries. Two types of nerve endings are present. It is alleged that one is sensory (associated with membranous pneumocytes) and the other is motor (associated with granular pneumocytes) (Hung et al. 1972).

Innervated epithelial corpuscles of granular, serotonin-producing cells are located in the bronchioles and extend into the alveolar walls in some species (Lauweryns et al. 1973). These bodies appear to be intrapulmonary neuroreceptor organs that secrete serotonin-containing granules and are modulated by the central nervous system.

INTERSTITIAL CELLS

Stellate-shaped cells resembling fibroblasts are sometimes encountered in the alveolar wall of mammalian lungs. They contain cytoplasmic fibrils, 3–8 nm in diameter, which bind fluorescein-conjugated antiactin antibodies. It thus appears that these cells may function as autoregulators of ventilation or blood perfusion, by contracting in response to hypoxia or substances such as epinephrine.

K CELLS

Distinctive granulated cells are sometimes encountered in bronchiolar epithelium. They are probably part of an amine precursor uptake and decarboxylation system and are analogous to Kulchitsky cells of the intestine. In primates they allegedly are the cell of origin of pulmonary "oat cell" or carcinoid tumors (Cutz et al. 1974).

PULMONARY EDEMA

To the veterinary clinician, pulmonary edema is a dramatic clinical entity with dire consequences for the patient. The head is held low, the nose is flecked with froth, and there are dyspnea and gasping. Wheezing, bubbly sounds of respiration are characteristic. To the pathologist, *pulmonary edema* is the accumulation of plasma protein filtrates in alveoli, due to altered hemodynamics or as an early peracute phase of inflammation. While (technically) it accompanies any focal inflammatory lesion, the diagnosis of pulmonary edema is used to imply a diffuse affection of large areas of the lung. Grossly, the lungs are doughy, heavy, firm, and foamy; fluid pours from the cut surface. Histologically, alveoli are filled with fluid that is high in content of albumin and which is coagulated by fixative (see Fig. 3.9). The greater the albumin content, the more intensely the fluid stains with eosin. Lymphatics are dilated and filled with fluid. In severe cases, fluid is present in the alveoli, the alveolar wall, and within the cells.

Pulmonary edema is brought about by excessive amounts of fluid leaving the capillary bed of the lung. There are two major reasons for the fluid exudation through the capillary: (1) circulatory failure-induced changes of pulmonary hemodynamics that result in a slow exudation of fluid into alveoli and (2) sudden diffuse and direct damage to the capillary endothelium. The second mechanism is usually a peracute stage of inflammation and, if the animal survives, it is followed by exudation of inflammatory cells and pneumonia. Both conditions are associated with marked capillary dilation, and the distinction between extreme hyperemia and pulmonary edema is often arbitrary (Table 7.1).

ALTERED PULMONARY HEMODYNAMICS

Hemodynamic pulmonary edema is a disturbance of normal fluid exchange in

Table 7.1. Mechanisms of pulmonary edema

Abnormal Pulmonary Hemodynamics
  Cardiac failure: elevated venous pressure, hypoxia, congestion
  Shock
  Renal disease: loss of plasma proteins
  Liver disease: failure in synthesis of plasma proteins
Defective Capillary Endothelium
  Direct damage to capillary endothelium in the alveolar wall (early inflammation)[a]
  Pulmonary elimination of circulating toxic chemicals ANTU, NH_4SO_4
  Viral replication: influenza pneumonitis
  Direct toxic injury: bacterial exotoxins
  Mast cell degranulation: anaphylaxis
CNS lesions inducing peripheral vasoconstriction (rare)

[a] "Inflammatory" edema is a transient early phase in the process of pneumonitis. We consider cases here in which edema is a dominant pathologic sign. The majority of lesions progress into overt inflammatory lesions.

the lung. Fluid collects in the alveolus and the interstitium of the wall without primary alteration of capillary endothelium. It is associated with conditions involving increased pulmonary venous pressure, inadequate lymph drainage, and systemic anoxia. Vascular stasis is prominent, and the condition may be referred to as "congestion and edema."

Cardiac failure is a cause of pulmonary edema in aged dogs. Fluid exudes into the alveolus because of increased pressure in the pulmonary venous system (see edema, Chapter 3). Pulmonary edema associated with cardiac failure is inevitably chronic. Lymph flow increases, lymphatics enlarge, and the alveolar walls thicken. Granular pneumocyte hyperplasia is common in spotty areas and these cells may line the alveoli. If passive hyperemia is prolonged, stasis of erythrocytes, leukocytes, and platelets occurs. Erythrophagocytosis, either intravascularly or following hemorrhage into the alveolus, causes the accumulation in the alveolus of "heart failure cells" (large macrophages filled with hemosiderin and free iron). Capillary hyperemia and stasis of blood combine to produce further injury to endothelium.

Hemorrhagic shock may be accompanied by pulmonary edema. Hemodilution follows blood loss and lowered plasma osmotic pressure (see shock, Chapter 3). The coexistence of these factors leads to pulmonary edema or "shock lung." Perivascular edema, swelling of endothelium, and sequestration of granulocytes in the lung capillary bed are the lesions seen (Pingleton et al. 1972; Ratliff et al. 1970). Severe kidney or liver disease may also sufficiently lower the plasma protein levels to cause fluid exudation into the alveoli.

NEURIGENIC PULMONARY EDEMA

Sympathetic nerves serve as vasodilators to pulmonary blood vessels. Life-threatening pulmonary edema and hemorrhage may result from severe trauma to the brain because of these connections. The edema is due to sympathetic vasomotor discharge from the medulla. This evokes potent systemic vasoconstriction that shifts large quantities of blood to the lungs. The consequent pulmonary arterial and venous hypertension is responsible for edema (Chen and Chai 1974).

PNEUMONITIS

Pneumonitis is inflammation of the lung. It is a broad category, including all inflammatory lesions, that is, interstitial pneumonitis, pneumonia, and lung abscesses. Unfortunately, the term pneumonia, because it is ingrained in clinical medicine, is also used as a general term for inflammation of the lung. The pathogenetic differences between pneumonia and pneumonitis, however, are real and significant. This distinction must be maintained, despite the disparity between clinical usage and anatomical definition.

Normally the lower respiratory tree is sterile. When bronchiolar ciliary-mucus and alveolar macrophage mechanisms falter or when the virulence of an organism is greater than the capacity of these systems to prevent invasion, infection of the respiratory lobule occurs. Respiratory infections are probably more frequent than infections of any other organ. The consequences are serious and often fatal.

The functional unit of the mammalian lung is the *acinus* (not the alveolus), which is the parenchymal unit connected to the first order respiratory bronchiole (Fig. 7.4).

This definition is not academic since diseases of the lung generally affect acinar units rather than alveoli.

INTERSTITIAL PNEUMONITIS

Interstitial pneumonitis or "alveolitis" is inflammation of the alveolar wall. It is reserved for those diseases that produce an inflammatory process in the alveolar wall, but that are not prone to progress to pneumonia. This pattern of lung damage is commonly seen in viral infections, chemical toxicity, and some allergic reactions.

VIRAL INFECTION

Influenza in swine, horses, and humans is characteristically accompanied by diffuse interstitial pneumonitis. Influenza virus initially replicates in epithelial cells of the upper respiratory tract. Infection spreads to bronchioles and then to endothelial cells and alveolar macrophages of the alveolar wall. Damage to the wall is accompanied by cell swelling and exudation of serous fluid and macrophages into the interstitial areas. The alveolar wall becomes thickened, and this is exaggerated by hyperplasia of granular pneumocytes. Infiltration of cells and fluid into the alveolus also occurs, but the reaction is sufficiently slow and limited so that removal follows. Surfactant, albumin, and fibrinogen combine in severe cases to produce hyalin membranes in the alveolus. Pulmonary edema occurs, but is not a serious consequence of the disease. When uncomplicated, the inflammatory process in influenza is not considered purulent. Secondary bacterial infection is common, however, and purulent bronchopneumonia is a serious complication of influenza. Viral infection paves the way for bacterial disease by destroying the mucociliary clearance mechanism, by inducing fluid to accumulate in the lung, and by a direct inhibition of phagocytosis by alveolar macrophages.

Other viral infections that begin as bronchiolitis, and also produce pneumonitis and predispose to bacterial infection, include canine distemper, hog cholera, and Newcastle disease. Viral infection of the lung accompanies several other systemic

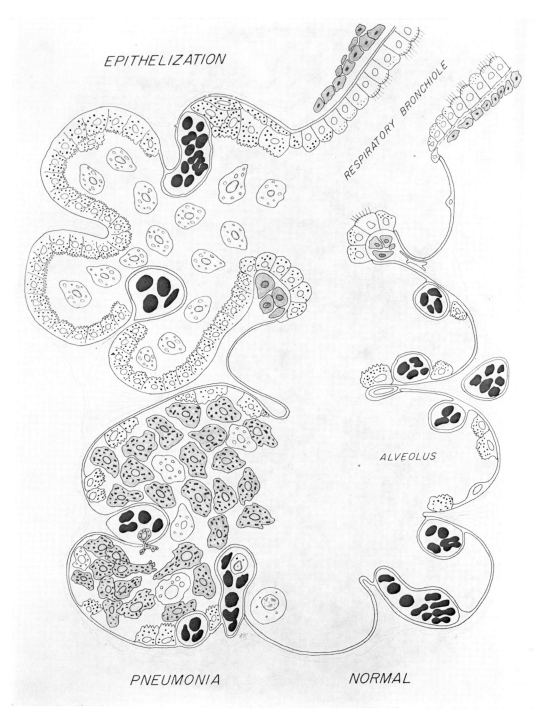

EPITHELIZATION

RESPIRATORY BRONCHIOLE

ALVEOLUS

PNEUMONIA

NORMAL

Fig. 7.4. Diagram of pulmonary acinus: normal and early and healing phases of pneumonia.

viral diseases, but pneumonitis is not a significant lesion of the process.

Mycoplasmosis is characterized by interstitial pneumonitis in some species, particularly porcine pneumonia. Mycoplasmas prefer to reside among cilia on the surface on the bronchiolar epithelium (as an extracellular infection). The first change in disease is inhibition of ciliary action. If cilia are destroyed, mycoplasmas readily enter alveoli where they are phagocytized by alveolar macrophages and the few neutrophils that exude. Granular pneumocytes react with extensive hyperplasia but do not phagocytize the organisms. Chlamydial infections of the lung are often characterized by interstitial pneumonitis. Organisms replicate within alveolar macrophages, which fill the alveoli causing histiocytic pneumonia.

ALLERGIC ALVEOLITIS

This may result when sensitized animals are exposed to large aerosols of particulate antigens. An inflammatory reaction is initiated by the complexing of these antigens to antibodies that are bound to mast cells and smooth muscle associated with the intrapulmonary vascular tree (see allergic alveolitis, Chapter 5).

TOXIC INJURY AND PNEUMONITIS

Diffuse injury to the pulmonary capillary bed with constriction of venules results in pulmonary edema when toxic chemicals are inhaled or are eliminated during exhalation. Inhalation of fumes from hot smoke and toxic chemicals is among the commonest causes of injury. In the early phases of the reaction, histamine and other vasoactive substances exert a rapid but brief effect. Interendothelial gaps occur in bronchiolar venules through which tracers can be demonstrated experimentally. The pathogenesis of more severe lesions is sustained by progressive vascular injury. Fibrin polymerizes in the edema fluid, obstructs lymphatic outflow, and seals alveolar wall pores. Fibrinolysis releases fibrin degradation products that cause increased capillary permeability and neutrophil exudation (Meyer and Ottaviano 1973).

Pulmonary edema and pneumonitis also result from the exhalation of circulating chemical toxins which are eliminated in the respiratory tract. Striking and usually fatal pulmonary edema follows the oral ingestion of alphanaphthathiourea (ANTU), which is used as a rodenticide. The crucial manifestation of ANTU poisoning is extreme swelling of endothelial cells (Cunningham and Hurley 1972). Perivascular and interstitial edema of the alveolar wall are marked. Fluid accumulates beneath the endothelial cells, separating them from their basement membranes and causing endothelial cytoplasm to herniate into the capillary lumen. Similar fluid accumulation may cause the membranous pneumocyte to herniate into the alveolus. Electrophoresis of fluid in the lung and trachea reveal it to be similar to plasma in protein content, which indicates the severity of the vascular damage.

Other substances associated with exhalation pulmonary edema include kerosene, turpentine, furniture polish, and lighter fluid. Their toxic components belong to the same group of aliphatic and aromatic hydrocarbons. Oral ingestion causes pulmonary edema and vascular damage during elimination via the lung ("hydrocarbon pneumonitis"). Experimental models of injury to the alveolar wall include damage induced by anthrax toxin (Beall and Dalldorf 1966), ammonium sulfate (Hayes and Shiga 1970), and staphylococcal enterotoxin (Finegold 1967).

The lesions of chronic toxic exhalation may be prolonged. Paraquat, a bipyridinium herbicide, evokes a slowly fatal pneumonic response following accidental poisoning in man and animals. The lesions seen at necropsy are focal areas of nonpurulent consolidation, with varying amounts of diffuse fibrosis throughout the lung. In the acute phases there are edema, hemorrhage, and destruction of the alveolar wall. The degenerative process in lung parenchyma is in capillary endothelium and alveolar pneumocytes (Brooks 1971). Severe swelling and vacuolation of these cells is followed by degeneration, necrosis, and denudation, leaving foci of naked basal laminae in the alveolar wall. The wall becomes thickened with fluid accumulation, and disorganization of collagen and ground substance occurs. Granular pneumocyte hyperplasia develops as a reparative phenomenon, but is inefficient in bridging damaged alveolar walls and insufficient to produce enough surfactant to maintain surface tension.

Accumulation of macrophages and a few neutrophils in the wall is followed by collapse of the heavy, nonfunctional parenchyma. The fatal outcome in most cases of accidental poisoning is progressive pulmonary fibrosis with extensive collagen deposition, fibroplasia, epithelization, and hyalin membrane formation.

PNEUMONIA

Pneumonia is the filling of the alveolus with cellular exudates. The severe and significant pneumonias of animals are predominantly bacterial in origin and are characterized by intense exudation of inflammatory cells, chiefly neutrophils, into the alveolus. The pattern of the inflammatory process depends upon the type and virulence of the bacteria involved. Predisposing factors such as chilling, intercurrent viral infection, inhalation of anesthetics, debility of old age, and unresponsiveness of the newborn lung may play important roles in initiating bacterial infection.

In chronic pneumonia, the exudation of macrophages and monocytes may be so extensive that the alveolar walls and alveoli are filled with closely packed alveolar macrophages (Fig. 7.5). This type of pneumonia, termed histiocytic pneumonia, is usually spotty in its distribution through the lung and is rarely associated with high morbidity (Farr et al. 1970).

BACTERIA IN THE LUNG

The main bactericidal property of the normal lung resides in the alveolar macrophages (Laurenzi et al. 1963). The effectiveness of macrophage lysosomes in proc-

essing particulate material determines in large part the outcome of the inhalation of bacteria. Particle size determines the accessibility of inhaled microorganisms to the respiratory unit. While large particles are trapped by the mucociliary apparatus, bacteria in the range of 0.5 to 3.0μ remain suspended and are carried to the alveoli. Most of these are quickly killed by macrophage lysosomes.

If animals are placed in an aerosol chamber and receive a large dose of bacteria (which are less than 4μ) for 30 min, large numbers of these same bacteria can be isolated from ground lung tissue (Kass et al. 1966; Lillie and Thompson 1972). Immediately after exposure there is a rapid decline in the number of viable bacteria that are culturable from lungs (Fig. 7.6). At 4 hrs about 85% are removed and at 6 hrs about 90%. The rate of clearance differs among organisms of different size. If bacteria are radioactively labeled the label does not disappear, indicating that bacteria are killed and remain in lung macrophages rather than being transported by blood and lymph out of the lung.

When highly pathogenic bacteria enter the lung, an inflammatory response is initiated. The mechanisms responsible for clearance of bacteria of low pathogenicity are distinct from the intense mechanisms involved in pneumonia. In the early stages of bacterial pneumonia, edema fluid fills the alveoli, and bacteria-laden macrophages migrate through the tissue (Baskerville et al. 1973). The alveolar wall becomes distended with fluid and its injured capillaries are dilated (Finegold 1969). As the capillary endothelium is damaged, fibrinogen exudes and fibrin polymerizes, which blocks the alveoli and draining lymphatics. Degranulation and degeneration of granular pneumocytes are responsible for high concentrations of surfactant within alveoli.

Fig. 7.5. Interstitial pneumonitis and early histiocytic pneumonia, cat. A. Hyperplastic granular pneumocytes contain inclusions, microvilli, and lipid globules. *Inset:* Histology. The alveolar walls are markedly thickened and filled with large round cells. Alveoli at bottom are filled with fluid and those at top with macrophages. B. Ultrastructure. Capillaries are dilated and filled with monocytes and erythrocytes. Granular pneumocytes are hyperplastic. Macrophages filled with phagosomes are present in the alveoli. C. Enlargement of macrophages showing large membrane-bound aggregates of membranes and small dense primary lysosomes (arrow).

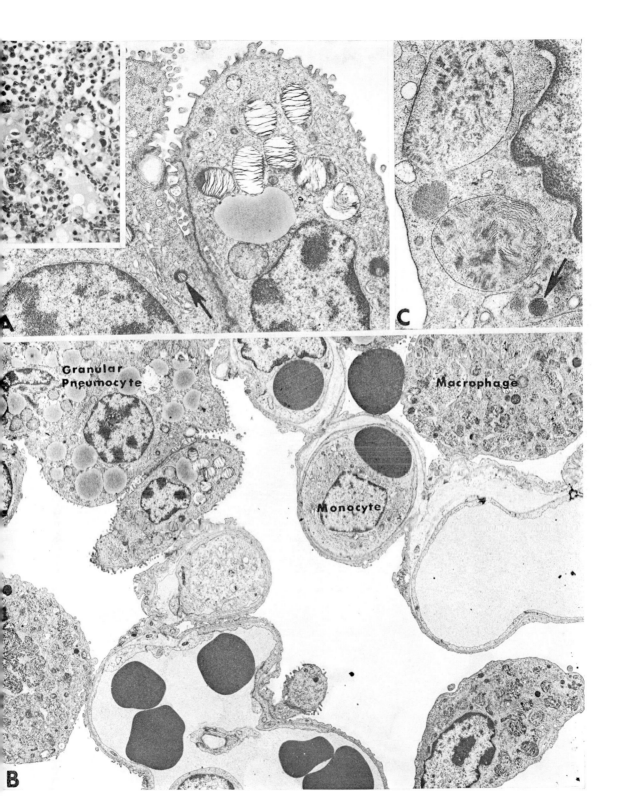

A

C

Granular
Pneumocyte

Macrophage

Monocyte

B

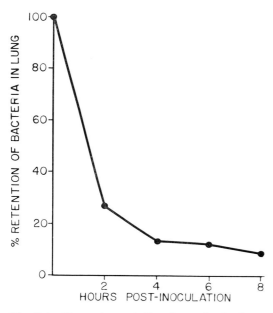

Fig. 7.6. Retention of live bacteria in lung after aerosol exposure. Determined by culture of lung tissue suspensions.

PURULENT PNEUMONIA

Pneumonia progresses through stages of hyperemia, serous exudation, and cellular infiltration. Each stage has characteristic gross, histologic, and ultrastructural appearances, but these are blurred together during the progression of the disease. In active, invasive bacterial pneumonia, neutrophilic granulocytes quickly dominate the reaction. These cells are present intravascularly and are seen with increasing frequency in the alveolus as the lesion ages (Fig. 7.7). Ultrastructurally neutrophils may contain bacteria, but the usual case is to find them degranulated within alveoli.

In the later stages of purulent pneumonia, neutrophils pack the alveolus. They are in varying stages of degeneration and differ markedly from normal cells in their structure. Fibrin is present throughout the lesions, especially in severe pneumonia. In general, little can be gained from the ultrastructural examination of tissues in this stage, for it is disorganized and necrotic. The tissue architecture is effaced and cell structures are masked by the massive accumulation of tissue debris.

The solid exudative reaction wherein inflammatory cells fill the terminal respiratory lobule is called consolidation. When consolidation is patchy, lobular, and centered around the bronchiolar tree, it is referred to as *bronchopneumonia*. The use of "bronchopneumonia" implies an aerosol origin of the causal agent. Consolidation of the lung occasionally involves entire lobes and may be referred to as *lobar pneumonia*. Lobar pneumonia, seen in overwhelming infections caused by *Mycoplasma* and *Pasteurella* spp., is usually severe, peracute, and fibrinous; it generally terminates fatally. In most cases, lobar pneumonia is a severe form of bronchopneumonia, but it may also be hematogenous in origin.

Bronchopneumonia usually begins by extension of purulent infection from the respiratory bronchiole into the terminal respiratory lobule. The filling of alveoli with edema fluid facilitates the flow of bacteria through the alveolar ducts and throughout the lobule. The pneumonic process may spread from one alveolus to another through the alveolar pores, which provide connection between adjacent alveoli. Exudate may also spread directly through the bronchiolar wall to produce peribronchiolar infection.

RECOVERY

If recovery occurs, the number of viable bacteria quickly drops. A few may remain and become the focus of microabscess formation. Hyperplasia of granular pneumocytes is the dominant characteristic of the lung recovering from an acute pneumonic process. Resolution of pneumonia depends on the extent of damage to the alveolar wall and on the fate of the invading organism. Persistence of bacteria of relatively low virulence may result in chronic multifocal pneumonia with lung abscesses. Severe inflammation of the alveolar wall is always followed by some degree of collagen deposition. If fibroplasia expands the wall to even a moderate degree, the parts of the lung so affected do not return to normal. Necrotic foci never become functional, and areas must repair by connective tissue deposition.

Epithelization of the remnants of the respiratory lobule occurs in some chronic

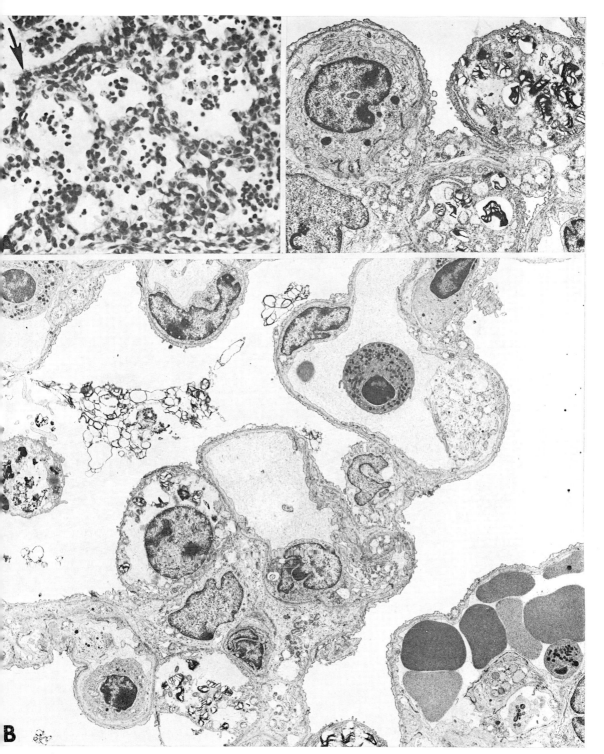

Fig. 7.7. Early purulent pneumonia, *Bordetella bronchiseptica*, 15-day-old pig. A. Histology. Alveolar walls are thickened by endothelial cell swelling and interstitial edema. Extensive hyperplasia of granular pneumocytes. Neutrophils and macrophages are in the alveoli. Terminal bronchiole, upper left (arrow). B. Ultrastructure. Hyperemia, debris in the alveolus, and increased numbers of granular pneumocytes. C. Contrast in granular pneumocyte (right) and a monocyte within a capillary (left).

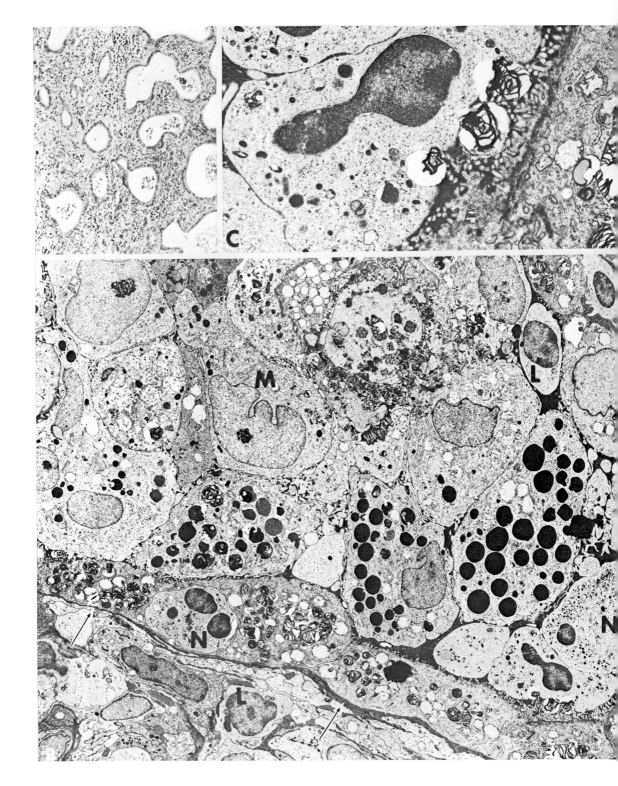

forms of pneumonia (Fig. 7.8). The epitheliallike cells lining the alveoli are granular pneumocytes and remarkably resemble the lining cells of the bronchiole (because they resemble the alveolar wall in the fetus the process is also called "fetalization"). Extreme examples of this type occur in rare, chronic lung diseases of ruminants termed pulmonary adenomatosis.

LUNG ABSCESSES

Abscesses in the lung most often are bronchiogenic in origin. That is, they are complications of bronchopneumonia or chronic bronchiolitis and bronchiectasis. Newly formed abscesses are foci of necrotic lung parenchyma and purulent exudate surrounded by a zone of acute inflammation, chiefly neutrophils. Older abscesses are encapsulated by a peripheral zone of connective tissue. The thickness and collagen content of the capsule correlates with the chronicity of the lesion.

Lung abscesses also arise by distribution in the blood of pyogenic bacteria, or emboli of bacterial colonies, or septic thrombi. Experimentally, they can be reproduced by the intravenous injection of bacteria-containing agar emboli. Direct penetration of the lung through the chest wall only rarely causes abscessation, for it is usually fatal due to hemorrhage or acute purulent pleuritis.

GANGRENE

Gangrenous pneumonia results from the aspiration of milk, oral medicaments, and other foreign substances that lodge in the bronchioles. Inhalation may cause diffuse deposition throughout the lungs. The reaction is especially severe if the inhaled material is contaminated with bacteria.

The aspiration of oils, kerosene, or vomitus is particularly bad, for these substances cause necrosis of large portions of the lung. When saprophytic bacteria contaminate affected areas, gangrene results and death invariably ensues.

EMPHYSEMA

Emphysema is overinflation of the alveoli. The alveoli are distended with air which cannot escape via the bronchioles or through the capillary bed. Focal areas of emphysema commonly accompany pneumonitis, pneumonia, and parasite infestation of the lungs. With few exceptions, however, the great significance of emphysema is when it occurs as a diffuse disease of the lung that progresses to cause general debility and cardiac failure. This occurs as peculiar syndromes in horses (Eyre 1972; Foley and Lowell 1966) and cattle (Moulton et al. 1963) and has been produced experimentally in laboratory rodents (Frasca et al. 1971, Pushpakom et al. 1970; Strawbridge 1960). Emphysema occurs in humans as a consequence of chronic bronchitis, and heavy cigarette smoking is involved in the high incidence of the disease.

In animals emphysema is common in lesions of pneumonia and inflammatory diseases of the lung. At the lung periphery, small areas of "collateral" emphysema alternate with foci of atelectasis. They represent alveoli that have expanded excessively due to pressure of the air inhaled to occupy the spaces vacated by adjacent atelectatic alveoli. Emphysema is also produced when bronchioles are plugged with mucus or purulent exudate. During inspiration the alveolus fills with air that cannot be removed during expiration because of the plug.

Senile emphysema is commonly seen in

Fig. 7.8. Consolidation, fibrosis, and epithelialization in chronic verminous pneumonia in a dog. A. Histology. Alveolar walls covered with cuboidal epithelium; interstitial areas expanded with collagen and inflammatory cells. B. Granular pneumocytes line basement membrane (arrows) of alveolar wall (cuboidal epithelium seen histologically). Note microvilli on luminal surfaces. Inflammatory cells packing alveolus (top) are eosinophils (with dark granules), neutrophils (N), macrophages (M), and small lymphocytes (L). C. Neutrophils fixed in process of phagocytizing granules from degenerating granular pneumocyte (right).

aged dogs. This is not truly emphysema, for there are no distension of alveoli, no bullae on the surface, and no enlargement of the lungs. The alveolar wall is thin and lacking in granular pneumocytes. There are ruptured alveoli and obvious breakage of the walls. The interstitium of the wall contains excess collagen, which is responsible for the lack of resilience of the lung parenchyma. The lesions are diffusely distributed and tend to be most severe at the periphery of the lung.

Emphysema is exaggerated by the forced breathing and gasping of dyspnea. This may be responsible for rupture of affected alveoli. In severe cases, large, thin-walled, air-filled bullae may develop and lead to fatal pneumothorax in mammals. The danger of diffuse emphysema, however, is the increased pulmonary pressure it produces and its effect on the right heart. Hypertrophy of the right heart accompanies diffuse emphysema; but, if the disease is prolonged and progressive, cardiac failure is inevitable.

ATELECTASIS

Atelectasis refers either to incomplete expansion of the lungs at birth or to collapse of a previously normal lung. In the newborn animal that has never breathed or has lived only a few minutes, the alveolar walls in the atelectatic areas do not markedly differ cytologically from those in the normal lung. The alveolar walls, which in the newborn contain many granular pneumocytes, are merely closely aligned. In the mature lung, foci of atelectasis are common in chronic pulmonary disease. Atelectasis occurs in all species except birds, where the rigid structure of the parabronchi prevent collapse of the alveoli.

Atelectasis is also used synonymously with "collapse" of the lung. Pressure of the lung due to fluid, pneumothorax, tumors, or abscesses drives out the air from the affected lung and the walls collapse against one another. Because the airflow is diminished and the affected lung parenchyma is in oxygen deficit, the capillaries dilate and the atelectatic area is hyperemic. The chronic vascular changes which ensue lead to thickening of the alveolar walls and progressive degenerative changes in

the pneumocytes. The deposition of fibrin and other plasma proteins and the lack of surfactant between the walls may promote fusion. Fibroplasia in the interstitium of the alveolar wall may cause irreversible injury (Fig. 7.9).

Obstructive atelectasis is due to the accumulation of material such as mucus in the bronchioles. The airway is fully obstructed. Air cannot enter the alveolus and it collapses. The amount of lung affected depends on the level of the airway obstructed.

CHRONIC DISEASE OF THE ALVEOLAR WALL

Chronic inflammatory disease of the lung may involve diffuse changes accompanying a systemic disturbance or focal lesions of repair superimposed over smouldering, slowly progressive acute inflammation. The hallmarks of the chronic process in the alveolar wall are: (1) mesenchymal thickening of the wall due to deposition of ground substance, collagen, and elastin; (2) granular pneumocytic epithelization; (3) hypertrophy of smooth muscle under the epithelial lining of the terminal bronchioles; and (4) peribronchial lymphoid hyperplasia. These reactions can accompany any chronic inflammatory focus in the lung; the components vary according to the irritant involved. Some of the diverse diseases so characterized are chronic bacterial pneumonia of the pig caused by Bordetella (Duncan et al. 1966), chronic progressive viral pneumonias of sheep (Ressang et al. 1968), and pyrrolizidine alkaloid poisoning in several species (Harding et al. 1964).

AGING

The alveolar wall of aged mammals is thinned and contains few granular pneumocytes. The interstitial areas contain increased amounts of collagen and deposits of basement membrane material and ground substance (Fig. 7.10). Bronchiectasis and breaks in the alveolar wall are common. These changes limit the capacity of the lung to completely recover from inflammatory disease. The changes of aging are accentuated by pathologic changes that accompany systemic diseases which com-

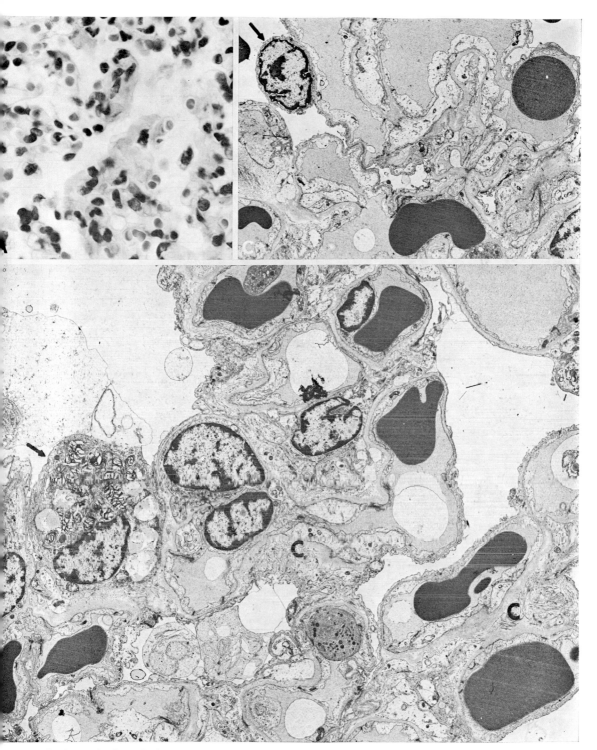

Fig. 7.9. Atelectasis, lung of dog was markedly compressed by large intrathoracic tumor. A. Histology. Alveoli are diminished or obliterated. Alveolar walls are hyperemic, thickened, and contain deposits of fibrin. B. Ultrastructure. Note distorted capillaries, deposits of collagen (C), and thickened basement membranes. Granular pneumocytes (arrow) are degenerate. C. Obliteration of alveolus and degeneration of membranous pneumocytes (arrow).

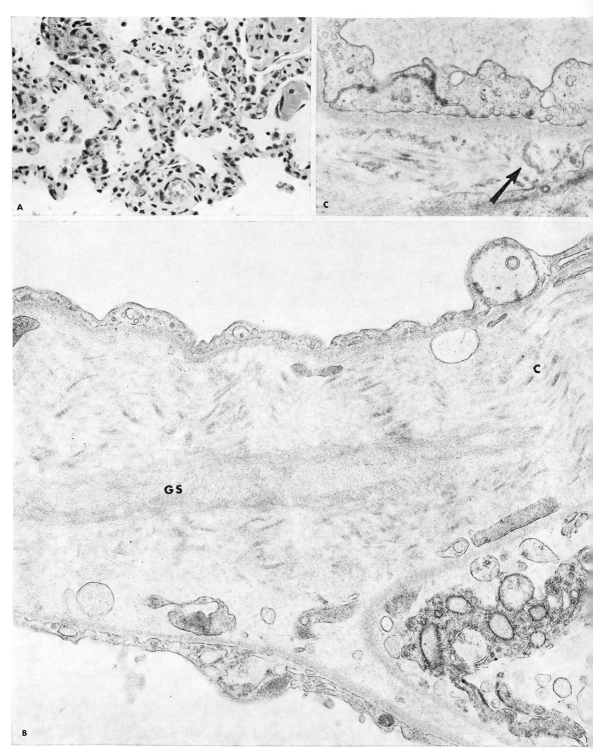

Fig. 7.10. Fibrosis of the alveolar walls in a dog with severe dyspnea, hypoxia, and chronic lung disease associated with hyperparathyroidism. A. Histology. Alveolar walls are thick and macrophages are present in the alveoli. Aggregates of organized fibrin are in alveoli. B. Deposition of collagen (C) and granular ground substance (GS) in the interstitium. Mitochondria are degenerate and protrude into the alveolus (a manifestation of severe hypoxia). Capillary (lower right) is necrotic. C. Endothelial cells in a capillary. The basement lamina is thickened and elastin (arrow) is present beneath it.

monly afflict older animals. Uremia, cardiac failure, liver disease (Popovic and Mullane 1972), and diseases involving hypercalcemia all have a degenerative effect on the alveolar wall.

FIBROSIS

Diffuse pulmonary fibrosis may result from inhalation or expiration of toxic substances that cannot be metabolized by the lung. Prolonged low levels of noxious chemicals in inspired air produce slow progressive degenerative changes accompanied by extensive diffuse fibroplasia of the alveolar wall interstitium. Early phases of aerogenic toxicity involve vacuolation and other degenerative changes in membranous pneumocytes and capillary endothelium. Hyperplasia of granular pneumocytes and epithelization occur as reparative processes. If toxicity continues there is progressive deposition of acidic mucopolysaccharides, collagen, and, in some cases, calcium crystals (Larsen 1959; Suzuki 1969).

Chronic pulmonary fibrosis can also be produced by toxins that arrive in the lung hematogenously and are eliminated during exhalation. Bleomycin, an intravenously administered anticancer agent, produces damage to the endothelium of the alveolar wall in this way. Endothelial cell swelling and separation cause movement of protein-rich fluid into the interstitium and subsequent slowly progressive fibrosis of the wall (Adamson and Bowden 1974).

Silica, which induces granulomas in the lung, exists in dust in amorphous and crystalline forms. The latter is particularly important in induction of fibrosing alveolitis. Following phagocytosis by alveolar macrophages, necrosis occurs due to damage by crystals of 0.5μ or less to lysosomal membranes (Allison et al. 1966). Hydrolytic enzymes leak into the interstitium of the alveolar wall producing lysis. Cycling of the silica which cannot be broken down results in prolonged destruction of macrophages. The silica and necrotic debris are finally walled off by a granulomatous reaction and collagen production throughout the lung is marked.

CALCIFICATION

Diffuse pulmonary calcification (pulmonary microlithiasis, pumice lung) is com-

monly seen in the dog: in young pups as a consequence of vitamin D toxicity and in aged dogs accompanying chronic renal insufficiency (uremia) and hyperparathyroidism. The lungs at necropsy are large, do not collapse, and have a granular, gritty feeling. Microscopically there are innumerable calcified concretions (calcospheres) in the alveolar wall throughout the lung. Despite this affection, signs of respiratory disease are often surprisingly few. If unresolved, however, diffuse calcification induces a slowly progressive interstitial fibrosis, with increasing dyspnea and respiratory difficulty.

The process of diffuse calcification of the lung is associated with elevations in blood calcium or hypercalcemia. It represents "metastatic" calcification as opposed to the dystrophic type that occurs in foci of injured lung parenchyma associated with necrosis. In the early stages, crystals of calcium are first deposited in foci of acidic mucopolysaccharide deposition and along elastic fibers (see Fig. 2.29). When calcium is being laid down rapidly, the basement membrane between the capillary endothelium and membranous pneumocytes is also a preferential site of deposition (Eggerman and Kapanci 1971). The calcified basement membrane is nodular, due to the capricious manner in which the mineral is deposited.

In advanced pulmonary calcification, calcium deposits are present throughout the alveolar wall. The alveolar wall progressively thickens, massive nodular deposits of concentric light and dark rings project into the alveolus and may become large enough to be seen grossly. Granular pneumocyte hyperplasia accompanies the deposition of calcium and adds to the thickness of the wall. This process is an attempt at repair and the granular pneumocyte is rarely affected by calcium deposition.

Diffuse pulmonary calcification also is a sequel of viral pneumonitis and pneumonia in some species. Varicella "pneumonia," a complication of severe cases of human chicken pox, is often followed by deposition of calcium in the lungs (Jones and Cameron 1969).

EPITHELIZATION

Chronic lung disease is often accompanied by proliferation of granular pneumocytes which line the alveolar spaces. Called *epithelization,* the process is the common response of the alveolar wall to chronic inflammation. Proliferation of the bronchiolar epithelium, particularly of its "Clara cells" (which closely resemble the granular pneumocytes), also occurs, and it is uncertain which cell type the response represents.

Epithelization reaches its extreme in a disease of sheep called pulmonary adenomatosis. Multiple foci of granular pneumocytes proliferate, allegedly under the stimulus of a virus, and form solid foci of neoplasticlike lesions. In some cases similar lesions are present in draining lymph nodes and it is believed that this condition represents a curious borderland case between hyperplasia and neoplasia.

PHYLOGENY OF THE RESPIRATORY ORGANS

GILLS

Fish and larval amphibia utilize gills (branchiae) for respiration and for the excretion of salt and nitrogenous wastes. Gas exchange can be accomplished through the epithelia of the pharynx, branchial cavity, and intestine in some species of stagnant swamp-dwelling fish (Jasinski 1973). Gills of the bony or teleost fishes consist of internal bony gill arches that are covered by an operculum. The blood from the heart enters the afferent branchial artery from the ventral aorta, perfuses through gill capillaries, returns to the efferent branchial artery, and goes directly to the dorsal aorta and the peripheral circulation.

The respiratory unit in fish is the *gill filament* which is attached to and projects outward from the concave surface of the bony gill arch. Gill filaments are lancet shaped and contain a border of long respiratory lamellae. The *lamella* is simply an extension of specialized capillaries from the efferent branchial arteriole which is covered by simple flattened respiratory epithelium (Fig. 7.11). In function, it is analogous to the alveolar wall in vertebrate lungs. Ultrastructurally, the unspecialized gill epithelial cells contain many pinocytotic vesicles but few other organelles (Morgan and Tovell 1973; Wright 1973).

Gills are also highly important in water and electrolyte balance. Freshwater teleost fishes such as perch and carp do not drink significant amounts of water but gain it by osmosis through the gill lamellae. They require salts which are actively taken in by absorptive chloride cells on the gills. Marine teleost fishes normally drink sea water and its salts are absorbed into the blood. To maintain electrolyte levels, the gills actively transfer salt from blood to sea water via specialized excretory "chloride" cells on the gill lamellae. Ultrastructurally, the chloride cells are distinguished by large amounts of endoplasmic reticulum (Philpott and Copeland 1963; Threadgold and Houston 1964) and repeating particles on the plasma membrane which extend into the cytoplasm (Ritch and Philpott 1969). The outward transport of sodium is due to a Na^+-K^+-activated ATPase in the plasma membrane (Forrest et al. 1973).

GILL DISEASE

Most known diseases of fish gills are caused by invasion of parasites of the gill epithelium (Molnar 1972). Gill flukes and many species of protozoa encyst within the respiratory lamellae, deform them, and cause degeneration and necrosis of adjacent structures. In epitheliocystis disease, the causal chlamydial organisms replicate in the epithelial cells of the gill lamellae. Cells become enlarged, fill with organisms, and desquamate (Wolke et al. 1970).

Hyperplasia of respiratory epithelial cells of the lamellae is a common response to infection. In myxobacterial disease clumps of bacteria aggregate on the lamellar surface. Hyperplasia begins in the lamellae at the distal end of the gill filament. Subsequent fusion of distorted lamellae results in large bulbous deformations in the filaments.

The nonrespiratory surface of the gills has columnar epithelium containing many goblet cells. Mucous hyperplasia with heavy deposition of mucus on the gills accompanies extensive injury. If prolonged, accumulations of slime may inhibit oxygen diffusion and cause respiratory difficulty.

Neoplasms of the gills have not been adequately studied and primary tumors have not been reported. Metastatic inva-

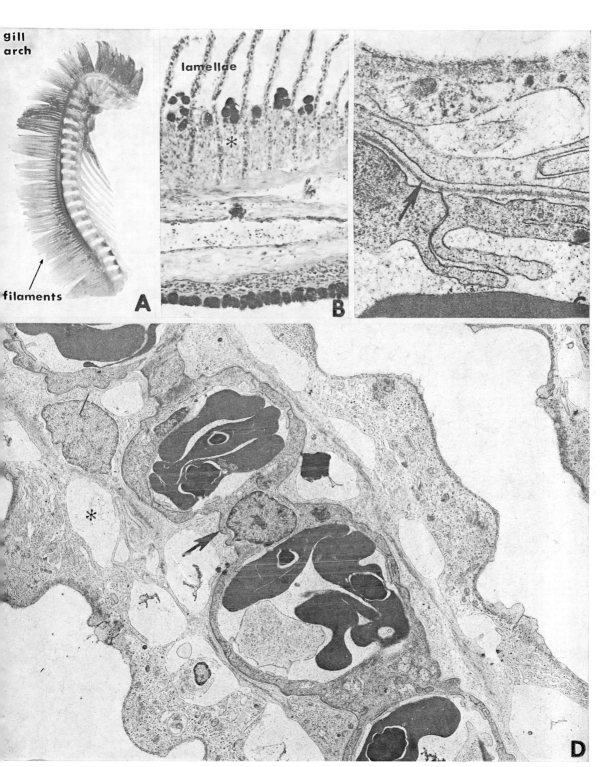

Fig. 7.11. Fish gill. A. Gill arch composed of bony arch and projecting filaments. B. Filament with surface lamellae. C. Ultrastructure of blood-water barrier, basement membrane (arrow). D. Emphysema of the lamella of a gill filament. Capillaries are dilated. Note pillar cell (arrow) and separated interepithelial cell junctions (asterisk).

sion by carcinomas occurs and tumor emboli lodge in the blood vessels of the gill filament interstitium (Ashley 1970). Infiltration and replication of thymic lymphosarcomas have been reported in trout gills.

Gills are normally red. Hyperemia, which is common in waters that are low in oxygen or are excessively warm, intensifies this color. Fish respond to anoxia by dilatation of the lamellar capillaries, increased rapidity of inhalation, and wider opening of the operculae. In very sick fish, gills are usually pale, indicating ischemia. Pallor develops rapidly after death or when gills are out of water.

Infarction of the gills may be due to intravascular parasites or to gas emboli that form when fish are swimming in very warm water containing many plants. Excessive oxygen is produced and causes gas bubbles to develop and lodge in the vascular system. Phycomycetes are the cause of a vascular disease called gill rot. Fungi grow into the veins of the gill filaments causing hemostases and infarction.

BRANCHIITIS

Inflammation of the gills is a response to microbial infection and some toxic injuries. Hyperemia and edema of the lamellae are followed by cell exudations. Leukocytes infiltrate the interstitial areas of the gill causing purulent *branchiitis*. Ballooning of the lamellae results from accumulation of exudate. Specialized "pillar cells" are intimately associated with the blood channels of the lamellae (Hughes and Weibel 1972). They are analogous to reticulum cells in mammalian lymphoid tissues and are phagocytic during the inflammatory process in fish gills.

Edema is a common response of the gill to injury. The lamellae become enlarged and swollen, particularly at the tips which become bulbous. Edematous lamellae are commonly seen in fish swimming in toxic water. DDT has been shown to cause swelling of lamellae with infiltration of leukocytes. If prolonged, dilatation and engorgement of the branchial vessels distend and distort the gill filament.

SWIM BLADDER AND AEROCYSTITIS

Air-filled swim bladders, which develop from an evagination of the foregut, are present in teleost fishes. The function is hydrostatic. Gas volume is regulated and affects the specific gravity of the fish. Gas enters the bladder hematogenously via a remarkable network of small arterioles and venules called the rete mirabilis or "red body." Gas is reabsorbed by specialized epithelium (Brooks 1970) or, in fish which have a patent duct connected to the gut, is bubbled out the mouth. Swim bladders are properly termed lungs when they function in gaseous exchange, as they do in lung fish.

Disease of the swim bladder results in the inability to maintain equilibrium; affected fish develop tumbling movements and tend to swim on the bottom. The swim bladder is compressed during enlargement of other abdominal organs. It may be ruptured by underwater explosions and by bringing deeply swimming fish species to the surface too quickly.

Infectious aerocystitis is a contagious disease of carp caused by a rhabdovirus (Bachman and Ahne 1973). It is particularly important in carp culture farms where the disease can produce severe losses. Lesions in the swim bladder are vascular in origin and include hyperemia and petechiation. Similar lesions develop in the brain and heart.

Purulent aerocystitis is bacterial and is generally due to *Aeromonas* or *Myxobolus* spp. Several protozoans, including the coccidium *Eimeria gadi,* encyst in the swim bladder and cause marked thickening of the wall due to deposition of developmental stages.

THE LUNG

The evolution of the lung is phylogenetically linked to climatic conditions in successive geological times. In the early Devonian period, when fish constituted the vertebrate fauna, the environment was alternately arid and wet with torrential rains. Heat in the atmosphere decreased the oxygen content of stagnant pools while also increasing the metabolic rate of aquatic animal life. The primordial lung evolved to cope with these hypoxic waters and to take advantage of the higher oxygen supply of air. The simplest lung (that of the lungfish), which phylogenetically occupies a position between fish and amphibia, consists of two simple muscular tubes lined by capillaries (Hughes and Datta Munshi 1968). Proceeding up the scale through amphibia there is progressive partitioning of this tube, resulting in double capillary beds. In mammals the walls are fused and the capillary bed ramifies through the interstitium, being exposed on either side. The dolphin, which must withstand drastic pressure changes of diving, has retained a double wall and dense connective tissue septa.

AMPHIBIANS AND REPTILES

The lungs of amphibians and reptiles are relatively simple paired sacs. Each contains one major respiratory duct (bronchus). The ciliated columnar epithelium of the bronchi with its mucous cells and subepithelial population of lymphoid cells is extremely important in the defense of the respiratory tract. In amphibians, gas exchange occurs not only through the lungs but through the skin and oral mucous membranes as well. Amphibian tracheas are short and their lungs differ in shape. Those of tailed species (salamanders) are elongate; those of the anurans (frogs and toads) are bulbous. Reptilian lungs show even more striking differences in shape. Reptilian tracheas are long and in some species are convoluted.

The lungs of frogs, toads, and salamanders are partitioned by thick interlobular septa into compartments appropriately termed alveoli. Capillaries ramify over the surface of the interlobular septa but do not penetrate the connective tissue lamellae and are thus in contact with only one alveolus. Capillary endothelial cells contain large numbers of dense, membrane-bound granules. A thin continuous layer of epithelial cells overlies the heavy carpet of respiratory capillaries. These membranous pneumocytes lie between the capillaries; their thin squamous cytoplasmic extensions are stretched over the vascular walls (Meban 1973).

Amphibian membranous pneumocytes are filled with ribosomes and a few large dense granules with an osmiophilic lamellar internal structure. These granules (which in birds and mammals are restricted to a more differentiated cell, the granular pneumocyte) contain lipopolysaccharides which are important in reducing surface tension in the lung (Dierichs 1973). In chronic inflammation the amphibian membranous pneumocyte proliferates and differentiates to cells with large numbers of lipopolysaccharide-filled granules. The alveolar wall becomes lined with these cells, a process called epithelization. Macrophages in amphibian lungs, like their mammalian counterparts, originate from circulating monocytes.

The mechanism of lung filling in frogs consists of compression rather than suction as in mammals. The frog fills the buccal cavity with air by contracting the buccal floor ("buccal cycle"). It blows the pulmonary contents through this fresh air in the buccal cavity without mixing and then, by closing the nostrils, pumps the fresh air into the lungs in a "ventilatory cycle" (Gans et al. 1969).

The lungs of reptiles are perfused via pulmonary arteries from a common ventricle. In snakes, the lungs are elongate and are divided into anterior alveolar and posterior saccular zones. The anterior lung has a higher ventilatory rate and blood flow; circulating microemboli are trapped preferentially in this zone (Read and Donnelly 1972).

Pathologic changes in amphibian and reptilian lungs are dominated by inflammatory conditions, particularly those due to nematodes and protozoa (Fig. 7.12). Focal granulomatous pneumonia is common but only rarely is the cause of death. Respiration through nonlung tissue makes compromised lung function of lesser importance than in birds and mammals.

BIRDS

The respiratory system of birds is the most complicated (and most efficient) in the animal kingdom. The main bronchus does not ramify as in mammals but passes through the entire lung, giving off groups of secondary bronchi. These in turn give rise to parabronchi (tertiary bronchi) which, in the large medial portions of the lung, anastomose with one another. The tortuous channels of respiratory capillaries and septal walls surround the parabronchi. The air spaces or "respiratory channels" communicate with the parabronchi via respiratory atria (King 1956). The epithelium of the parabronchi is highly reactive in hypoxic and inflammatory disease of the avian lung (Länsimies and Karkola 1973).

The septal wall, as seen ultrastructurally, is lined with thin membranous pneumocytes which cover the respiratory capillaries and interstitium of the wall (Fig. 7.13).

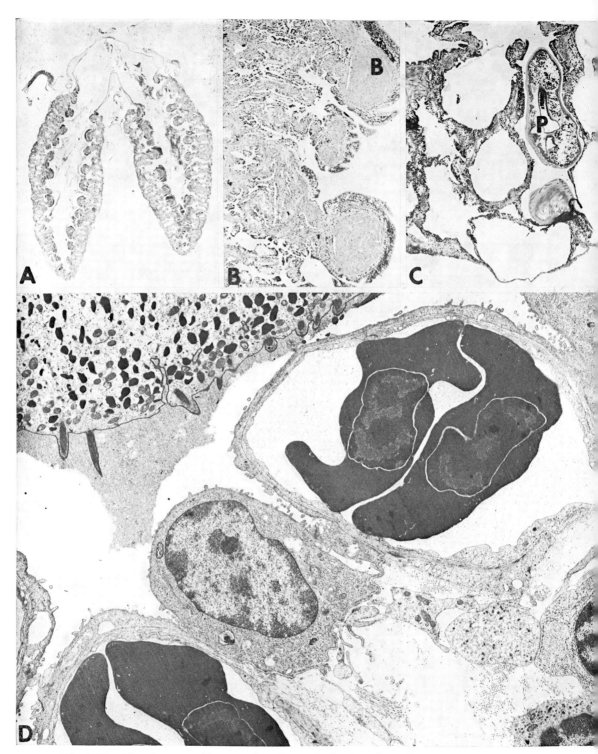

Fig. 7.12. Verminous emphysema, frog lung. A. Section through entire lungs. B. Histology of bronchial wall. Note large muscular bands (B). C. Blockade of bronchiole by nematode parasite (P). D. Ultrastructure of parasite-alveolar wall interface. Membranous pneumocyte (center) is separated by two capillaries. Parasite at upper left.

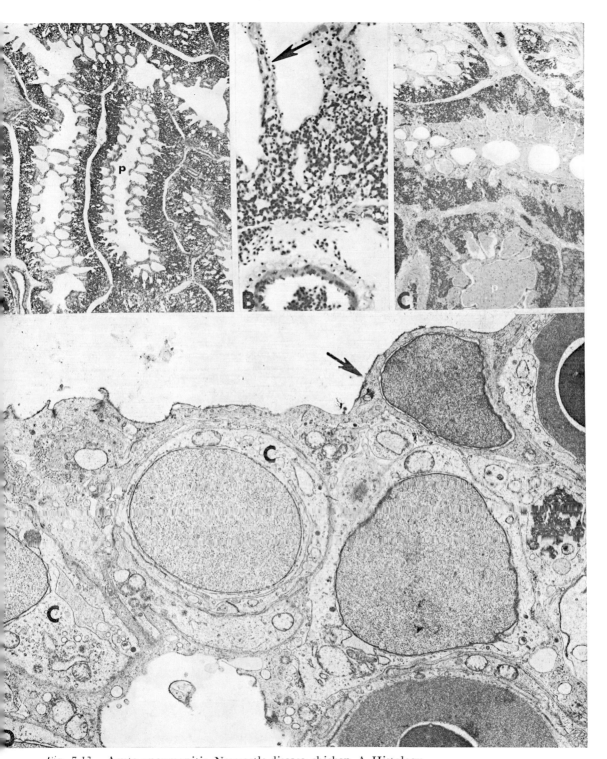

Fig. 7.13. Acute pneumonitis, Newcastle disease, chicken. A. Histology of airways. Parabronchus (p). B. Enlargement showing wall of respiratory atrium (arrow), septal walls of air spaces (center), and pulmonary artery. C. Severe pulmonary edema with necrosis of the parabronchi. D. Ultrastructure. Note membanous pneumocyte (arrow), capillary (C).

Granular pneumocytes, which contain dense laminar inclusions, are sparse but occur regularly at the surface of the septal wall (Adamson and Bowden 1973). They are the source of tension-reducing lipopolysaccharides which cover the membranous pneumocytes and can be seen as dense, irregular, amorphous strands (Petrik and Riedel 1968; Tyler and Pangborn 1964). Distinctive membrane-bound dense inclusions appear also in the nongranular pneumocytes at the time of hatching and their excretion is stimulated by air breathing (Jones and Radnor 1972).

The most striking difference of the avian respiratory tract is the elaborate system of air sacs and air spaces within the central areas of the bones. All of these connect to the lungs. On inhalation, air passes completely through the lung and into the air sacs. During exhalation it passes back again and more completely fills the air channels. Air sacs are poorly vascularized and do not function directly in gaseous exchange.

Normal air sacs are thin sheets of squamous mesothelial cells which are supplied by a delicate base of blood vessels and fibrous connective tissue (Carlson and Beggs 1973). Large portions of the air sac membranes are avascular. The early response to injury or infection is serous or fibrinous exudation. The mesothelial membrane rapidly undergoes metaplasia to form cuboidal cells and also columnar cells. Many of the latter form mucus and some are ciliated.

A bird with a blocked trachea can still breathe if a connection is made between one of its pneumatized bones and the outside air. John Hunter, in 1758, demonstrated this capacity: ". . . I cut the wing through the os humeri . . . and [on] tying of the trachea . . . found that the air passed to and from the lungs by the canal in this bone."

REFERENCES

Adamson, I. Y. R. and Bowden, D. H. The intracellular site of surfactant synthesis. Autoradiographic studies on murine and avian lung explants. *Exp. Mol. Path.* 18: 112, 1973.

———. The pathogenesis of bleomycin induced pulmonary fibrosis in mice. *Am. J. Path.* 77:185, 1974.

———. Derivation of type 1 epithelium from type 2 cells in the developing rat lung. *Lab. Invest.* 32:736, 1975.

Allison, A. C., Harington, J. S. and Birbeck, M. An examination of the cytotoxic effects of silica on macrophages. *J. Exp. Med.* 124:141, 1966.

Ashley, L. M. Pathology of fish fed aflatoxins and other antimetabolites. *Symp. Dis. Fish and Shellfish.* S. F. Snieszku, ed., p. 366. Spec. Publ. 5, Am. Fish. Soc., Wash., D.C., 1970.

Askin, F. B. and Kuhn, C. The cellular origin of pulmonary surfactant. *Lab. Invest.* 25: 260, 1971.

Asmundsson, T. and Kilburn, K. H. Mucociliary clearance rates of various levels in dogs' lungs. *Am. Rev. Resp. Dis.* 102:388, 1970.

Asmundsson, T., Kilburn, K. H. and McKenzie, W. N. Injury and metaplasia of airway cells due to SO_2. *Lab. Invest.* 29:41, 1973.

Bachmann, P. A. and Ahne, W. Isolation and characterization of agent causing swim bladder inflammation in carp. *Nature* 244:235, 1973.

Bang, B. G. and Bang, F. B. Experimentally induced change in nasal mucous secretory systems and their effect on virus infection in chickens. *J. Exp. Med.* 130:105, 1969.

Baskerville, A. et al. Further studies on experimental bacterial pneumonia: Ultrastructural changes produced in the lungs by *Salmonella cholerae-suis*. *Brit. J. Exp. Path.* 54:90, 1973.

Beall, F. A. and Dalldorf, F. G. The pathogenesis of lethal effect of anthrax toxin in the rat. *J. Inf. Dis.* 116:377, 1966.

Bernstein, J. et al. Mucopolysaccharide in the pulmonary alveolus. *Lab. Invest.* 21:420, 1969.

Bienenstock, J., Johnston, N. and Perey, D. Y. E. Bronchial lymphoid tissue. *Lab. Invest.* 28:686, 1973.

Bowden, D. H. et al. The origin of the lung macrophage. *Arch. Path.* 88:540, 1969.

Breeze, R. G. et al. Fog fever in cattle. *J. Comp. Path.* 85:147, 1975.

Brooks, R. E. Ultrastructure of lung lesions produced by ingested chemicals. *Lab. Invest.* 25:536, 1971.

———. Ultrastructure of the physostomatous swim bladder of rainbow trout *(Salmo gairdineri). Zt. Zellf.* 106:473, 1970.

Buckingham, S. et al. Phospholipid synthesis in large pulmonary alveolar cell. Its relation to pulmonary surfactants. *Am. J. Path.* 48:1027, 1966.

Carlson, H. C. and Beggs, E. C. Ultrastructure of the abdominal air sac of the fowl. *Res. Vet. Sci.* 14:148, 1973.

Chen, H. I. and Chai, C. Y. Pulmonary edema and hemorrhage as a consequence of systemic vasoconstriction. *Am. J. Physiol.* 227:144, 1974.

Chevalier, G. and Collet, A. J. In vivo incorporation of choline-^{3}H, leucine-^{3}H and galactose-^{3}H in alveolar type II pneumocytes in relation to surfactant synthesis. *Anat. Rec.* 174:289, 1972.

Colacicco, S. and Scarpelli, E. M. Pulmonary surfactants: Phospholipid or lipoprotein. *Fed. Proc.* 29:661, 1970.

Cunningham, A. I. and Hurley, J. V. Alpha-naphthyl-thiourea-induced pulmonary oedema in the rat. *J. Path.* 106:25, 1972.

Curtain, C. C., Clark, B. C. and Duffy, J. H. The origins of the immunoglobulins in the mucous secretions of cattle. *Clin. Exp. Immun.* 8:335, 1971.

Cutz, E. et al. Endocrine cells in rat fetal lungs. *Lab. Invest.* 30:458, 1974.

Dahlgren, S. E. and Dalen, H. Ultrastructural observations on chemically induced inflammation in guinea pig trachea. *Virch. Arch. B* 11:211, 1972.

Dierichs, R. Elektronenmikroskopische Untersuchungen an der Froschlunge. I. Darstellung der Alveolar-Grenzschicht (Surfactant). *Zt. Zellf.* 137:533, 1973.

Duncan, J. R., Ramsey, F. K. and Switzer, W. P. Pathology of experimental *Bordetella bronchiseptica* infection in swine: Pneumonia. *Am. J. Vet. Res.* 27:467, 1966.

Eggerman, J. and Kapanci, Y. Experimental pulmonary calcinosis in the rat. Ultrastructural and morphometric studies. *Lab. Invest.* 24:469, 1971.

Eyre, P. Equine pulmonary emphysema. *Vet. Rec.* 91:134, 1972.

Farr, G. H., Harley, R. A. and Hennigar, G. R. Desquamative interstitial pneumonia. An electron microscopic study. *Am. J. Path.* 60:347, 1970.

Finegold, M. J. Interstitial pulmonary edema. *Lab. Invest.* 16:912, 1967.

———. Pneumonic plague in monkeys. *Am. J. Path.* 54:167, 1969.

Flodh, H. and Magnusson, G. Genesis of foam cells. *Virch. Arch. B* 12:360, 1973.

Foley, F. D. and Lowell, F. C. Equine centrolobular emphysema. *Am. Rev. Resp. Dis.* 93:17, 1966.

Forrest, J. N. et al. Sodium transport and sodium-potassium-ATPase in gills. Effect of cortisol. *Am. J. Physiol.* 224:709, 1973.

Frasca, J. M. Electron microscopic observation of the bronchial epithelium of dogs. *Exp. Mol. Path.* 9:363, 1968.

Frasca, J. M. et al. Electron microscopic observations on pulmonary fibrosis and emphysema in smoking dogs. *Exp. Mol. Path.* 15:108, 1971.

Gans, C., de Jongh, H. J. and Farber, J. Bullfrog *(Rana catesbiana)* ventilation: How does the frog breathe? *Science* 12:1223, 1969.

Giddens, W. E. and Fairchild, G. A. Effects of sulfur dioxide on the nasal mucosa of mice. *Arch. Envir. Hlth.* 25:166, 1972.

Godleski, J. J. and Brain, J. D. The origin of alveolar macrophages in mouse radiation chimeras. *J. Exp. Med.* 136:630, 1972.

Goldenberg, V. E., Buckingham, S. and Sommers, S. C. Pilocarpine stimulation of granular pneumocyte secretion. *Lab. Invest.* 20:147, 1969.

Gould, V. E. and Smuckler, E. A. Alveolar injury in acute carbon tetrachloride intoxication. *Arch. Int. Med.* 128:109, 1971.

Harding, J. D. J. et al. Experimental poisoning by *Senecia jacobaea* in pigs. *Vet. Path.* 1:204, 1964.

Hayes, J. A. and Shiga, A. Ultrastructural changes in pulmonary edema produced experimentally with ammonium sulfate. *J. Path.* 100:281, 1970.

Hughes, G. M. and Datta Munshi, J. S. Fine structure of the respiratory surfaces of air breathing fish, the climbing perch *Anabus testudineus* (Bloch). *Nature* 219:1382, 1968.

Hughes, G. M. and Weibel, E. R. Similarity of supporting tissue in fish gills and the mammalian reticuloendothelium. *J. Ult. Res.* 39:106, 1972.

Hung, K.-S. et al. Innervation of pulmonary alveoli of the mouse lung. *Am. J. Anat.* 135:477, 1972.

Jasinski, A. Air-blood barrier in the respiratory intestine of the pond-loach *Misgurnus fossilis* L. *Acta Anat.* 86:376, 1973.

Jones, A. W. and Radnor, C. J. P. The development of the chick tertiary bronchus. II. The origin of the surface lining system. *J. Anat.* 113:325, 1972.

Jones, E. L. and Cameron, A. H. Pulmonary calcification in viral pneumonia. *J. Clin. Path.* 22:361, 1969.

Kass, E. H., Green, G. M. and Goldstein, E. Mechanisms of antibacterial action in the respiratory system. *Bact. Rev.* 30:488, 1966.

Kikkawa, Y., Motoyama, E. K. and Gluck, L. Study of the lungs of fetal and newborn rabbits. *Am. J. Path.* 52:177, 1968.

Kikkawa, Y. et al. Mucopolysaccharide in the pulmonary alveolus. II. Electron microscopic observations. *Lab. Invest.* 22:272, 1970.

King. A. S. The structure and function of the respiratory pathways of *Gallus domesticus*. *Vet. Rec.* 66:544, 1956.

Länsimies, E. and Karkola, K. Enzyme histochemical studies of the lung of domestic fowl. *Acta Path. Micro. Scand. A* 81:159, 1973.

Larsen, K. A. Diffuse progressive interstitial fibrosis of the lungs. *Acta Path. Micro. Scand.* 45:167, 1959.

Laurenzi, G. A. et al. Clearance of bacteria by the lower respiratory tract. *Science* 142:1572, 1963.

Lauweryns, J. M., Cokelaere, M. and Theunynck, P. Serotonin producing neuroepithelial bodies in rabbit respiratory mucosa. *Science* 180:410, 1973.

Lieberman, P. et al. Effect of antigen variation on production of antibody in canine tracheal secretions. *J. Immun.* 107:1349, 1971.

Lillie, L. E. and Thompson, R. G. The pulmonary clearance of bacteria by calves and mice. *Can. J. Comp. Med. Vet. Sci.* 36:129, 1972.

Livingston, C. W. et al. Pathogenesis of mycoplasmal pneumonia in swine. *Am. J. Vet. Res.* 33:2249, 1972.

Lüllmann, H., Lüllman-Rauch, R. and Reil, G. H. A comparative ultrastructural study of the effects of chlorphentermine and triparanol in rat lung and adrenal gland. *Virch. Arch. B* 12:91, 1973.

Lüthgen, W. Untersuchungen zum Nachweis von Antikörperchen in Tracheal-exudate des Huhnes nach experimenteller Infektion mit Newcastlevirus. *Zt. Immun.* 144:273, 1972.

Mahaffey, L. W. and Rossdale, P. D. A convulsive syndrome in newborn foals resembling pulmonary syndrome in the newborn infant. *Lancet* 1:1223, 1969.

McCarthy, C., Reid, L. and Gibbons, R. A. Intra-alveolar mucus removal by macrophages with iron accumulation. *J. Path.* 87:39, 1964.

Meban, C. The pneumocytes in the lung of *Xenopus laevis*. *J. Anat.* 114:235, 1973.

Meyer, E. C. and Ottaviano, R. The effect of fibrin on the morphometric distribution of pulmonary exudative edema. *Lab. Invest.* 29:320, 1973.

Molnàr, K. Studies on gill parasitosis of the grasscarp *(Ctenopharyngodon idella)* caused by *Dactylogyrus lamellatus* Achmerov 1952. IV. Histopathologic studies. *Acta Vet.* 22:9, 1972.

Morgan, M. and Tovell, P. W. A. The structure of the gill of the trout, *Salmo gairdneri*. *Zt. Zellf.* 142:147, 1973.

Moulton, J. E., Cornelius, C. E. and Osborn, B. I. Acute pulmonary emphysema in cattle. *J.A.V.M.A.* 142:133, 1963.

Petrik, P. and Riedel, B. A continuous osmiophilic noncellular membrane at the respiratory surface of the lungs of fetal chickens and of young chicks. *Lab. Invest.* 18:54, 1968.

Philpott, O. W. and Copeland, D. F. Fine structure of the chloride cells from three species of Fundulus. *J. Cell Biol.* 18:389, 1963.

Pingleton, W. W. et al. Effects of steroid pretreatment on development of shock lung. *Lab. Invest.* 27:445, 1972.

Popovic, N. A. and Mullane, J. F. Effects of biliary obstruction on pulmonary ultrastructure in the rat. *Am. J. Path.* 68:97, 1972.

Potter, C. W., Shore, S. L. and McLaren, C. Immunity to influenza in ferrets. *J. Inf. Dis.* 126:387, 1972.

Pushpakom, R. et al. Experimental papain-induced emphysema in dogs. *Am. Rev. Resp. Dis.* 102:778, 1970.

Ratliff, N. B. et al. The lung in hemorrhagic shock. *Am. J. Path.* 58:353, 1970.

Read, J. and Donnelly, P. Stratification of blood flow in the elongated lungs of the carpet python. *J. Appl. Physiol.* 32:842, 1972.

Ressang, A. A., de Boer, G. F. and de Wijn, G. C. The lung in Zwoegerziekte. *Vet. Path.* 5:353, 1968.

Ritch, R. and Philpott, W. Repeating particles associated with an electrolyte transport membrane. *Exp. Cell Res.* 55:17, 1969.

Schneeberger, E. E. Development of peroxisomes in granular pneumocytes during pre- and post-natal growth. *Lab. Invest.* 27:581, 1972.

Schneeberger, E. E., Keeley, E. and Burger, E. J. Intravascular macrophages in cat lung after open chest ventilation. *Lab. Invest.* 22:361, 1970.

Spicer, S. S. et al. Histochemistry of mucosubstances in the canine and human respiratory tracts. *Lab. Invest.* 25:483, 1971.

Stephens, R. J. et al. Early response of lung to low levels of ozone. *Am. J. Path.* 74:31, 1973.

Strawbridge, H. T. G. Chronic pulmonary emphysema (an experimental study). *Am. J. Path.* 37: 309, 1960.

Suzuki, Y. Fenestration of alveolar capillary endothelium in experimental pulmonary fibrosis. *Lab. Invest.* 21:304, 1969.

Threadgold, L. T. and Houston, A. H. An electron microscope study of the "chloride cell" of *Salmo salar* L. *Exp. Cell Res.* 34:1, 1964.

Tyler, W. S. and Pangborn, J. Laminated membrane surface and osmiophilic inclusions in avian lung. *J. Cell Biol.* 20:157, 1964.

Ungar, J. and Wilson, G. R. Monocytes as a source of alveolar macrophages. *Am. J. Path.* 11:681, 1935.

Wang, N. S. et al. Accelerated appearance of osmiophilic bodies in fetal lungs following steroid treatment. *J. Appl. Physiol.* 30:362, 1971.

Wolke, R. E., Wyand, D. S. and Khairallah, L. H. A light and electron microscopic study of epitheliocystis disease in the gills of Connecticut striped bass *(Morone saxatilis)* and white perch *(Morone americanus).* *J. Comp. Path.* 80:559, 1970.

Wright, D. E. The structure of the gills of the elasmobranch, *Scyliorhinus canicula* (L.), *Zt. Zellf.* 144:489, 1973.

CHAPTER EIGHT

Kidney

Urine is the collective product of many nephrons functioning together. The degree to which urine reflects renal damage depends not only upon the type of nephron injury but upon the distribution of that injury within both kidneys. Acute renal failure, for example, may result from the total affection of all nephrons even though the injury has produced only subtle cytopathology. In contrast, severely destructive focal damage to the kidney may result in limited changes in urine if only a few nephrons are affected. In addition to disease that begins in the kidney, renal failure may also result from failure of blood to reach the kidney, and from blockade of the excretory system for the removal of urine (Table 8.1).

Below we consider the anatomical pathology of the kidney, stressing the location of injury and how the kidney reacts to correct structural damage. Unless otherwise specified, the mammalian kidney is referred to. While models of disease have been chosen that produce selective injury

Table 8.1. Causes of renal failure

Prerenal: Reduced renal blood flow and glomerular filtration
  Cardiac failure
  Water and sodium depletion (vomiting and diarrhea)
  Shock
Renal: Pathology of the kidney
  Glomerulopathy
  Tubule disease
  Renal vascular and interstitial disease
Postrenal: Obstruction of the urinary tract
  Calculi
  Prostatic hypertrophy
  Neoplasms
  Congenital stricture

to the glomeruli, tubules, vascular supply, or interstitium, it is to be remembered that disease of one portion of the kidney ultimately affects the other parts. The total function of the kidney is dependent upon the integrity of the various portions of the nephron. Even in defined glomerular diseases, the indices of renal function can be often shown to correlate better with secondary tubule changes than with glomerular lesions.

GLOMERULI

Glomerular filtrate is formed in the urinary spaces of the renal glomerulus by the filtration of plasma through the glomerular filtration barrier. It passes into the proximal convoluted tubules where reabsorptive and secretory phenomena begin its modification to urine. The glomerular filtration barrier consists of: (1) fenestrae within the endothelial cells of the glomerular capillaries, (2) basement membrane, and (3) epithelial slit pores produced by gaps in the foot processes of the visceral epithelial cells. Each of these sites plays a role in the passage of fluid and electrolytes and the selective retention of plasma proteins and other macromolecules.

ENDOTHELIAL CELLS

Endothelial cells of the glomerular capillaries have thin, fenestrated cytoplasm (Fig. 8.1). The basement membrane is thicker than in most capillaries and, in many species, it progressively thickens with age (Østerby 1971). The basement membrane does not surround the entire capil-

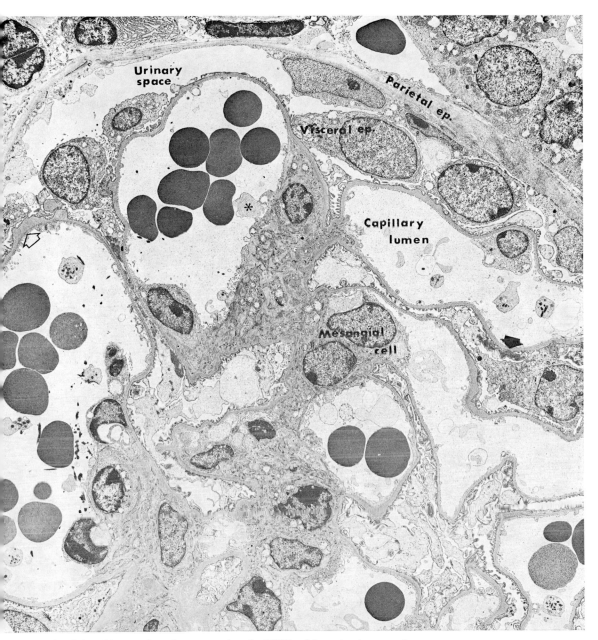

Fig. 8.1. Glomerulus of a mouse (strain NZB) with early changes of membranous glomerulonephritis. The capillary lumens contain erythrocytes, platelets, and fibrin. Note the relation of the capillary basement membrane to the dense mesangium at center. Parietal and visceral epithelium of Bowman's capsule are at top. Granular deposits have been trapped beneath the capillary endothelium (asterisk) and below the capillary basement membrane (open arrow). Dense deposits are present in the fused foot processes of some visceral epithelial cells (dark arrow).

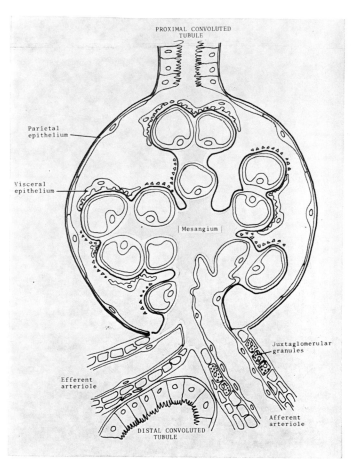

Fig. 8.2. Diagram of renal glomerulus.

lary, as in most vessels, but covers it as the serosa does the intestine (Fig. 8.2). The capillary wall adjacent to the mesangium may be penetrated by a mesangial cell; that is, a limb of the mesangial cell occasionally extends through the endothelial cell into the capillary lumen.

EPITHELIAL CELLS

Epithelial cells interdigitate between and cover the outer surfaces of the glomerular capillaries. Their cytoplasmic volume is large and they contain many fibrils, large Golgi complexes, and small amounts of rough endoplasmic reticulum. They have long, thick cytoplasmic processes that ramify outward from the cell center. Each process contains many small terminal foot processes which, as seen by scanning electron microscopy, give the cell a fernlike appearance. The spaces between the foot processes at their zone of contact with the capillary basement membrane are called *slit pores.* The slit pore or diaphragm is actually a continuous junctional band 30–45 nm wide

Fig. 8.3. A.–B. Acute exudative glomerulitis, horse, acute equine viral arteritis. Glomerulus is enlarged and hyperemic. A. Swollen epithelial cells (ep) are pressed together and obliterate urinary space. Endothelial cell (en). C.–E. Renal papillary area of dog, excess mucopolysaccharide (mps) deposition. C. Histology of collecting tubules (note swollen cells) separated by dilated lymphatics (lym) and interstitial cells (arrow). D. Ultrastructure of mps. E. Stellate interstitial cells with granular mps material and collagen (c).

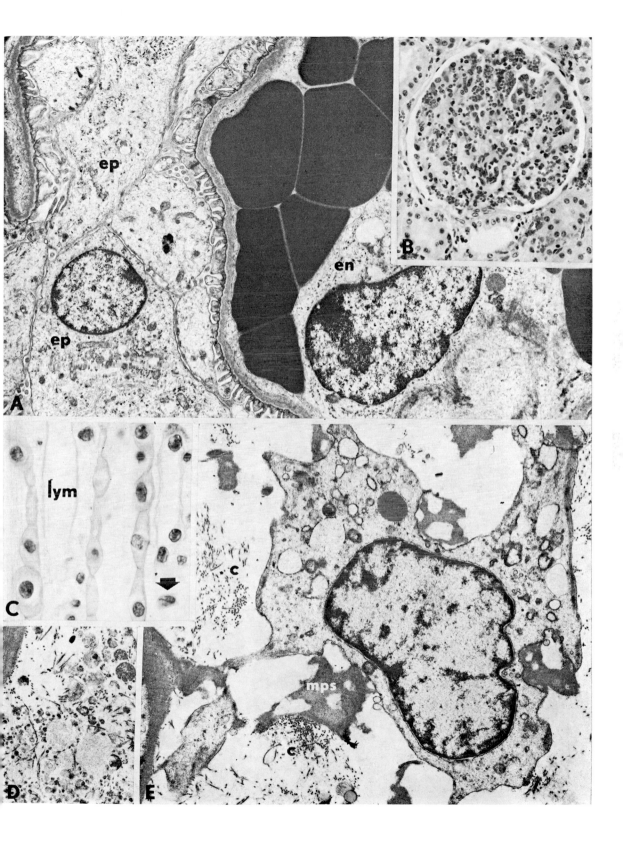

that covers all slits formed by the foot processes of the epithelial cell (Radewald and Karnovsky 1974).

Any process causing cell swelling of the glomerular epithelial cells tends to obliterate the urinary spaces by compressing the foot processes against the basement membrane (Fig. 8.3). In nephrosis and some types of proteinuria, the terminal foot processes swell selectively, causing the fernlike arrangement to become distorted and stubby (Arakawa and Tokunaga 1972). The epithelial cell is concerned with protein transport, and the abnormalities of this transport that occur in proteinuria cause dense protein granules to appear in the foot process.

MESANGIAL CELLS

Mesangial cells and their associated basement membranes extend from the vascular pole of the glomerulus throughout the capillary tuft. They are specialized cells concerned with the uptake of macromolecular material passing the filtration barrier and contain granules and dense arrays of cytoplasmic fibrils. Mesangial cells phagocytize both endogenous and exogenous substances. They constitute a protective unit for the filtration apparatus, which fails when its maximum is exceeded. The mesangial reaction is conspicuous in chronic glomerular injury. Mesangial cells proliferate and appear to secrete basement membrane material.

GOMERULAR FILTRATION BARRIER

The glomerular filtration barrier is comparable in structure and function in differ-ent mammalian species (Fig. 8.4). Based upon size comparisons with the albumin molecule, this slender diaphragm is the filtration barrier to the plasma proteins. For the dog, the critical threshold of permeability is between the molecular size of albumin (69,000 MW) and hemoglobin (68,000 MW). Thus, in the normal kidney, circulating hemoglobin passes freely into the glomerular filtrate, while albumin is retained in the blood. Permeability may vary among individual animals, and various conditions alter glomerular filtration.

Experimental studies that trace the passage of various sized molecules through the filtration barrier indicate that the basement membrane is a coarse prefilter and the epithelial filtration slit pore is the final definitive barrier (Venkatachalam et al. 1970). The mechanism by which the slit pore excludes molecules the size of albumin and above is unclear. Physiologic data indicate the filtration barrier behaves as a membrane with pores of 7–8 nm diameter but the actual slit pore diameter is 20–30 nm, far too wide to account for molecular sieving. A sialoprotein coat which is demonstrable on the epithelial cell surface with colloidal iron stains or ruthenium red may narrow the slit pore and explain the variance (Michael et al. 1970).

The integrity of the basement membrane is essential to glomerular function. Focal discontinuities or gaps are produced by neutrophil proteases in some types of acute glomerulonephritis. This leads to exudation of fibrinogen and fibrin polymers into the urinary spaces and mesangium, and may cause destruction of glomeruli if fibroplasia and mesangial cell proliferation are not prevented.

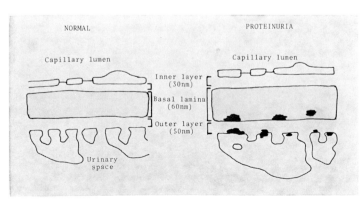

Fig. 8.4. Diagram of renal glomerular filtration barrier.

Experiments involving the sequential examination of the glomerulus at various times after the intravenous injection of small protein molecules reveals that these molecules readily pass through the barrier into the glomerular filtrate. The transient high levels of protein in the blood are rapidly eliminated through capillary fenestrae, basement membrane, and slit pore.

Protein molecules are also taken up by mesangial cells, where they persist long after removal from other sites in the glomerulus (Oliver and Essner 1972). Proteins in the glomerular filtrate enter the tubules, where they absorb to the microvilli of the proximal convoluted tubule cells. They are taken up at the luminal surface, concentrated into "protein absorption droplets" in the cytoplasm, and are eliminated at the infoldings of the basal surface of the epithelial cell. When the absorptive capacity of the tubule mechanism is overloaded, the protein molecules pass through the nephron and appear in urine (*proteinuria*).

Large protein molecules occur in the blood in diseases characterized by lysis of erythrocytes or muscle cells (myoglobinemia or hemoglobinemia). They pass the glomerular capillaries by crossing the endothelial cell in vacuoles, not through fenestrae (Menefee et al. 1964), and traverse the basement membrane without markedly altering the dense lamina. In passage through the slit pore, however, the foot processes are markedly deformed and fuse together, obliterating the slit pores. Protein aggregates accumulate in the pores, epithelial cells, and urinary spaces. Like small protein molecules, they empty into the nephron, producing protein droplets in the proximal tubules and resulting in proteinuria. In summary, large proteins that spill over the glomerular filter induce damage to the epithelial cell foot process, which alters the filtration process in the kidney. These changes fortunately are reversible and, if the condition causing proteinuria is corrected, the renal glomerulus returns to normal structure and function.

The glomerular filtration barrier may be damaged directly by inflammatory, degenerative, or immunologic reactions. Toxic injury to the renal glomerulus most often affects the epithelial cells. Foot processes fuse, slit pores are destroyed, and intercellular junctions are narrowed and lengthened (Sternberg 1970; Venkatachalam et al. 1970). If large tracer protein molecules (which are normally stopped at the filtration barrier) are injected intravenously in animals rendered "nephrotic" by glomerular damage, they permeate freely into the urinary spaces. Although the epithelial cell with its foot processes fused provides a solid cell barrier at the distal side of the filter, protein molecules are transferred by transepithelial migration. When examined ultrastructurally, proteins are seen in conspicuous cytoplasmic vacuoles. The vacuoles begin as basal pockets in the epithelial cells adjacent to the basement membrane, become intracytoplasmic, and discharge their contents into the urinary space. The uptake of these macromolecules by the epithelial cells in toxic injury indicates their role in the conservation of protein. Although the basement membrane is not noticeably altered structurally in many acute toxic injuries, there are marked changes in permeability which indicate decreased function.

The relation between proteinuria and changes in the glomerular visceral epithelial cell is constant. Proteinuria accompanies such diverse conditions as congestive heart failure, cirrhosis of the liver, and exceptionally strenuous exercise. Glomerular changes are due to (not the cause of) protein molecules passing the glomerular filter.

TUBULES

PROXIMAL CONVOLUTED TUBULES

The epithelial cells of the proximal convoluted tubules make up much of the renal cortical mass. These cells reabsorb more than 80% of the water of the glomerular filtrate. They shunt glucose and sodium across the luminal cell membrane by active transport, an energy-requiring process (Fig. 8.5). Diffusion of chloride accompanies sodium transport and the reabsorption of NaCl and glucose carries the water across the nephron passively, that is, by osmotic diffusion. Urea, uric acid, creatinine, and phosphates are not significantly reabsorbed.

Cells of the proximal tubular epithe-

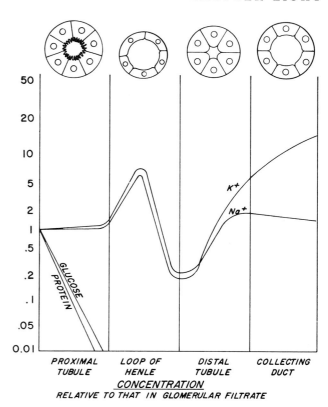

Fig. 8.5. Changes in glucose, protein, potassium, and sodium in passage through the nephron.

lium differ from tubule cells in the lower nephron in having tall microvilli of the luminal plasma membrane (the brush border), a vacuolar system below the plasma membrane, and prominent lysosomes in the cytoplasm. Peroxisomes are present in the basal portions of proximal tubule cells (Beard and Novikoff 1969). Microvilli are long and slender in epithelial cells near the glomerulus and are progessively shorter and broader on the lower portions of the proximal tubule. They are associated with large amounts of alkaline phosphatase, which plays a role in the reabsorption process. Disaccharidases are present along the microvillous border and function in glucose transport. Cilia have been reported in epithelial cells of the proximal convoluted tubule in some types of renal disease (Wesson and Duckett 1973).

Microvilli are highly sensitive to injury and anoxia and react by becoming ballooned and by shedding globules of various sizes into the tubule lumen. Nephrotoxins such as mercury and amphotericin B dam-

age the tubule in this way and cause loss of water, glucose, and sodium that are normally absorbed.

The vacuoles below the luminal plasma membrane originate as invaginations in the membrane. They are associated with reabsorption and increase markedly during reabsorption of substances from glomerular filtrate. For example, they are prominent in experimental glucose infusion (Maunsbach et al. 1962).

Protein spillover into the glomerular filtrate is followed by reabsorption in the cells of the proximal convoluted tubule. Large round hyalin (eosinophilic) protein absorption droplets are seen histologically. Ultrastructurally, protein absorption droplets are dense, membrane-bound bodies. They represent secondary lysosomes which form following endocytosis of protein. Hyalin droplets are present in the proximal tubules in myoglobinuria, after multiple blood transfusions, and in hemoglobinuria. Protein droplets are commonly present in the rat which normally excretes some albumiin in the glomeruli (Logothetopoulos and Weinbren 1955).

The proximal convoluted tubules appear to be the chief site of synthesis of erythrogenin, the precursor of erythropoietin. The anemia that usually accompanies severe renal disease can be explained, in part, by a deficiency of erythrogenin production.

LOOPS OF HENLE

In mammals, a significant number of nephrons (the long nephrons), have a special anatomical arrangement for concentrating urine. A portion of the nephron, the loop of Henle, dips deeply down into the tips of the papillae. It is accompanied by special capillary loops, the vasa rectae. This peritubular capillary bed is a "low pressure" bed (in contrast to the higher pressure of the glomerulus) and blood is very sluggish in moving through it. There is no lymphatic drainage of the medullary area.

There is a correlation in different species between the ability to produce a concentrated urine and the number and length of long nephrons. Fish and amphibia lack long nephrons but birds have some long types. In desert mammals, such as gerbils, the nephrons are almost all of the long variety. In the beaver and other aquatic animals, the nephrons have chiefly short loops of Henle.

Ultrastructurally, the epithelial cells of the loops are small and narrow (Bulger and Trump 1966; Osvaldo and Latta 1966). Compared to the proximal tubules, they contain few organelles. Mesenchymal cells are present in the interstitium and are the source of mucopolysaccharides that accumulate in the medulla and papillae in some aged animals. Interstitial tissue of the medulla is rich in albumin which exudes through the descending limb. Granule-containing cells also occur in the interstitial spaces and it is believed that they play a role in blood pressure regulation (Gloor and Neiditsch-Halff 1965; Muehrcke 1970).

By the retransport of sodium and chloride again and again from the lumen of the ascending to the descending loops of Henle (via the interstitium), water is removed in the highly permeable descending limb.

This "countercurrent" osmotic multiplier mechanism functions in both the loops of Henle and the vasa rectae. The descending limb of the loop is highly permeable both to water and to sodium and chloride. The ascending limb has a strong transport mechanism to move these ions into the interstitium but is relatively impermeable to water. Tubule fluid in transit through the loops therefore passes through a hyperosmotic medulla. High urea and sodium concentrations in the interstitium allow water to be removed in the descending limb. In the ascending limb, the impermeability to water allows the tubular fluid to become progressively more dilute.

Low blood sodium (hyponatremia), acting via sodium-sensing mechanisms in the macula densa, increases renin synthesis and secretion by the juxtaglomerular cells. This results in increased plasma angiotensin which stimulates increased blood pressure by peripheral vasoconstriction. Angiotensin also circulates in the blood to the adrenal cortex where it stimulates aldosterone secretion in the zona glomerulosa. Aldosterone, circulating back to the kidney, acts specifically on the ascending loop of Henle to increase the rate of Na^+ reabsorption.

Small autonomic nerves ramify through the renal cortex, and adrenergic and cholinergic termini have been demonstrated in close association with both proximal and distal tubules (Müller and Barajas 1972). It is probable that the nervous system can influence sodium reabsorption in this way.

DISTAL TUBULES

In the distal tubules, reabsorption of water is controlled by the antidiuretic hormone (ADH, vasopressin) which originates in the posterior pituitary. ADH causes the otherwise impermeable tubules to become permeable to water (and, in the frog, increased permeability of the skin). Exposure to the high osmolarity of the renal papilla causes water to be removed from the tubule. Increased permeability of the distal tubule epithelial cell is due to changes in the hormone-sensitive luminal surface of the collecting tubule epithelial cells. When absorption occurs, the cells become swollen and have large vacuoles in the cytoplasm

(Ganote et al. 1968). Opening of the intercellular junctions (except at tight junctions) appears to facilitate reabsorption of water. It is alleged that ADH acts by stimulating the formation of cyclic AMP which directly increases the permeability of the tubule membrane.

ADH is packaged in secretory granules within nerve cell bodies in the hypothalamic supraoptic nucleus. Granules pass down the axon and into the posterior pituitary where they are stored and eventually taken up by capillary endothelium. During dehydration and other hypovolemic conditions, depletion of granules in the hypothalamic neurons can be detected (Omachi 1971).

Diabetes insipidus, which in dogs is characterized by excessive thirst, water intake, and urine formation (of low specific gravity), is a result of either a deficiency of ADH or failure of renal distal tubules to respond to ADH (nephrogenic diabetes insipidis). The most common cause is pressure from expanding tumors, which disturbs synthesis in hypothalamic nuclei and destroys neurosecretory pathways in the neurohyophysis. In a series of 27 canine pituitary neoplasms, 25 individuals had evidence of diabetes insipidis. Ultrastructural examination of the supraoptic nuclei revealed lack of granules and other cytoplasmic evidence of disturbed function (Koestner and Capen 1967). *Nephrogenic diabetes insipidis,* which results from the failure of the distal tubules to respond to ADH, has been reported in the dog (Lage 1973).

H^+ secretion and acidification of urine are prime functions of the distal tubule and are immediate responses in the defense of blood pH. The kidney thereby regulates acid-base balance by regulating the concentration of bicarbonate in plasma. The renal acidification process reclaims all filtered bicarbonate and excretes an amount of acid (H^+) equal to that produced endogenously. Both bicarbonate reabsorption and acid excretion are mediated by a single tubular operation: the exchange of H^+ (secreted) for Na^+ (reabsorbed).

In the proximal convoluted tubule lumen, the secreted H^+ spent in titrating HCO_3^- to H_2CO_3 is not excreted in urine as acid. The H_2CO_3 dissociates to H_2O and CO_2. Carbonic anhydrase located in the microvillous border of the proximal tubule cell reduces the concentration of luminal H_2CO_3 by catalyzing this dissociation. In the distal tubule, the H^+ secretory process further titrates the residual bicarbonate and the major urinary buffers: NH_3 and $Na_2HPO_4 \rightarrow NH_4^+$ and NaH_2PO_4.

During metabolic acidosis, bicarbonate is titrated to extinction in the proximal nephron and excess acid is present in the filtrate. The distal secretion of H^+ adds to the increased net H^+ excretion. Urine pH decreases and net acid excretion increases, the classic indices of renal acidification.

The distal tubule also secretes K^+. In general, as Na^+ is reabsorbed K^+ is secreted. Aldosterone promotes Na^+ absorption at the expense of K^+ loss. K^+ deficiency states are fairly common and are seen in severe diarrhea and vomiting, hyperadrenocorticoidism, and any cause of renal tubular acidosis. The tubular defects are manifested as vacuolation of the distal tubules and diminished tubular function.

NEPHRITIS

Inflammation develops in the kidney in distinct patterns which vary according to the agent involved and to its route of entry. The separation of glomerulonephritis, interstitial nephritis, and pyelonephritis (Table 8.2) is somewhat artificial since the signs of disease and the lesions that result overlap considerably. Any of these may be acute, subacute, or chronic. Clini-

Table 8.2. Classification of nephritis

Glomerulonephritis		
Exudative	Serous	
	Purulent	
	Fibrinopurulent	
Embolic	Thrombotic	
	Crystalline	
	Lipidic	
Proliferative	Fibroplastic	
Deposition	Membranous (basement membrane)	
	Glomerulosclerotic (collagen)	
	Amyloidotic	
Interstitial nephritis	Purulent	
	Lymphocytic or Plasmacytic	
	Granulomatous	
Pyelonephritis	Purulent	

cal signs depend upon which stage of disease is present and to what extent the total mass of the kidney is involved.

The gross appearance of the kidney at necropsy indicates the progress of the disease process. In acute nephritis, the kidney is usually hyperemic, enlarged, swollen, and wet. The cut surface bulges from the capsule and individual tiny red glomeruli may be visible. In severe nephritis, especially involving vascular tissue, scattered petechiae may be present. Pus and fatty degeneration of tubules impart gray-yellow streaks through the cortex and medulla.

Chronic nephritis, in contrast, is characterized by pale, hard, shrunken kidneys with irregular scarred surfaces. Cysts are often present, and fibrotic bands extend through the parenchyma. The cortex is thinned and the pelves are apt to be flecked with solid yellow and white foci. The pelvis and the renal end of the ureter are thickened and distorted when pyelonephritis or hydronephrosis is involved in the kidney disease.

GLOMERULONEPHRITIS AND OTHER GLOMERULOPATHIES

EXUDATIVE GLOMERULITIS

Acute *serous glomerulitis* is a common lesion in systemic viral diseases. Acute infectious canine hepatitis, hog cholera, equine viral arteritis, Newcastle disease, and the hemorrhagic fevers of primates are examples in which viruses replicate in the endothelial and epithelial cells of the glomerulus. Fluorescent antibody tests are useful in localizing infected cells (Cheville et al. 1970). Ultrastructurally, hyperemia, edema, and severe swelling of endothelial cells are common. Virions are difficult to locate in infected cells, except for adenovirus infection where they are located in nuclei of endothelial and mesangial cells (Wright et al. 1973). In all cases, mesangial hypertrophy and hyperplasia are present as secondary effects. Despite cellular degeneration and the accumulation of edema in the mesangium, the filtration capacity of the kidney is rarely abnormal.

Viral infections in the kidney are rarely recognized as glomerulonephritis except where capillaries are sufficiently damaged to destroy the glomeruli. The outcome of the infection is not determined in the kidney but in other organs. If the animal survives, viruses are cleared from the renal parenchyma and are no longer shed into the urine. In rare instances of chronic viral infection, viruses may persist in the kidney, and the animal intermittently excretes infectious virus in the urine. If the virus is present in the glomerulus, membranous glomerulonephritis may result from the deposition of antigen-antibody complexes (see immunopathologic disease, Chapter 5).

Purulent glomerulonephritis occurs as a specific lesion in some systemic bacterial diseases, notably swine erysipelas. Purulent lesions of the glomeruli are seen in infections involving Streptococci, Toxoplasma, and Salmonella. Organisms localize in the glomerulus during bacteremia, where they cause exudation of fluid and granulocytes. Focal necrosis of capillaries initiates fibrin deposition with destruction of individual glomeruli. Ultrastructurally, these glomerular lesions are dominated by degranulate neutrophils, necrotic debris, fibrin, and erythrocytes.

Septic thrombi originating from infected mammae, uteri, and umbilical cords may lodge in glomeruli and initiate fibrinopurulent inflammation. Fibrinous glomerulonephritis is also characteristic of toxemic disorders, including toxemia of pregnancy in some species. These are often associated with systemic derangements of the coagulation system and are more properly considered as thrombotic glomerulopathy.

PROLIFERATIVE GLOMERULONEPHRITIS

Proliferative glomerulonephritis may be defined as inflammation with increase in the cellularity of the glomerulus. The proliferating cells are chiefly endothelial and visceral epithelial cells. While proliferation of these cells is a component of most types of glomerulonephritis, as a distinct lesion (not dominated by membranous or exudative changes) it is rare. Generally, it tends to be seen in subacute reactions in association with infectious lesions. Specific proliferative glomerulonephritis occurs in chickens with chronic infection with *Streptococcus zooepidemicus*. Subtle proliferative glomerulonephritis is encountered in ruminants, for which the cause is not known (Lerner and Dixon 1968).

MEMBRANOUS GLOMERULONEPHRITIS

Membranous glomerulonephritis is due to abnormal thickening of the glomerular basement membrane. The condition is rarely inflammatory and membranous *glomerulopathy* would be the appropriate term if "glomerulonephritis" were not so firmly rooted in texts on renal pathology. Membranous glomerulonephritis is due to excessive synthesis of basement membrane material or to the trapping and deposition of macromolecular materials. It is commonly seen in aged animals, where both these factors are operative.

The glomerular basement membrane thickens progressively with age. The glomeruli of old animals usually have a uniformly increased width of the dense lamina and granular densities in the epithelial cell foot processes. These changes are related to pathologic turnover and synthesis of basement membrane material by the epithelial cell. Corticosteroids act on the glomerular basement membrane to increase synthesis of polysaccharides (Misra and Berman 1972).

Membranous glomerulonephritis has been described in reptiles, birds, and many mammalian species (Kurtz et al. 1972; Murray et al. 1971; Slauson et al. 1971). It is associated with toxemia of pregnancy in sheep (Ferris et al. 1969), chronic interstitial nephritis in dogs, canine diabetes mellitus (Bloodworth 1965; Ricketts 1962), and chronic viral infections in several species. Most of these diseases are associated with depression of the reticuloendothelial system, which in a sense includes the glomerular mesangium. The failure of mesangial cells to process macromolecules that pass the capillary results in the pro-

gressive accumulation of those substances within the basement membrane.

Diffuse membranous glomerulonephritis accompanies chronic systemic diseases characterized by tissue breakdown and hyperproteinemia. The lesions begin as thickening of capillary loops and mesangium by an increase in basement membrane material. The initial thickening of the dense lamina of the basement membrane and expansion of the mesangium is followed, in the subacute stages, by proliferation of mesangial and epithelial cells.

The classic example of this renal lesion is the membranous glomerulopathy associated with purulent pyometra in the bitch with cystic hyperplasia of the endometrium (Fig. 8.6). This is an infectious process superimposed upon hormonal imbalances due to persistence of a corpus luteum. Luteal tissue may persist after parturition or may be a consequence of abnormal estrus and pseudopregnancy. In either case, the secreted progesterone confers an extraordinary susceptibility to infection upon the uterus by inducing hyperplasia of the glandular epithelium with dilatation and retention of secretions, inhibition of myometrial contraction, and maintenance of a closed cervical canal. Thick, foul-smelling exudates distend the uterus and drip from the vaginal orifice. Extrauterine lesions of pyometra are related to intermittent bacteremia and include diffuse reticuloendothelial hyperplasia, hepatic granulomas, anemia, glomerulopathy, and adrenal cortical hyperactivity.

If the uterine condition is not corrected, nodular deposits of granular material accumulate in the glomerulus below the endothelium, in the dense layer of the basement membrane, and adjacent to the foot process of the epithelial cell. There are swelling of endothelial cells and fusion of epithelial foot processes. Thickened basement membranes also form around the

Fig. 8.6. A. Membranous glomerulonephritis in a dog with chronic purulent metritis and cystic endometrial hyperplasia. Visceral and parietal epithelium in close apposition obliterate exterior urinary space Extensive accumulation of basement membrane material (bm) thickens the basement membrane and the capsule. Deposits of dense granular material (arrow) in the basement membrane. Erythrocytes (e). *Inset:* Histology. B. Enlargement. Fenestrae (arrow) in endothelial cell, granular bm material and dense deposits in foot processes (asterisk). C. Chronic membranous glomerulonephritis, dog, periodic acid-Schiff stain.

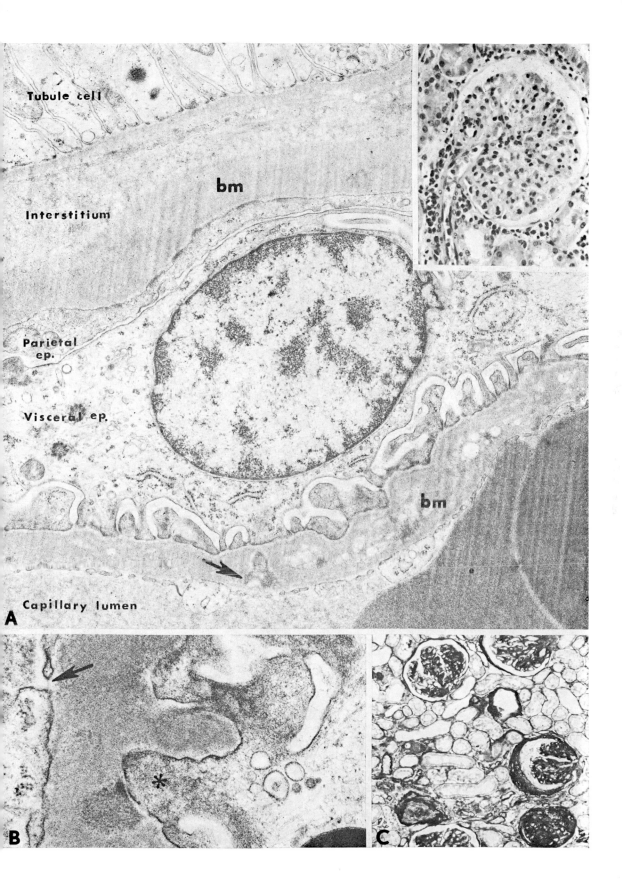

Tubule cell

bm

Interstitium

Parietal ep.

Visceral ep.

bm

Capillary lumen

A

B

C

collecting tubules and there are changes elsewhere in the nephron. Affected dogs invariably have reduced concentrating ability and often have depressed glomerular filtration (Asheim 1965). If the pyometra and metritis are corrected and the intermittent bacteremia stopped, the renal glomerular lesions regress (Obel et al. 1964).

The lesions described above for membranous glomerulonephritis are an integral part of the renal syndrome in dogs diagnosed clinically as "chronic interstitial nephritis." Although this term is probably a misnomer as regards the origin of the process, it is useful in the differentiation of renal disease in the dog. The disease is characterized by membranous glomerulopathy, tubular dilatation and atrophy, plasmacyte infiltration, and fibrin deposition in the interstitium. The cause is not known. Affected dogs have polydipsia, polyuria, and slight proteinuria. During the disease, which lasts a few months to 1–2 years, blood urea nitrogen increases; the animals die in uremia. The glomerular basement membranes are markedly thickened with occasional subendothelial and epithelial deposition of dense granular material (Fig. 8.7). Immunofluorescent studies have demonstrated the presence of immunoglobulins and complement in the deposits (Krohn et al. 1973) and this suggests that complement-fixing antigen-antibody complexes may be present in damaged glomeruli.

The glomerular deposition of immune complexes is implicated in several chronic viral infections (see glomerulonephritis, Chapter 5). In Aleutian disease, chronic hog cholera, and equine infectious anemia, dense, irregular, lumpy, globular deposits of antigen-antibody complexes are deposited within the basement membrane. A high incidence of membranous glomerulonephritis is seen in chronic lymphosarcoma and this, too, may be related to viral infection.

RENAL AMYLOIDOSIS

Renal amyloidosis is the disease resulting from the deposition of amyloid fibrils in tissue (see amyloid, Chapter 5). Amyloid produces its most disastrous effect in the kidney, where it causes uremia by massive accumulation in the glomerulus. This is a prominent lesion in amyloidosis in aged animals, particularly the dog, cat, and hamster.

Deposition of amyloid within the kidney also occurs around the tubules and arterioles. Renal peritubular amyloid is deposited between the tubule epithelial cell and its basement membrane. Fibrils are occasionally present between and within tubular epithelium (Cohen and Shirahama 1971).

In the glomerulus, amyloid accumulates chiefly in the mesangial matrix and along the adjacent basement membrane (see Fig. 5.25). In rare instances, it has also been reported in subendothelial, subepithelial, and even intravascular locations. The occurrence of amyloid in the mesangium would lead one to believe that it was of plasma origin, for this is the known position of plasma-borne macromolecular material. For the following reasons, however, it appears that amyloid is formed in situ: (1) there is an intimate relationship between the cell membrane and amyloid fibrils; (2) mesangial cells containing amyloid have the property of protein-synthesizing cells (elaborate endoplasmic reticulum with abundant free ribosomes); and (3) the fibrils are regular in array and the cell membrane is indistinct at sites of formation (Shirahama and Cohen 1967). This does not preclude the phagocytosis of amyloid as part of accompanying resorption in amyloidosis.

THROMBOTIC GLOMERULOPATHY

When capillary endothelial cells in the renal glomerulus are destroyed, platelets

Fig. 8.7. Severe membranous glomerulopathy. A. Cat, feline infectious peritonitis. Thickening of capillary basement membrane with dense nodular deposits (arrow). Aggregates of fibrin (F) within the capillaries. Dense membrane-bound granules (G) in epithelial cells. B. Swollen (light) and necrotic (arrow) epithelial cells. Total fusion of foot processes. Note intertwined cytoplasmic processes of light and dark cells.

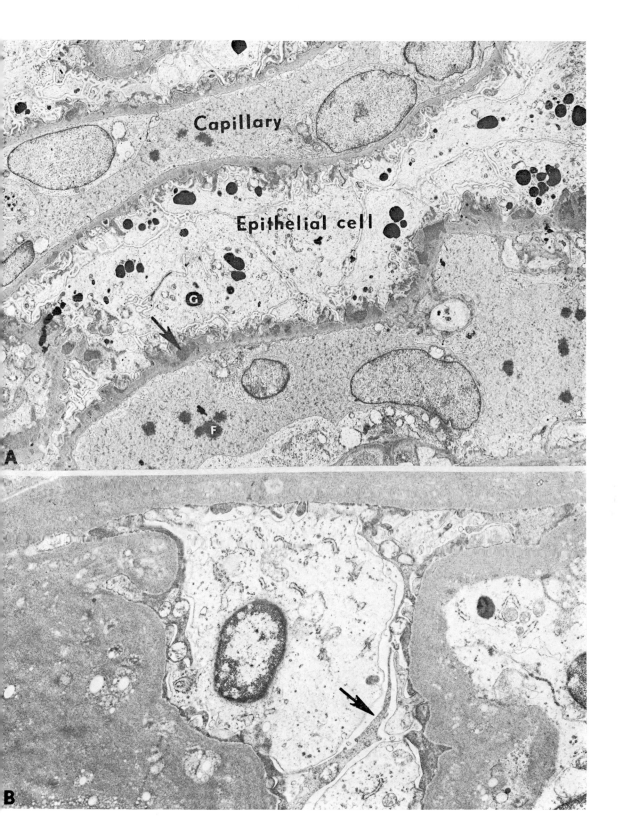

and fibrin cover the defects over the basement membrane. In some situations, capillary destruction is so extensive that thrombi develop and occlude glomeruli. *Thrombotic glomerulopathy* is the chief cause of death in disseminated intravascular coagulation, associated with many severe systemic diseases (see coagulation, Chapter 3).

Thrombotic glomerulopathy is a cause of acute renal disease in septicemic bacterial infections. *Hemophilus* spp. are a common causal factor in swine, cattle, and humans. The microscopic changes in the glomerular vessels consist of fibrinous thrombi and the deposition of platelets in the vascular lumen. In most cases, there is fibrinoid necrosis of the muscular arteries of the kidney (Nordstoga and Fjolstad 1967). Thrombotic glomerulopathy is also seen in some severe viral infections of the kidney, and should not be confused with immunologically induced glomerulopathy, even though the two processes may coexist.

Thrombotic glomerulonephritis is characteristic of toxemic disorders, including the toxemia of pregnancy in some species. In hamsters and humans these are associated with systemic derangements of the coagulation system (Galton and Slater 1966). Fibrinolytic activity in vascular structures may be enhanced and aid in clearance of fibrin (Humair et al. 1969) but these diseases often prove fatal due to renal disease (Vassali et al. 1963).

Although the occurrence of thrombotic glomerulopathy is probably frequent, its significance as a cause of death is not common. A potent fibrinolytic mechanism operates in the kidney (Myhre-Jensen 1971), and when thrombotic processes are developing, they are suppressed. Only when severe systemic afflictions overwhelm the fibrinolytic mechanism does thrombotic glomerulopathy ensue. These lesions may be responsible for acute renal failure with uremia, but are reversible if appropriate treatment is given (Courtecuise et al. 1967).

LIPID GLOMERULOPATHY

Lipid glomerulopathy is a rare lesion reported only in dogs. The disease involved is fatal and at postmortem examination the renal cortex is peppered with small yellow foci. Microscopic examination reveals these to be lipid-filled glomeruli. Mesangial cells are expanded by large amounts of neutral lipid globules (Fisher and Fisher 1954). The cause of the lesion is not known, but similar lipid glomerulopathy has been produced experimentally in rabbits by inducing hyperlipidemia (Wellmark and Volk 1971). Mucopolysaccharide glomerulopathy associated with storage disease has been reported in humans (Scott et al. 1973).

INTERSTITIAL NEPHRITIS

The interstitium of the kidney reacts to any disease process, and interstitial nephritis is a component of primary disease of the glomeruli and tubules. Here, however, we discuss only those reactions that begin in the interstitium and its vascular tissue, and in which the disease is largely dominated by lesions at this site.

Focal purulent interstitial nephritis develops following the dissemination of pyogenic bacteria to the kidney. *Escherichia coli, Corynebacterium pyogenes, Streptococcus* sp., and *Shigella* sp. are among the organisms commonly cultured from these lesions in animals. The suppurative process involves the replication of bacteria in the interstitium; vasculitis, exudation of granulocytes, and destruction of tubular epithelium are consequent lesions.

Neutrophils, macrophages, and debris are present in and obliterate the renal tubules. In most instances, these lesions are subclinical, resolve without permanent injury, and are discovered incidentally months or years later as nodules of lymphoid tissue or small connective tissue scars. Foci of purulent inflammation may also arise from lodging of septic emboli in the interstitial areas, and chronic abscess formation is often a consequence.

Diffuse interstitial nephritis is common in many species of animals, and particularly in the dog and cat. Often the causal agent remains unidentified, but the inflammatory reaction is obvious and can be related to changes in the urine. Leptospirosis is one of the diseases commonly associated with acute interstitial nephritis (McIntyre and Montgomery 1952; Monlux 1948). Leptospires arrive in the kidney hematogenously and produce an acute vasculitis in the capillaries and lymphatics of the intertubular areas of the cortex. The inflammatory process that arises is seen as edema of the interstitium followed by plasmacyte infiltration (Fig. 8.8). Necrosis of tubules may occur, with inspissation of granulocytes and cell debris. Lesions tend to be multifocal in character and sites of damage depend upon localization of the leptospires. These bacteria do not persist in the interstitium, but migrate into the tubules. They associate intimately with the microvilli of the proximal convoluted tubule, where they replicate and are shed into the urine. At this site they are effectively separated from antibodies and exuding plasmacytes, and a chronic "carrier" condition may persist.

Dogs with acute leptospirosis rarely develop chronic lesions, but chronic interstitial nephritis may follow acute disease. Intermittent healing and acute disease produce a shrunken, irregular white kidney, prone to renal failure. Fibroplasia and collagen deposition result in scarring and contraction. Leptospirosis, however, is not responsible for the far more common condition discussed previously as chronic interstitial nephritis in the dog. Many dogs with this syndrome have antibody titers against leptospires, but the causal relationship of the organism to renal disease is not established.

PYELONEPHRITIS

Pyelonephritis is inflammation of the renal pelves and parenchyma. It is a suppurative condition arising from an ascending urogenous bacterial infection, and is consistently associated with similar lesions in the ureter and bladder. The lesions are present in the lower nephrons and interstitium and radiate toward the cortex from the initial foci of infection in the pelvic areas.

The major route whereby bacteria enter the kidney is in retrograde travel from the bladder, a pathway facilitated by vesiculoureteral reflux. The opportunity for infection is frequent but bacterial colonization of the renal pelvis is not. Whether or not infection occurs depends upon the ability of the pelvic or tubular epithelium to resist infection. One mechanism by which gram negative bacteria adhere to epithelial cells is through their filamentous appendages called pili. These play a role in pathogenesis by allowing firm adhesion to cell surfaces and are factors of virulence in different organisms. Virulent *Proteus* sp. have longer and more functional pili than their avirulent counterparts (Silverblatt 1974). Once attached by pili, bacteria cross the epithelial barrier by direct penetration of epithelial cells, passage between epithelial cells, and migration through necrotic foci in the pelvis.

In some types of pyelonephritis the causal bacterium has a defined tropism for the epithelium of the urinary tract. Infection of cattle with *Corynebacterium renale* is an example (Jones and Little 1925). The bacteria will produce pyelonephritis when inoculated intravenously and, while this indicates the special tropism for the urinary tract, it does not imply that naturally occurring infection results from this route. Within the kidney, the bacterium appears to attach to the epithelium of the lower nephron but the finite pathogenesis of the disease has not been examined.

In most species that develop bacterially induced suppurative pyelonephritis, the infection is nonspecific and there are predisposing factors that lead to generalized disease of the lower urinary system (Brumfitt and Heptinstall 1960). Some of these include congenital urinary stricture, nephrocalcinosis, and lesions that depress the voiding of urine. Ascending pyelonephritis is readily reproduced experimentally by damaging the ureter. In the dog, diabetes mellitus, gout, and immunosuppressive treatment may also promote urinary infections.

In pyelonephritis, the renal pelvis is affected initially and the infection spreads to the renal parenchyma via the collecting ducts. It ultimately spreads to the tubules and interstitium. Pyelonephritis is a relapsing disease in the dog and cat. Repeated attacks of acute suppuration lead to chronic fibroplasia and scarring in medullary areas. Blockage of the lower nephron chokes off the flow of urine, causing the upper tubules and urinary spaces of the glomeruli to dilate and become cystic.

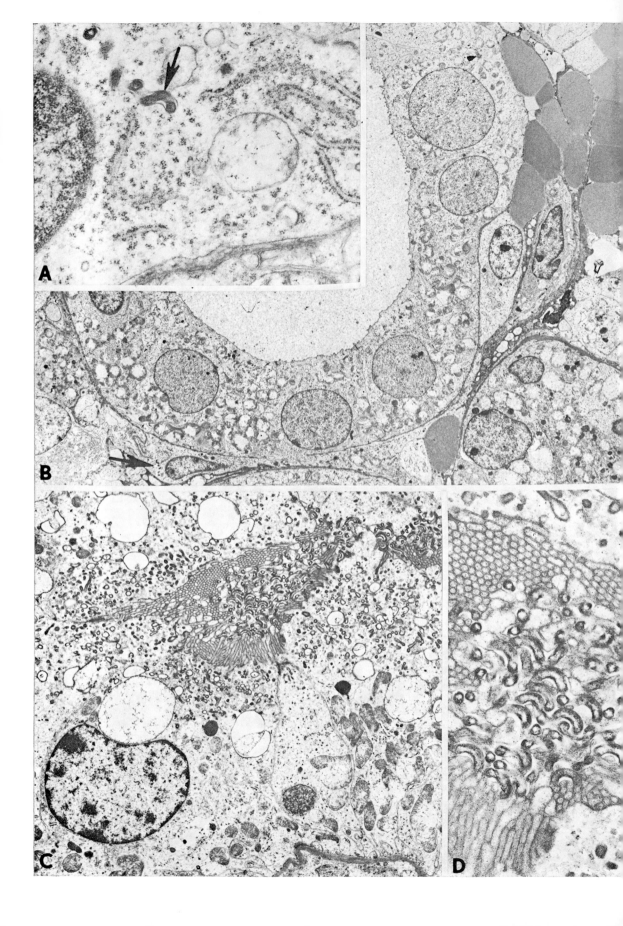

In severe involvement, hydronephrosis may complicate the renal lesion.

NEPHROSIS

Nephrosis is classically applied to degenerative disease of the kidney, in direct contrast with inflammatory renal disease. "Nephrosis" is also used by human clinicians in reference to patients with a triad of albuminuria, hypoproteinemia, and edema who lack signs of renal failure and hypertension, but this usage bears no relation to nephrosis as it is to be used here.

It is the highly sensitive tubules that are seriously affected by toxins, metabolic poisons, and changes in blood levels of electrolytes and oxygen. Nephrosis is one of the hazards of chemotherapy, especially with toxic parasiticides and antibiotics. The clinical signs of nephrosis relate to the degenerative process in the tubules, and oliguria (or anuria) indicates severe, diffuse disease. Renal tubular disease also occurs when tubule lumens are obstructed by cell debris or are compressed by severe intertubular edema.

Cytologic evidence of nephrosis includes the spectrum of changes from cell swelling to necrosis and desquamation of tubule cells. Early changes include disappearance of microvilli and development of lysosomes and residual bodies within the cytoplasm. Glomeruli are often remarkably free of damage. Damage to the tubule epithelium, particularly that of the proximal convoluted tubule, accompanies severe fever and toxemia and is seen chiefly as fatty degeneration (Trump and Bulger 1967). These nonspecific changes may be accompanied by albuminuria and cell sediments in the urine. Vacuolar degeneration occurs in severe electrolyte imbalance, especially during severe potassium deficiency (Wilson et al. 1969).

Regeneration of tubular epithelial cells is evident in most chronic cases of nephrosis. Pleomorphic, deeply staining cells line the denuded tubular basement membranes (Oliver 1953). Some cells are greatly enlarged and mitotic figures are present. Other cells persist as thin, narrow cells that do not regain normal function. Regenerating proximal tubule epithelial cells have fewer cytoplasmic organelles, lack typical microvilli, and consist of large numbers of ribosomes (Nagle et al. 1972).

TOXIC TUBULAR DEGENERATION

Renal tubular epithelial cells are exquisitely sensitive to poisons. Injury usually results from a direct effect upon organelles such as the plasma membrane, endoplasmic reticulum, or mitochondria. The initial locus of injury is often obscured, however, by secondary effects in the damaged kidney. Vascular changes, reduced blood flow, and ischemia may be superimposed upon tubule injury and exaggerate the signs of disease. We consider below only a few models of tubule injury that may lead to progressive renal failure. Other experimental models include nephrotoxicity due to carbon tetrachloride (Stroker et al. 1968), methoxyfluorane (Koset et al. 1972), aminonucleoside (Feldman and Fischer 1959), staphylococcal enterotoxin (Normann et al. 1969), and burn tissue injury (Ericsson and Rammer 1972).

AMPHOTERICIN B

Several antibiotics, used therapeutically against bacterial infections, are associated with toxic injury to the renal tubules. One of these is amphotericin B, used to combat systemic fungal infections. Amphotericin B combines with sterols in the plasma membrane of the fungal cells and causes leakage of cytosol. Unfortunately, the same mechanism operates on the renal tubule cells of the animal undergoing treatment. The lytic effect has also been demonstrated on cholesterol-rich lysosomal membranes of kidney cells (Weissmann et al. 1966).

At high dosage, amphotericin B causes distal tubule injury and renal ischemia in humans and dogs (Wertlake et al. 1965).

Fig. 8.8. Acute leptospirosis, pig. A. Enlargement of leptospira within cistern (arrow). B. Cell swelling, distal tubular epithelium, intense hyperemia, and leptospires in the peritubular fibroblasts (arrow). C. and D. Leptospires intertwined among the microvilli of proximal convoluted tuble.

Direct injury to the distal tubular epithelial cell leads to excessive potassium, bicarbonate, and water loss in urine. Increased tubular epithelial cell permeability allows loss of potassium and entrance of hydrogen ions back into the cell. Hypokalemia and metabolic acidosis develop and, if renal disease is progressive, lead to death. At necropsy kidneys show tubule degeneration, peritubular fibrosis, nephrocalcinosis, and glomerular sclerosis. Other than cell swelling, no ultrastructural lesions have been described in the early phases of degenerating tubule cells.

Acute potassium deficiency, the initial deficit in amphotericin B toxicity, produces multiple secondary derangements in mammalian kidneys. The best established defect is in renal concentrating power. Vacuolation of proximal tubular epithelial cells is a prominent change, and medullary areas are severely affected. Lysosomes develop in the nephron, and dilatation and epithelial proliferation are usually present. Kaliopenic nephropathy has not been adequately documented in domestic animals, but experimental disease in laboratory rodents has been widely used as a model (McDonald et al. 1962; Muehrcke and Rosen 1964).

MERCURY

As a model for tubule damage induced by heavy metals, we examine mercury poisoning. Mercury is excreted by the glomeruli and concentrated in the tubules where it causes massive necrosis. Organomercurials from seed preservatives are responsible for poisoning when outdated seeds are fed to domestic mammals. Toxic mercury effluents from industrial pollutants poison fish and other aquatic animals. Humans may be affected by eating meat from these animals.

In the kidney, organic mercury compounds are converted to inorganic mercury which is concentrated to high levels. Inorganic mercury (such as $HgCl_2$) selectively damages the straight portion (pars recta) of the proximal tubule (Gritzka and Trump 1968; Rodin and Crowson 1962). Intracellularly, mercury is reported to concentrate in the endoplasmic reticulum. Detoxifying enzymes are present at these sites, and in experimental studies on the rat kidney this is the presumptive site of conversion of methyl to inorganic mercury. Mercurials cause the inhibition of enzymes by complexing with sulfhydryl groups on the active sites of the enzyme.

The lesions of mercury poisoning characteristically involve every nephron. Initially, there are loss of brush borders, dispersion of ribosomes, and reduplication of smooth endoplasmic reticulum. Swelling of mitochondria and fatty degeneration are later changes and necrosis is the end result (Ganote et al. 1974; Klein et al. 1973). Necrotic cells which detach and block the tubule lumens may produce anuria. If the animal survives, the tubular epithelium recovers and becomes lined with dense, low epithelial cells that cannot concentrate urine. Oliguria is characteristic. In time, the cells slowly develop into functional tubule cells.

OTHER HEAVY METALS

Other heavy metals are associated with tubular injury at different sites. Gold salts, used in the treatment of human rheumatoid arthritis, may cause tubule damage and proteinuria. The mitochondrion is the site of gold accumulation. These organelles are destroyed and expelled into the tubular lumen (Stuve and Galle 1970). Uranium poisoning damages the renal tubules. The mitochondrion, through alterations of the calcium-transport mechanism, becomes a locus for calcium deposition (Carafoli et al. 1971). Massive increase of mitochondrial calcium leads to mitochondrial swelling, clarification of the matrix, and death of the cell.

PROTEIN ABSORPTION

When hemoglobin passes into the glomerular filtrate, it accumulates as reddish eosinophilic protein droplets in the proximal convoluted tubules. Hemoglobin enters the apical absorption vacuoles by pinocytosis and is transferred to lysosomes where hydrolytic breakdown occurs (Ericsson 1965). If solutions containing hemoglobin are infused intravenously in an experimental animal, hemoglobinuria develops within 1 hr. Droplets (which stain for hemoglobin and acid phosphatase) progressively develop and reach a peak at 4 hrs. They soon begin to disappear and are absent at 24 hrs. Massive accumulation of hemoglobin is sometimes seen in renal failure and the lesions are termed hemoglobinemic nephrosis. Hemoglobin by itself is not injurious, however, and other processes such as circulatory failure and bacterial endotoxin are required for serious injury to the kidney (Hoffmeister et al. 1965).

In severe icterus, bilirubin collects in a similar manner in the proximal convoluted tubules. Swelling of affected cells occurs (De Vos et al. 1972) but there is little or no impairment of function. "Cholemic nephrosis" as seen in man has not been described in the kidneys of animals. Renal melanosis occurs in cattle but the nature of the pigment is not clear (Winter 1966).

ANOXIC NEPHROSIS

The common denominator of this diverse subtle group of injuries is diminished renal circulation. It may be seen in shock, severe burns, trauma, and in sudden massive obstruction of the intestine. Tubulorrhexis, the essential lesion, is scattered randomly throughout the kidney. Other lesions are often superimposed; it is usually difficult to interpret the changes in anoxic injury to the renal tubule.

OTHER TUBULAR DEFECTS

Cystinuria is a familial metabolic renal tubular disease reported in humans and dogs. It occurs in Dachshunds and in Scottish and Irish terriers. The defect is in the kidney and its capacity to take up cystine. No definitive structural changes are present although ultrastructural evidence of cystine crystals has been described in human cystinuria (Witzelben et al. 1972). In dogs, plasma levels of cystine are normal but there are increased concentrations of cystine (and lysine and arginine) in the urine (Tsan et al. 1972). There is a predisposition to stone formation and male dogs may develop pure cystine calculi in the urinary bladder.

Dalmation dogs excrete urates due to a tubular resorptive defect. Urates are not absorbed from the glomerular filtrate. There is no deficiency of uricase or in the rate of urate metabolism (Kessler et al. 1959). Urate calculi may develop but urates are not deposited in the kidney.

END STAGE KIDNEY AND RENAL FAILURE

Because renal functions are interdependent upon all portions of the nephron, progressive chronic renal disease evolves into the end stage kidney. Kidney structure is radically altered; it is often impossible to interpret the primary causal mechanism. Glomerular disease enhances tubular disease and vice versa. These organs are no longer kidneys in the conventional sense but a collection of distorted nephrons deviating chaotically from normal. There is wide diversity of nephron function and the urine is a composite product of these highly abnormal nephrons. For practical purposes, the pattern of injury is limited to the dog and cat which are fortunate enough to survive to old age but unfortunate in being nursed through long chronic terminal illness.

Structurally, the end stage kidney is distorted by deposition of connective tissue. Large segments of the parenchyma are atrophic, particularly the tubules. Tubular epithelium which remains is hyperplastic and embedded in a meshwork of collagen, ground substance, and tubular remnants (Fig. 8.9). Glomerulosclerosis is invariably superimposed on any primary lesions in the glomeruli. Vasculitis and vascular degeneration are prominent. The media of the arterioles is enlarged by hyalin changes and, in cases of acidosis and hyperparathyroidism, calcium deposits are present (Scarpelli et al. 1960).

The pathways of all severely destructive diseases of the kidney lead to uremia. In the dog and cat, the commonest causes are chronic interstitial nephritis and chronic progressive amyloidosis. Hydronephrosis and pyelonephritis also cause uremia, but less frequently.

Azotemia is the retention of nitrogenous wastes in the blood. It develops from the inability of the kidney to excrete these substances (or through their failure to reach

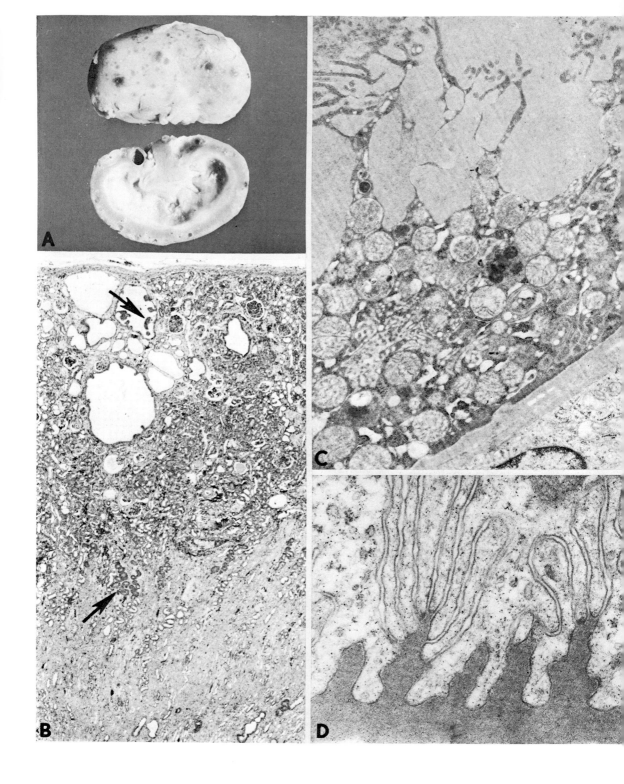

Table 8.3. Mechanisms in chronic uremia in the dog

Depression of	Leads to		Pathology
Glomerular filtration	PO$_4$ retention ⎤ ⟶ Parathyroid hyperplasia ⟶ Bone resorption ⟶		OSTEOPOROSIS
	SO$_4$ retention	and Hypocalcemia	
	H$^+$ retention		
	Urea retention ⎱ ⟶ Acidosis ══════════════════		ACIDOSIS
Tubular secretion & reabsorption	NH$_4^+$ retention ⎰ ⟶ Hyperammonemia		
	K$^+$ retention ⟶ Hyperkalemia		CARDIAC DYSFUNCTION
	Na$^+$ loss ⟶ Hyponatremia		
Tubular detoxification	⟶ Toxin accumulation		ANEMIA VASCULAR DAMAGE

the kidney, as in circulatory failure). When azotemia becomes symptomatic, the condition is termed uremia. The retention of nitrogenous wastes is reflected in elevations of blood urea nitrogen (BUN); this laboratory test is customarily taken as an index of renal function even though urea is not directly responsible for all the signs of uremia.

UREMIA

Uremia is the complex systemic disease syndrome brought about by decreased glomerular filtration and failure of tubular resorption and secretion (Table 8.3). There are: (1) failure to conserve water (volume regulation), (2) electrolyte imbalance, (3) acid-base imbalance, and (4) failures in the excretion of urea and other nonprotein nitrogenous wastes. As the tubules fail to resorb water, urine volumes may remain large until shortly before death. Failure to absorb sodium and to secrete ammonia leads to progressive metabolic acidosis.

Vomiting, weakness, congestion of mucous membranes, and paleness and coolness of the skin are seen in animals with uremia. Neurologic signs range from drowsiness to coma. The abnormal electroencephalographic changes in dogs are related to increased Ca^{++} content to the brain (Guisado et al. 1975). An ammonia odor of the breath is common. In dogs, ulceration and inflammation of the tongue and oral mucosa are nearly always present. "Uremic gastritis," a striking lesion occasionally encountered in dogs, is due to severe edema, hemorrhage, necrosis, and calcification of the gastric mucosa. Lesions of the intestinal tract are also common, although they are more subtle. In some species, colitis is prominent (Nairn and Williams 1955). The pleura and other serous membranes may be thickened with edema and effusions of serum and fibrin.

No single substance has been identified as the "uremia toxin" that acts at a cellular level. Urea, ammonia, creatinine, and guanidine (or its derivatives) have all waxed and waned as culprits. It now appears that the "toxin" is a circulating dialyzable protein that affects cAMP levels and the sodium pump to produce diminished plasma membrane function, which is in

Fig. 8.9. End stage kidney, dog. A. Severe pyelonephritis and secondary degeneration, renal parenchyma. Cortex is thinned and contains multiple cystic spaces. Pelvic areas are dilated. B. Histology. Changes include: cystic dilatation of proximal convoluted tubules with papillary proliferation of epithelium (top arrow), scarring and atrophy of glomeruli, interstitial deposition of collagen and mucopolysaccharides, and hyperplasia of regenerating epithelium of the collecting ducts (lower arrow). C. Ultrastructure of a necrotic proximal convoluted tubule, lumen filled with albumin precipitates. D. Extension of basement membrane material into canalicular system of proximal tubule cell.

turn responsible for anemia, lymphocytopenia, and vascular damage.

GASTROINTESTINAL LESIONS

In the gastrointestinal lesions of uremia, epithelial cell proliferation is enhanced. In the gastric mucosa the mitotic index is enhanced in all types of cells: parietal cells, surface epithelium, and gland cells (Wegener et al. 1971). Increased proliferation is due to shortening of the G1 phase. Gastric HCl, which is neutralized by ammonia in uremia, is not essential for mucosal proliferation.

The basis of the later lesions of edema and hemorrhage in the gastrointestinal tract is destruction of arterioles, capillaries, and venules. It is alleged that ammonia is split from urea at epithelial surfaces in relation to blood vessels and the endothelium is injured. Fibrinoid destruction of the arterioles leads to infarction of affected areas with necrosis and ulcer formation. Vascular lesions tend to occur throughout the uremic animal but their association with the disease is not fully explained. Foci of cell degeneration and necrosis are found in the myocardium, skeletal muscles, liver, and pancreas. It appears that enteric bacteria and their endotoxins may enhance the intestinal lesions of uremia (Carter et al. 1966).

LUNG

Pulmonary hyperemia and edema (and attendant dyspnea) are common manifestations of uremia. Acidosis depresses membrane transport mechanisms and this may explain injury to the alveolar wall. Lung function is also hyperactive in efforts to eliminate CO_2. Diffuse calcium deposition in the alveolar wall may lead to solid, gritty, pale lungs ("pumice lungs").

HEART

Hyperkalemia and hypocalcemia are the commonest and most significant of the electrolyte imbalances (Wirth 1962). They may influence myocardial contractility and be responsible for a twitching phenomenon of skeletal muscle.

BONE

The osteoporosis or "renal osteodystrophy" that occurs in canine uremia is of complex cause. Acidosis suppresses bone matrix formation by osteocytes, and osteoclastic resorption leads to removal of mineral at a greater rate than its surrounding matrix. Affected bones become osteoporotic and soft and are responsible for the term "rubber jaw syndrome." Although hypocalcemia occurs in uremia and does contribute to osteoclastic resorption, the changes in bone are independent of parathyroid hormone levels (Delling and Donath 1973). The kidney is necessary for synthesis of the active metabolite of vitamin D (1, 25-dihydroxycholecalciferol). Failure of damaged tubular mitochondria to produce this hormone prevents the intestinal epithelium from synthesizing the Ca^{++}-binding protein required for Ca^{++} absorption. This contributes to the hypocalcemia-hyperparathyroidism-osteodystrophy pathway in uremia (Weisbrode et al. 1974).

BLOOD

Anemia is invariably present in uremia and is due both to shortened life span of erythrocytes and to diminished erythropoiesis. The latter is caused by low plasma levels of erythropoietin. The kidney, a potent source of erythropoietin (the vascular endothelium is allegedly the site of formation and activation), is damaged sufficiently to affect its synthesis. Destruction is not caused by an intrinsic property of the uremic erythrocyte. In humans, transfusion of uremic erythrocytes into normal patients allows normal survival; normal erythrocytes transfused into uremic patients have shortened life spans (Stewart 1967).

LYMPHOID SYSTEM

Atrophy of lymphoid tissue is commonly found in long-standing uremia. Immunoreactivity is depressed, allegedly due to a failure of interaction of antibody with antigen (Kroe and Yazquez 1967). The depression of cell-mediated reactivity in human uremia enhances the survival of persons with kidney transplants.

REFERENCES

Angus, K. W. et al. Mesangiocapillary glomerulonephritis in lambs. *J. Comp. Path.* 84:319, 1974.

Arakawa, M. and Tokunaga, J. A scanning electron microscope study of the glomerulus. *Lab. Invest.* 27:366, 1972.

Asheim, A. Pathogenesis of renal damage and polydipsia in dogs with pyometra. *J.A.V.M.A.* 147:736, 1965.

Beard, M. E. and Novikoff, A. B. Distribution of peroxisomes (microbodies) in the nephron of the rat. A cytochemical study. *J. Cell Biol.* 42:501, 1969.

Bloodworth, J. M. B. Experimental diabetic glomerulosclerosis. II. The dog. *Arch. Path.* 79:113, 1965.

Brumfitt, W. and Heptinstall, R. H. Experimental pyelonephritis. *Brit. J. Exp. Path.* 41:552, 1960.

Bulger, R. E. and Trump, B. F. Fine structure of the renal medulla. *Am. J. Anat.* 118:685, 1966.

Carafoli, E. et al. A study of Ca^{2+} metabolism in kidney mitochondria during acute uranium intoxication. *Lab. Invest.* 25:516, 1971.

Carter, D. et al. The role of microbial flora in uremia. II. Uremic colitis, cardiovascular lesions, and biochemical observations. *J. Exp. Med.* 123:251, 1966.

Cheville, N. F., Mengeling, W. L. and Zinober, M. R. Ultrastructural and immunofluorescent studies of glomerulonephritis in chronic hog cholera. *Lab. Invest.* 22:458, 1970.

Cohen, A. S. and Shirahama, T. Ultrastructural studies of renal peritubular amyloid experimentally induced in guinea pigs. II. Tubular epithelial cells. *Arthr. Rheum.* 14:429, 1971.

Courtecuise, V., Habib, R. and Monnier, C. Nonlethal hemolytic and uremic syndrome in children: An electron microscope study of renal biopsy from six cases. *Exp. Mol. Path.* 7:327, 1967.

Delling, G. and Donath, K. Morphometrische, elektronenmikroskopische und physikalischchemische Untersuchungen über die experimentelle Osteoporose bei chronischer Acidose. *Virch. Arch. A* 358:321, 1973.

De Vos, R., De Woolf-Peeters, C. and Desmet, V. Electron microscopy of the tubule cells of rat kidney after experimental bile duct ligation. *Exp. Mol. Path.* 16:353, 1972.

Ericsson, J. L. E. Transport and digestion of hemoglobin in the proximal tubule. II. Electron microscopy. *Lab. Invest.* 14:16, 1965.

Ericsson, J. L. E. and Rammer, L. Renal morphology in burned rats. *Acta Path. Micro. Scand.* 80:671, 1972.

Feldman, J. D. and Fisher, E. R. Renal lesions of aminonucleoside nephrosis as revealed by electron microscopy. *Lab. Invest.* 8:371, 1959.

Ferris, T. F. et al. Toxemia of pregnancy in sheep. *J. Clin. Invest.* 48:1643, 1969.

Fisher, E. R. and Fisher, B. Glomerular lipidosis in the dog. *Am. J. Vet. Res.* 15:285, 1954.

Galton, M. and Slater, S. M. Naturally occurring fatal disease of the pregnant golden hamster. *Proc. Soc. Exp. Biol. Med.* 120:873, 1966.

Ganote, C. E., Reiner, K. A. and Jennings, R. B. Acute mercuric chloride nephrotoxicity. *Lab. Invest.* 31:633, 1974.

Ganote, C. E. et al. Ultrastructural studies of vasopressin effect on isolated perfused renal collecting tubules of the rabbit. *J. Cell Biol.* 36:355, 1968.

Gloor, F. and Neiditsch-Halff, L. A. Die interstitiellen Zellen des Nierenmarkes der Ratte. *Zt. Zellf.* 66:488, 1965.

Gritzka, T. L. and Trump, B. F. Renal tubular lesions caused by mercuric chloride electron microscopic observations. *Am. J. Path.* 52:1225, 1968.

Guisado, R. et al. Changes in the EEG in acute uremia. *J. Clin. Invest.* 55:738, 1975.

Hoffmeister, F. S., Regelson, W. and Wilkin, H. Acute renal failure. *Lab. Invest.* 14:1506, 1965.

Humair, L., Potter, E. V. and Kwaan, H. C. The role of fibrinogen in renal disease. I. Production of experimental lesions in mice. *J. Lab. Clin. Med.* 74:60, 1969.

CHAPTER NINE

Intestine

H. W. MOON, D.V.M., Ph.D.

Highly differentiated epithelial cells are the unique cytological feature of the intestinal mucosa. This discussion will consider them as an independent cell population. However, they are structurally and functionally integrated with ingesta, secretory products, and alimentary flora on their luminal aspects as well as with the mesenchymal elements of the lamina propria at their bases. Examples of this integration will be apparent.

NORMAL EPITHELIUM

Intestinal epithelium is composed of a variety of epithelial and mesenchymal cells that vary in proportion to one another and somewhat in structure and function within each cell type. These variations depend upon species, age, and location within the tract as well as the nature of any superimposed pathologic state. Furthermore, intestinal epithelium is in a constant state of migration and replacement. Normally, epithelial cell loss occurs principally and continuously from surface epithelium. In the small intestine this occurs at the tip of the villus from the extrusion zone (Fig. 9.1). The constant migration and loss of epithelial cells require constant proliferation to produce new cells and this proliferation occurs in the crypts. Thus there is a gradient within the epithelium such that the oldest, most differentiated epithelial cells are at the surface, which in small intestine is the tip of the villus. Those cells on more proximal por-

H. W. Moon is veterinary pathologist with the National Animal Disease Center, Ames, Iowa, and professor of Veterinary Pathology, Iowa State University.

tions of the villus are younger and less differentiated, while the proliferating pool of undifferentiated cells is confined to the crypts (Trier 1968).

RATE OF EPITHELIAL CELL REPLACEMENT

This rate is sometimes considered to be a constant with complete replacement occurring every 2–4 days. However, the normal replacement rate varies with species, age, and location in the intestine. For example, replacement in small intestine requires 7–10 days in newborn pigs but only 2–4 days in 3-wk-old pigs (Moon 1971). A similar acceleration in replacement rate occurs at about 3 wks of age in rats and mice (Grey 1968; Koldovsky et al. 1966). This postnatal acceleration is at least partly an adaptation to the microflora, because replacement remains comparatively sluggish in germ-free mice and pigs even after the immediate neonatal period (Abrams et al. 1963a; Moon et al. 1973b). It is not known whether the microflora cause accelerated replacement by direct cytotoxicity (Ranken et al. 1971) or indirectly as the result of chronic inflammation of the lamina propria. Endocrine changes as the result of adaptation to the flora probably also accelerate replacement at this time (Herbst and Sunshine 1969). Replacement is further accelerated in some pathologic states such as salmonellosis of mice (Abrams et al. 1963b), transmissible gastroenteritis of swine (Thake et al. 1973), celiac sprue, and ulcerative colitis of humans (Eastwood and Trier 1973; Trier and Browning 1970). There are several mechanisms that act

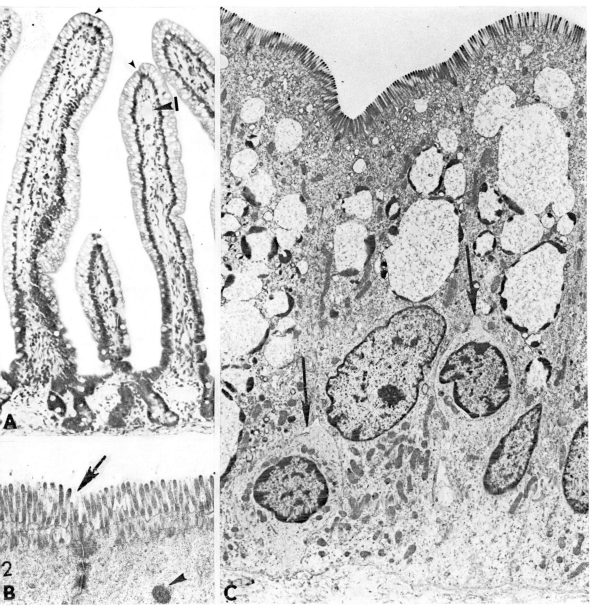

Fig. 9.1. Normal epithelium. A. Ileum, 13-day-old pig. Note cell
volume, vacuolation, and staining differences from new cells in crypts
to mature cells at the extrusion zones (arrow). Large dilated lacteal
in villous lamina propria (l). B. Microvilli (M), absorptive cells, rabbit
cecum. Note spherical bodies (large arrow). Terminal web (2), lysosome
(small arrow). C. Ultrastructure of A. Vacuolated absorptive cells near
tip of villus. Large supranuclear vacuoles have dense precipitates on
their limiting membranes (material taken from lumen by endocytosis).
Vesicles and tubules in terminal web. Lymphocytes are in lateral
intercellular spaces (arrows).

alone or in combination to change the replacement rate. For example, accelerated replacement would occur if the number of proliferating crypt cells were increased, or if the rate at which individual cells proliferate were accelerated (i.e., a reduction in time required for a single proliferating cell to synthesize DNA, divide, and for a daughter cell to reenter DNA synthesis). Reduction in villus size also accelerates replacement by reducing the number of nonproliferating cells to be replaced. In addition, villous epithelium regulates the proliferation of crypt cells by feedback inhibition (Galjaard et al. 1972). The inhibitory substances are referred to as *chalones,* and chalone production is apparently directly proportional to the number of villous epithelial cells. Thus normally crypt proliferation can be considered to be at a chalone-inhibited rate. Reduction in villus size would be expected to result in accelerated replacement by reducing the number of cells to be replaced and by increased proliferation because of reduced chalone inhibition.

MAJOR CELL TYPES

Cells of several distinctly different structural and functional types occur in intestinal epithelium. Absorptive epithelial cells and their precursors, the undifferentiated crypt epithelial cells, are present throughout the intestinal tract and are more numerous than the others. Furthermore, the major digestive and absorptive functions of the epithelium depend upon the integrity of these two highly integrated cell types. Thus they are the major cell types in intestinal epithelium.

UNDIFFERENTIATED CRYPT EPITHELIAL CELLS

These are the most numerous crypt epithelial cells and are the progenitors for other epithelial cells. They occur throughout the crypts or start near the base and

extend nearly to the mouth of the crypt, depending upon species and location within the intestine (Fig. 9.2). In addition to their location and proliferative activity, undifferentiated crypt cells can be recognized by their sparse short irregular microvilli, reasonably straight lateral membranes with multiple desmosomes at their apex, numerous free ribosomes and polyribosomes, and by their numerous membrane-bound apical secretory granules (Fig. 9.3). These cells are equipped to divide, synthesize protein, and secrete into the intestinal lumen. There is good evidence that one substance secreted by one type of secretory granule in these cells is secretory antibody (IgA) (Allen et al. 1973; Atkins et al. 1971; Schofield and Atkins 1970). This antibody is probably synthesized locally in the lamina propria by plasma cells. It is not known whether the secretory piece of IgA is added to the molecule during transit through undifferentiated cells or whether this addition occurs later, in the intestinal lumen. Presumably, undifferentiated cells have little or no absorptive capacity. As they migrate toward the villi their microvilli elongate, become more numerous and regular, and develop a full complement of digestive and absorptive enzymes. Near the crypt mouth there is cessation of proliferation, completing the metamorphosis to the mature absorptive cells of surface epithelium.

ABSORPTIVE EPITHELIAL CELLS

These tall columnar cells are characterized by numerous long, regular microvilli along their luminal borders. The microvilli have a surface glycocalyx (Fig. 9.3) that consists in part of digestive and absorptive enzymes (Ito 1969; Johnson 1969). Microvilli and glycocalyx become more extensive as the cell matures in its migration toward the villous tip or surface of the epithelium. Microvilli are more numerous, regular, and elongated on villous absorp-

Fig. 9.2. A. Normal crypt epithelium from pig jejunum. Lumen and microvilli (1), undifferentiated cells (2), undifferentiated cells in mitosis (3), secretory granules at the apex of undifferentiated cells (4), portions of goblet cells (5), enterochromaffin cell (6). Note close apposition of cells. B. Paneth cells, crypt-base, normal rabbit jejunum. Cytoplasm dominated by large apical secretion granules and lamellae of rough ER. Crypt lumen (1), lysosome (2).

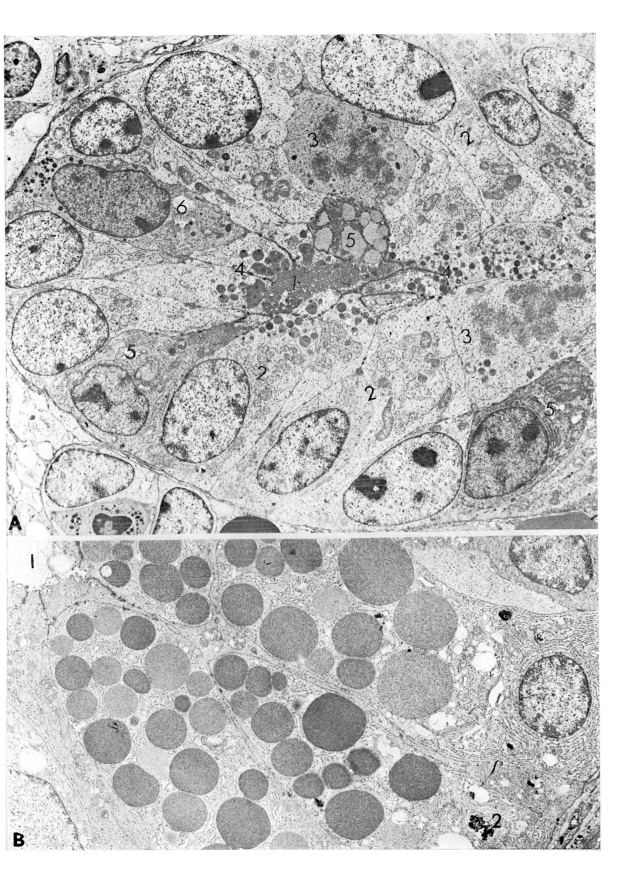

A

B

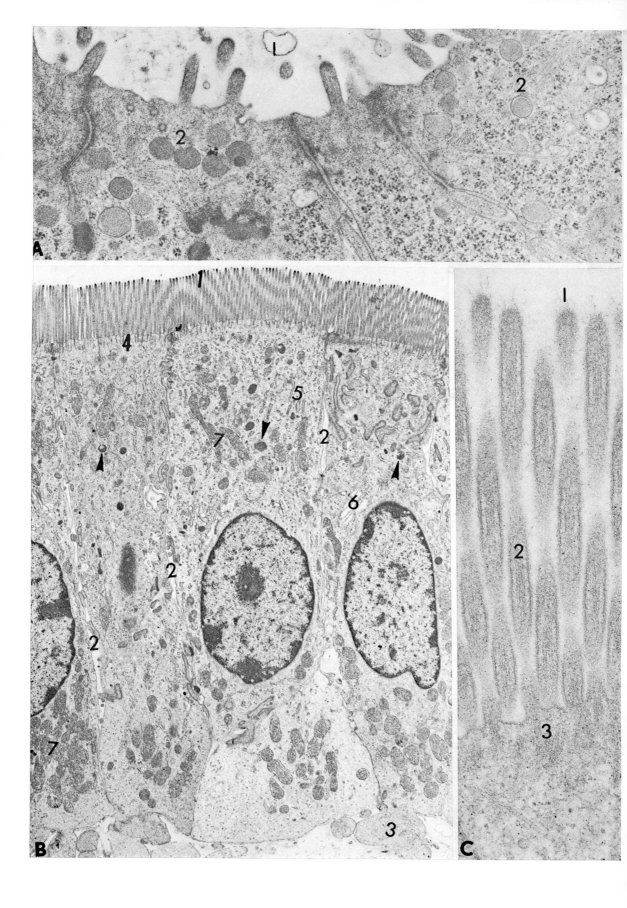

tive cells of small intestine than on surface absorptive cells in the colon. In addition, colonic epithelial cells have numerous small spherical bodies dispersed among their microvilli (Donnellan 1965). The significance of these bodies is unknown, but those unfamiliar with normal structure could confuse them with virus particles (Fig. 9.1). The area immediately beneath the microvilli is called the terminal web and is relatively free of organelles except for filaments that extend into the cores of the microvilli. The remainder of the cytoplasm contains numerous mitochondria, occasional lysosomes, rough endoplasmic reticulum, and vesicles. Absorptive cells interdigitate extensively along their lateral borders and usually have a single desmosome in their apical junctional complex. The lateral intercellular space, between the apical junctional complexes and the basement membrane of absorptive cells, does not occur in normal crypt epithelium. This space becomes progressively more prominent as the cells move toward the extreme surface or villous tip. Most absorbed materials, such as water or lipid, move into the lateral intercellular space on their way to blood and lymph (Loeschke et al. 1970; Tomasini and Dobbins 1970). The prominence of the lateral intercellular space depends both upon stage of cellular differentiation and physiologic state of the particular field examined.

Under some conditions, absorptive cells develop invaginations of their apical membranes that connect or merge with tubules in the terminal web and eventually with vesicles and large vacuoles in the cytoplasm (Fig. 9.1). In neonatal mammals, cells with this apical tubular and vacuolar system dominate the villous epithelium for hours, days, or weeks depending upon species and location in small intestine (Clarke and Hardy 1970; Kraehenbuhl and Campiche 1969). This system is involved in macromolecular uptake and the absorption of colostral and milk antibody from the intestinal lumen during passive immunization of the newborn. There is also evidence that this pinocytotically active epithelium serves as a portal of entry for bacteria and viruses during the neonatal period (Staley et al. 1969; Worthington and Graney 1973).

Epithelial cell differentiation occurs continuously throughout the life of the cell. Vacuolated villous absorptive cells in the ileum of the pig demonstrate that epithelial cell replacement rate influences the degree of differentiation and thus the cytology of the epithelium. Absorptive cells differentiate to vacuolated absorptive cells with marked pinocytotic capacity at about 4 days post–DNA synthesis (Moon et al. 1973a). Thus maximally differentiated (vacuolated) absorptive cells dominate the ileal epithelium during the first 2–3 wks of life when replacement is sluggish. However, with accelerated epithelial replacement after this period, cells are sloughed before they reach this stage of differentiation.

Absorptive cells on the distal portions of villi in proximal small intestine of newborn pigs and rats have pseudopodlike cytoplasmic processes extending through the epithelial basement membrane into the lamina propria (Kraehenbuhl and Campiche 1969) (Fig. 9.3). These also disappear when the host is about 3 wks old. It has been suggested that they facilitate macromolecular exchange between epithelial and mesenchymal elements in the mucosa during maturation (Mathan et al. 1972). The apical position of nuclei and

Fig. 9.3. A. Normal rabbit jejunum, crypt lumen, and apical portions of undifferentiated cells. Luminal blebs of cell cytoplasm (1). Microvilli are short, sparse, and irregular. Junctional complexes have multiple desmosomes. Secretion granules (2) and free ribosomes are numerous. B. Normal absorptive cells, proximal portion, jejunal villus, young pig. Microvilli (1) are numerous, long, and regular. Lateral cell membranes interdigitate extensively but lateral intercellular spaces are apparent (2). Basal cytoplasmic processes (3) extend through the basement membrane into lamina propria. Terminal web (4), rough endoplasmic reticulum (5), Golgi apparatus (6), mitochondria (7), lysosomes (arrows). C. Higher magnification of microvilli from cell showing glycocalyx (1), and central filaments (2), which extend into the terminal web as rootlets (3).

subnuclear position of the Golgi complex in villous absorptive cells in newborn pigs (Staley et al. 1968) are additional cytologic variations that occur in the neonate only and could be confused with pathologic processes.

MINOR CELL TYPES

EPITHELIAL CELLS

Goblet cells occur both in crypt and villous epithelium (Fig. 9.2). Presumably their only important functional contribution is mucus secretion. They do have a few apical microvilli in addition to their characteristic mucous granules and prominent rough endoplasmic reticulum. Discharged goblet cells appear shrunken with dilated ER and dark cytoplasm; they may contain some small mucus droplets.

Paneth cells occur at or near the bases of the crypts in small intestine (Fig. 9.2). They are prominent in primates and rodents but do not occur in cattle, cats, dogs, or pigs. Their functional significance is not well understood; however, they are both phagocytic and secretory (Erlandsen and Chase 1972a,b). In histologic sections they are recognized by their distribution and large acidophilic granules. Ultrastructurally, large secretory granules nearly fill their cytoplasm; nuclei are basal; and there are prominent lamellar arrays of rough ER, numerous lysosomes, and a few irregular microvilli. The lysosomal debris may be phagocytosed material or accumulated autophagic material. Paneth cells are longer lived than most intestinal epithelial cells (Troughton and Trier 1969).

Enterochromaffin cells (argentaffin cells) occur throughout the alimentary tract mostly in crypts (Fig. 9.2). They are endocrine cells and can be further classified on the basis of granule type and content: that is, whether they contain serotonin, catecholamine, gastrin, secretin, or enteroglucagon (Forssmann et al. 1969). Enterochromaffin cells tend to be triangular in outline, with most of their small heterogeneous secretory granules between the nucleus and broad aspect of the cell which is near the basement membrane. This arrangement coupled with their endocrine function suggests that the secretory products are liberated into tissue and eventually enter the blood, in contrast to other intestinal epithelial cells that secrete their products into the intestinal lumen.

Enterochromaffin cell neoplasms occur in humans and rarely in animals. Some humans with enterochromaffin cell tumors develop a carcinoid syndrome characterized by circulatory and respiratory malfunction and watery diarrhea. These signs are presumably caused by complex secretory products released from the neoplastic cells into the blood.

MESENCHYMAL CELLS

Lymphocytes are common in the intercellular spaces between epithelial cells and are referred to as theliolymphocytes (Fig. 9.1). They increase in numbers during the neonatal period and during chronic inflammation, presumably in response to exposure to antigens. It is not known if theliolymphocytes are entrapped in and slough with the epithelium, or migrate back into the lamina propria, or if they migrate through the epithelium into the intestinal lumen.

Polymorphonuclear leukocytes (neutrophils) are seen occasionally in normal epithelium and are numerous during some inflammatory processes. In inflammation they are also numerous in the lamina propria and in the intestinal lumen. Thus they are considered to be merely passing through the epithelium. They can do this readily when the epithelial cells separate at their apical tight junctions during inflammation. They move through epithelium into the intestinal lumen in large numbers during certain immune reactions and there are numerous neutrophils in the intestinal lumen normally (Bellamy 1973). They can phagocytize bacteria in the lumen: the lysosomal enzymes liberated by degenerating neutrophils may also influence bacteria in the intestinal lumen (Fig. 9.4).

Globule leukocytes are mononuclear cells named for their large eosinophilic cytoplasmic granules (Fig. 9.5). Ultrastructurally, the globules are membrane bound, the cells have pseudopods, and they are located in the intercellular spaces of the epithelium. Globule leukocytes are nearly all in epithelium and can be seen throughout

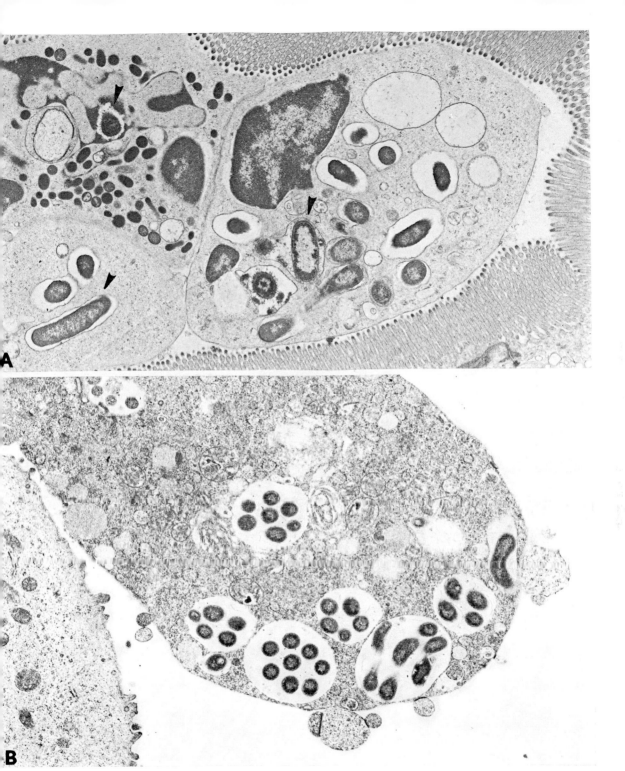

Fig. 9.4. A. Jejunum, newborn pig after exposure to enterotoxigenic *E. coli*. Neutrophils, in lumen surrounded by microvilli, contain *E. coli* (arrows), and are in various stages of degranulation. Fuzzy surface of some *E. coli* is an early degenerative change. B. Degenerate absorptive cells sloughed from surface of cecal epithelium, rabbit, acute cecocolitis. Cytoplasmic vesicles contain numerous bacteria *(Vibrio* sp.) and bits of flagellae. Microvilli missing except remnants on cell at left.

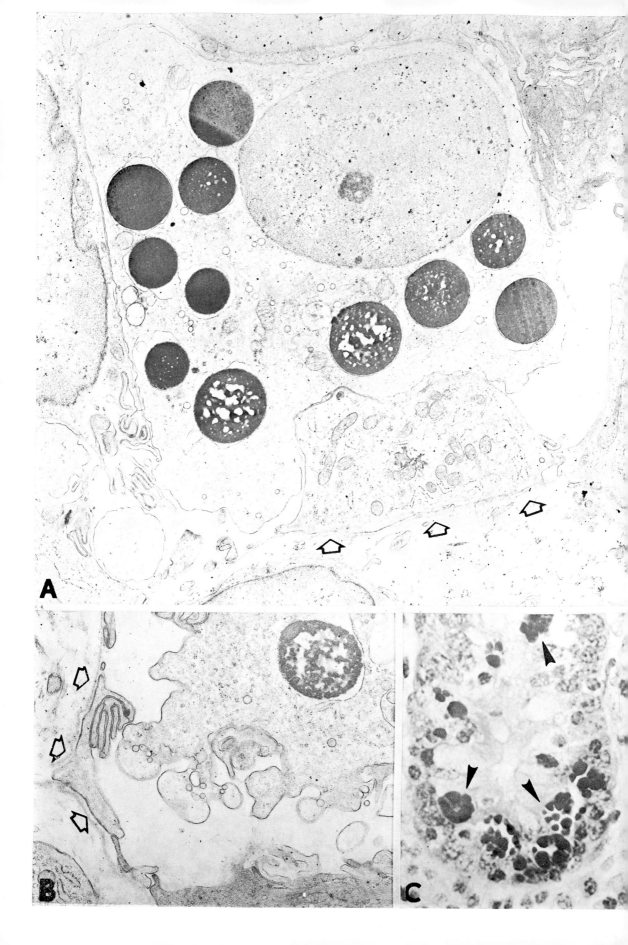

the intestinal tract of animals in which they occur. They increase in number during the neonatal period and during parasite infestations in some species. The content of the globules is similar to that of Paneth cell granules and there is some evidence the globular content can be discharged into the intestinal lumen (Takeuchi et al. 1969). There is confusion as to whether globule leukocytes arise from plasma cells, lymphocytes, or mast cells. The functional significance of these cells remains unknown. A tumor of globule leukocytes in the ileum of a cat has been reported (Finn and Schwartz 1972).

Mast cells in intestinal epithelium are rare (Dobbins et al. 1969).

DISEASES OF EPITHELIUM

This discussion emphasizes some of the principal features of epithelial pathology by selecting a disease that illustrates the feature to be discussed. Some diseases are characterized by destruction and loss of a specific cell type, while others may affect several types of epithelial cells. In some cytolytic processes the early target may be rather selective but as the lesion progresses there may be nonselective extension to all elements of the mucosa, submucosa, and even the tunica muscularis. Not all intestinal diseases are characterized by cell destruction. Some are characterized by primary abnormalities of subcellular organelles while the affected target cells remain viable. Furthermore, some diseases are characterized by profound functional alterations with little or no associated morphologic abnormality.

DISEASES OF ABSORPTIVE CELLS

VIRAL-INDUCED CELL DESTRUCTION

Transmissible gastroenteritis of swine (TGE) is an acute disease characterized by vomiting, diarrhea, dehydration, and high mortality in newborn pigs. The disease is caused by a coronavirus that grows in and destroys absorptive cells in the small intestine. The virus does not affect crypt epithelium nor lamina propria, and these latter elements remain viable (Pensaert et al. 1970; Thake 1968). Degenerate absorptive cells are rapidly sloughed, and there may be temporary areas of microulceration. Lost cells are replaced by others migrating from the less injured villous base or virus-free crypt epithelium. These cells become cuboidal to squamous as they expand to cover the cell-depleted area. In addition, the lamina propria contracts, greatly reducing villous length and thus the surface area to be covered by epithelium. The resultant lesion at this state (Fig. 9.6) is referred to as *villous atrophy* because of the reduction in surface area, volume, and absorptive cell population of the villi. Viral particles can be found among microvilli or within cytoplasmic vesicles of absorptive cells. Lipid accumulates in the cytoplasm and mitochondria; occasional profiles of endoplasmic reticulum may be distended. In addition to degenerative changes, the surface epithelial cells that remain on the remnants of villi are incompletely differentiated; that is, they have the sparse short irregular microvilli, numerous free ribosomes, and deficient enzyme profile characteristic of crypt epithelium or epithelium from the villous base. These incompletely differentiated cells are delivered to the surface because cell loss and epithelial migration occur more rapidly than differentiation (Thake 1968; Thake et al. 1973).

In contrast to villous epithelium, the continuous demand for cells results in hyperplasia of crypt epithelium and expansion of the crypt cell population. As the virus disappears the hyperplastic crypts rebuild the villi in a matter of days. Thus because of lack of damage to crypt epithelium and lamina propria the lesion of transmissible gastroenteritis is rapidly and completely reversible (Hooper and Haelterman 1969; Moon et al. 1973b).

The functional deficit resulting from this lesion is referred to as *malabsorption*.

Fig. 9.5. Globule leukocytes. A. In intercellular space of villous epithelium, cat. Epithelial basement membrane (arrows). Leukocyte separated from basement membrane by portion of an absorptive cell. B. Globule leukocyte has several pseudopodia (Micrograph, A. Takeuchi). C. Histology. Globule leukocytes (arrows), jejunal crypt, goat.

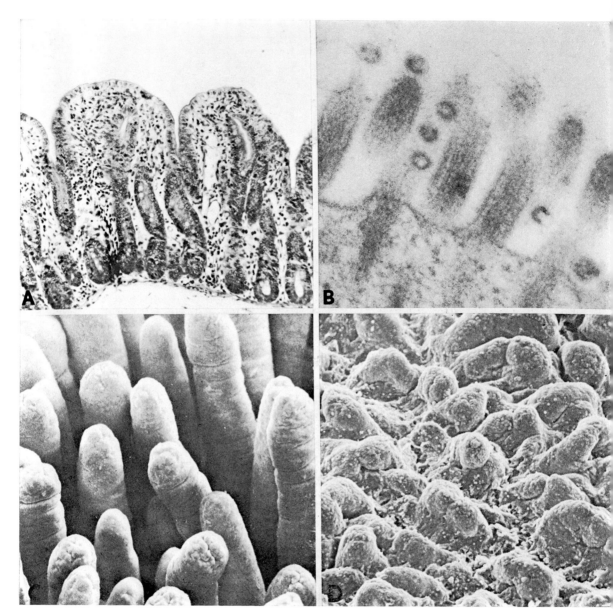

Fig. 9.6. Pig jejunum, transmissible gastroenteritis. A. Histology.
Villi are atrophic; crypts are hyperplastic. B. Ultrastructure. Virus
particles are interspersed among the short microvilli of this absorptive
cell; glycocalyx is intact (Micrograph, D. Thake). C. and D. Scanning
electron micrographs of normal (C) and atrophic (D) villi in transmissible gastroenteritis (Micrographs, K. Rhoades).

In reality, both digestive and absorptive capacities of the mucosa are reduced because of diminished villous surface area and diminished numbers of absorptive cells, as well as diminished functional capacity of the incompletely differentiated cells remaining. Ingesta and normal alimentary secretions are unabsorbed, and they undergo bacterial degradation and fermentation in the intestine. This degradation increases the osmolality of the intestinal contents and fluid is drawn into the intestine by the resultant osmotic gradient (Hooper and Haelterman 1966). Absorptive cells in the large intestine are not affected by this virus. Because of the pathology in the small intestine, however, the material presented to the large intestine is qualitatively abnormal and its quantity exceeds the absorptive capacity of the large intestine. Thus much of the fermented ingesta and the enteroluminal fluids generated by them are excreted as the watery feces characteristic of this diarrheal disease.

Selective absorptive cell damage or destruction also occurs in other viral diseases such as epizootic diarrhea of infant mice, neonatal calf diarrhea caused by a reolike virus, and lethal intestinal virus infection of mice (Adams and Kraft 1967; Biggers et al. 1964; Mebus et al. 1971). It also occurs in such bacterial diseases as human food poisoning caused by staphylococcal enterotoxin and in anoxic or chronic inflammatory lesions of intestine (Kent and Moon 1973).

INTRACELLULAR BACTERIA AND
CELL DESTRUCTION

Shigellosis (bacillary dysentery) is an acute bacterial colitis of monkeys, chimpanzees, and humans. The disease usually does not affect the small intestine and bacteremia is rare. The ability of Shigella to cause enteric disease depends upon their capacity to penetrate, multiply within, and destroy epithelial cells (LaBrec et al. 1964). Absorptive cells are much more susceptible to this invasion than crypt cells are. The cell destruction results in flattened epithelium and microulceration. There is also hemorrhage and acute exudative inflammation of the lamina propria. It is not clear to what extent the inflammation is secondary to epithelial cell damage and to products released from the damaged bacteria-infested surface epithelial cells or what proportion is caused by the occasional bacteria that reach the lamina propria. It is clear that the bacteria principally inhabit colonic epithelial cells and have little tendency to expand beyond them. In the dysentery of shigellosis, feces contain abundant fresh blood and mucus in contrast to the watery feces characteristic of damage to absorptive cells in small intestine.

Shigella occur intracellularly within membrane-lined vacuoles in the cytoplasm of the epithelial cells. Some infected cells become shrunken, dark, and pyknotic; others become swollen and pale with dilated ER, mitochondria, and nuclei. Lipid droplets and lysosomal debris accumulate in the cytoplasm, and cells separate from the basement membrane, pile up, become rounded, separate at the apical junctional complexes, and slough (Takeuchi 1971). It is not clear to what extent flattening of surface cells and abbreviation of microvilli are a result of juvenile incompletely differentiated cells migrating to the surface. As in TGE, there is crypt hyperplasia and one expects rapid regeneration upon removal of the agent.

Some other bacterial diseases seem to follow this model. For example, in *swine dysentery*, spirochetes *(Treponema hyodysenteriae)* invade and cause damage to colonic surface epithelium similar to that seen in shigellosis (Glock and Harris 1972). In addition, Vibrio have been seen within absorptive cells in the large intestine of rabbits with diarrheal disease (Moon et al. 1974) (Figs. 9.4 and 9.7) and certain strains of *E. coli* associated with dysentery in man cause disease in a Shigellalike manner (DuPont et al. 1971).

In contrast to Shigella, Salmonella rapidly move deep into the mucosa and become septicemic. During their initial penetration of epithelial cells they cause focal degeneration of microvilli but little else, even though they actually enter the absorptive cells (Takeuchi 1971). On the other hand, some protozoa, such as Coccidia, also cause enteric disease by penetration of, multiplication within, and destruction of intestinal absorptive cells.

The growth phase of Coccidia occurs in

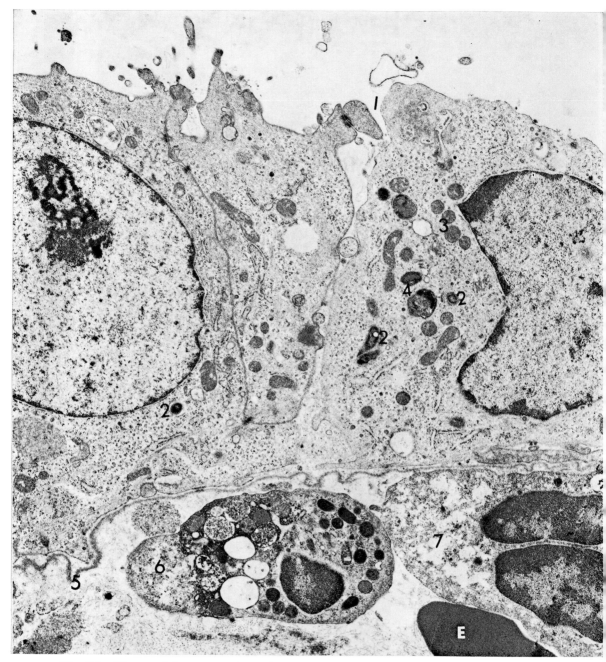

Fig. 9.7. Flattened degenerate absorptive cells in cecal epithelium,
rabbit, acute vibrionic cecocolitis. Microvilli are sparse and degenerate.
Apical junctional complexes are open and dilated (1). Intracellular
Vibrio sp. (2), mitochondria (3), lysosome (4), intact basement
membrane (5), polymorphonuclear leukocyte (6), macrophage or
degranulated neutrophil (7), erythrocyte (E).

host epithelial cells and is responsible for the clinical signs of disease: diarrhea and bloody feces. Sporozoites, which develop within the oocyte, emerge when the thick durable oocyst wall is disrupted in the intestine of the newly infected host (Fig. 9.8). Within the intestinal absorptive cells, the feeding sporozoites are termed trophozoites and reside within a membrane-bound parasitophorous vacuole. By the process of schizogony, trophozoites give rise to many new cells called merozoites (Fig. 9.9). Merozoites break out of the infected cell and may either begin new cycles of schizogony or initiate sexual division by developing into macro- or microgametocytes. Pathogenicity of coccidial isolates is related to their tendency to sustain asexual cycles of schizogony, the process that extensively destroys intestinal epithelium.

The intracellular replication of Coccidia leads to increased epithelial cell loss and crypt cell hyperplasia of the parasite-laden intestinal mucosal epithelium. Depending on the balance between accelerated loss and replacement of epithelial cells that is reached, crypt epithelium may be hyperplastic and villi atrophic or both elements may be hyperplastic (Fernando and McCraw 1973; Kent and Moon 1973). The anticipated functional consequence is malabsorption accompanied by exudation.

Cryptosporidia are other sporozoan parasites that invade intestinal epithelium in several host species and cause changes similar to those seen in coccidiosis (Vetterling et al. 1971). These parasites inhabit the extreme apex of the epithelial cells where they are attached to the absorptive cell surface by a highly specialized attachment zone (Fig. 9.10). In severe infections, microulceration of the mucosa occurs and leads to edema and hemorrhage.

ABNORMALITIES OF MICROVILLI AND GLYCOCALYX

The brush border may be functionally deranged but structurally normal in specific enzyme deficiencies such as lactase deficiency or deficiency of other disaccharidases (Christopher and Bayless 1971; Crane 1966). In lactase deficiency, as it occurs in humans, milk consumption leads to abdominal discomfort and diarrhea because lactose cannot be digested and thus is not absorbed. Even though absorptive cells are morphologically intact in this disease, the pathophysiology of the diarrhea is similar to that in TGE where absorptive cells are destroyed. In both diseases, the unabsorbed lactose remains in the intestinal lumen and is carried along to the colon, where it undergoes microbial fermentation to organic acids and gas. Lactose in the lumen of the small intestine and the fermentative products in the colon increase the osmotic pressures of these fluids, and thus instead of absorption more fluid is drawn into the intestinal lumen osmotically, causing a diarrhea. It is thought that the fermentative products might also exert a further cathartic effect by stimulating colonic peristalsis and mucus secretion. The syndrome is sometimes referred to as lactose intolerance because other substances are digested and absorbed normally by the otherwise normal brush border; thus diets free of lactose cause no problem. In some individuals lactase deficiency is a congenital enzyme defect; however, in many human populations lactase levels in intestine normally decline during childhood and most adults are intolerant of large oral loads of lactose. Similarly swine intestine at birth has high lactase and low sucrase and maltase content (Hartman et al. 1961). Thus sucrose and maltose are not well utilized by the neonate and diets rich in these disaccharides fed early in the neonatal period result in diarrhea. Later in life they are well tolerated because as lactase levels decline with age, sucrase and maltase levels increase. Hereditary glucose and galactose malabsorption in man apparently has similar mechanisms, but instead of digestive enzyme (disaccharidase) deficiency, here apparently an enzyme involved in the transport of monosaccharide from brush border into the cell is deficient. Thus this disease operates specifically at the absorptive rather than digestive level (Meeuwisse and Dahlquist 1968).

Neomycin can also cause brush border disease, enzyme deficiency, and malabsorption. Toxic amounts of this drug cause fragmentation of microvilli and disruption of the glycocalyx (Cain et al. 1968). The generalized structural abnormality of the brush border in neomycin toxicity con-

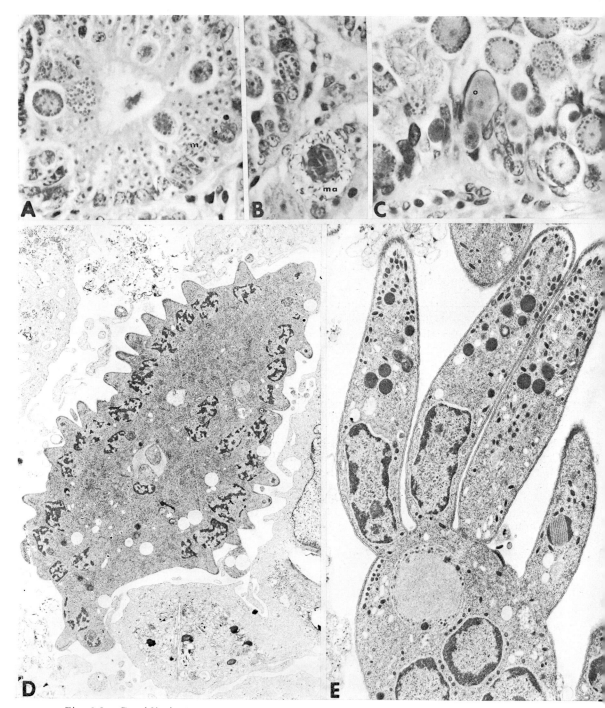

Fig. 9.8. Coccidiosis. A.–C. Histology of infected intestinal epithelial cells. Oocyst (o), merozoite (m), macrogamete (ma). D. Ultrastructure of trophozoite with merozoite buds and multiple nuclei. E. Merozoites budding from the mother blastophore (Micrographs, G. Kelley).

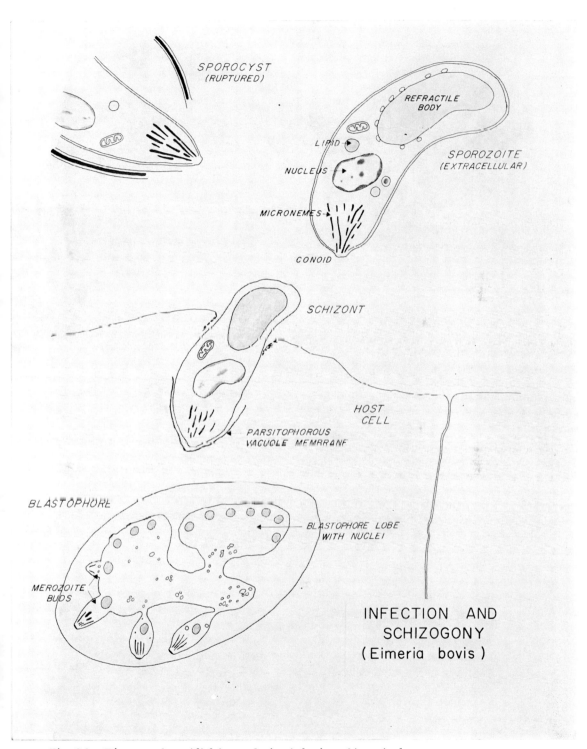

SPOROCYST
(RUPTURED)

REFRACTILE
BODY

LIPID

NUCLEUS

SPOROZOITE
(EXTRACELLULAR)

MICRONEMES

CONOID

SCHIZONT

HOST
CELL

PARSITOPHOROUS
VACUOLE MEMBRANE

BLASTOPHORE

BLASTOPHORE LOBE
WITH NUCLEI

MEROZOITE
BUDS

INFECTION AND
SCHIZOGONY
(Eimeria bovis)

Fig. 9.9. Diagram of coccidial forms during infection of intestinal epithelial cell.

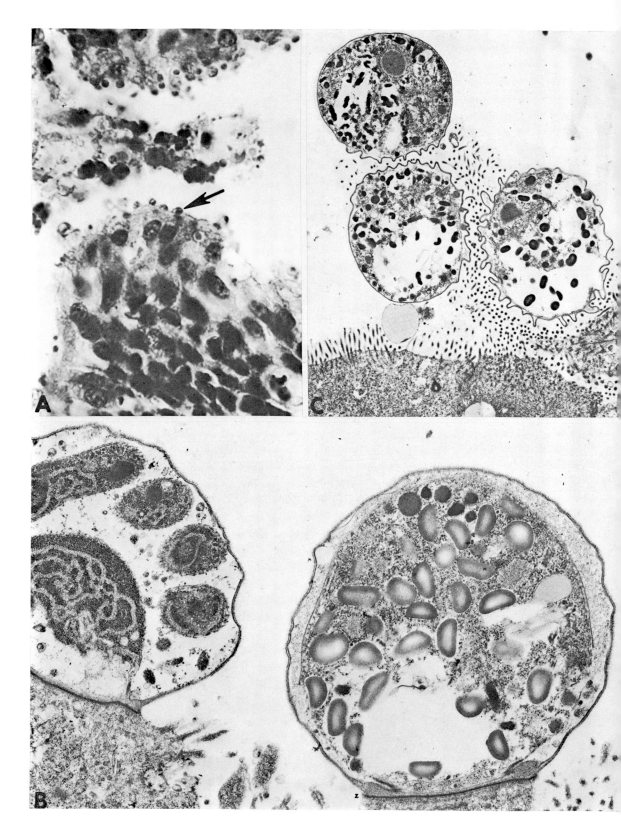

trasts with the morphologically normal microvilli in the specific enzyme deficits mentioned above. Thus in contrast to the hereditary enzyme deficiencies, one would expect malabsorption in neomycin deficiency to be generalized rather than confined to specific substrates.

Degeneration of microvilli and effacement of the brush border is a characteristic early step in attachment to and invasion of absorptive cells by Shigella, E. coli, and other bacteria (Staley et al. 1969; Takeuchi 1971) (Figs. 9.4 and 9.7). The affected areas are widely scattered on villous absorptive cells and the extent of decreased absorptive capacity resulting from the focal damage to microvilli in these infections is unknown. The destruction and loss of absorptive cells and enterotoxin-mediated secretion of fluid by the mucosa are probably more important in diseases caused by these bacteria than the degenerative changes in microvilli.

DISEASES OF UNDIFFERENTIATED CRYPT CELLS

VIRAL-INDUCED CELL DESTRUCTION

In contrast to TGE, the target cells for infection and destruction by the parvovirus of feline panleukopenia are the rapidly proliferating and undifferentiated crypt epithelial cells (Kent and Moon 1973). Thus in feline panleukopenia, as villous absorptive cells are sloughed from the tips of the villi they are not replaced by new cells from the crypts. Eventually both crypts and villi become depleted of cells because migration and cell shedding from the tips of the villi continue; absorptive capacity is eventually impaired, as in TGE. Thus both diseases are manifested by diarrhea resulting from lack of absorptive cells. However, pathogenesis of the lesion differs, because in TGE these cells are destroyed directly but in feline panleukopenia normal cell losses are not replaced.

RADIATION

Intestinal radiation injury, like panleukopenia virus, destroys crypt but not villous epithelium and leads to decreased absorptive capacity because of diminished replacement of epithelial cells, thus the lesions of intestinal radiation injury are similar to those in feline panleukopenia.

DISEASES IN WHICH EPITHELIAL TARGET CELLS ARE UNKNOWN OR NOT SPECIFIC

BACTERIAL ENTEROTOXINS

Human cholera and enteric enterotoxic colibacillosis of pigs, calves, lambs, and humans are acute enteric diseases characterized by a profuse watery diarrhea which can result in fatal dehydration and acidosis even though the causative bacteria and their toxins are confined to the intestinal epithelium. These diseases are caused by certain strains of E. coli and Vibrio cholerae that produce specific exotoxins referred to as E. coli enterotoxin and cholera enterotoxin or choleragen. The distinguishing feature of these enterotoxins is that local enteroluminal exposure to them causes the small intestine to secrete water and electrolytes. When this secretion exceeds colonic absorption, diarrhea results. In contrast to many enteric diseases, there may be little or no cytopathology associated with the profound functional abnormality of the intestinal mucosa caused by these enterotoxins (Moon 1974; Moon et al. 1971). Discharge of goblet cell mucus can be demonstrated, but other organelles of epithelial cells as well as the capillaries and lymphatics in the lamina propria remain morphologically normal. In order to understand the mechanism of such diseases, the pathologist needs to know both the cytology and electrolyte transport mechanisms of the epithelium.

Sodium ions (Na^+) are constantly

Fig. 9.10. Cryptosporidiosis, goose intestine. A. Histology. Organisms attached to the surface of the intestinal absorptive cells (arrow). B. and C. Ultrastructure of cryptosporidia. Note attachment zone (z) to epithelial cells and the thin rim of epithelial cell cytoplasm surrounding the parasite on the lower right (Micrographs, J. Proctor).

pumped out of normal epithelial cells at their lateral borders into the lateral inter-cellular space (Fig. 9.11). Therefore Na⁺ concentration within the cells is kept low. However, the membrane of the microvillous border of the cell is permeable to Na⁺, and Na⁺ from the intestinal lumen constantly enters the cell by diffusion from an area of high to an area of low Na⁺ concentration. This Na⁺ in turn is pumped out into the intercellular space. Sodium in the intercellular space either diffuses across the basement membrane into the vessels of the lamina propria to be carried away thus contributing to net Na⁺ absorption, or diffuses through the apical junctional complexes between cells back into the intestinal lumen thus reducing net Na⁺ absorption. Water transport is entirely passive and moves with electrolyte transport in response to the osmotic gradients generated by electrolyte transport. Therefore net Na⁺ absorption also results in net water absorption. The movement of electrolytes into the cell across the plasma membrane of the microvillous border is thought to be controlled by cyclic 3′-5′ adenosinemonophosphate (cAMP). Increased cAMP decreases electrolyte entry into the cell and thus electrolyte and water absorption. However, back diffusion from the intercellular space through the apical junctional complexes continues, resulting in net secretion of electrolyte and water into the intestinal lumen. Furthermore, elevated cAMP stimulates active secretion of Cl⁻

by epithelial cells. In normal intestine this entire process is usually regulated so that absorption exceeds secretion. However, enterotoxins from *V. cholerae* and *E. coli* cause elevated cAMP levels in epithelial cells and thus result in intestinal secretion by altering normal control mechanisms, not by causing structural damage (Schultz and Frizzell 1972).

There is evidence that crypts are the principal site of this secretory process (Roggin et al. 1972). However, the electrolyte and water transport phenomena affected are thought to be principally functions of absorptive cells. Thus there is confusion as to whether undifferentiated, absorptive, or even goblet cells are the principal targets of the enterotoxins.

In addition to their enterotoxigenicity the *E. coli* and *V. cholerae* associated with these diseases have special attributes of virulence which enable them to colonize the small intestine. They adhere to the apical surface of villous absorptive cells (Fig. 9.12) and overcome the washout effects of peristalsis which would otherwise carry them harmlessly down to the enterotoxin-resistant colon. In contrast to the *Shigella* and penetrating strains of *E. coli* discussed earlier, they have little tendency to invade the epithelial cells to which they adhere. Furthermore, these bacteria have no particular propensity to cause septicemia (Bertschinger et al. 1972).

Many of the *E. coli* strains associated with enteric enterotoxic colibacillosis of

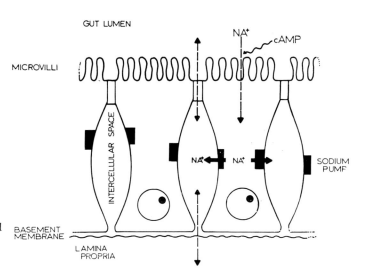

Fig. 9.11. Sodium transport across intestinal epithelium. Diffusion (broken arrow); unidirectional active transport by sodium pump (solid arrow); cAMP inhibition of sodium entry into cell (crooked arrow.)

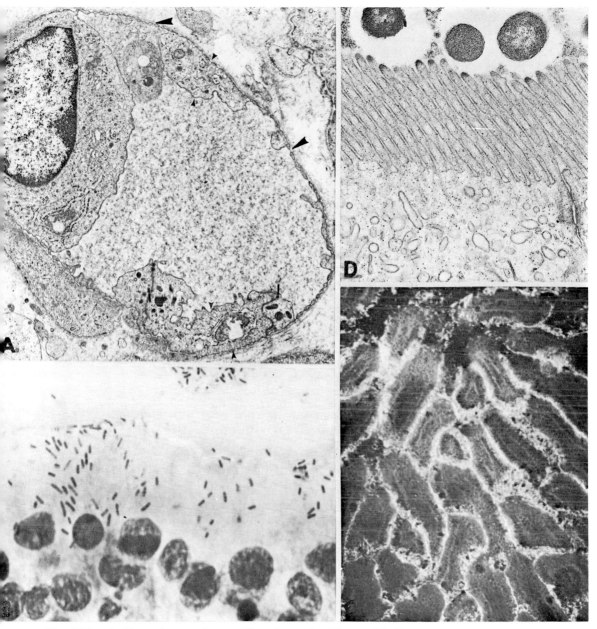

Fig. 9.12. A. Normal-appearing capillary beneath villous epithelium, pig jejunum 16 hrs after exposure to cholera enterotoxin. Fenestrae (large arrows), plasmalemmal vesicles (small arrows), and intercellular junctions (1) of endothelial cells are intact. B. *E. coli* adhering to villous epithelium of jejunum, newborn pig. C. Fluorescent antibody-stained section, heavy continuous layer of *E. coli* along surface of epithelium. D. Ultrastructure. Organisms separated from absorptive cell microvilli by lucent region.

pigs possess a surface antigen designated as K88. The K88 antigen occurs as a fine filamentous network of fimbriaelike protein strands that surround the bacterial cell and confer adhesive capacity to those strains that possess it (Jones and Rutter 1972; Stirm et al. 1967). Presumably adherence is the result of physical-chemical interactions between the filamentous K88 network of the bacterium and the filamentous glycocalyx network of the absorptive cell. It is thought that *V. cholerae* and those strains of *E. coli* that lack K88 antigen but still adhere to absorptive cells do so via K88-like surface structures.

The genetic information for both enterotoxin and K88 production by *E. coli* is mediated by plasmids rather than the bacterial chromosome. Each is located on a separate plasmid which can be transmitted from one bacterial strain to another during sexual conjugation. The plasmid mechanism apparently offers a method for the dissemination of these virulent attributes among *E. coli* in nature (Smith and Lingood 1971).

Clostridium perfringens type C also causes enteric disease in newborn pigs, lambs, and calves via an enterotoxin which the causal bacteria liberate in the intestine. The early stages of this disease are also characterized by adhesion of the causal bacteria to absorptive cells in the small intestine (Arbuckle 1972). In contrast to the enterotoxins of *V. cholerae* and *E. coli*, the enterotoxin of *Cl. perfringens* type C (beta toxin) is markedly cytotoxic. The early lesion caused by this toxin is necrosis of villous absorptive cells. With time the necrotic process extends nonselectively to involve all elements of lamina propria, crypt epithelium, submucosa, and even tunica muscularis. The usual end result of this process is a sharply defined segmental lesion in the jejunum, characterized by hemorrhage, necrosis, and fibrin exudation involving the full thickness of the intestinal wall (Barnes and Bergeland 1970). Certain type A strains of *Cl. perfringens* associated with human food poisoning also produce an enterotoxin (Duncan et al. 1968). The toxin is also active in the intestine of domestic animals (Hauschild et al. 1970) and in the future it may be shown to cause spontaneous disease in animals.

The lesion produced by type A enterotoxin has not been completely characterized but it differs from that produced by the type C strains.

SEPARATION OF APICAL JUNCTIONAL COMPLEXES

The apical portions of the junctional complexes between epithelial cells are characterized by fusion of plasma membranes between adjacent cells (Trier 1968). This region is sometimes referred to as the tight junction or zonula occludens and serves as a barrier to macromolecular movement across the epithelium (Fig. 9.3). However, as mentioned when discussing intestinal secretion, there is evidence that electrolytes and water can cross the tight junction by diffusion. Presumably fusion at the tight junction is reversible, because normal epithelial cells do slough individually. Furthermore, cells from several crypts normally migrate onto one villus, and not all epithelial cells migrate at the same rate. Such migratory patterns could not occur with membrane fusion between cells unless the tight junctions could be opened and reestablished.

In certain parasitic diseases such as gastric ostertagiasis in cattle (Murray 1969) and intestinal Nippostrongylus infestation (Murray et al. 1971) as well as other inflammatory lesions, the tight junctions are opened pathologically and permit macromolecules to move through them. This has been proposed as a route for the delivery of massive amounts of serum antibody to the intestinal lumen in parasite infestations. In some inflammatory diseases, diarrhea is thought to be explained by the *leaky membrane* concept. That is, exaggerated loss of fluid to the intestinal lumen is thought to occur via open (Fig. 9.7) or defective tight junctions resulting in increased ultrafiltration of electrolytes or exudation of serum. Increased filtration pressures in the absence of mucosal inflammation may also open this route for macromolecule transport in some protein-losing enteropathies (Finco et al. 1973). Enteric diseases in which tight junctions are defective might also be complicated by movement of toxic macromolecules from the intestinal lumen to the blood.

NEOPLASIA

Adenomas and carcinomas of intestinal epithelium are less common than epithelial neoplasms in other systems in animals. They are most frequently encountered in aged dogs and cats, with the colon having the greater incidence in the former and the small intestine in the latter (Brodey and Cohen 1964; Hayden and Nielsen 1973). The low incidence of colonic neoplasia contrasts with humans, in whom colonic cancer is a leading cause of death. Diets high in fat red meat are thought to cause cancer of the colon in humans by changing colonic flora so that it either actively synthesizes carcinogens de novo from food residue, or releases preformed carcinogens in the colon by deconjugation of substances normally excreted in bile in their relatively noncarcinogenic conjugated glucuronide form (Reddy et al. 1974).

The maturation arrest characteristic of neoplastic cell populations has been recognized in adenomas of the human colon (Kaye et al. 1973). Mature epithelial cells were infrequent even at the mucosal surface in adenomas. Instead, undifferentiated crypt cells extended along the crypts toward the mouths, and the remainder of the epithelium was comprised chiefly of cells intermediate between undifferentiated and mature absorptive or goblet cells. Some characteristics of these immature cells were short sparse irregular microvilli, straight lateral membranes with few intercellular interdigitations and numerous desmosomes, sparse rough endoplasmic reticulum, numerous free ribosomes, and continued proliferative activity (Kaye et al. 1971). There is evidence that such adenomatous epithelium extends across the surface of the mucosa and rather than sloughing at this point, as in normal mucosa, proliferates back down into adjacent crypts, undermining and replacing normal epithelium as it goes (Lane and Lev 1963). Malignant transformation occurs in adenomatous epithelium and results in atypical cells qualitatively different from those seen in normal epithelium. The atypical cells may have bizarre nuclei, lack any evidence of differentiation, form giant cells, and extend through the basement membrane (Kaye et al. 1973).

In contrast to what might be expected in a proliferative lesion, neoplastic human colonic epithelial cells actually proliferate at subnormal rates with marked prolongation of the G_2 or postsynthetic premitotic phase of the cell cycle (Lipkin 1971). Thus neoplastic growth occurs because of an increased proportion of cells remaining in the proliferative cycle. This is additional evidence of arrested maturation.

DISEASES OF LAMINA PROPRIA

The lamina propria is composed of mesenchymal tissue and its unique features are related chiefly to its integration with epithelium and to the functional characteristics of the intestinal mucosa. Morphologically, diseases of the lamina propria resemble similar processes in well-vascularized lymphoreticular tissues elsewhere in the body.

DISEASES OF VASCULATURE

Endothelial cells of blood capillaries in villous lamina propria have fenestrae which are more numerous at the venous than at the arterial end of the capillary (9.12). Such capillaries tend to be polarized with fenestrae in that portion subjacent to the epithelium and with endothelial cell nuclei on the opposite side of the vessel (Casley-Smith 1971). In the healthy mucosa and in experimental cholera (Yardley and Brown 1973), macromolecules cross the endothelium via these fenestrae and the plasmalemmal vesicles of the endothelial cells.

INCREASED CAPILLARY PERMEABILITY

Inflammatory lesions of the mucosa are characterized by increased capillary permeability. This is caused at least in part by separation of the tight junctions between endothelial cells both in the nematode-induced, immune-mediated, mast cell–associated, macromolecular leak characteristic of Nippostrongylus infestation of rats, and in experimental mustard oil–induced enteritis (Hurley and McQueen 1971; Murray et al. 1971). It may be that transport via fenestrae and plasmalemmal vesicles is also enhanced in such inflammatory lesions, further contributing to increased capillary permeability, within the intestinal mucosa.

LYMPHANGIECTASIA

Syndromes referred to as *protein-losing enteropathies* are frequently characterized by lymphangiectasia in the intestinal mucosa and marked transudation of protein into the intestinal lumen (Finco et al. 1973). The causes of the syndromes in humans and dogs are unknown; however, massive infiltration of the lamina propria by macrophages laden with *Mycobacterium paratuberculosis* in Johne's disease is one cause of protein-losing enteropathy in cattle (Nielsen and Andersen 1967). Lymphangiectasia probably occurs because of obstruction of lymph flow by lesions in the submucosa and mesenteric lymph nodes, such as granulomatous lymphangitis and lymphadenitis in Johne's disease, rather than as the result of primary damage to mucosal lacteals.

DISEASES OF LYMPHORETICULAR TISSUE

INFILTRATIVE PROCESSES

Canine histiocytic ulcerative colitis (granulomatous colitis of Boxers) is a disease of unknown cause and genetic predisposition characterized by progressive ulcerative colitis and chronic dysentery in young Boxer dogs (Russell et al. 1971; Van Kruiningen 1967). Canine histiocytic ulcerative colitis, Johne's disease of ruminants, intestinal tuberculosis, and Whipple's disease of man (Dobbins and Ruffin 1967) are all characterized by chronic inflammation of the lamina propria leading to a massive accumulation of macrophages, along with other cells of chronic inflammation, in the lamina propria. The latter three diseases are caused by bacteria which persist and probably multiply within macrophages, thus accounting for the progressive infiltrative nature of the lesions. However, the cause of canine histiocytic ulcer-

ative colitis is not known, and it is not clear whether the periodic-acid-Schiff staining macrophages which characterize this disease accumulate autophagic debris, specific causal infectious agents, or both (Gomez et al. 1974). The cause of this disease, the reasons Boxers are predisposed to it, and whether the primary inborn defect is in epithelium, lamina propria, or both seem to be useful areas for research that would significantly enhance our understanding of chronic inflammatory diseases of intestine.

Malignant lymphoma and amyloidosis are additional infiltrative processes of the lamina propria that may lead to mucosal malfunction.

Researchers do not know to what extent infiltrative lesions of the lamina propria cause malabsorption merely by occupying space and physically impairing diffusion in the mucosa and to what extent mucosal malfunction in these diseases is the result of epithelial changes or increased vascular permeability for any of these diseases. In view of the functional integration between elements of the mucosa and the complex nature of these diseases, it seems useful to assume that all three processes are involved to varying degrees in space-occupying lesions of the lamina propria (Kent and Moon 1973).

NECROTIZING PROCESSES

Such diseases as bovine virus diarrhea and feline panleukopenia which cause necrosis and cellular depletion of lymphoreticular tissues in other systems do so in the intestinal lamina propria as well. At the current state of our knowledge it does not seem useful to speculate whether or not such lesions in the lamina propria contribute to the digestive malfunctions characteristic of these diseases.

PATHOGENESIS AND CONSEQUENCES OF DIARRHEA

Diarrhea is defined as the excretion of abnormally fluid feces and is usually accompanied by increased volume of feces and increased frequency of defecation. It is a sign common to many enteric diseases but is not specific for primary enteric malfunction in that it occurs consistently in some primary gastric, pancreatic, and endocrine diseases as well. This discussion has indicated several mechanisms by which primary enteric diseases lead to diarrhea: (1) malabsorption, or malabsorption accompanied by bacterial fermentation, leading to osmotic diarrhea as in TGE of swine, (2) hypersecretion by a structurally intact mucosa as in enteric enterotoxic colibacillosis, and (3) exudation in diseases characterized by increased capillary and/or epithelial permeability such as shigellosis or the chronic protein-losing enteropathies. It seems probable that all three mechanisms are involved in some diseases. Intestinal hypermotility, resulting in decreased transit time and thus malabsorption, with a functionally normal intestinal mucosa, is often cited as an additional mechanism leading to diarrhea. There is no well-documented specific disease where

this has been shown to be the primary mechanism. It may occur; however, decreased transit time probably occurs when intestinal contents become abnormally fluid as the result of one of the three mechanisms above, even if propulsive muscular contractions remain normal or decrease. Increased intestinal fluid may also cause secondary hypermotility. The subject has not received enough study for useful generalization, but numerous fragmentary bits of evidence suggest that intestinal motility is decreased in some diarrheal diseases.

The systemic consequences of diarrhea are dehydration, acidosis, and electrolyte imbalance, and these are all interrelated (Fig. 9.13). Dehydration leads to hypovolemia and hemoconcentration, inadequate tissue perfusion, anaerobic glycolysis, hypoglycemia, and keto-acidosis (Tennant and Ewing 1971). Acidosis also occurs because of inadequate renal excretion of H^+ and absorption of HCO_3^-. This is probably a comparatively late effect of inade-

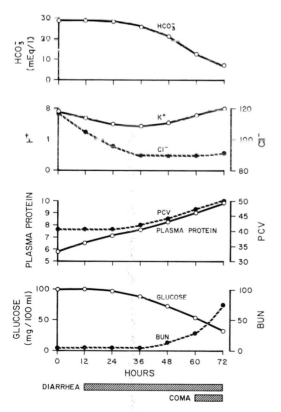

Fig. 9.13. Blood values during fatal enteric infection and diarrhea. Note acidosis, hyperpotassemia, hypochloridemia, hypoglycemia (due to shift to anaerobic glycolysis), and terminal renal failure. Increase in packed cell volume (PCV) and plasma proteins is relative due to loss of fluid from plasma (after Tennant et al. J.A.V.M.A. 161:993, 1972).

quate renal perfusion. Direct massive losses of HCO_3^- in fecal fluids also contributes to and may be the major cause of acidosis. Acidosis leads to decreased blood and tissue pH, and thus myriad vital enzyme systems are not maintained at their pH optima. Furthermore, intracellular H^+ increases and intracellular K^+ decreases; hyperkalemia frequently results. This intracellular K^+ deficit accompanied by an extracellular K^+ excess interferes with neuromuscular control of myocardial contraction. This results in further deficits in tissue perfusion, more severe acidosis, etc.,

in the classical vicious cycle of shock. In many cases death ultimately appears to be the direct result of cardiotoxic hyperkalemia (Fisher and McEwan 1967; Moon et al. 1970). Even though plasma K^+ is elevated, total body K^+ may be depleted because of excess renal and fecal excretion. In acute diarrhea of horses and in other species with prolonged diarrhea or after fluid therapy that does not adequately restore depleted total body K^+, hypokalemia occurs and can also lead to cardiac failure (Tasker 1971; Tennant and Ewing 1971).

REFERENCES

Abrams, G. D., Bauer, H. and Sprinz, H. Influence of normal flora on mucosal morphology and cellular renewal in the ileum. A comparison of germ-free and conventional mice. *Lab. Invest.* 12:355, 1963a.

Abrams, G. D. et al. Cellular renewal and mucosal morphology in experimental enteritis. *Lab. Invest.* 12:124, 1963b.

Adams, W. R. and Kraft, L. M. Electron-microscopic study of the intestinal epithelium of mice infected with the agent of epizootic diarrhea of infant mice (EDIM virus). *Am. J. Path.* 51:39, 1967.

Allen, W. D., Smith, C. G. and Porter P. Localization of intracellular immunoglobulin A in porcine intestinal mucosa using enzyme-labelled antibody. *Immunology* 25:55, 1973.

Arbuckle, J. B. R. The attachment of *Clostridium welchii (Cl. perfringens)* type C to intestinal villi of pigs. *J. Path.* 106:65, 1972.

Atkins, A. M., Schofield, G. C. and Reeders, T. Studies on the structure and distribution of immunoglobulin A—containing cells in the gut of the pig. *J. Anat.* 109:385, 1971.

Bellamy, J. E. C. Neutrophil emigration into the lumen of the porcine small intestine. Ph.D. dis., Univ. of Saskatchewan, Saskatoon, 1973.

Bergeland, M. E. Clostridial infections. In *Diseases of Swine.* H. W. Dunne and A. D. Leman, eds., Iowa State Univ. Press, Ames, 1975.

Bertschinger, H. U., Moon, H. W. and Whipp, S. C. Association of *Escherichia coli* with small intestinal epithelium. I. Comparison of enteropathogenic and nonenteropathogenic strains in pigs. *Inf. Immun.* 5:595, 1972.

Biggers, D. C., Kraft, L. M. and Sprinz, H. Lethal intestinal virus infection of mice (LIVIM). An important new model for the study of the response of the intestinal mucosa to injury. *Am. J. Path.* 45:413, 1964.

Brodey, R. S. and Cohen, D. An epizootiologic and clinicopathologic study of 95 cases of gastrointestinal neoplasms in the dog. *Proc. 101st Ann. A.V.M.A.*, p. 167, 1964.

Cain, G. D., Reiner, E. B. and Patterson, M. Effects of neomycin on disaccharidase activity of the small bowel. *Arch. Int. Med.* 122:311, 1968.

Casley-Smith, J. R. Endothelial fenestrae in intestinal villi: Differences between the arterial and venous ends of capillaries. *Microvascular Res.* 3:49, 1971.

Christopher, N. L. and Bayless, T. M. Role of the small bowel and colon in lactose-induced diarrhea. *Gastroenterology* 60:845, 1971.

Clarke, R. M. and Hardy, R. N. Structural changes in the small intestine associated with the uptake of polyvinyl pyrrolidone by the young ferret, rabbit, guinea-pig, cat and chicken. *J. Physiol.* 209:669, 1970.

Crane, R. K. Enzymes and malabsorption: A concept of brush border membrane disease. *Gastroenterology* 50:254, 1966.

Dobbins, W. O. and Ruffin, J. M. A light and electron-microscopic study of bacterial invasion in Whipple's disease. *Am. J. Path.* 51:225, 1967.

Dobbins, W. O., Tomasini, J. T. and Rollins, E. L. Electron and light microscopic identification of the mast cell of the gastrointestinal tract. *Gastroenterology* 53:268, 1969.

Donnellan, W. L. The structure of the colonic mucosa. The epithelium and subepithelial reticulohistiocytic complex. *Gastroenterology* 49:496, 1965.

Duncan, C. L., Sugiyama, H. and Strong, D. H. Rabbit ileal loop response to strains of *Clostridium perfringens*. *J. Bact.* 95:1560, 1968.

DuPont, H. L. et al. Pathogenesis of *Escherichia coli* diarrhea. *New Engl. J. Med.* 258:1, 1971.

Eastwood, G. L. and Trier, J. S. Epithelial cell renewal in cultured rectal biopsies in ulcerative colitis. *Gastroenterology* 64:383, 1973.

Erlandsen, S. L. and Chase, D. G. Paneth cell function: Phagocytosis and intracellular digestion of intestinal microorganisms. I. *Hexamita muris*. *J. Ult. Res.* 41:296, 1972a.

———. Paneth cell function: Phagocytosis and intracellular digestion of intestinal microorganisms. II. Spiral microorganisms. *J. Ult. Res.* 41:319, 1972b.

Fernando, M. A. and McCraw, B. M. Mucosal morphology and cellular renewal in the intestine of chickens following a single infection of *Eimeria acervulina*. *J. Parasit.* 59:493, 1973.

Finco, D. R. et al. Chronic enteric disease and hypoproteinemia in 9 dogs. *J.A.V.M.A.* 163:262, 1973.

Finn, J. P. and Schwartz, L. W. A neoplasm of globule leucocytes in the intestine of a cat. *J. Comp. Path.* 82:323, 1972.

Fisher, E. W. and McEwan, A. D. Death in neonatal calf diarrhea. II. The role of oxygen and potassium. *Brit. Vet. J.* 123:4, 1967.

Forssmann, W. G. et al. The endocrine cells in the epithelium of the gastrointestinal mucosa of the rat. *J. Cell Biol.* 40:692, 1969.

Galjaard, H., VanDerMeer-Fleggen, W. and Giesen, J. Feedback control by functional villus cells on cell proliferation and maturation in intestinal epithelium *Exp. Cell Res.* 72:197, 1972.

Glock, R. C. and Harris, D. L. Swine dysentery. II. Characterization of lesions in pigs inoculated with *Treponema hyodysenteriae* in pure and mixed culture. *Vet. Med./ Small An. Clin.* 67:65, 1972.

Gomez, J. A., Russell, S. W. and Trowbridge, J. O. Canine histiocytic ulcerative colitis. *Lab. Invest.* (submitted) 1974.

Grey, R. D. Epithelial cell migration in the intestine of the young mouse. *Develop. Biol.* 18:501, 1968.

Hartman, P. A. et al. Digestive enzyme development in the young pig. *J. An. Sci.* 20: 114, 1961.

Hauschild, A. A. W., Nilo, L. and Dorward, W. J. Response of ligated intestinal loops in lambs to an enteropathogenic factor of *Clostridium perfringens* type A. *Can. J. Micro.* 10.999, 1970.

Hayden, D. W. and Nielsen, S. W. Canine alimentary neoplasia. *Zentr. Vetmed. A* 20:10, 1973.

Herbst, J. J. and Sunshine, P. Postnatal development of the small intestine of the rat. *Pediat. Res.* 3:27, 1969.

Hooper, E. E. and Haelterman, E. O. Concepts of pathogenesis and passive immunity in transmissible gastroenteritis of swine. *J.A.V.M.A.* 149:1580, 1966.

———. Lesions of the gastrointestinal tract of pigs infected with transmissible gastroenteritis. *Can. J. Comp. Med. Vet. Sci.* 33:29, 1969.

Hurley, J. V. and McQueen, A. The response of the fenestrated vessels of the small intestine of rats to application of mustard oil. *J. Path.* 105:21, 1971.

Ito, S. Structure and function of the glycocalyx. *Fed. Proc.* 28:12, 1969.

Johnson, C. F. Hamster intestinal brush-border surface particles and their function. *Fed. Proc.* 28:26, 1969.

Jones, G. W. and Rutter, J. M. Role of the K88 antigen in the pathogenesis of neonatal diarrhea caused by *Escherichia coli* in piglets. *Inf. Immun.* 6:918, 1972.

Kaye, G. I., Pascal, R. R. and Lane, N. The colonic pericryptal fibroblast sheath. *Gastroenterology* 60:515, 1971.

Kaye, G. I. et al. Comparative electron microscopic features of normal, hyperplastic, and adenomatous human colonic epithelium. *Gastroenterology* 64:926, 1973.

Kent, T. W. and Moon, H. W. The comparative pathogenesis of some enteric diseases. *Vet. Path.* 10:414, 1973.

Koldovsky, O., Sunshine, P. and Kretchmer, N. Cellular migration of intestinal epithelium in suckling and weaned rats. *Nature* 212:1389, 1966.

Kraehenbuhl, J. P. and Campiche, M. A. Early stages of intestinal absorption of specific antibodies in the newborn. *J. Cell Biol.* 42:345, 1969.

LaBrec, E. H. et al. Epithelial cell penetration as an essential step in the pathogenesis of bacillary dysentery. *J. Bact.* 88:1503, 1964.

Lane, N. and Lev, R. Observations on the origin of adenomatous epithelium of the colon. *Cancer* 16:751, 1963.

Lipkin, M. Proliferation and differentiation of normal and neoplastic cells in the colon of man. *Cancer* 28:38, 1971.

Loeschke, K., Bentzel, C. J. and Csaky, T. Z. Asymmetry of osmotic flow in frog intestine: Functional and structural correlation. *Am. J. Physiol.* 218:1723, 1970.

Mathan, M., Hermos, J. A. and Trier, J. A. Structural features of the epithelio-mesenchymal interface of rat duodenal mucosa during development. *J. Cell Biol.* 52:577, 1972.

Mebus, C. A. et al. Pathology of neonatal calf diarrhea induced by a reo-like virus. *Vet. Path.* 8:490, 1971.

Meeuwisse, G. W. and Dahlquist, A. Glucose-galatose malabsorption. *Acta Paed. Scand.* 57:273, 1968.

Moon, H. W. Epithelial cell migration in the alimentary mucosa of the suckling pig. *Proc. Soc. Exp. Biol. Med.* 137:1651, 1971.

———. Pathogenesis of enteric diseases caused by *Escherichia coli*. *Adv. Comp. Med. Vet. Sci.* 18:179, 1974.

Moon, H. W., Kohler, E. M. and Whipp, S. C. Vacuolation: A function of cell age in porcine ileal absorptive cells. *Lab. Invest.* 28:23, 1973a.

Moon, H. W., Nielsen, N. O. and Kramer, T. T. Experimental enteric colibacillosis of the newborn pig: Histopathology of the small intestine and changes in plasma electrolytes. *Am. J. Vet. Res.* 31:103, 1970.

Moon, H. W., Norman, J. O. and Lambert, G. Age-dependent resistance to transmissible gastroenteritis of swine (TGE). I. Clinical signs and some mucosal dimensions in small intestine. *Can. J. Comp. Med. Vet. Sci.* 37:157, 1973b.

Moon, H. W., Whipp, S. C. and Baetz, A. L. Comparative effects of enterotoxins from *Escherichia coli* and *Vibrio cholerae* on rabbit and swine small intestine. *Lab. Invest.* 25:133, 1971.

Moon, H. W. et al. Intraepithelial Vibrio associated with acute typhlitis of young rabbits. *Vet. Path.* 11:313, 1974.

Murray, M. Structural changes in bovine ostertagiasis associated with increased permeability of the bowl wall to macromolecules. *Gastroenterology* 56:763, 1969.

Murray, M., Jarrett, W. F. H. and Jennings, F. W. Mast cells and macromolecular leak in intestinal immunological reactions. *Immunology* 21:17, 1971.

Nielsen, K. and Andersen, S. Intestinal lymphangiectasia in cattle. *Nord. Vetmed.* 19:31, 1967.

Pensaert, M., Haelterman, E. O. and Burnstein, T. Transmissible gastroenteritis of swine. *Arch. Ges. Virusforsch.* 31:321, 1970.

Ranken, R., Wilson, R. and Baelmear, P. M. Increased turnover of intestinal mucosal cells of germfree mice induced by cholic acid. *Proc. Soc. Exp. Biol. Med.* 138:270, 1971.

Reddy, B. W., Weisburger, J. A. and Wynder, E. L. Fecal bacterial β-glucuronidase: Control by diet. *Science* 182:416, 1974.

Roggin, E. M. et al. Unimpaired response of rabbit jejunum to cholera toxin after selective damage to villus epithelium. *Gastroenterology* 63:981, 1972.

Russell, S. W., Gomez, J. A. and Trowbridge, J. O. Canine histiocytic ulcerative colitis. The early lesion and its progression to ulceration. *Lab. Invest.* 25:509, 1971.

Schofield, G. C. and Atkins, A. M. Secretory immunoglobulin in columnar epithelial cells of the large intestine. *J. Anat.* 107:491, 1970.

Schultz, S. F. and Frizzell, R. A. An overview of intestinal absorptive and secretory processes. *Gastroenterology* 63:161, 1972.

Smith, H. W. and Lingood, M. A. Observations on the pathogenic properties of the K88, Hly and Ent plasmids of *Escherichia coli* with particular reference to porcine diarrhea. *J. Med. Micro.* 4:467, 1971.

Staley, T. E., Wynn Jones, E. and Corley, L. D. Attachment and penetration of *Escherichia coli* into intestinal epithelium of the ileum in newborn pigs. *Am. J. Path.* 56:371, 1969.

Staley, T. E., Wynn Jones, E. and Marshall, A. E. The jejunal absorptive cell of the newborn pig: An electron microscopic study. *Anat. Rec.* 161:497, 1968.

Stirm, S. et al. Episome-carried surface antigen K88 of *Escherichia coli. J. Bact.* 93:740, 1967.

Takeuchi, A. Penetration of the intestinal epithelium by various microorganisms. *Curr. Topics Path.* 54:1, 1971.

Takeuchi, A., Jervis, H. R. and Sprinz, H. The globule leucocyte in the intestinal mucosa of the cat. *Anat. Rec.* 164:79, 1969.

Tasker, J. B. Fluids, electrolytes, and acid-base balance. In *Clinical Biochemistry of Domestic Animals.* J. J. Kaneko and C .E. Cornelius, eds., Academic Press, New York, 1971.

Tennant, B. C. and Ewing, G. O. Gastrointestinal function. In *Clinical Biochemistry of Domestic Animals.* J. J. Kaneko and C. E. Cornelius, eds., Academic Press, New York, 1971.

Thake, D. C. Jejunal epithelium in transmissible gastroenteritis of swine. *Am. J. Path.* 53:149, 1968.

Thake, D. C., Moon, H. W. and Lambert, G. Epithelial cell dynamics in transmissible gastroenteritis of neonatal pigs. *Vet. Path.* 10:330, 1973.

Tomasini, J. T. and Dobbins, W. O. Intestinal mucosal morphology during water and electrolyte absorption. *Am. J. Dig. Dis.* 15:226, 1970.

Trier, J. S. Morphology of the epithelium of the small intestine. In *Handbook of Physiology*, Section 6, *Alimentary Canal*, Vol. 3, p. 1125. C. F. Code, ed., William Wilkins, Baltimore, 1968.

Trier, J. S. and Browning, T. H. Epithelial cell renewal in cultured duodenal biopsies in celiac sprue. *New Engl. J. Med.* 283:1245, 1970.

Troughton, W. D. and Trier, J. S. Paneth and goblet cell renewal in mouse duodenal crypts. *J. Cell Biol.* 41:251, 1969.

Van Kruiningen, H. J. Granulomatous colitis of boxer dogs: Comparative aspects. *Gastroenterology* 53:114, 1967.

Vetterling, J. M., Takeuchi, A. and Madden, P. A. Ultrastructure of *Cryptosporidium wrairi* from the guinea pig. *J. Protozool.* 18:248, 1971.

Worthington, B. B. and Graney, D. O. Uptake of adenovirus by intestinal absorptive cells of the suckling rat. *Anat. Rec.* 175:37, 1973.

Yardley, J. H. and Brown, G. D. Horseradish peroxidase tracer studies in the intestine of experimental cholera. *Lab. Invest.* 28:482, 1973.

CHAPTER TEN

Endocrine Glands

The science of endocrinology was born early in the twentieth century through experiments by Bayliss and Starling which showed the presence and action of secretin. They coined the word "hormone" after demonstrating release of this substance from the stomach, its conveyance by the circulating blood to the pancreas, and its stimulation in the discharge of pancreatic juice. *Hormones* are now considered as those chemical messengers synthesized by localized aggregates of cells (usually ductless glands) carried by blood to specific target tissues or organs.

When parenchymal cells of endocrine glands are injured, they undergo cell swelling, loss of glycogen, and fatty degeneration as do other rapidly metabolizing cells. Injury to the process of hormone formation is reflected in organelles concerned with synthesis and release: the endoplasmic reticulum, Golgi complex, and secretory granules. Pathologic changes that occur in the endocrine glands are reflected not only in their parenchymal cells but in the target cells stimulated by their secretion. Furthermore, many of the endocrine glands are under trophic control of the pituitary gland and complex cell changes can sometimes be detected in this organ.

The course of most endocrine disease is made more complex by secondary interacting feedback mechanisms. For example, parathyroid hormone is secreted in response to hypocalcemia, and calcitonin from the thyroid parafollicular cells in response to hypercalcemia. When blood calcium levels are drastically diminished, multiple cycles of secretion of these two hormones may be required before plasma calcium levels return to normal and are sta-

bilized. This may cause the lesions in bone, the target organ, to be difficult to evaluate.

In examining cells taken from animals with endocrine disease, it is imperative to know at what stage of the process the tissue was taken. Hypertrophy and hyperplasia are the response of endocrine glands to stimulation. Their parenchymal cells therefore are expected to be heavily granulated and to contain large active cytocavitary networks and Golgi complexes. This is indeed the case after a simple cycle of stimulation-hypertrophy. In the earliest phase, cells may be degranulate although organelles remain small. Endocrine cells tend to discharge their granules explosively on an immediate stimulatory response, while synthesis of new hormone and regranulation may take several hours.

In long-term hyperplasia, the endocrine cells may be heavily granulated or virtually devoid of granules. Prolonged stimulation usually leads to diverse reactivity among the cells of a gland, but it is common to find many cells with few granules and shrunken cytoplasm: evidence of exhaustion and inability to react to further stimulation for hormone release.

ADRENAL CORTEX

Only vertebrates have corticosteroid hormones; they are not detectable in Amphioxus or other invertebrates. Secretion of the adrenal cortex is stimulated and controlled by the pituitary, and all vertebrates have an adrenocorticotrophic hormone (ACTH). Among different species the action is similar; mammalian ACTH will stimulate secretion in the cortical cells of fish and other species. Cyclic AMP functions as an intracellular mediator of the rapid action of ACTH to enhance adrenocortical steroidogenesis (Nussdorfer and Mazzocchi 1972). ACTH produces an increase in cyclic AMP by stimulating adenyl cylcase in adrenal cortical cells.

The adrenal cortex of mammals is divided into three zones, each of which secretes a dominant specialized variant of corticosteroid: zona glomerulosa, minerocorticoids; zona fasciculata, glucocorticoids; and zona reticulata, androgenic hormones. Although their functions overlap, the secretory products are chemically different and have strikingly different physiologic effects (Table 10.1). Bird adrenals lack the mammalian type of zonation but central and peripheral areas appear to react differently to different stimuli. Amphibian and reptilian adrenal cortices are diffuse and their various functions have not been isolated into distinct zones.

The closely packed arcades of columnar cells at the periphery of the adrenal constitute the *zona glomerulosa*. Its product, *aldosterone,* affects the renal tubules by stimulating excessive sodium-for-hydrogen and sodium-for-potassium exchange. Aldosterone also stimulates sodium efflux in the gills of teleost fishes, in the nasal gland of marine birds, and in the skin and bladder of amphibians.

Hypertrophy of the zona glomerulosa occurs in a variety of diseases, demanding increased aldosterone secretion; cardiac failure with sodium retention is one example. Hypertrophy is difficult to detect grossly or microscopically as an increase in width of the layer. In the dog adrenal the zona glomerulosa has a normal thickness of 10% of the radius of the gland. Because

it is outermost, it represents 30% of the gland mass (Nichols and Hennigar 1964). An increase in width of 9% at the periphery results in a 96% increase in mass of the gland.

When adrenocortical cells are stimulated by ACTH to secrete, there are progressive decreases in cytoplasmic steroid lipid bodies, increases in smooth endoplasmic reticulum, and reduplication of mitochondrial cristae (Giacomelli et al. 1965). Mitochondria are actively engaged in synthesis of steroid hormones and exhibit striking changes when stimulated by ACTH. Cristae become bulbous and appear as small rings within the mitochondrion when they are cut in cross section. Rough endoplasmic reticulum transforms into smooth in response to ACTH (Fig. 10.1). The gerbil, whose adrenal gland in relation to body weight is one of the largest, contains large membranous whorls which transform to smooth endoplasmic reticulum in response to stress (Nickerson 1972). During rapid secretion, the adrenocortical cell cytoplasm may evert into blebs which project into the sinusoidal lumen through fenestrae in the endothelial cells (Penney et al. 1972).

On withdrawal of ACTH the adrenal cortex atrophies and regressive changes occur in its cells. Mitochondria become disoriented and enlarged, and inclusions develop within the matrix (Fig. 10.2). Some of the affected cells condense, separate from their neighbors, and fragment. The cellular pieces are ingested by sinusoidal lining cells (apoptosis) and are degraded within phagolysosomes (Wyllie et al. 1973). These changes are apt to be seen in diseases involving pituitary dysfunction, hypophysectomy (Volk and Scarpelli 1966), and hyperthyroidism (Moore and Callas 1972). If ACTH is injected into the affected ani-

Table 10.1. Biologic activity of adrenal corticoids

| | Corticosteroids | | | |
| | Glucocorticoids | | Mineralcorticoids | |
Biological Activity	Hydrocortisone	Corticosterone	Deoxy-corticosterone	Aldosterone
Gluconeogenesis	++++	++	0	+
Antiinflammatory	++++	0	0	0
Antiinsulin	++++	++++	+	+
Increases renal blood flow	++++	+	+	+
Lymphoid lysis	+++ ++	++	+	0
Sodium retention	+	+	++++	++++ (20X)

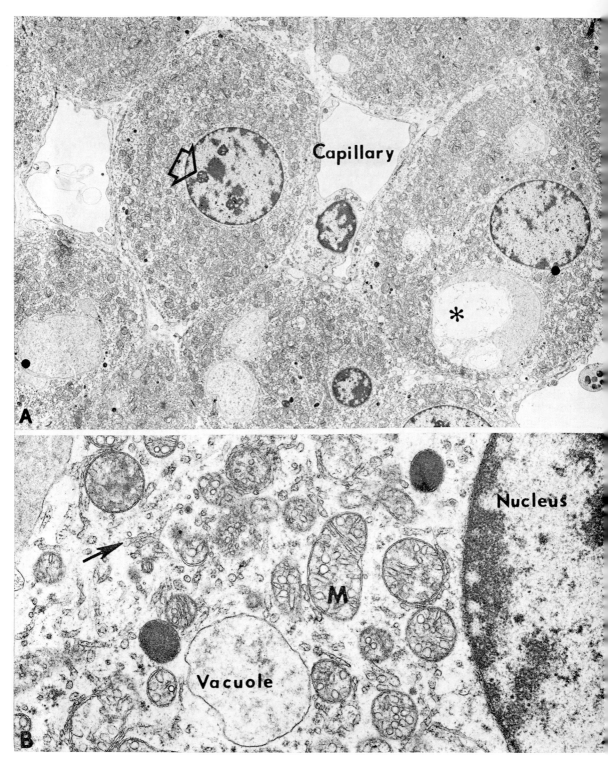

Fig. 10.1. Acute depletion of adrenal cortex, sheep, anaphylaxis.
A. Cells are vacuolated (asterisk) and depleted of granules. Note
relation of parenchymal cells to capillary, multiple nucleoli (arrow).
B. Higher power. Mitochondria (M), fragmented smooth endoplasmic
reticulum (arrow).

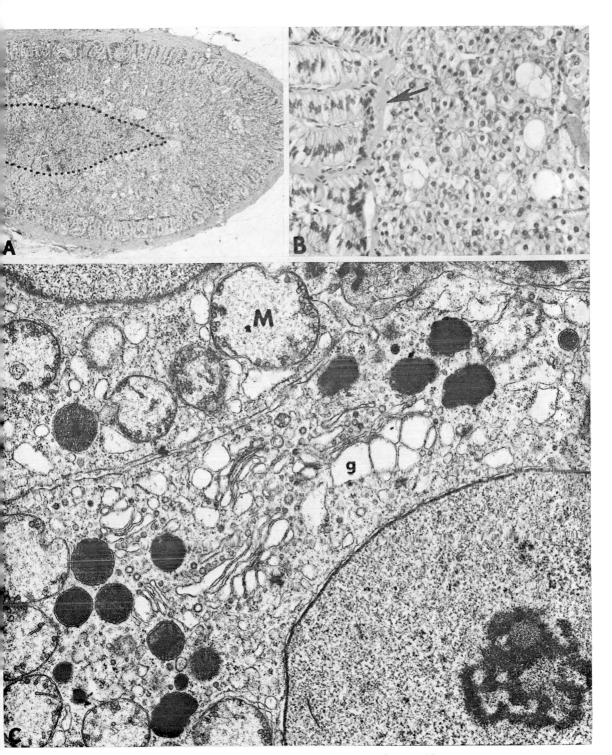

Fig. 10.2. Chronic depletion of adrenal cortex, aged dog, corticosteroid therapy. A. Adrenal is small, capsule is thickened, and zona fasciculata is reduced and vacuolated. Corticomedullary junction (dotted line).
B. Vacuolation of zona fasciculata and deposition of hyalin (arrow).
C. Ultrastructure of cell in zona fasciculata. Mitochondrial cristae are disorganized (M). Golgi complex (g) is vacuolated and surrounded by vesicles and dense granules.

mals, mitochondrial structure returns to normal and cell enlargement occurs. The presence of excess adrenocorticoids, most often due to therapy, suppresses ACTH release, which may cause atrophy of adrenocortical cells (Nickerson 1973).

STRESS AND THE ADRENAL GLAND

Adrenalectomy in experimental animals obliterates the capacity to make homeostatic adjustments in response to injury, hemorrhage, increased metabolism, and changes in the surrounding environment. These influences are crudely lumped as "stress" because they alter the requirements for maintenance of metabolic activity. The adrenal gland plays a leading role in these adaptive adjustments. For example, when animals are stressed, an immediate need for glucose is furnished by epinephrine-induced glycogenolysis and by the capacity of glucocorticoids to promote glucose formation from noncarbohydrate precursors. Adrenal corticosteroids also play crucial roles in restoration of blood volume and regulation of kidney function.

Acute stress results in marked depletion of steroid lipid granules and lipids from cells of the adrenal cortex. Grossly, the glands are small, buff colored, and may contain small scattered hemorrhages. We have seen massive hemorrhages in the adrenals of horses which were trapped in fencing and developed shock during efforts to free themselves. If the stressor is removed, the adrenal rapidly regranulates and normal levels of lipid develop. If, on the other hand, a chronic lower level of stress is applied, hyperplasia of the adrenal cortex develops. The width of the gland is gradually increased and it is composed of actively secreting cells. Immense adrenals may be found in animals exposed to long periods of severe cold, especially if they are on a low plane of nutrition.

ADRENAL CORTEX IN ELECTROLYTE IMBALANCE

The zona glomerulosa hypertrophies and secretes increased amounts of aldosterone in response to angiotensin. This can be demonstrated experimentally by sodium-deficiency stimulation of the juxtaglomerular apparatus or by the intravenous injection of renin. Electrolyte metabolism is thereby regulated independently of the pituitary.

The zona glomerulosa is thickened in dogs with pulmonary hypertension, ascites, and sodium retention due to heartworm blockade of the pulmonary artery (Nichols and Hennigar 1964). The juxtaglomerular apparatus is highly granular in these dogs; this is a reflection of the increased production and secretion of renin in response to sodium loss. The angiotensin which results from renin activity directly stimulates the zona glomerulosa of the adrenal cortex. The ascites and edema, manifestations of sodium retention, are relieved by the administration of aldosterone antagonists.

This situation also occurs in congestive heart failure in dogs in which widening of the zona glomerulosa, increased aldosterone levels in plasma, and ascites are characteristic. In experimentally induced heart disease, these lesions are reproduced (Davis et al. 1957).

ADRENAL CORTEX AND INFECTION

Adrenocortical function plays a protective role against infection, and the normal pituitary-adrenal response is necessary for survival of the animal with septicemia. In adrenalectomized mice maintained on graded doses of cortisone and inoculated with pneumococci, survival was greatest in groups whose maintenance cortisone most closely resembled the normal. Mortality progressively increased toward the extremes of hypo- and hyperadrenocorticism (Kass and Finland 1958).

In acute generalized infection the major corticosteroid hormones are elevated and appear to be stimulated early (Beisel and Rapaport 1969). Increases have even been reported in the incubation and prodromal stages of disease. It is only in the late stages of disease that high levels are seen, however. In chronic disease, such as tuberculosis, adrenal cortical secretion is usually depressed. The fetal adrenal cortex undergoes hyperplasia during infection and elevated levels of adrenocorticoids are considered a mechanism of abortion (Osburn et al. 1972).

Severe, overwhelming, complicated in-

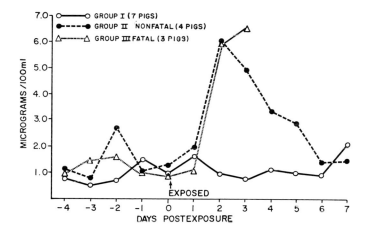

Fig. 10.3. Plasma hydrocortisone levels in pigs with erysipelas: I. controls, II. survivors, III. animals that died. (From Wood et al. 1971)

fections are associated with increasing levels of plasma corticoids. In swine erysipelas, plasma hydrocortisone levels are progressively elevated to death (Fig. 10.3). In survivors, they return to normal during the recovery phase (Wood et al. 1971). In addition to increased secretion, slower rates of corticoid clearance may also be important, especially with liver impairment or shock. Hemorrhage and necrosis of the adrenal may occur in overwhelming infections in some species. In most instances it is probable that hemorrhage and necrosis simply represent a local manifestation of disseminated intravascular coagulation in the presence of shock. It appears that hyperactivity of the cortex also precipitates necrosis because a functional cortex is necessary in the development of hemorrhage following toxin injection, and structural changes are reduced by treatment with drugs that depress endogenous adrenal hyperactivity. Radioactively labeled endotoxin (bacterial lipopolysaccharide-C^{14}) accumulates in the cortex in higher concentrations than in other tissue (Jones and Carter 1955).

HYPERADRENOCORTICISM OF DOGS

The syndrome of *hyperadrenocorticism* in dogs is a bilateral adrenal cortical hyperplasia with secretion of excessive amounts of adrenocorticosteroid hormones. Clinically, dogs exhibit abdominal enlargement, muscle weakness, obesity, and alopecia. Clinical signs also include polydipsia, polyphagia, and imbalance of heat

regulation. The disease is comparable mechanistically to Cushing's syndrome of hyperadrenocorticism in humans (Capen et al. 1967a; Rijnberk et al. 1968).

Adrenal glands of affected dogs are enlarged and contain extracapsular and juxtamedullary nodules of hyperplastic cells. The diffuse increase in width of the cortex which often is present is due to hyperplasia of the zona fasciculata; the zona glomerulosa is usually normal or atrophic (Kelly et al. 1971). Cytologically, the enlarged, polygonal hyperplastic adrenal cortical cells are filled with mitochondria, lipid globules, and vacuoles. They cannot be differentiated ultrastructurally from normal cells of the zona fasciculata. Rare, functional tumors of the adrenal cortex are known to be associated with canine hyperadrenocorticism. Hyperadrenocorticism may also be caused by ACTH-secreting tumors of the pituitary (Capen and Koestner 1967). Transient signs of hyperadrenocorticism may be iatrogenic, that is, a result of the therapeutic use of ACTH or cortisone.

ADRENAL MEDULLA

The *granular chromaffin cells* of the adrenal medulla secrete catecholamines, are derived from neurectoderm, and are innervated by preganglionic sympathetic fibers. They are colored brown by chrome salts, and this *chromaffin reaction* results from the oxidation and polymerization of the catecholamines epinephrine and norep-

pituitary, and thyroid gland proper may, therefore, result in disturbances in thyroid function.

THYROXIN

The major circulating thyroid hormones are thyroxin and triiodothyronine, which are bound to thyroglobulin, the storage form of thyroid hormones. The thyroid gland is able to efficiently concentrate iodide from the blood. Iodide is actively taken into the follicular epithelial cell, where it is oxidized to higher valence and iodinates thyroglobulin-bound tyrosine (the initial step in thyroglobulin synthesis). Thyroperoxidase, which is responsible for iodination, is bound to the plasma membrane and forms iodoproteins at the luminal surface of the follicular epithelial cells (Tice and Wollman 1972).

A defect in the iodide-concentrating capacity causes an animal to be hypothyroid. The glandular epithelium is hyperplastic, its I^{131} uptake is abnormal, and there are low levels of thyroxin in serum. Among mammals there are significant differences in iodide uptake. Even within species differences occur. The Basenji breed of dog differs from others in having a perpetually active thyroid in which there is rapid and continual I^{131} turnover (Nunez et al. 1972).

When trapping of iodine is inhibited, thyroid function is depressed. Iodine itself, in massive quantities, inhibits organic binding. More important are chemical inhibitors. The antihelminthic phenothiazine, which contains large amounts of iodine, is known to depress thyroid function in lambs. Thiocyanate, periodate, and nitrate are similarly known to prevent iodine binding and to be goitrogenic. Thiourea, which inhibits the peroxidase-induced oxidation of iodide to iodine, is used therapeutically as an antithyroid substance in fattening cattle. It causes hyperplasia of follicular epithelium although the changes in bovine thyroids appear to be variable (Griem 1973). Antithyroid substances are important causes of disturbances of growth and development.

Thyroxin is required for normal growth and development. The lack of it results in runted adult animals called, in humans, cretin dwarfs. The cause is the depression of metabolic activity in growing cells. A striking example is the failure of tadpoles to metamorphose after thyroidectomy. They may grow to very large size but do not change from tadpole to frog (Bohrod and Merritt 1963). In contrast, precocious metamorphosis results from thyroxin injection. This model was reported in the early 1900s (feeding tadpoles bits of horse thyroid). Since changes were induced long before they normally occur, the froglets were about one-third the size of normal adult frogs.

Thyroxin activity on target cells is implicated in protein synthesis, oxidative phosphorylation, and stimulation of mitochondrial protein synthesis. The widespread effect on cell metabolism has been investigated in liver cells of animals given large doses of thyroxin or triiodothyronine. There are decreases in cell size, volume of smooth endoplasmic reticulum, glycogen, and numbers of mitochondria. The membrane surfaces including the cristae of mitochondria are increased, however (Reith 1973). Microbodies are increased in number.

The selective action of thyroxin depends upon interaction of the hormone with specific protein receptors that are unique to certain cells. This is the basis for target cell specificity. Autoradiographic studies have localized thyroxin on the plasma membrane, mitochondrial membranes, and the membranes of the cytocavitary system of stimulated target cells (Manuelidis 1972).

THYROID FOLLICULAR CELLS

The cuboidal follicle cells are joined laterally by junctional complexes. The free luminal surface bears small numbers of short, irregular microvilli. The nuclei are large and the cytoplasm bears lysosomes, membrane-bound vacuoles of colloid, and phagolysosomes. It is important to differentiate the newly formed *apical granules* that discharge colloid into the lumen and *colloid droplets* that take up colloid from the lumen to degrade it. The size and development of the secretory apparatus depends upon the activity of the cell.

Hyperplastic cells are taller and have

large amounts of endoplasmic reticulum and large Golgi complexes. There are greater numbers of microvilli on the cell surface and increased numbers of lysosomes and phagolysosomes in the cytoplasm.

Atrophy of the thyroid follicular epithelium, which results from decreased endocrine stimulation, produces thinning of the epithelial layer. The follicular colloid becomes less dense and more basophilic. Within the cytoplasm there is dilatation of the endoplasmic reticulum with small precipitates in the cisternae (Fig. 10.5). Both colloid droplets and apical granules are increased and large dense lipofuscin granules accumulate.

Normal follicles are surrounded by a very thin smooth basement lamina (about 50 nm thick). In the thyroids of aged animals, especially those with thyroid disease, the basement lamina is thickened, sometimes sufficiently to retard the flow of thyroid hormones to the vascular system. The fenestrated capillary endothelium below the follicular epithelium is rarely altered, although occasionally inflammatory lesions will block the fenestrae. Deposits of calcium salts are commonly found in thickened basement laminas.

GOITER

Goiter is enlargement of the thyroid. Despite this clear definition, goiter is used clinically to equate only with noninflammatory, nonneoplastic enlargement of the thyroid. The basic lesion of hyperplasia may or may not be associated with hyperfunction.

The common cause of thyroid hyperplasia is iodine deficiency. As a result of the lack of iodine, thyroxin output is decreased; there is compensatory increase in pituitary TSH secretion and consequent hyperplasia of thyroid epithelium. The iodine-deficient goiters of animals are usually euthyroid. *Hyperthyroidism,* characterized by thyroid enlargement and increased metabolic activity (and responding to treatment with iodine) is uncommon in most animal species. It is the most important thyroid disease of humans. Hyperthyroid syndromes have been reported in fish (Hamre and Nichols 1926), birds, dogs (Krook 1957), and other mammals. In most, the critical evidence involving metabolic changes has not been provided. Parakeets have a high incidence of hyperplastic goiter (Blakemore 1963) and the incidence, which may be 85%, is reduced by supplementation of diets with iodine.

Hypothyroidism, or decreased function, is documented by demonstrating diminished I^{131} uptake by radioactive scanning, atrophic thyroid epithelium in biopsy, and decreased levels of thyroxin in plasma. A response to thyroxin therapy is expected. Syndromes of congenital hypothyroidism-hyperplastic thyroid are seen in ruminants, pigs, and horses. Hypothyroidism of aged dogs, which accompanies thyroid atrophy, is more common.

ATROPHY

Atrophy of follicular epithelium occurs secondary to deficiency of pituitary secretion of thyroid stimulating hormone. It is most commonly seen in aged, obese, and lethargic dogs. In their thyroids, the epithelium is thinned and the follicles are irregular and filled with colloid of varying density. Some follicles rupture and coalesce, forming colloid cysts. Colloid and proteins of plasma origin may seep into interfollicular areas. Amyloid fibers are sometimes deposited in interfollicular areas as part of systemic amyloidosis.

THYROIDITIS

Thyroiditis is rare although it may accompany any severe systemic infectious disease. Granulomas and abscesses do occur, especially in tuberculosis and other granulomatous diseases. Autoimmune thyroiditis probably occurs in dogs and cats but has only been adequately documented in the mutant obese strain of chickens (see immunologic disease, Chapter 5).

PARAFOLLICULAR CELLS

The parafollicular cells of the mammalian thyroid gland secrete the hypocalcemic hormone *calcitonin*. These cells are located between the thyroid follicles and function independently of the thyroid epithelial cells. Ultrastructurally, the parafol-

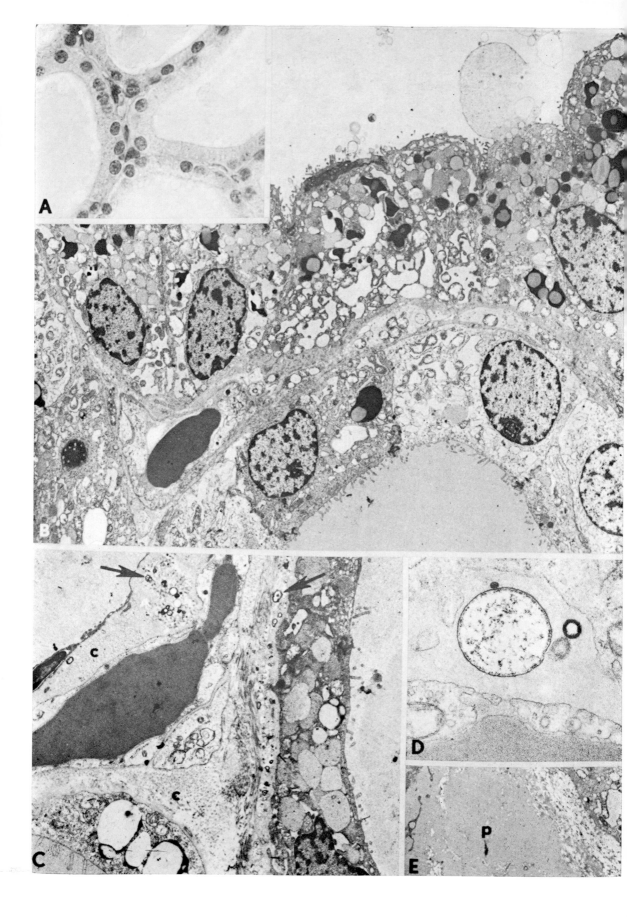

licular cells contain large numbers of dense membrane-bound granules which are the source of calcitonin (Fig. 10.6).

Early suggestions of parafollicular localization of calcitonin resulted from the observations that the number and distribution of the granules were responsive to the concentration of calcium in plasma (Bauer and Teitelbaum 1966). Experimental hypercalcemia in the dog resulted in rapid degranulation of parafollicular cells. Parafollicular cells of cows made hypercalcemic by the administration of vitamin D had reduced numbers of secretory granules; parafollicular cell hyperplasia developed after chronic hypercalcemic stimulation of 30 days (Capen and Young 1969).

Calcitonin was localized structurally in the cytoplasm of parafollicular cells by immunofluorescent studies. Its presence was shown to be confined to the secretory granules of parafollicular cells in the pig thyroid gland. No label was found in the endoplasmic reticulum or Golgi complex (De Grandi et al. 1971).

Mammalian parafollicular cells are derived from ultimobranchial origin during embryonic development. Cells in the ultimobranchial body of some amphibians and reptiles are analogous to the mammalian parafollicular cells. Teleost fishes lack paratollicular cells as such. High levels of plasma Ca^{++} are regulated by the paired *corpuscles of Stannius* which are attached to or embedded in the kidney. Their hypocalcemic secretion is not characterized but its activity is demonstrable. "Stanniectomy" produces hypercalcemia in seawater or other water where Ca^{++} is present (Pang et al. 1973). Fish in seawater are in constant danger of calcium overload and the hypocalcemic mechanism of the corpuscles of Stannius prevent this. Freshwater fish, however, tend to be in danger of calcium depletion. The hypercalcemic mechanism, analogous to the mammalian parathyroid, has not been established but it appears that the pituitary may so function.

The concentration of ionized calcium in plasma is the stimulus for calcitonin secretion. During hypercalcemia the parafollicular cells are induced to release calcitonin. The action of this hormone is mainly on bone, where it acts to inhibit both matrix and mineral resorption (Fig. 10.7). Osteocytes of animals given calcitonin experimentally show signs of output of calcium apatite crystals. Star-shaped aggregates of crystals may be seen around these cells.

The inhibition of bone matrix resorption by calcitonin is independent of, and in direct opposition to, the action of parathyroid hormone. Complex interactions between these two hormones may lead to complex tissue lesions. For example, during hypocalcemia-induced parathyroid hormone secretion, plasma calcium may be raised and secondary oversecretion of calcitonin occurs. This inhibits osteolysis (induced by parathyroid hormone) which in turn begins the cycle anew.

Ultimobranchial neoplasms of the thyroid are common in bulls. They are composed of poorly differentiated parafollicular or C cells with occasional secretion granules and numerous microfilaments in the cytoplasm (Black et al. 1973b). Amyloid fibrils can be found in the interstitium. These neoplasms contain calcitonin activity which can be released in response to infusions of calcium. The high incidence in bulls and low incidence in cows is theorized to be due to the high intake of calcium in the diet of this species coupled with the lack of an outlet for it (via lactation) in the bull. The long-term effect of calcitonin thereby is on the bone and affected bulls have ankylosing spondylosis, vertebral osteosclerosis, and degenerative osteoarthropathy which causes decreased breeding ability (Wilke et al. 1970; Young et al. 1971).

In humans, the medullary carcinoma of the thyroid is a tumor of parafollicular cells which produce calcitonin. Despite

Fig. 10.5. Thyroid. A. and B. Follicles, aged dog. Note large dense secretion granules. ER cisternae are enlarged and distorted. C. Severe atrophy with deposition of calcium (arrows) and collagen (c) below epithelium, dog. Note remnant of atrophic epithelium (top left). D. Spherical deposits of calcium between follicular epithelial cell (top) and capillary endothelium (bottom). E. Plasma protein (p) in interfollicular spaces, dog.

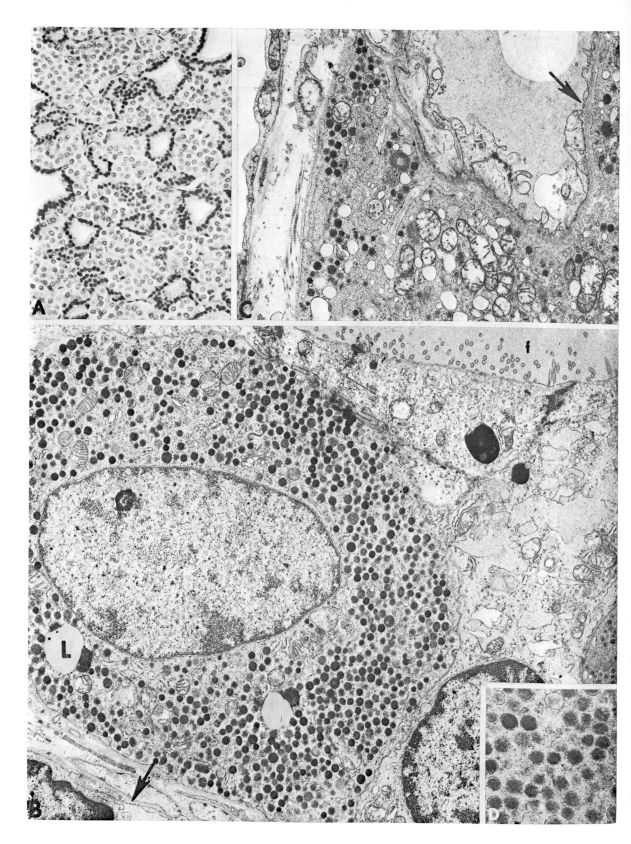

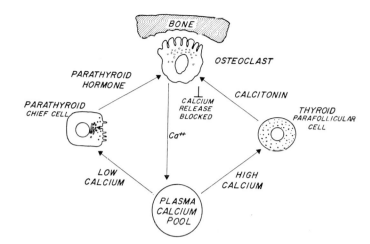

Fig. 10.7. Calcium pool.

this functional activity, patients with this tumor rarely have osteomalacia as an accompanying lesion.

ULTIMOBRANCHIAL FOLLICLES

The third anatomical structure identified in the thyroid is the ultimobranchial follicle, a remnant of the ultimobranchial body of the embryo. Cysts develop from these structures, especially in ruminants. Ultrastructurally, the follicular epithelial cells are granular and typical of actively secreting cells (Tashiro 1963). They contain acidic mucopolysaccharides and the luminal surface stains heavily with Alcian Blue.

PARATHYROID

PARATHYROID HORMONE AND PLASMA CALCIUM

The parathyroids control the concentration of calcium ion in plasma by secreting parathyroid hormone (PTH). PTH mobilizes Ca^{++} from the skeleton, increases renal excretion of phosphorus (by suppressing tubular reabsorption), and augments the rate of absorption and excretion of calcium from the intestine. PTH is secreted in response to low levels of ionic calcium in plasma (hypocalcemia). It causes Ca^{++} to be removed from bone matrix to replenish the circulating calcium pool (Fig. 10.7). The Ca^{++} mobilizing activity of PTH is mediated through the activation of adenyl cyclase; PTH also regulates the rate at which the renal tubule cell forms 1,25-dihydroxycholecalciferol, the active form of vitamin D_3.

PTH is synthesized by ribosomes on the endoplasmic reticulum of parathyroid chief cells as a larger precursor termed proparathyroid hormone. The primary structure and amino acid sequence of bovine PTH have been determined and fragments have been synthesized which stimulate target cells in bone and kidney. Highly sensitive radioimmunoassay techniques are available to measure plasma PTH but it is important to recognize that hormone heterogeneity, due to chemically distinct types of secreted PTH that differ in structure, may give rise to differences in quantitation.

PARATHYROID HORMONE AND BONE RESORPTION

PTH induces elevations in plasma calcium by increasing osteolysis. For exam-

Fig. 10.6. C-cell hyperplasia, thyroid, dog. A. Histology. Thyroid follicles are separated by C cells. B. Ultrastructure. Large granular C cell lies below thyroid follicle lumen (f). Note lipofuscin bodies (L) and fenestrated endothelium (arrow). C. Capillaries within (upper) and outside of (left) aggregate of C cells. Note fenestrae (arrow). D. Granules.

ple, when PTH is given to cows, bone resorption is increased 5-fold by osteoclastic activity on the trabecular surfaces of bone (Rowland et al. 1972). Osteolysis is the absorption and destruction of bone in which bone matrix is modified and bone calcium salts are lost. Bone matrix resorption is reflected in elevated levels of urinary hydroxyproline (Black and Capen 1971).

PTH causes increased osteolysis both by osteoclasts and osteocytes. Osteoclasts located on bone surfaces are stimulated in some unknown way to increase in numbers and activity. Bone-resorbing osteoclasts have active ruffled plasma membranes (brush borders) where they abut the bone matrix. The active and vigorous pinocytotic action of this border has been demonstrated in time-lapse motion picture studies of bone in vitro. Ultrastructurally, the plasma membrane consists of repeating units along the cytoplasmic surfaces that contain fine bristlelike structures of 15–20 nm which project perpendicularly into the cytoplasm (Kallio et al. 1971). These specialized areas of the plasma membrane, which are involved in active ion exchange, are structurally different from those that border the nonbone related surfaces of the osteoclast.

Deep in bone, the osteoblasts are also transformed into osteocytes which secrete proteases and collagenases that resorb bone. In osteocytic osteolysis the surrounding bone matrix becomes less dense and is nearly devoid of mineral (Matthews and Martin 1971).

PARATHYROID GLAND STRUCTURE

Mammalian parathyroid glands are composed of *chief cells* in groups or clusters which are surrounded by a basement membrane and collagen fibrils. Chief cells, especially during hyperplasia, may assume a true acinar or follicular grouping with a lumen containing granular amorphous material. The cell surfaces around the lumen contain microvilli and rare cilia which project outwards. Parathyroid chief cells have an intimate association with fenestrated capillaries which allows rapid cell-to-blood exchange of PTH.

Chief cells may be light or dark depending on the state of their activity (Table 10.2). The terms light and dark are confusing, since the structural appearance of the cell may be misleading in regard to cell function. Large, vacuolated, "water-clear" cells develop in some species with parathyroid hyperactivity. They are probably a variant of light chief cell even though they are structurally different (Roth and Capen 1974). The mitochondria-rich oxyphil cells, found in adults of some species, have small Golgi complexes and are probably not associated with secretory activity.

Table 10.2. Cytology of the parathyroid gland chief cells

Cell Type	Occurrence	Characteristics
Active chief cell (Dark chief cell[a])	Actively secreting cell in normal parathyroid gland.	Cytoplasm is electron-dense due to crowded organelles. There is little glycogen or lipid.
Inactive chief cell (Light chief cell)	Predominates in the normal parathyroid gland of most species.	Cuboidal shape, simple intercellular connections, electron-transparent cytoplasm, and few organelles. Golgi complex is small and there are many lipid globules and lipofuscin bodies.
Hyperactive chief cell (Hypertrophic light cell)	Chronic stimulation. Examples: renal and nutritional imbalances.	An electron-transparent cell with evidence of a rapidly developing protein synthetic machinery. Golgi complex is large and endoplasmic reticulum is increased in quantity.
Atrophic chief cell (Atrophic dark cell)	Chronic suppression. Examples: high calcium diets and excessive dietary vitamin D.	Dark, condensed cell with contracted organelles. Nucleus is pyknotic.

[a] The terms light and dark as applied in classic histologic description are misleading in terms of cell function and are best avoided.

The dense membrane-bound granules in the chief cell cytoplasm contain the PTH (MacGregor et al. 1973). Immunofluorescent studies on sections of parathyroid tissue from cattle, rats, and humans have localized fluorescein-labeled anti-PTH globulin in granule-containing areas of the cell (Hargis et al. 1964).

In any individual gland the chief cells are in various stages of secretory activity. The number of secretory granules varies among species, but in general there are fewer numbers of granules in chief cells than in most polypeptide hormone-secreting cells. Parathyroid glands of cows contain more numerous secretory granules than other animal species (Capen et al. 1968).

Parathyroid hypertrophy occurs when the demands of plasma calcium are increased persistently. For example, large parathyroid glands are found in prepartum (for fetal bone growth) and postpartum (for milk production) cows. The laying hen has large parathyroids and bones with thin cortices (Nevalainen 1969). The parathyroids of these long-term hypocalcemic animals are dominated by actively secreting chief cells. Ultrastructurally, the important changes are: reduplication of the endoplasmic reticulum, enlargement of the Golgi complex with formation of prosecretory granules, alignment of mature secretory granules along the cell surface, and granule secretion by exocytosis (Capen 1971) (Figs. 10.8 and 10.9). Persistent hypocalcemic stimulation may lead to vacuolation and accumulation of glycogen in the cytoplasm. In response to long-term hypercalcemia, most of the chief cells are either inactive or atrophic. They are cuboidal and their cytoplasm is more transparent than normal.

PRIMARY HYPERPARATHYROIDISM

Excessive production of PTH in the absence of hypocalcemia occurs, in dogs, as a result of neoplastic alteration in the parathyroids. Parathyroid adenomas are most often unilateral, spherical, encapsulated tumors composed of well-differentiated chief cells. Carcinomas tend to be nodular and their component cells less differentiated. Ultrastructurally, tumor cells contain few granules but many free ribosomes and much fragmented endoplasmic reticulum.

The clinical sequel of functional parathyroid neoplasms is debilitating bone disease. Plasma calcium tends to be high and plasma phosphorus low (Table 10.3). Neoplastic cells function autonomously (not in response to hypocalcemia) and the excessive levels of plasma PTH are responsible for excessive Ca^{++} resorption from bone, enhanced renal tubular resorption of Ca^{++} from the glomerular filtrate (decreased renal excretion and low urinary calcium), suppression of renal tubular phosphate resorption, and increased intestinal absorption of Ca^{++}.

The bone lesions are due to subperiosteal resorption of Ca^{++} and may be seen as thin dense bone cortices, osteoporosis, or fibrous osteodystrophy, depending upon the chronicity of the disease and the age of the animal. Metastatic calcification, due to hypercalcemia, causes mineralization in the kidney (nephrocalcinosis) and lung (pumice lung).

Primary hyperparathyroidlike syndromes, termed pseudohyperparathyroidism, occur in dogs with neoplasms that secrete peptides with activity resembling PTH. Any nonendocrine malignant tumor that has not metastasized to bone may be implicated in this hypercalcemic-hypophosphatemic state but pseudohyperparathyroidism is most often associated with malignant lymphoma (Osborne and Stevens 1973).

HYPOCALCEMIC DISEASE AND SECONDARY HYPERPARATHYROIDISM

The persistent depression of plasma levels of calcium leads to secondary parathyroid hypertrophy and hyperplasia. The parathyroids are enlarged bilaterally and the chief cells are in an active state of secretion. A few of the varying mechanisms and manifestations of secondary hyperparathyroidism are discussed below.

NUTRITIONAL DEFICIENCY

Dietary deficiency of calcium may, in animals with immature skeletons, result in parathyroid hyperplasia. Nutritional secondary hyperparathyroidism occurs relatively commonly in cats, dogs, horses,

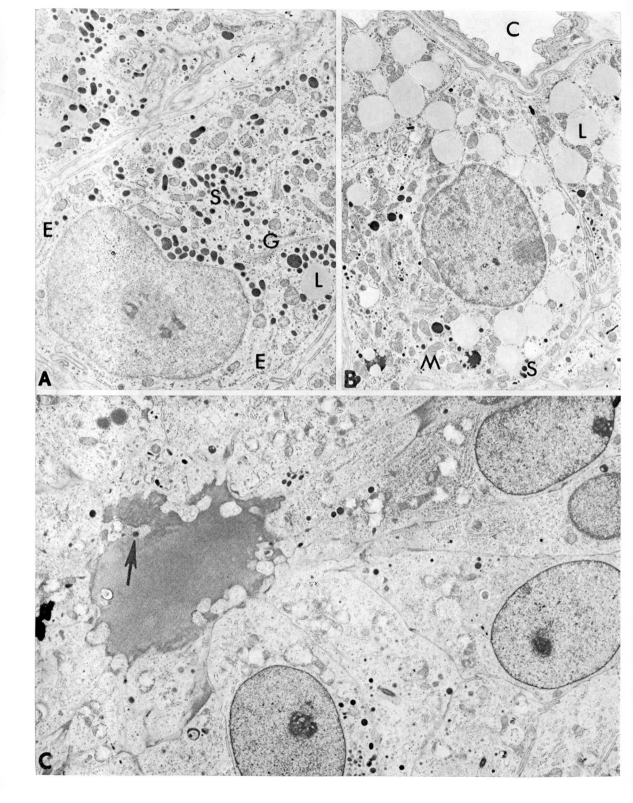

Table 10.3. Calcium and phosphorus levels expected in parathyroid disease

Disease	Serum Ca	Serum P
Primary hyperparathyroidism (neoplasm)	High[a]	Low
Renal secondary hyperparathyroidism	Low[b] or low normal	High
Nutritional secondary hyperparathyroidism		
Early	Low	High
Compensated	Normal	Normal
Low phosphorus osteomalacia		
Early	Low	Low
Compensated	Normal	Low

[a] Other causes of hypercalcemia: vitamin D toxicity, leukemic syndromes.

[b] Other causes of hypocalcemia: milk fever (cow), acute pancreatitis with fat necrosis, protein-losing gastroenteropathy.

primates, birds, and reptiles. It is manifested as severe bone disease and is usually complicated by other deficiencies (Capen and Rowland 1968; Rowland et al. 1968). Experimentally, young kittens placed on a diet of beef heart and distilled water develop hypocalcemia in 1 wk. The diet provides large amounts of phosphorus but is severely deficient in calcium. Ultrastructural examination of the parathyroid glands of affected kittens reveal that they are dominated by actively secreting chief cells. Alterations consisted of hypertrophy and reduplication of organelles concerned with PTH secretion. The excess PTH levels were reflected in generalized osteitis fibrosa. Naturally occurring bone disease due to dietary deficiency of calcium is a relatively common problem since unsupplemented, all-meat diets are still common in a number of animal species. The syndrome of hypocalcemia-parathyroid hyperplasia-bone disease can also be secondary to deficiencies of vitamin D or to excesses of phosphorus.

Dietary excess of phosphorus (in proportion to calcium) may cause secondary hyperparathyroidism indirectly by virtue of the ability of hyperphosphatemia to decrease blood calcium levels. The resultant decrease in plasma calcium directly stimulates parathyroid hyperplasia which eventually leads to generalized fibrous osteodystrophy. The most notable example among animals is nutritional secondary hyperparathyroidism of the horse which is, according to its appearances, variously called osteodystrophy fibrosa, bran disease, or bighead. The parathyroids are hyperplastic in direct relation to the hypocalcemia and the gland is dominated by hypertrophic light chief cells (Krook and Lowe 1964). Ultrastructurally, these cells are enlarged and markedly vacuolated (Fujimoto et al. 1967). Osteoclastic resorption is especially prominent in the skull bones but also occurs in the ribs and metaphases of the long bones. The leading feature is the transformation of bone into a fibrous tissue of high collagen content with rebuilding of bone in a more primitive pattern rather than highly organized haversian systems. This nutritional secondary hyperparathyroidism is reproduced experimentally by feeding excessive amounts of phosphorus in relation to calcium. The resultant hypocalcemia slowly produces parathyroid hyperplasia and osteoclastic resorption.

RENAL FAILURE AND SECONDARY
HYPERPARATHYROIDISM OF DOGS

A syndrome of renal disease, hyperphosphatemia, hyperparathyroidism, and osteodystrophy occurs in dogs. The causes include chronic interstitial nephritis, congenital renal hypoplasia, and any terminal renal disease (Platt 1951). In severe, end-stage renal disease, the kidney fails to ex-

Fig. 10.8. Parathyroid. *Top:* Chief cells from bovine parathyroids (Micrographs, C. Capen). A. Active chief cell with numerous secretory granules (S), endoplasmic reticulum (E), and Golgi complexes (G). Lipid globules (L) are uncommon. B. Inactive chief cells with numerous lipid globules. Secretory granules are sparse and plasma membranes are straight. Note capillary (C), mitochondria (M). C. Chief cells in acinar arrangement, canine parathyroid hyperplasia. Ribosomes and endoplasmic reticulum are prominent; secretory granules are sparse. Note granule in a filopodium projecting into dense luminal material (arrow).

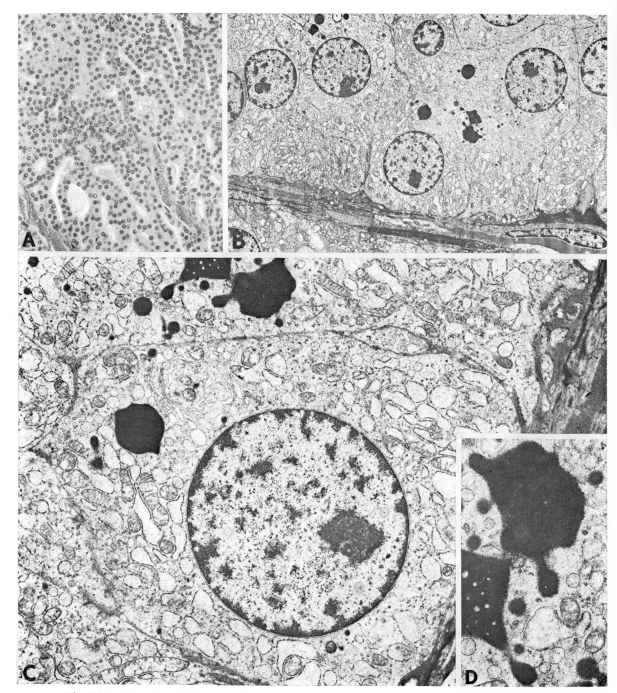

Fig. 10.9. Parathyroid hyperplasia, dog. A. Histology. B. Ultra-structure, low power. Endoplasmic reticulum is dilated and few granules are present. C. Chief cell filled with dilated endoplasmic reticulum. Few secretory granules. Those present are large, pleomorphic, and appear to have fused (see D).

crete normal amounts of phosphorus from plasma to urine. The accumulation of phosphorus in plasma depresses plasma calcium and this in turn induces parathyroid hyperplasia and secretion of PTH (Shimamura and Morrison 1971). The progressive hypocalcemia and hyperphosphatemia lead to increased destruction of cortical and trabecular bone and the formation of new poorly formed bone which is not functionally arranged. Affected dogs characteristically have bones that are soft and bowed.

The high levels of plasma phosphorus are related both to the failure of phosphorus to pass the damaged renal glomerulus and to the failure of the altered renal tubule to respond to PTH (which normally suppresses phosphate resorption and enhances calcium resorption). Thus, despite increased plasma PTH, phosphorus does not pass into the glomerular filtrate in sufficient amounts and that which does is resorbed. The calcium which manages to pass into the glomerular filtrate is not preferentially resorbed. To complicate the disease, the hyperphosphatemia leads to excretion of large amounts of phosphorus into the gut where they combine with calcium to deprive the animal of its dietary source.

Parathyroid hyperplasia secondary to renal damage was established experimentally in dogs by removal of one kidney and partial destruction of the other. Phosphate overload induced by chronic intravenous infusion of phosphorus-containing solutions will accomplish the same results. Hypocalcemia, not hyperphosphatemia, was established as the cause of the parathyroid and bone lesions. Diets low in phosphorus help to prevent hyperparathyroidism in dogs with renal disease (Slatopulsky et al. 1971).

PARTURIENT PARESIS OF CATTLE

Calcium homeostasis is especially important in the dairy cow which secretes about 1 g/kg of calcium in the milk. At parturition, the sudden needs of lactation must adapt the plasma calcium balance to this drain. Plasma levels of calcium drop from preparturient amounts of 10–12 mg to 7–9 mg/100 ml. In some individuals, calcium drops below 5 mg/100 ml of plasma; these cows develop the characteristic syndrome of tetany (spasm of skeletal muscle), collapse, and unconsciousness known as *parturient paresis* or milk fever.

The mechanism whereby hypocalcemia induces parathyroid hormone secretion (which stimulates bone resorption for calcium release) is too sluggish to meet the explosive demands for calcium brought on by lactation. Animals may die if they are not treated by giving solutions of calcium intravenously.

The parathyroid glands of affected cows have evidence of increased secretory activity, and elevated PTH levels have been measured in plasma (Capen and Young 1967). The hyperactive chief cells, which predominate in the parathyroids, have large Golgi complexes containing many prosecretory granules and lamellar arrays of endoplasmic reticulum. Mature secretory granules may be diminished in number (due to accelerated secretion) and those present in chief cells are concentrated along the plasma membrane bordering perivascular spaces.

Cows fed high calcium diets, especially if the diet is alkaline, are prone to develop milk fever near parturition. Chief cells in cows fed large amounts of calcium are inactive or atrophic (Black et al. 1973c). Their ability to secrete parathyroid hormone in response to a hypocalcemic challenge is significantly reduced when compared to cows fed prepartum diets with the required amounts of calcium and phosphorus. Prepartum diets low on calcium, conversely, reduce the incidence of milk fever near parturition and chief cells in the parathyroids are predominately in the actively synthesizing stage of the secretory cycle.

In milk fever, severe hypocalcemia develops in spite of hyperparathyroidism and elevated levels of immunoreactive PTH in plasma occur. Treatment with large doses of exogenous PTH does not elevate plasma calcium. Thus there is failure of PTH to stimulate bone resorption sufficiently to replenish blood calcium lost in the milk. This is due not only to the sluggish response of chief cells in cows on high calcium diets but also to suppression of osteoclastic and osteocytic activity in bone by other humoral factors.

Bone turnover (particularly resorption) is low in cows with parturient paresis (Rowland et al. 1972). The reason for the low bone turnover is uncertain but an inappropriate secretion of calcitonin prepartum in certain cows may be one factor that contributes to the inability of the elevated levels of PTH to rapidly mobilize calcium from skeletal reserves and to maintain blood levels during the critical period near parturition. Parafollicular cells in cows with parturient hypocalcemia appear to have discharged much of their stored secretory product and the thyroid content of calcitonin activity is reduced to about 15% of control cows (Capen and Young 1967). The outpouring of adrenal corticosteroid and estrogens that also occurs near parturition may suppress bone resorption and contribute to the development of milk fever.

PRIMARY BONE DISEASE WITH HYPOCALCEMIA

Bone disease characterized by extensive subperiosteal and endosteal bone formation may be accompanied by hypocalcemia and secondary parathyroid hyperplasia. Leukosis virus–induced osteopetrosis of chickens has been shown to induce actively secreting parathyroid cells (Dent et al. 1971; Youshak and Capen 1970). Chickens normally have a high rate of calcium metabolism and the kinetics of plasma calcium in osteopetrosis have not been determined. It is probable that plasma calcium levels and parathyroid secretion are altered in diseases such as metastatic neoplasms of bone and hypertrophic pulmonary osteodystrophy.

HYPERCALCEMIC DISEASE

HYPERVITAMINOSIS D

Vitamin D is required to maintain an active calcium transport mechanism in the intestinal mucosa. *Hypervitaminosis D* is characterized by elevated levels of calcium and phosphorus in serum and urine and decrease in the amounts of parathyroid glandular parenchyma (Capen et al. 1968). Parathyroid cells are shrunken and atroph-

ic; there is evidence of depressed parathyroid hormone synthesis as a result of elevated plasma calcium levels. Secretory granules are concentrated at the cell periphery and there are swelling and vacuolation of mitochondria. If vitamin D–induced hypercalcemia is prolonged, calcium-phosphorous crystals (hydroxyapatite) are deposited in certain tissues such as vessel walls, gastric mucosa, lung, and kidney. Damage to the kidney is severe and may cause uremia and death (Scarpelli et al. 1960).

HIGH CALCIUM DIETS

Large amounts of calcium in the diet lead to a continued source of plasma calcium from the intestine. Because the parathyroid activity is not required to periodically raise plasma calcium levels, the chief cells become atrophic. Organelles associated with hormone synthesis and secretory granule formation are poorly developed (Black et al. 1973a). It appears that these animals have a diminished capacity to respond to the explosive requirements for calcium during parturition when compared with those whose PTH-bone resorption mechanism is active.

ENDOCRINE PANCREAS

The pancreatic islets of mammals are small collections of granular cells interspersed among a labyrinth of anastomosing capillaries. The three major types of islet cells can be differentiated histochemically (Table 10.4). Ultrastructural differentiation depends upon differences in size, shape, and electron density of their granules (Fig. 10.10). If the granules are removed, the islet cells cannot be told apart, for cytologically they are similar. The function of the islets is the regulation of blood glucose levels, which takes place as a result of the secretion of insulin by their β-cells. The α- and δ-cells appear to regulate insulin release by mutually counteractive influences on the β-cells.

Phylogenetically, the first isolated endocrine pancreas is found in the cyclostomes. They do not have an exocrine pancreas but have well-defined β-cell–containing en-

Table 10.4. Cell types in mammalian pancreatic islets

Cell	Secretion	Granule	
		Ultrastructure	Histochemistry
Alpha	Glucagon	High electron density Uniform	Argyrophilia (Bodian procedure)
Beta	Insulin	Protein crystalline structure Pleomorphic	Aldehyde-fuchsin stain Immunofluorescent stain
Delta	Gastrin	Low electron density Larger than α and β granules	Argyrophilia (Hellerstrom procedure)

docrine foci adjacent to the bile duct, within the liver, or disseminated along the intestine. Fish, amphibia, and reptiles have an exocrine pancreas with interspersed endocrine cells. These cells exist in a wide spectrum of anatomic associations with the pancreas and intestine. As soon as α- and δ-cells appear in the phylogenetic scheme, the islets show a close association with an exocrine pancreas. It is believed that this intimate structural relationship promotes the mutual regulation between glucagon, gastrin, secretin, and pancreatic-enzyme-stimulated water and protein secretion. Birds have a high percentage of α-cells and characteristic α-, β-, and δ-cells. In mammals, a wide variety of anatomic variations have been reported related to diverse climatic conditions; that is, differences in arctic, desert, and marine species (Falkmer and Patent 1972).

Blood flow through the mammalian islet is rapid and does not appear to be influenced by secretion of islet cells. Endothelial cells are fenestrated and permit rapid exchange of insulin and other secretions (Fig. 10.10). Pathologic changes in islet vessels have not been adequately examined. The capillaries are separated from the islet cells by two basement membranes: one around the capillary, the other around the islet cell. In hyalinization and amyloidosis of the islets, the space between these basement membranes is increased and probably affects insulin secretion.

Both adrenergic and cholinergic nerves have been demonstrated in islet cells in several mammals, but their role in insulin secretion is not clear. The nerve fibers are absent in the islets of spiny mice, which have a defective insulin secretory mechanism (Orci et al. 1970).

BETA CELLS

The beta cell is the most numerous granule cell in the islets (except in birds). The beta granules are the source of insulin. This was first known by correlation of the granularity of β-cells with levels of insulin determined by bioassay. Insulin has been structurally localized in the granules by the fluorescent antibody technique and by localization of a specific reaction product over β-granules by use of peroxidase-labeled antibodies to insulin (Misugi et al. 1970). Aldehyde fuchsin, the classical and accepted histologic stain for insulin, is not specific but attaches to the sulfonic acid groupings of insulin in the granules. Beta cells are able to replicate and increase the mass of the islet although the mitotic potential is low.

INSULIN

Insulin facilitates the entry of glucose and other hexoses across the plasma membrane by depressing the critical level for entry and exit from the cell (see glycogen, Chapter 2). It stimulates glucose entrance into the metabolic pool by stimulating phosphorylation of glucose to glucose-6-phosphate. Insulin also prevents the overproduction of glucose by inhibiting the action of glucose-6-phosphatase in the liver.

Flux of glucose across the plasma membrane of insulin-sensitive cells (adipose, skeletal, and cardiac myocytes) occurs by passive transport and involves a carrier-mediated transport system. Insulin binds to sites on the plasma membrane and markedly accelerates glucose transport. (Insulin sensitivity is regulated by pituitary and

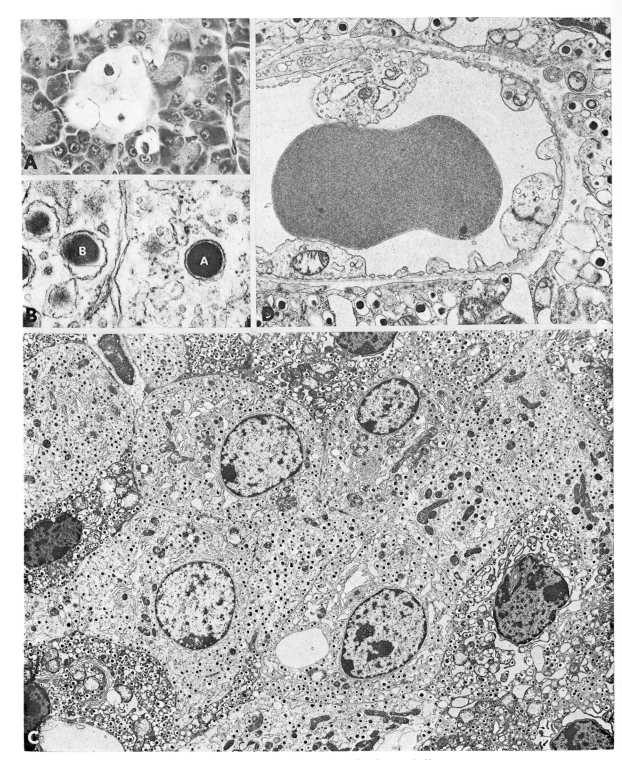

Fig. 10.10. Vacuolation in pancreatic islets. A. Histology. Cell
swelling and hydropic degeneration, dog with diabetes mellitus.
B. Ultrastructure of α- and β-granules. C. Degeneration and vacuolation
of β-cells, obese Db mouse with diabetes. D. Fenestrated capillary in
an islet, surrounded by β-cells.

adrenal hormones and other factors.) Insulin is degraded in the liver by insulinase.

Insulin synthesis begins with the formation of proinsulin within the endoplasmic reticulum. Proinsulin is transferred to the Golgi complex where conversion of insulin occurs. Immature β-granules may occur in this organelle. Mature β-granules are inclosed in smooth membranous sacs and released into the cytoplasm. Insulin is released by exocytosis. Beta granules move to the plasma membrane, fuse with it, and are extruded into the extracellular space. Current theory indicates that glucose initiates the entrance of calcium into the β-cells. Calcium triggers microtubules which are associated with the granules and which pull them to the surface of the cell (Orci et al. 1973).

BETA-CELL DEGENERATION

Vacuolation of β-cells is a classic lesion in acute diabetes of dogs and humans. Affected cells in dogs are filled with glycogen deposits and large, clear, membrane-bound vacuoles. They are devoid of β-granules (Volk and Lazarus 1963). These lesions have been studied in a wide array of experimentally induced diabetes. Beta-cell degranulation and degeneration can be induced by specific drugs such as alloxan (an oxidation product of uric acid), streptozotocin, and cyproheptadine (Lazarus and Shapiro 1973). Encephalomyocarditis virus causes β-cell necrosis and lymphoid cell infiltration in mice (Craighead and McLane 1968; Müntefering 1972; Wellmann et al. 1972). Partial pancreatectomy combined with growth hormone injections is a common model for inducing β-cell exhaustion. Immunologically induced diabetes may result from injection of large doses of exogenous insulin in rabbits (Lee et al. 1969).

BETA-CELL NEOPLASMS

Syndromes of hyperinsulinism and hypoglycemia and neurologic disease occur in dogs with pancreatic islet cell tumors. Cells of the tumor structurally resemble β-cells (Capen and Martin 1969). Functional islet neoplasms that secrete gluca-gon and gastrin have been studied in humans (Munger 1972).

ALPHA CELLS

Alpha cells are the source of glucagon (Baum et al. 1962). They can be differentiated in some species because of the relatively high electron density of cell granules. Alpha granules are also less pleomorphic than β-granules. They are interspersed with β-cells in most species although they tend to be located centrally in the horse. Birds have a high content of α-cells and some such as the duck have separate α-cell islets. Specific α-cell degranulation is a reaction to hyperglycemia and can be experimentally induced with several chemicals; it is analogous mechanistically to β-cell degranulation. Lysosomal digestion of α-granules (granulolysis) occurs as a response to hyperglycemia and is the structural representation of the cessation of glucagon release.

GLUCAGON

This hormone antagonizes insulin by increasing glycogenolysis. It converts inactive phosphorylase to the active form with consequent glycogenolysis and hyperglycemia.

DELTA CELLS

Delta-cell granules have low electron density and are usually larger than the α- and β-granules. Gastrin has been identified histochemically in δ-cells (Lomsky et al. 1969). Gastrin is probably a response from inhibition of insulin release found in extracts of δ-cells. Glucose-stimulated insulin release is inhibited by gastrin.

DIABETES MELLITUS

Diabetes mellitus, hereafter called diabetes, is classically considered pathologic hyperglycemia (Table 10.5), that is, the persistence of hyperglycemia during fasting (with or without glycosuria). Glucose is eliminated by the kidney and glycosuria causes osmotic diuresis, polyuria, and polydipsia. Carbohydrate and lipid metabolisms are abnormal and these lead to

Table 10.5. Milestones in research on diabetes mellitus

1674	Willis recognizes "sweetness" of urine in humans with "diabetes or pissing evil."
1869	Langerhans discovers islands of endocrine cells among the acinar cells of the pancreas.
1889	Von Mehring demonstrates that pancreatectomy of dogs results in diabetes mellitus.
1893	LaGuesse localizes endocrine function in islets.
1900s	Weichselbaum, Opie et al. describe classic lesions of islet cells in comatose diabetic humans including: vacuolation, insulitis, fibrosis, and hyalinization.[a]
1907	Lane subdivides islet cells into 2 types on basis of granule solubility in alcohol.
1914	Homans demonstrates hydropic degeneration in islets of experimental diabetes in dogs and cats which progressed with the duration of disease.
1921	Banting and Best discover insulin activity in pancreatic homogenates.
1943	Dunn discovers alloxan-induced β-cell necrosis leads to diabetes mellitus.
1964	Synthesis of insulin molecule by scientists in U.S., Germany, and China.

[a] They also noted that islet lesions could not be found in many diabetics, and that islet lesions were occasionally present in nondiabetics.

emaciation and ketosis. Due to the effectiveness of insulin in combating hyperglycemia, it is inferred that abnormal insulin production is involved mechanistically in diabetes.

A more modern definition would be that diabetes is a relative or actual deficiency in peripheral insulin action (not necessarily in pancreatic islet insulin output) that leads to a decreased utilization of carbohydrate for energy and other biochemical abnormalities and metabolic shifts. This broadens the concept of diabetes to include pathologic insulin synthesis, insulin transport, and insulin utilization. The hypotriglyceridemia that occurs in chronically insulin-deficient animals is due to a lipoprotein removal defect (of both dietary and endogenous fats) and is characterized by retention of very low density lipoproteins (liposomes) in the Golgi complex (Reaven and Reaven 1974).

The cause of diabetes in animals is nearly always β-cell destruction in the islets. In rare cases the β-cells are normal and diabetes results from the suppression of insulin activity by some nonpancreatic factor. Whatever the case, the pancreas is always involved in diabetes. If not the primary cause when islets are destroyed, it is affected by the elevated levels of blood glucose.

When the concentration of glucose in the circulating blood exceeds the renal threshold, glucose passes the glomerular filter. In most cases of diabetes mellitus, the high concentration of glucose in the glomerular filtrate overloads the reabsorptive mechanism of the proximal convoluted tubule. Glucose is retained in the tubular fluid, where it restricts the isosmotic reabsorption of water in the proximal tubules. This causes the distal tubule fluid volume to be greater than normal. The reabsorptive capacity of the distal tubule is overloaded and this results in diuresis. The end result is polyuria. Large amounts of urine containing detectable amounts of glucose are passed by the diabetic animal.

In its total spectrum of pathologic carbohydrate and lipid metabolism, diabetes represents a set of complex syndromes of differing etiology but with one common denominator—hyperglycemia.

DIABETES MELLITUS IN DOGS

In naturally occurring diabetes mellitus in dogs, a presumptive diagnosis based upon polyuria, polydipsia, and weight loss is substantiated by detection of elevated blood sugar levels. Blood glucose levels may exceed 1500 mg per 100 ml and are a reflection of insulin deficiency (Manns and Martin 1972). Insulin is undetectable in plasma by most assay techniques and does not increase upon intravenous glucose injection (see Fig. 2.23). Treatment with exogenous insulin reduces the hyperglycemia, but oral medication with glucagon antagonists is without effect (Berkow and Ricketts 1965).

Diabetes in dogs is associated most commonly with acute pancreatic necrosis. It may also accompany chronic interstitial fibrosing pancreatitis and neoplastic destruction of the pancreas. It is presumed in all these instances that destruction of islets is the cause of hypoglycemia. Indeed, vacuolation, degranulation and, in older dogs, hyalinization can be seen in the cells of the islets. Vacuolar degeneration with accumulation of glycogen is typical of the acute phases of diabetes.

Nonpancreatic lesions are dominated by centrolobular fatty degeneration of the liver and deposition of glycogen and lipids in the kidney (Dixon and Sanford 1962; Gepts and Toussaint 1967). Glycogen appears in the distal convoluted tubule and loop of Henle. In the glomerulus the mesangium is enlarged and the basement membranes of the capillaries are thickened. The initial lesion in diabetic glomerulopathy in dogs is probably the excessive production of basement membrane material in the mesangium and basement membranes (Bloodworth 1965; Ricketts 1962). Retinopathy and lenticular opacity occur in chronic canine diabetes (Patz and Maumenee 1962). In late stages the activity of the reticuloendothelial system is depressed (Drachman et al. 1966).

DIABETES IN OTHER ANIMALS

Spontaneous diabetes has been reported and described in cats, cattle, sheep, buffalo, pigs, horses, chickens (Langslow and Freeman 1972), newts, monkeys (Howard 1972; Kirk et al. 1972), wild rodents (Wise et al. 1972), and fish. In most instances an associated causal factor was not discerned and the course of the hyperglycemia was not adequately examined.

In cats, amyloidosis of the islets of Langerhans is a lesion associated with diabetes (Johnson and Stevens 1973). Amyloid is deposited throughout the islet and destroys its architecture. Unfortunately, the cell origin of the islet amyloid is not established in cats or humans (Westermark 1973). It is not established whether the amyloid is a cause or result of the diabetic state.

A syndrome of atrophy of the dorsal musculature of cultured carp in Japan known as *Sekoke* is reportedly a manifestation of spontaneous diabetes. Beta cells in the pancreas are degranulate and filled with glycogen and Golgi vesicles (Nakamura et al. 1971).

GENETIC DIABETES IN MICE

Several inbred mutant strains of mice are known to develop diabetes sponta-neously. These are the diabetic mutant strain (db/db), the obese-hyperglycemic strain (ob/ob), and spiny mice. Other strains are the Wellesley-hybrid mouse, the New Zealand obese (NZO) mouse, the KK mouse, and the yellow obese mouse. Models of diabetes have also been described in Chinese hamsters and Egyptian sand rats.

The db/db strain develops diabetes at an early age. There are intense hyperplasia of the islets, elevations in blood glucose, and hyperglycemia (Coleman and Hummel 1967). The mice become progressively more obese. In late stages, the islets are exhausted and the β-cells are degranulate and filled with vacuoles. Thickening of the glomerular mesangium and capillary basement membrane develops (Like et al. 1972).

The ob/ob strain develops diabetes at 3–4 wks of age. Pancreatic islet hyperplasia with β-cell degranulation, hyperinsulinemia, hyperglycemia, and obesity are characteristic. Disease reaches a peak at 8–9 months, after which islet hypertrophy and fibrosis occur and the obesity and hyperglycemia regress. Insulin resistance in muscle cells has been noted.

The desert sand rat (*Psammomys obesus*) is normally lean and subsists on vegetation in Middle Eastern deserts. On high caloric laboratory diets these rats develop obesity, hyperinsulinemia, and, in some individuals, diabetes. Obesity is associated with accelerated triglyceride secretion and increased adipocyte size.

PITUITARY

When the brain of a mammal is removed from the calvarium, the pituitary stalk breaks and the gland remains embedded between its bony depression in the sphenoid bone and its cover of dura mater. A shelf of dura, the diaphragma sellae, extends over the top of the gland and prevents its removal with the brain in many species. By carefully cutting the dura that envelops the pituitary, it can be extracted from its dural enclosure.

Grossly, the pituitary contains two distinct portions. The lighter posterior lobe resembles the brain in color. The anterior lobe is larger and darker in most species.

The short hollow stalk or infundibulum contains an extension of the third ventricle. Under the dissecting microscope, the pars intermedia is seen as a dark vascular line on the deep wall of the hypophyseal cleft (the residual lumen of Rathke's pouch).

Microscopically, the pituitary has two major subdivisions: the *neurohypophysis,* which develops embryologically as a downgrowth from the diencephalon; and the *adenohypophysis,* which forms from an outpouching on the roof of the mouth. These subdivisions, in turn, are divided into characteristic parts.

The anterior lobe, the most significant structure endocrinologically, is known to secrete seven distinct hormones. Its parenchymal cells are traditionally classified according to their avidity for crude histologic stains as chromophobes and chromophils. *Chromophobes* are small, poorly granular cells which are precursors of the chromophil cells. *Chromophils* are the functioning cells of the anterior pituitary and are differentiated into specific hormone-secreting cells. On a crude histologic basis they are divided into acidophils and basophils.

Granules of the chromophil cells are formed in the Golgi complex and exist in the cytoplasm as dense membrane-bound bodies. Under stimulation by releasing hormones which arrive from the hypothalamus via the portal system, granules are released by exocytosis (Nakayama et al. 1970; Pelletier 1973). Specific hormones have been identified by the use of peroxidase-labeled antibodies (Mendoza et al. 1973). Hormone secretion is mediated by the adenyl cyclase system (Pelletier et al. 1972). As granules pass the plasma membrane, they lose density and quickly disintegrate. Degranulation of specific cells can be induced experimentally by castration, thyroidectomy, and induction of hypertension (Rosa and D'Angelo 1972).

The *pars intermedia* is poorly developed in mammals and consists of irregular aggregates of follicles and pale cells. In fish and amphibia the pars intermedia produces a melanocyte-stimulating hormone (MSH) that causes aggregated pigment granules in cells of the skin to disperse and thereby imparts a deepened coloration to the skin.

The *pars tuberalis* is not known to secrete hormones but provides a framework for vascular structures of the hypophyseal-portal system. Parenchymal cells are present but their function is not known.

The *pars nervosa* stores the neurosecretory hormones oxytocin and antidiuretic hormone. These hormones are synthesized in nerve cell bodies in the hypothalamus and granules pass down axons of the hypothalamo-hypophyseal tract and are stored in the pars nervosa. *Pituicytes* are modified glial cells that serve a supporting function. Large amorphous hyaline eosinophilic *Herring bodies* are terminal bulb formations of hypothalamic fibers which increase with aging (Bodian 1966; Dellman and Rodriquez 1970). They are large bulbous sacs filled with neurosecretory vesicles, mitochondria, and ribosomes. They contain large lysosomal inclusions which develop from the progressive aggregation of neurosecretory granules (Erkocak 1973).

NEUROSECRETION

Hormones are synthesized by neurons of the hypothalamus which directly affect secretion of the pituitary. They are transmitted to the pituitary by two mechanisms: neural and vascular.

The *posterior pituitary hormones,* oxytocin and antidiuretic hormone (ADH), are packaged in secretory granules within nerve cell bodies located in the hypothalamic supraoptic nucleus. They pass down the axon of the neuron and into the posterior pituitary where they are taken up by capillary endothelium. Secretory granules can be identified ultrastructurally in the perikaryon of hypothalamic nuclei, in axons of the brain substance, and in axon terminals within the posterior pituitary (Cannata and Morris 1973; Sloper and Bateson 1965). Granules become depleted during demands for secretion of these hormones. For example, dehydration stimulates ADH secretion and depletes neurosecretory granule deposits in the posterior lobe and median eminence. Destructive lesions of this hypothalamic-neurohypophyseal tract may result in diabetes insipidus or disturbed renal function (Asheim 1963). Oxytocin acts on smooth muscle of the uterine wall during parturition and, on release by the stimulation of nursing, causes milk letdown by inducing mammary gland periacinar myoepithelial cells to contract.

In contrast to neural secretion, the *hypothalamic releasing factors,* which induce synthesis and secretion of cells of the anterior pituitary, are secreted by neurons directly into local capillaries. These vessels carry the factors through the portal veins to the endocrine cells in the anterior pituitary. This vascular mechanism of neurosecretion depends upon the integrity of the special capillary network at the base of the hypothalamus which penetrates directly into the anterior lobe of the pituitary.

INFLAMMATION

The pituitary suffers inflammatory effects in many severe systemic diseases. This is especially true in severe neurotropic viral infections such as hog cholera, foot-and-mouth disease, infectious equine anemia, and bovine pseudorabies. The neurohypophysis may be severely altered but the adenohypophysis is rarely so. Suppurative inflammation may occur in several species by embolization or primary infection. *C. pyogenes* infection of the pituitary of cattle is one example.

OTHER DISORDERS

Genetically determined pituitary dysfunction is associated with prolonged gestation in cattle. In the Jersey and Guernsey breeds, aplasia occurs as an autosomal recessive characteristic. In Holsteins, failure of acidophil differentiation is blamed.

Minor developmental defects are commonly found incidentally in the postmortem examination of aged animals. Cysts may arise by distention of the hypophyseal lumen or by persistence of the craniopharyngeal duct. They contain fluid which varies from clear and watery to mucinous.

Atrophy of the pituitary is a result of pressure of cysts or neoplasms. Atrophy may be severe without disruption of hypophyseal function. Ablation of the pituitary in mammals is unsuccessful if even minute portions of the gland are left by the surgeon.

NEOPLASMS

Neoplasms of the pituitary are encountered in dogs, horses, and parakeets but are rare in other species. They may arise from any portion of the gland but in most species certain varieties are characteristic. The tumors are usually quite vascular and the endothelial cells are often abnormal. Acidophil and basophil adenomas may be functional and the clinical manifestations depend upon which hormone is being synthesized (Dingemans 1973). Functional tumors are usually well vascularized and ultrastructurally the cells are packed with dense secretory granules.

Adenomas are most commonly reported in the dog. Individual tumors are classified as chromophobe, acidophil, and basophil adenomas. Chromophobe tumors are the the most common and basophil tumors are the most rare (Capen et al. 1967a). Chromophobe adenomas with ultrastructural evidence of actively secreting corticotrophs often are associated with a syndrome of hyperadrenocorticism in dogs (Capen and Koestner 1967). The ultrastructure of acidophil adenomas differs from that of chromophobe adenomas. The single reported tumor consisted of two types of cells: one densely granular, the other only poorly granular. Secretion granules were consistently larger than in the chromophobe adenomas (Capen et al. 1967b).

Tumors of the pars intermedia are reported in horses and dogs. They appear to begin as areas of nodular hyperplasia and usually are not functional tumors. However, certain adenomas of the pars intermedia may be associated with a syndrome of hyperadrenocorticism in dogs. Because they invade the neurohypophysis they are causes of disturbed water balance.

DIABETES INSIPIDUS

Diabetes insipidus is characterized by excessive thirst, water intake, and urine formation (of low specific gravity). The basis of the disease is deficiency of the anti-diuretic hormone (ADH). This may result from disturbed synthesis in the hypothalamic nuclei or destruction of storage and transfer mechanisms in the neurohypophysis. An associated disturbance of heat regulation and appetite indicates hypothalamic injury.

The cause of diabetes insipidus is usually a neoplasm which compresses the hypothalamus (Loeb 1966). Cranial trauma is also a cause (Henry and Sieber 1967). In dogs the shallow sella turcica allows expansion with compression of adjacent neurons. In a series of pituitary neoplasms in old dogs, 25 of 27 tumor-bearing animals had manifestations of diabetes insipidus (Capen et al. 1967a). Ultrastructural changes

in the hypothalamus were found in neurons of the supraoptic nuclei. The secretory apparatus was impaired. The neurons were lacking granules, the Golgi complex was small, and there were vesiculation and loss of ribosomes in the endoplasmic reticulum (Koestner and Capen 1967).

Diabetes insipidus occurs as a hereditary disease in mutant strains of chickens (Dunson et al. 1972), mice (Naik 1970), and rats (Sokol and Valtin 1965). In chickens, ADH activity of the neurohypophysis is reduced but no changes are present in hypothalamic nuclei and the defect resembles mammalian nephrogenic diabetes insipidus. The defect in rodents involves deficiency of the neurosecretory apparatus.

REFERENCES

Abrahams, S. J. and Holtzman, E. Secretion and endocytosis in insulin-stimulated rat adrenal medulla cells. *J. Cell Biol.* 56:540, 1973.

Asheim, A. Renal function in dogs with pyometra. I. Studies of the hypothalamic-neurohypophyseal system. *Acta Vet. Scand.* 4:281, 1963.

Bauer, W. C. and Teitelbaum, S. L. Thyrocalcitonin activity of particulate fractions of the thyroid gland. *Lab. Invest.* 15:323, 1966.

Beisel, W. R. and Rapaport, M. I. Inter-relations between adrenocortical function and infectious illness. *New Engl. J. Med.* 280:541, 1969.

Berkow, J. W. and Ricketts, R. L. Spontaneous diabetes mellitus in dogs. *J.A.V.M.A.* 146:1101, 1965.

Black, H. E. and Capen, C. C. Urinary and plasma hydroxyproline during pregnancy, parturition, and lactation in cows with parturient hypocalcemia. *Metabolism* 20:337, 1971.

Black, H. E., Capen, C. C. and Arnaud, C. D. Ultrastructure of parathyroid glands and plasma immunoreactive parathyroid hormone in pregnant cows fed normal and high calcium diets. *Lab. Invest.* 29:173, 1973a.

Black, H. E., Capen, C. C. and Young, D. M. Ultimobranchial thyroid neoplasms in bulls. *Cancer* 32:865, 1973b.

Black, H. E. et al. Effect of a high calcium prepartal diet on calcium homeostatic mechanisms in thyroid glands, bone, and intestine of cows. *Lab. Invest.* 29:437, 1973c.

Blakemore, D. K. The incidence and aetiology of thyroid dysplasia in budgerigar *(Melopsittacus undulatus). Vet. Rec.* 75:1068, 1963.

Bloodworth, J. M. B. Experimental diabetic glomerulosclerosis. II. The dog. *Arch. Path.* 79:113, 1965.

Bodian, D. Herring bodies and neuro-apocrine secretion in the monkey. *Bull. Johns Hopkins Hosp.* 118:282, 1966.

Bohrod, M. G. and Merritt, D. Antithyroid effect of lathyrogenic agents in tadpoles. *Arch. Path.* 75:75, 1963.

Cannata, M. A. and Morris, J. F. Changes in the appearance of hypothalamus-neurohypophyseal neurosecretory granules associated with their maturation. *J. Endocrin.* 57:531, 1973.

Capen, C. C. Fine structural alterations of parathyroid glands in response to experimental and spontaneous changes of calcium in extracellular fluids. *Am. J. Med.* 50:598, 1971.

Capen, C. C. and Koestner, A. Functional chromophobe adenomas of the canine adenohypophysis. *Vet. Path.* 4:326, 1967.

Capen, C. C. and Martin, S. L. Hyperinsulinism in dogs with neoplasia of the pancreatic islets. *Vet. Path.* 6:309, 1969.

Capen, C. C. and Rowland, G. N. Ultrastructure evaluation of the parathyroid glands of young cats with experimental hyperparathyroidism. *Zt. Zellf.* 90:495, 1968.

Capen, C. C. and Young, D. M. Fine structural alterations in thyroid parafollicular cells of cows in response to hypercalcemia induced by vitamin D. *Am. J. Path.* 57:365, 1969.

———. The ultrastructure of the parathyroid glands and thyroid parafollicular cells of cows with parturient paresis and hypocalcemia. *Lab. Invest.* 17:717, 1967.

Capen, C. C., Cole, C. R. and Hibbs, J. W. Influence of vitamin D on calcium metabolism and the parathyroid glands of cattle. *Fed. Proc.* 27:142, 1968.

Capen, C. C., Martin, S. L. and Koestner, A. Neoplasms in the hypophysis of dogs. *Vet. Path.* 4:301, 1967a.

———. The ultrastructure and histopathology of an acidophil adenoma of the canine adenohypophysis. *Vet. Path.* 4:348, 1967b.

Coleman, D. L. and Hummel, K. P. Studies with the mutation diabetes in the mouse. *Diabetologia* 3:238, 1967.

Craighead, J. E. and McLane, M. R. Diabetes mellitus: Induction in mice by encephalomyocarditis virus. *Science* 162:913, 1968.

Davis, J. O. et al. Increased aldosterone secretion in dogs with right-sided congestive heart failure and in dogs with thoracic inferior vena cava constriction. *J. Clin. Invest.* 36:689, 1957.

De Grandi, P. B., Kraehenbuhl, J. P. and Campiche, M. A. Ultrastructural localization of calcitonin in the parafollicular cells of pig thyroid gland with cytochrome C-labeled antibody fragments. *J. Cell Biol.* 50:446, 1971

Dellman, H.-D. and Rodriquez, R. Herring bodies: An electron microscopic study of local degeneration and regeneration of neurosecretory axons. *Zt. Zellf.* 111:293, 1970.

Dent, P. B. et al. Abnormalities of calcium metabolism in advanced osteopetrosis. *Lab. Invest.* 24:118, 1971.

Dingemans, K. P. The development of TSH producing pituitary tumors in the mouse. *Virch. Arch.* B 12:338, 1973.

Dixon, J. and Sanford, J. Pathological features of spontaneous canine diabetes mellitus. *J. Comp. Path.* 72:153–64, 1962.

Drachman, R. H., Toot, R. K. and Wood, W. B., Jr. Studies on the effect of experimental nonketotic diabetes mellitus on antibacterial defense. *J. Exp. Med.* 124:227, 1966.

Dunson, W. A. et al. Hereditary polydipsia and polyuria in chickens. *Am. J. Physiol.* 222.1107, 1972.

Erkocak, A. Etude au microscope électronique de la neurohypophyse du rat normal ou après surrénalectomie bilatérale. *Acta Anat.* 84:178, 1973.

Falkmer, S. and Patent, G. J. Comparative and embryological aspects of the pancreatic islets. In *Handbook of Physiology*, Sec. 7, Vol. 1. John Field, ed., p. 1, 1972.

Fetter, A. W. and Capen, C. C. Ultrastructural evaluation of the parathyroid glands of pigs with experimental turbinate osteoporosis (atrophic rhinitis). *Lab. Invest.* 24:292, 1971.

Fujimoto, Y. et al. Electron microscopic observations of the equine parathyroid glands with particular reference to those of equine osteodystrophia fibrosa. *Jap. J. Vet. Res.* 15:37, 1967.

Gepts, W. and Toussaint, D. Spontaneous diabetes in dogs and cats: A pathological study. *Diabetologia* 3:249–65, 1967.

Giacomelli, F., Wiener, J. and Spiro, D. Cytological alterations related to stimulation of the zona glomerulosa of the adrenal gland. *J. Cell Biol.* 26:499, 1965.

Greim, W. Pathologisch-histologische Veränderungen von Schilddrüsen bei Rindern und Kaninchen nach Verfütterung von Methylthiouracil. *Berl. Muench. Tieraerztl. Wsch.* 86:50, 1973.

Hamre, C. and Nichols, M. S. Exophthalmia in trout fry. *Proc. Soc. Exp. Biol. Med.* 26:63, 1926.

Hargis, G. K. et al. Cytologic detection of parathyroid hormone by immunofluorescence. *Proc. Soc. Exp. Biol. Med.* 117:836, 1964.

Henry, W. B. and Sieber, S. E. Traumatic diabetes insipidus in a dog. *J.A.V.M.A.* 146: 1317, 1967.

Howard, C. F. Spontaneous diabetes in *Macaca nigra*. *Diabetes* 21:1077, 1972.

Johnson, K. H. and Stevens, J. B. Light and electron microscopic studies of islet amyloid in diabetic cats. *Diabetes* 22:81, 1973.

Jones, R. S. and Carter, Y. Incorporation in adrenal cortex of C^{14} labeled fractions of *Klebsiella pneumoniae*. *Proc. Soc. Exp. Biol. Med.* 90:148–53, 1955.

Kallio, D. M., Garant, P. R. and Minkin, C. Evidence of coated membranes in the ruffled border of the osteoclast. *J. Ult. Res.* 37:169, 1971.

Kass, E. H. and Finland, M. Corticosteroids and infections. *Adv. Int. Med.* 9:45–80, 1958.

Kelly, D. F., Siegel, E. T. and Berg, P. The adrenal gland in dogs with hyperadrenocorticism. *Vet. Path.* 8:385, 1971.

Kirk, J. H., Casey, H. W. and Harwell, J. F. Diabetes mellitus in two Rhesus monkeys. *Lab. An. Med.* 22:245, 1972.

Koestner, A. and Capen, C. C. Ultrastructural evaluation of the canine hypothalamic-neurohypophyseal system in diabetes insipidus associated with pituitary neoplasms. *Vet. Path.* 4:513, 1967.

Krook, L. Spontaneous hyperthyroidism in the dog. *Acta Path. Micro. Scand.* 122(1):41, 1957.

Krook, L. and Lowe, J. E. Nutritional secondary hyperparathyroidism in the horse. *Vet. Path.* 1:(1), 1964.

Langslow, D. R. and Freeman, B. M. Partial pancreatectomy and the role of insulin in carbohydrate metabolism in *Gallus domesticus*. *Diabetologia* 8:206, 1972.

Lauper, N. T. Pheochromocytoma. *Am. J. Cardiol.* 30:197, 1972.

Lazarus, S. S. and Shapiro, S. H. Comparison of morphologic changes in nuclei of rabbit pancreatic islet β-cell induced by Streptozotocin, alloxan, and in vitro necrosis. *Lab. Invest.* 29:90, 1973.

Lee, J. C. et al. Experimental immune diabetes in the rabbit. *Am. J. Path.* 57:597, 1969.

Like, A. et al. Studies in the diabetic mutant mouse. *Am. J. Path.* 66:193–244, 1972.

Loeb, W. Adenoma of the pars intermedia associated with hyperglycemia and glycosuria in two horses. *Cornell Vet.* 56:623, 1966.

Lomsky, R., Langr, F. and Vortel, V. Immunohistochemical demonstration of gastrin in mammalian islet of Langerhans. *Nature* 223:618, 1969.

Lucht, U. and Maunsbach, A. B. Effects of parathyroid hormone on osteoclasts in vivo. An ultrastructural and histochemical study. *Zt. Zellf.* 141:529, 1973.

MacGregor, R. R. et al. Studies on the subcellular localization of proparathyroid hormone and parathyroid hormone in the bovine parathyroid gland. *Endocrinology* 93: 1387, 1973.

Manns, J. G. and Martin, C. L. Plasma insulin, glucagon and nonesterified fatty acids in dogs with diabetes mellitus. *Am. J. Vet. Res.* 33:891–85, 1972.

Manuelidis, L. Studies with electron microscopic autoradiography of thyroxin^{125}I in organotypic cultures of the CNS. *Yale J. Biol. Med.* 45:501, 1972.

Matthews, J. L. and Martin, J. H. Intracellular transport of calcium and its relationship to homeostasis and mineralization. An electron microscopic study. *Am. J. Med.* 50: 589, 1971.

Mendoza, D., Arimura, A. and Schally, A. V. Ultrastructural and light microscopic observations of rat pituitary LH-containing gonadotrophs following injection of synthetic LH-RH. *Endocrinology* 92:1153, 1973.

Misugi, K. et al. The pancreatic beta cell demonstration with peroxidase-labeled antibody technique. *Arch. Path.* 89:97, 1970.

Moore, N. A. and Callas, G. The effects of hyperthyroidism on the fine structure of the zona fasciculata of the rat adrenal cortex. *Anat. Rec.* 174:451, 1972.

Munger, B. L. The biology of secretory tumors of the pancreatic islets. In *Handbook of Physiology*, Sec. 7, Vol. 1. John Field, ed., p. 305, 1972.

Müntefering, H. Zur pathologie des Diabetes mellitus der weissen Maus bei der EMC-virusinfektion. *Virch. Arch. A* 356:207, 1972.

Naik, D. V. Pituitary-adrenal relationships in mice with hereditary nephrogenic diabetes insipidus with special emphasis on the neurohypophysis and pars intermedia. *Zt. Zellf.* 107:317, 1970.

Nakamura, M., Yamada, K. and Yokote, M. Ultrastructural aspects of the pancreatic islets in carps of spontaneous diabetes mellitus. *Experientia* 27:75, 1971.

Nakayama, I., Nickerson, P. A. and Skelton, E. R. An electron microscope study of the changes in ACTH- and FSH-producing cells during development of methylandrostenediol hypertension in the rat. *Am. J. Path.* 58:377, 1970.

Nevalainen, T. Fine structure of the parathyroid gland of the laying hen *(Gallus domesticus)*. *Gen. Comp. Endocrin.* 12:561, 1969.

Neve, P. and Dumont, J. E. Time sequence of ultrastructural changes in the stimulated dog thyroid. *Zt. Zellf.* 103:61, 1970.

Nichols, J. and Hennigar, G. Effects of pulmonary hypertension on adrenal and kidneys of dogs infected with heart worms *(Dirofilaria immitis)*. *Lab. Invest.* 13:800, 1964.

Nickerson, P. A. Adrenocortical cells in rats bearing a corticosterone secreting tumor. *Virch. Arch. B* 13:297, 1973.

———. Effect of testosterone, dexamethazone and hypophysectomy on membranous whorls in the adrenal gland of the Mongolian gerbil. *Anat. Rec.* 174:191, 1972.

Nunez, E. A., Belshaw, B. B. and Gershon, M. D. A fine structural study of the highly active thyroid follicular cell of the African Basenji dog. *Am. J. Anat.* 133:463, 1972.

Nussdorfer, G. G. and Mazzocchi, G. A stereologic study of the effects of ACTH and cyclic 3',5'-AMP on adrenal cortical cells of intact and hypophysectomized rats. *Lab. Invest.* 26:45, 1972.

Orci, L. et al. Insulin release by emiocytosis. *Science* 179:82, 1973.

Orci, L. et al. Ultrastructural changes in A-cells exposed to diabetic hyperglycaemia. *Diabetologia* 6:199, 1970.

Osborne, C. A. and Stevens, J. B. Pseudohyperparathyroidism in the dog. *J.A.V.M.A.* 162:125, 1973.

Osburn, B. I., Drost, M. and Stabenfeldt, G. H. Response of fetal adrenal cortex to congenital infections. *Am. J. Obst. Gyn.* 114:622, 1972.

Pang, P. K. T., Pang, R. K. and Sawyer, W. H. Effects of environmental calcium and replacement therapy on the killfish *Fundulus heteroclitus* after the surgical removal of the corpuscle of stannius. *Endocrinology* 93:705, 1973.

Patz, A. and Maumenee, A. E. Studies on diabetic retinopathy in a dog with spontaneous diabetes mellitus. *Am. J. Ophth.* 54:532, 1962.

Pelletier, G. Secretion and uptake of peroxidase by rat adenohypophyseal cells. *J. Ult. Res.* 43:445, 1973.

Pelletier, G. et al. Ultrastructural changes accompanying the stimulatory effect of N[6]-monobutyryl adenosine 3'5' monophosphate on the release. *Endocrinology* 91:1355, 1972.

Penney, D. P., Averill, K. and Olson, J. Projections of adrenocortical cells into sinusoidal lumina. *Am. J. Anat.* 135:135, 1972.

Platt, H. Chronic canine nephritis. *J. Comp. Path.* 61:197, 1951.

Reaven, E. P. and Reaven, G. M. Mechanisms for development of diabetic hypertriglyceridemia in streptozotocin-treated rats. *J. Clin. Invest.* 54:1167, 1974.

Reith, A. The influence of triiodothyronine and riboflavin deficiency on the rat liver with special reference to mitochondria. *Lab. Invest.* 29:216, 1973.

Ricketts, H. T. Renal glomerular lesions in diabetic dogs. *Diabetes* 11:150, 1962.

Rijnberk, A., der Kindern, P. J. and Thijssen, J. H. H. Spontaneous hyperadrenocorticism in the dog. *J. Endocrin.* 41:397, 1968.

Rosa, C. G. and D'Angelo, S. A. The ultrastructure of the thyrotropic cells during thyrotropin rebound in the adenohypophysis of the rat. *Am. J. Anat.* 135:33, 1973.

Roth, S. I. and Capen, C. C. Ultrastructural and functional correlations of the parathyroid glands. *Int. Rev. Exp. Path.* 13:161, 1974.

Rowland, G. N., Capen, C. C. and Nagode, L. A. Experimental hyperparathyroidism in young cats. *Vet. Path.* 5:504, 1968.

Rowland, G. N. et al. Microradiographic evaluation of bone from cows with experimental hypervitaminosis D, diet-induced hypocalcemia and naturally occurring parturient paresis. *Calc. Tiss. Res.* 9:179, 1972.

Scarpelli, D. G., Tremblay, G. and Pearse, A. G. E. A comparative cytochemical and cytologic study of vitamin D induced nephrocalcinosis. *Am. J. Path.* 36:331, 1960.

Shimamura, T. and Morrison, A. B. Secondary hyperparathyroidism in rats with an experimental chronic renal disease. *Exp. Mol. Path.* 15:345, 1971.

Slatopulsky, E. et al. On the pathogenesis of hyperparathyroidism in chronic experimental renal insufficiency in the dog. *J. Clin. Invest.* 50:492, 1971.

Sloper, J. C. and Bateson, R. G. Ultrastructure of neurosecretory cells in the supraoptic nucleus of the dog and rat. *J. Endocrin.* 31:139, 1965.

Smith, U. et al. Exocytosis in the adrenal medulla demonstrated by freeze-etching. *Science* 179:79, 1973.

Sokol, H. W. and Valtin, H. Morphology of the neurosecretory system in rats homozygous and heterozygous for hypothalamic diabetes insipidus. *Endocrinology* 77:692, 1965.

Tashiro, M. Electron microscopic observations of the cyst of ultimobranchial origin found in the thyroid gland of the dog. *Nagoya J. Med. Sci.* 25:159, 1963.

Tice, L. W. and Wollman, S. H. Ultrastructural localization of peroxidase activity in some membranes of the typical thyroid epithelial cell. *Lab. Invest.* 26:23, 1972.

Volk, B. W. and Lazarus, S. S. Ultramicroscopic evolution of β-cell ballooning degeneration in diabetic dogs. *Lab. Invest.* 12:697, 1963.

Volk, T. L. and Scarpelli, D. G. Mitochondria gigantism in the adrenal cortex following hypophysectomy. *Lab. Invest.* 15:707, 1966.

Wellmann, K. F. et al. Fine structure of pancreatic islets of mice infected with the M variant of the encephalomyocarditis virus. *Diabetologia* 8:349, 1972.

Westermark, P. Fine structure of islets of Langerhans in insular amyloidosis. *Virch. Arch. A* 359:1, 1973.

Wilkie, B. N. et al. Ultimobranchial tumors of the thyroid and pheochromocytoma in the bull. *Vet. Path.* 7:126, 1970.

Wise, P. H. et al. The diabetic syndrome in the tuco-tuco *(Ctenomys talarum)*. *Diabetologia* 8:165, 1972.

Wood, R. L., Whipp, S. C. and Witzel, D. A. Plasma glucose, hydrocortisone, and insulin levels in acute swine erysipelas. *Cornell Vet.* 61:596, 1971.

Wyllie, A. H. et al. Adrenocortical cell deletion and the role of ACTH. *J. Path.* 111:85, 1973.

Young, D. M., Capen, C. C. and Black, H. E. Calcitonin activity in ultimobranchial neoplasms from bulls. *Vet. Path.* 8:19, 1971.

Youshak, M. M. and Capen, C. C. Fine structural alterations in parathyroid glands of chickens with osteopetrosis. *Am. J. Path.* 61:257, 1970.

CHAPTER ELEVEN

Muscle Cells

CARDIAC MYOCYTES

The performance of the heart as a pump is dependent upon the contractile function of the cardiac myocyte sarcomere. The sarcomere extends from one Z line to the next. Its striated character is due to the presence of actin and myosin filaments which insert between and overlap each other (Fig. 11.1). During contraction, the ends of the actin filaments slide deeply into the A band between the myosin filaments. Z lines, to which the actin filaments are attached, are drawn closer together, shortening the myofibril. During relaxation, actin filaments are withdrawn from the A band and the sarcomere is lengthened. The sarcoplasmic reticulum takes up, stores, and releases calcium for the excitation of contraction.

Structural analysis of the pathologic sarcomere (see Fig. 2.3) is concerned with the integrity of the myofilaments, the apposition of Z lines, the structure of the sarcoplasmic reticulum, and the length of the individual sarcomeres. Sarcomere length is a function of ventricular filling pressure and changes in filament extension are characteristic of the failing heart.

Cardiac myofilaments are not organized into discrete myofibrils as in skeletal muscle. They exist as cylindrical bundles incompletely subdivided into irregular fascicles by deep incisures and fusiform clefts of sarcoplasm. Each cell (myocyte or myofiber) is separated by an intercalated disk, the integrity of which is also essential in contractility. In degenerative disease of the cardiac myocyte, abnormal twisting and gapping may occur between membranes.

MYOCARDITIS

Inflammation of the heart accompanies many systemic infectious diseases. Myocyte damage in inflammatory heart disease may occur in two ways. (1) Direct destruction of the myocyte is by intracellular microbial replication or by the production of the potent toxins that cause cell lysis. In many infectious diseases, these lesions are accompanied by the attack of lymphocytes and plasmacytes which are attracted to antigen-containing sites on the cell membrane. (2) The indirect effects of acute exudative inflammation are on the vascular and interstitial tissues. Most infections damage blood vessels and result in exudation of fluid and cells through the damaged capillary bed. Capillary stenosis due to endothelial cell swelling (augmented by pressure of perivascular fluid) may induce focal ischemia of the myocardium. Many inflammatory lesions of the myocardium are not striking histologically, however, and in acute disease often go unnoticed. They generally resolve without permanent structural damage to the heart.

Chronic infection of the heart is fortunately rare but can be disastrous. *Chronic myocarditis* is most often associated with the production of proliferative lesions of the endocardium of the heart valves. If the organisms persist, as they do in streptococcal and erysipelothrix infections of swine, large fibrinous lesions on the valve may obstruct blood flow and induce indirect damage by increases in workload.

CARDIOMYOPATHY

Degenerative cardiomyopathy is used as an umbrella term covering an unrelated

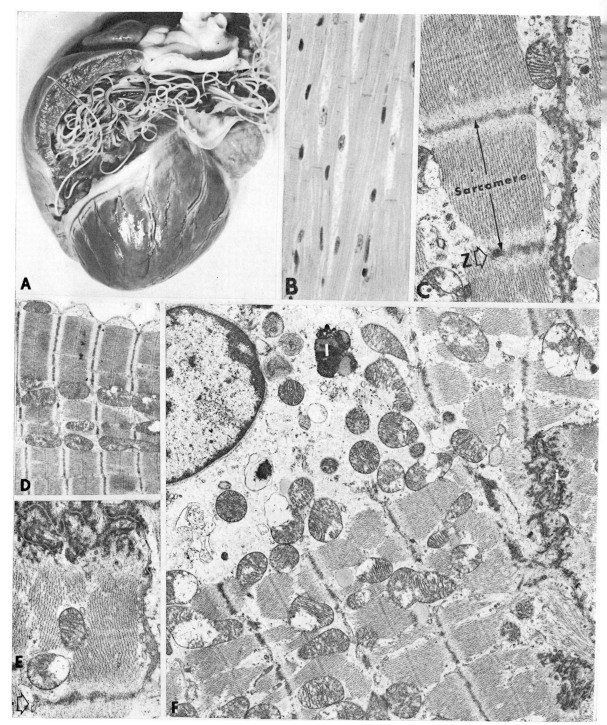

Fig. 11.1. Right ventricular myocardial hypertrophy with dilatation, obstruction by heartworms, dog. A. Right wall, markedly thickened. B. Histology. C. and D. Ultrastructure of sarcomere and Z line. E. Tubule system. Sarcoplasmic reticulum (arrow). F. Disruption of intercalated disk (i) and attachment of microfibrils. Mitochondria are enlarged. Expansion of paranuclear space. Lipofuscin pigment (l).

group of slowly progressive insidious diseases that directly affect the cardiac myocyte. Most are rare and, except for the hereditary diseases, are ill defined. The heart lesions are known to be augmented by other metabolic changes such as cold stress, adrenalin secretion, thyroid deficiency, and hypoxia.

The hallmark of cardiomyopathy is primary degeneration and necrosis of the cardiac myocyte. The cellular reaction is due to proliferation of sarcolemmal nuclei with little or no inflammatory component. Necrotic cells may persist and become mineralized.

HEREDITARY CARDIOMYOPATHY

Hereditary cardiomyopathy usually occurs in newborn animals. Heart lesions are an integral part of some muscular dystrophies (Forbes and Sperelakis 1972), glycogen storage diseases (Garancis 1968), and lipodystrophies. In glycogenosis in the dog (Mostofa 1970), large deposits of glycogen particles distort the normal myofilament structure. The hamster (strain B10) is afflicted with a hereditary cardiomyopathy which leads to cardiomegaly, cardiac failure, and systemic signs of heart failure (edema, liver congestion). Defective genesis of myofilaments in the newborn hamster leads to necrosis of the myofibril (Bajusz et al. 1969; Paterson et al. 1972). Electrolyte disturbances including elevated calcium and decreased magnesium are progressive and accompanied by degenerative changes in the mitochondria and sarcoplasmic reticulum.

ELECTROLYTE CARDIOMYOPATHY

Electrolyte cardiomyopathy accompanies depletion of such electrolytes as magnesium and potassium (Heggtveit and Nadkarni 1971). Depletion of magnesium may be a common denominator in the early pathogenesis of myocyte necrosis which occurs in animals dying of different causes. Experimental magnesium depletion is characterized by small spotty foci of degeneration and necrosis in affected hearts. Ultrastructural lesions consist of swelling and vacuolization of mitochondria; giant forms may be present and there is elongation and disorganization of cristae. This is fol-

lowed by deposition of dense material in the matrix and by calcification. Separation of intercalated disks and fragmentation of myofibrils occur in necrosis.

In potassium deficiency, mitochondria appear to be fairly well preserved (Emberson and Muir 1969). Inhibition of fluid with disorientation of the sarcoplasmic reticulum and myofibrils indicate that alteration of membrane permeability is induced by the electrolyte imbalance.

NUTRITIONAL CARDIOMYOPATHY

Nutritional cardiomyopathy occurs in starvation, protein deficiency, fatty acid and choline deficiencies, and several specific vitamin deficiencies. Fatty degeneration of the cardiac myocyte is a common finding; it is nonspecific, for it is also seen in extreme obesity. Vitamin E deficiency, especially when complicated by high fat diets, results in degeneration and necrosis of both skeletal and cardiac myocytes. The lesion is caused by the lack of the depressant effect of vitamin E on oxidation in mitochondria. Enlargement and degeneration of mitochondria are accompanied by degeneration of other components of the myocyte.

TOXIC CARDIOMYOPATHY

The action of most myocardial poisons involves the exquisitely sensitive mitochondria. The precise mechanisms are often complex and multiple toxic effects occur. Reserpine, for example, exerts a direct toxic action on the mitochondrion but it also depletes the myocardium of serotonin and catecholamines and these secondary effects exaggerate the primary injury.

Toxic concentrations of potassium, copper, and iron are associated with naturally occurring cardiomyopathy. Mitochondrial lesions have also been induced with common drugs such as reserpine, digitalis, thyroxin, β-adrenergic blocking agents, and the antimalarial drug plasmocid (D'Agostino 1963; Gardell et al. 1970; Hagopian et al. 1972; McCallister and Page 1973). Venoms of some reptiles are known to produce foci of myocardial necrosis (Yarum and Braun 1971). Cobalt toxicity induces mitochondrial degeneration by depression of respiratory activity via inhibition of pyruvate and α-ketoglutarate dehydrogenase.

Of the plant toxins that cause cardiac myocyte necrosis in grazing animals, that of coffee senna *(Cassia occidentalis)* is best known. Mitochondrial damage is the primary structural lesion and there are subsequent myofibrillar degeneration, necrosis of myocytes, and congestive heart failure (Read et al. 1968). In cattle and horses, myocyte destruction leads to myoglobinuria, hyperkalemia, and release of enzymes such as glutamic oxaloacetic transaminase into the bloodstream.

RADIATION CARDIOMYOPATHY

Radiation-induced myocardial disease is practically limited to human patients receiving large doses of therapeutic, antineoplastic radiation. Tissue injury results from vascular lesions. Early changes of endothelial cell swelling and altered capillary permeability are followed by basement membrane reduplication, platelet aggregation, and phagocytosis (Khan and Ohanian 1973).

OXYGEN-DEFICIT CARDIOMYOPATHY

Most tissues remove about 25% of blood oxygen during the flow of blood through the capillaries. The myocardium removes 75% and is exquisitely sensitive to oxygen deprivation. Myocardial cells may be injured during asphyxiation, severe anemia, severe hypotension, or any vascular lesion causing myocardial ischemia. The extent to which hypoxia affects the cardiac myocyte depends upon the type, severity, and duration of oxygen deficiency.

The immediate cytopathologic change in the acutely hypoxic cardiac myocyte occurs in the mitochondria: they are swollen, their matrix is clarified, and the cristae are fragmented (cristolysis). Glycogen deposits, disorganization of myofilaments (appearing as smudging of the A and I bands), vacuolation of the sarcoplasmic reticulum, and irregularities of the Z band are subsequent changes. Separation of intercalated disks is seen in severe damage and indicates drastic changes in contractility.

Cell membrane changes in injured myocytes permit enzymes such as the transaminases to leak out of the cell. They appear in high levels in serum and the ischemic myocyte may be shown to be enzyme-deficient histochemically. Enzyme levels in serum reliably reflect a severe degree of myocardial damage.

Cell membrane damage also permits the entrance of water, electrolytes, and plasma proteins into the cell. Ischemic myocytes from experimental myocardial infarcts in the dog contain large amounts of albumin, globulin, and fibrinogen which appear bound to the damaged muscle filaments (Kent 1967). In irreversible injury the electrolyte composition of the myocyte begins to resemble the interstitial fluid. Increases in cell calcium occur and calcium appears to be preferentially located in the mitochondrial matrix (Shen and Jennings 1972).

It is difficult to demonstrate these finite changes in tissue from clinical disease and much of the information comes from the experimental production of hypoxia. Models for the experimental induction of ischemic myocardial damage usually involve: (1) asphyxiation, (2) sudden hypotension induced by bleeding, or (3) occlusion of the coronary artery either by ligation or by gradually narrowing mechanical cuffs. Changes in the myocardium have been detected by 1 hr with 20% reduction in coronary flow (De La Iglesia and Lumb 1972).

HYPOXIC DISEASE

Asphyxia following experimental clamping of the trachea rapidly leads to cardiac dilation, heart stoppage, and death. As seen in movies of the living heart in rabbits, this acute hypoxic cardiac dilation begins in the atria within seconds and spreads to the ventricles (Büchner 1971). If oxygenation is permitted, the ventricle rapidly returns to normal size. The cardiac dilation correlates with an hypoxia-induced mitochondrial degeneration and a fall in ATP and high energy phosphate concentrations in heart muscle homogenates. Upon regression of dilatation, mitochondria and their electron-transfer systems return to normal.

Severe ischemia of the myocardium,

even though transient, may produce disseminated myocyte necrosis. Severe hypotension which characterizes the shock state following extensive hemorrhage causes small disseminated zonal lesions throughout the myocardium (Martin and Hackel 1963). Certain individual cells are destroyed, allegedly due to their particular stage of metabolic activity at the time of injury. If hypotension is intense and prolonged, the process becomes irreversible and zonal lesions develop into large segmental areas of necrosis. If hypotension is transient the myocardium returns to normal and the necrotic cells are broken down and processed by leukocytes and sarcolemmal cells. Dead cells accumulate calcium, and foci of necrosis may heal leaving tiny areas of mineral within a connective tissue scar. These calcified areas are found most commonly in the ventricles in mammals but occur in the anterior heart more commonly in fishes and birds (Prior et al. 1968).

Dogs that suffer prolonged epileptic seizures with interruption of breathing contain these small disseminated necrotic foci throughout the ventricular myocardium. They are analogous to the focal lesions in man that are considered relics of angina pectoris (Büchner 1971). Hypertrophied hearts which have outgrown their vascular supply are particularly prone to this pattern of heart necrosis, which is also augmented in shock, severe anemia, and other forms of chronic hypoxia.

In the dog, these lesions have been produced experimentally. A large quantity of blood was removed, sufficient to result in severe systemic oxygen debt. Eight minutes were allowed to elapse and the blood was replaced. Although the dogs recovered normally, foci of necrosis were present in the heart and other organs when they were killed 4 days later (Weaver et al. 1972).

CARDIAC VASCULAR (ISCHEMIC) DISEASE

When the lumen of an artery within the heart is narrowed, the myocardium supplied by its ramifications is affected. The result may vary from diffuse fibrosis to infarction and depends upon the extent of vascular narrowing. Only the dog has been sufficiently studied to provide reliable information on cardiac vascular disease. It

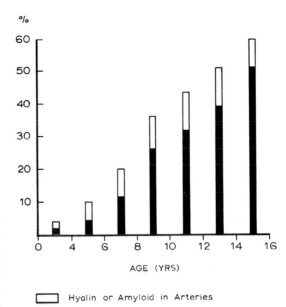

Fig. 11.2. Incidence of heart disease in the dog (from Jönsson).

is plain that as dogs age they become increasingly susceptible to arterial disease and its associated lesions of the myocardium (Fig. 11.2.)

Acute obstruction of coronary arteries due to emboli (usually thrombi) results in *infarction*—ischemia of large segments of the myocardium and necrosis of myocytes. The clinical outcome depends upon the size of the infarct and the seriousness of the underlying disease causing the embolization. Myocardial infarction precipitated by atherosclerosis of the coronary artery is a burden of aging humans, but is rare in dogs and presumably in other animals.

Coronary artery ligation has been used experimentally as a model for myocardial ischemia (Brachfeld and Schever 1967). The biochemical events in the myocardium which followed restriction of coronary flow were: oxygen consumption depressed 45%, glucose consumption increased 91% (glucose extracted from heart muscle increased 500%), and lactate increased in the venous outflow. It is clear, therefore, that myocardial ischemia is accompanied by accelerated glycolysis. Anaerobic glucose breakdown (glycolytic cycle) is insignificant as an energy source in the normal cardiac myocyte. However, when energy supplied by oxygen utilization in the mitochondria is insufficient, the myocyte oxidizes glucose to pyruvate and lactate, which provide a supplemental source of energy. In myocardial ischemia, this augmentation may generate enough energy to be of critical importance. In vitro, glucose has a sparing effect on hypoxic myocardial cells. In dogs, infusion of glucose-potassium-insulin solution protects against myocyte necrosis during myocardial infarction (Sybers et al. 1973). Local acidosis occurs in ischemic heart muscle. This, when superimposed upon oxygen-deficit, has profound effects on the function of the heart.

Chronic vascular obstruction slowly but progressively constricts the arterial supply to the myocardium, producing myocardial atrophy. There is disappearance of myocardial cells with concomitant fibroplasia of the interstitium. The end result is diffuse scarring of the myocardium and markedly altered function. Obstruction of the lymphatics of the heart augments these chronic changes.

EXCESS WORKLOAD

The capacity of the heart to deal with transient increases in workload is enormous, provided adequate intervals occur for recovery of nutritive and electrolyte levels. Permanent elevations in workload which produce heart disease may result from congenital heart defects and a wide variety of diseases that produce increased peripheral resistance to the outflow of blood from the heart (Table 11.1). Compared to direct injury to the heart, these diseases are often complex and produce their effects upon the heart by several different mechanisms. Severe anemia, for example, causes an increased workload because of decreased oxygen-carrying capacity of blood; it also predisposes the myocardium to ischemic injury.

Extensive lung disease has a profound influence on the heart. The force required to pump blood through the pneumonic lung markedly increases heart work. Acute diffuse purulent pneumonia may thereby directly cause acute heart failure. Heart damage due to chronic diffuse lung disease is more complex because increased

Table 11.1 Cardiac failure: Mechanisms of cardiac myocyte damage

Myocyte destruction (direct)
  Myocarditis: inflammation (nonspecific or specific myocyte damage)
  Myocardiopathy: primary myocyte degeneration (nutritional, genetic disorders)
  Vascular disease: ischemia—acute (infarction) or chronic

Excessive workload (indirect)
  Anoxia: anemia, high altitude disease, chronic diffuse lung disease
  Chamber obstruction: heartworms, valve lesions, tumors
  Obstructive lung disease: pulmonary embolism, pulmonary fibrosis
  Constrictive lesions: pericarditis, hydropericardium, hemopericardium
  Congenital heart defects: septal defects, patent ductus

workload is accompanied by secondary, hypoxic effects on the heart.

Severe anemia is commonly overlooked as a cause of heart disease. Hemoglobin below 50% endangers the myocardium and results in clinical signs of weakness, dyspnea, tachycardia, and electrocardiographic changes. Anemia in these cases is accompanied by cardiac hypertrophy. If untreated, it may develop into dilatation with fatty degeneration and necrosis of cardiac myocytes (Paplanus et al. 1958).

CARDIAC ENLARGEMENT: HYPERTROPHY AND DILATATION

The cardial sign of heart disease is cardiac enlargement. If the heart works against a sustained overload, it eventually becomes unable to deliver a normal output of blood. With development of myocardial fatigue, slight dilatation occurs due to stretching of individual myocardial cells, presumably as a result of overfilling during diastole. The increase in ventricular volume is associated with increase in length of the sarcomere (Leyton and Sonnenblick 1971). The myocardium responds by myocyte hypertrophy, that is, by enlargement of individual myofibers. Hypertrophied myocytes provide increased energy (although less efficiently) for production of the necessary output. Hypertrophy may enable the heart to maintain sufficient output without further dilatation, and in hearts examined during this stage the chambers appear relatively normal in size.

In time the myocardium again fails, which again produces dilatation leading to more hypertrophy, and so on until the cycle is unable to compensate for increases in workload. The chain of events involved in dilatation-hypertrophy may be accelerated or prolonged depending on the severity of damage to the heart. In some instances, marked hypertrophy is present with little dilatation, particularly in the left ventricle. In others, little hypertrophy is seen but there is remarkable dilatation with an enlarged flabby heart.

Of the animal species, only dogs have been examined clinically and experimentally in sufficient numbers for data on cardiac enlargement to be valid. The normal heart weight/body weight ratios in dogs range from 5 to 11. Differences are those of differing breeds. Racing Greyhounds in good condition may exceed this range. In cardiac enlargement the heart weight/body weight ratio increases.

Cytopathic changes in cardiac myocyte hypertrophy occur chiefly in two organelles: mitochondria and myofilaments. Mitochondria of the cardiac myocyte can rapidly enlarge in response to increased workloads and enlargement is characteristic of early hypertrophy of myocardium (Bozner and Meessen 1969; McCallister and Brown 1965). Autophagy may accompany severe hypertrophy but lysosomal enzymes measured in homogenates of failing dog hearts do not differ from normal (Stoner et al. 1973).

Sarcomeres in hypertrophic myocardium may be overstretched, normal, or contracted. The presence of supercontracted sarcomeres (< 1.5 nm) indicates extensive change. The myocyte enlarges in hypertrophy by the addition of new myosin filaments to the muscle fiber. New sarcomere units appear to be added since Z to Z distances do not markedly change. The Z bands become irregular and thickened in the cat (Fawcett 1967) and dog (Munnell and Getty 1968). It is theorized that Z band material (tropomyosin) spreads through the new sarcomere and acts as a structural scaffold for assembly of actin and myosin filaments. Although some myocytes may split and enlarge, hyperplasia

does not appear to be an effective mechanism of growth in cardiac enlargement.

Hypertrophied hearts are prone to failure. In the normal heart, each myofibril is accompanied by a capillary. Hyperplasia of capillary endothelial cells occurs in cardiac hypertrophy (Mandache et al. 1973), but as fiber size increases the vascular supply does not do so accordingly. It has been demonstrated that the relative amount of fluid which can circulate within the heart decreases progressively with hypertrophy. The metabolizing mass of the myofiber enlarges markedly but the cell membrane and its relation to the capillary do not. When the hypertrophied heart reaches a critical size, there thus may be overgrowth beyond the capillary supply and unseating of the heart valves. Biologically, then, in chronic hypertrophy the heart is set up for hypoxic injury.

As a model of right-sided disease with hypertrophy, we examine the effect of mechanical obstruction of the right ventricle and pulmonary artery by heart worms in the dog (Fig. 11.3). Affected dogs are submitted for necropsy because of weakness, anorexia, and progressive respiratory difficulty. Clinical pathologic examination reveals microfilaria of *Dirofilaria immitis* in the blood and radiologic examination shows a markedly enlarged heart with dense areas distributed throughout the lungs. At necropsy, the myocardial walls are thickened and the chambers are often enlarged. The lungs are large, pale, meaty, and do not collapse. Fluid is usually present in the abdominal and thoracic cavities. The pathologic diagnoses include: (1) cardiac hypertrophy with obstruction of the right ventricle and pulmonary artery; (2) chronic multifocal granulomatous pneumonitis due to embolization of adult parasites and microfilaria present in the capillary bed of the lung; (3) bronchiectasis with mucous hyperplasia; and (4) centrolobular fatty degeneration of the liver with foci of necrosis and fibrosis.

In heart worm cases, disastrous increases of workload on the right heart occur by several mechanisms. First, there is mechanical obstruction of blood flow by adult parasites. Microfilaria are sucked from the blood of infected dogs by mosquitoes and are transmitted as larvae to other dogs,

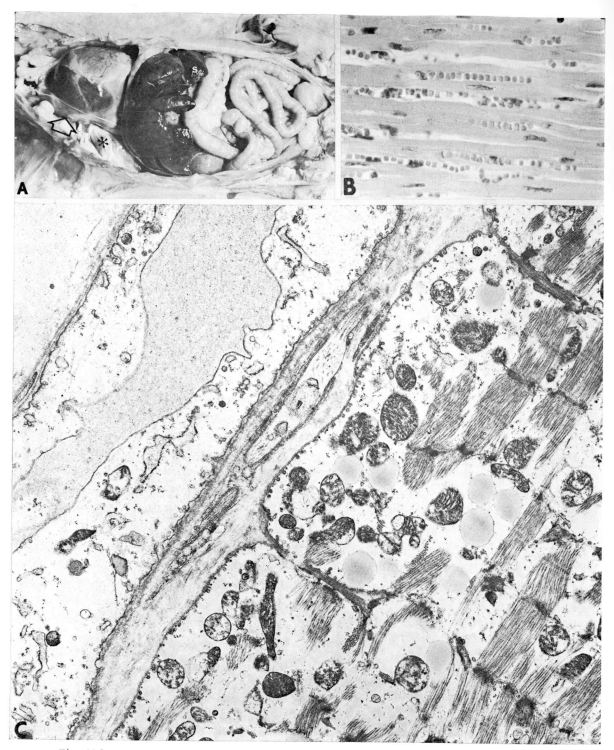

Fig. 11.3. Congestive heart failure, old dog. Heart fills large portion
of thoracic cavity (arrow); vena cava and right atrium markedly
enlarged. Spleen (s), lung (asterisk). B. Histology. Left myocardium.
Hyperemia and lengthening of myocytes. Myofibers not distinct. C.
Ultrastructure of myocytes. Disorganization of myofibrils and
organelles, lipid accumulation (fatty degeneration), and cell swelling.
Endothelial cells are swollen. Edema in perivascular areas (top left).

where they develop within the right ventricle and pulmonary artery to adult worms. Second, pulmonary arterial vascular lesions develop and shed thrombotic emboli into the pulmonary capillary bed. This leads to chronic inflammatory disease of the lung with hemosiderosis, alveolar wall fibrosis, and focal granulomatous lesions. Last, live microfilaria shed into the pulmonary capillary bed. These factors, when combined, initiate the cycle of pulmonary edema–heart failure. Fluid accumulates in the alveolar wall; fibrosis and emphysema develop. These, in turn, increase the heart workload and so on. The failing right heart cannot pump sufficient blood to the lung. Death may occur during cardiac hypertrophy due to sudden embolization of microfilaria and thrombi, or it may not occur until cardiac failure and severe dilatation have developed.

Chronic myocardial hypertrophy due to increased cardiac work has been studied experimentally in three models: (1) production of aortic stenosis by placing a band around the ascending aorta, (2) chronic swimming experiments in rodents (Pelosi and Agliati 1968), and (3) production of renal hypertension. Progressive hypertrophy of heart muscle due to aortic stenosis in dogs illustrates that the ratio of mitochondria to myofilament decreases in waves. Dogs (whose normal ratio is 0.42) show increased values at 3 to 6 days postsurgery. Decreased ratios develop and persist until the 25th wk, when elevated values are again found (Onishi et al. 1969). Biochemical data suport the structural changes; that is, ATP values recover and relapse accordingly.

Three stages in experimental overload are therefore hypothesized: (1) an initial stage due to sudden increase of pressure work of left ventricle with increase in mitochondrial volume, decreases in high energy phosphates, and marked increase in protein synthesis; (2) a stabilized state of hyperactivity where myocytes and mitochondria appear normal and with normal values of high energy phosphates; and (3) insufficiency with chronic hypertrophy of heart muscle (Meerson 1969).

CARDIAC FAILURE

When the myocardium is no longer able to compensate for increases in workload, the chambers of the heart dilate and degeneration of cardiac myocytes can be detected. The pathologic changes vary according to the causal mechanism involved. In the slowly failing heart, secondary factors such as ischemia, aging, and endocrine imbalances may be superimposed upon the primary structural alterations of the myocardium. In the ventricular walls a spectrum of change from relatively normal myocytes to total fibrosis may exist. Degenerate myocytes may alternate with bands of fibrous interstitium.

The myofilaments of the degenerate cardiac myocyte are often disoriented with smudging and fraying at the Z line. The perinuclear pale zones are enlarged and lipofuscin bodies are generally prominent. In heart failure, there may be increased numbers of mitochondria but their total mass may be less (Bishop and Cole 1969). Although mitochondria appear to function normally (Walker and Bishop 1971), they fail to supply sufficient energy.

The two sides of the heart usually do not fail together. In early heart disease, distinct syndromes of right or left failure occur although failure of one cannot exist long without producing excess strain on the other.

RIGHT HEART DISEASE

Any obstruction of the pulmonary blood flow results in selective hypertrophy of myocytes in the right ventricle and ultimately in changes in the right atrium. In the dog, in addition to heart worms, lesions of the right atrioventricular valve and diffuse lung disease are causes of right heart disease. *Cor pulmonale* is the clinical term applied to right ventricular strain produced by diffuse pulmonary disease. Diseases such as chronic emphysema, pneumonia, and pulmonary fibrosis notably affect the right heart. Cor pulmonale also results from pressure atelectasis due to tumors. Hypoxic cor pulmonale of cattle occurs in brisket disease (Alexander et al. 1960). The extent of right ventricular hypertrophy is traditionally believed to be directly related to the extent of loss of lung parenchyma and its capillary bed. The degree of muscular hypertrophy of pulmonary arterioles, however, is probably a more reliable index of heart damage.

LEFT HEART DISEASE

The heart's more powerful force is generated by the left ventricular myocardium and the clinical signs that accompany disease of the heart are more readily apparent because of its failure. Diffuse heart disease is therefore generally manifested as left-sided failure.

END STAGE HEART

Congestive heart failure is the clinical syndrome resulting from the inability of cardiac output to keep pace with venous return. It is the final common pathway for several types of heart disease. Retention of water and sodium ions (allegedly from decreased renal blood flow and adrenal cortical mechanisms) may result in overhydration with increased blood volume. This distends the venous bed so that the heart chambers cannot keep up with the amount of blood delivered. The venous bed is distended further and fluid begins to accumulate in the tissues (Wallace and Hamilton 1962).

The signs of congestive heart failure are the secondary effects of failing circulation due to stasis and congestion. Lesions are extensive in the lung and liver. They are rare in the kidneys, brain, and subcutis, although lesions of anoxia and fluid exudation do occur in these organs.

Dogs with congestive heart failure eventually develop edema of the legs and abdomen, anemia, emaciation, and progressive deterioration. They have, in some cases, been treated for several years with digitalis for cardiac failure. In those that die, there is massive enlargement of the heart with extreme distention of the vena cavae and atria (Fig. 11.3). Fluid is present in the subcutis and in all body cavities. The liver and spleen are enlarged and the bone marrow is often red throughout. In summary, the histopathologic diagnoses usually include: (1) myocardial degeneration with edema and hyperemia of the capillary bed, (2) centrolobular degeneration of the liver with fibrosis and hyperplasia of Kupffer cells due to erythrophagocytosis, (3) engorgement of the splenic red pulp, and (4) pulmonary fibrosis with fluid in the alveoli.

In the lungs of dogs with cardiac failure, blood dams up and the increased pressure in the pulmonary veins is transmitted to the capillaries. Fluid accumulates in the alveolar wall and overflows into alveoli (pulmonary edema). The lesions seen postmortem include capillary dilatation (hyperemia), hemorrhage into scattered alveoli, and eosinophilic granular debris in the alveoli. In long-standing cases, there are collagen fibers in the alveolar wall and iron-laden macrophages ("heart failure cells") in the alveoli. These result from erythrophagocytosis due to stasis in the capillary bed.

Backing up of blood in the liver produces hepatomegaly and striking lesions of the parenchyma. "Nutmeg liver" results from congestive, red accentuation of centrolobular areas which are surrounded by pale fatty hepatocytes. If heart failure is sudden and severe, the sinusoids become engorged with blood and sinusoid rupture with hepatocyte necrosis results ("hemorrhagic cardiac necrosis"). In chronic forms, the centrolobular areas slowly become fibrotic and these lesions are called *cardiac sclerosis* (or cardiac cirrhosis). Abnormalities of portal system congestion are also responsible for ascites.

SMOOTH MUSCLE VASCULAR MYOCYTES

Arteries, like the heart, are subject to disease caused by direct microbial, toxic, or immunologic injury. They are also affected secondarily at sites of severe inflammatory lesions. The anatomical relationships of the intimal, medial, and adventitial tunics are important in the evaluation of structural changes in the pathogenesis of arterial disease.

Arterial lesions are often exaggerated due to endothelial damage of the vasa vasorum. The arteriole supplying the muscular artery breaks into capillary plexuses in the deep layer of the tunica adventitia and does not penetrate deeply into the media. Myocytes situated deeply depend upon diffusion via the lumen of the artery for sustenance. Hypoxia therefore may predispose myocytes of the large muscular arteries to injury. Significant numbers of mast cells are present in the adventitia of younger animals and may be involved in histamine-mediated reactions.

Contraction and dilatation of muscular arteries, which influence blood distribution and pressure, are regulated by vasoconstrictor and vasodilator nerves of the autonomic nervous system. These nerves terminate in the superficial one-third of the media. Myocytes are normally in a state of contraction referred to as tone. The degenerate myocyte cannot maintain contraction and this failure places excessive workloads on adjacent cells and areas of the vascular wall.

The arterial wall changes structurally during vasoconstriction. Endothelial cells assume teardrop shapes and their nuclei protrude into the lumen. Smooth myocytes become short and thick and have deeply indented borders. Elastic fibers develop a pleated appearance. The endothelium and muscle cells adhere tightly to the elastic membrane and their conformation follows its convolutions. Within the endothelial cells the thicker microfilaments are not contractile but the small microfilaments appear to shorten during vasoconstriction.

The site of action in the arterial wall of neural and humoral factors, particularly adrenalin, is considered to be myofilaments of the smooth myocyte. Adrenalin acts directly on this cell to induce vasoconstriction. Angiotensin II, a powerful vasoconstrictor, has been shown to induce widespread structural changes in both endothelium and muscle. There are increases in the number and size of pinocytotic vesicles and widening of intercellular spaces. Isotope-labeled angiotensin II localizes in the nuclear areas of affected endothelial and smooth muscle cells and probably acts mechanistically upon the nucleus (Robertson and Khairallah 1971). Angiotensin-induced sustained elevation in arterial pressure has been shown to induce damage to arterial walls. Then endothelium, which provides a barrier protecting the media, develops focal defects. These permit the escape of plasma proteins into the wall and amorphous dense deposits can be seen displacing smooth muscle cells.

Hyperplasia of arterial smooth muscle cells is occasionally encountered. A striking example is a massive idiopathic hyperplasia of the pulmonary arteries of cats. The cause is not known and the lesions are as common in pathogen-free cats as in ordinary cats. They are associated with increased pulmonary vascular resistance and decreased cardiac output.

ARTERITIS

Nonspecific arteritis is a component of all acute inflammatory lesions. Damage is secondary to and correlates directly with the inciting cause. These lesions are most striking in foci of purulent inflammation where destruction of the vascular wall is characterized by edema and infiltration of neutrophils. Lymphocytic arteritis involving the adventitia is seen in several subacute and chronic viral infections but is apt to be a periarteritis.

Specific types of arteritis occur in a wide variety of systemic infectious diseases. Damage may be due to direct effect of a microbial organism or its toxin on any component of the vascular wall. For example, Newcastle disease virus extensively destroys endothelial cells and also replicates within the myocytes of the media. Endothelial cells are sloughed and cell swelling expands the width of the arterial wall (Fig. 11.4). As the affected myocyte degenerates, shrinks, and dies, plasma proteins exude into the empty spaces, mix with ground substance and collagen, and form an eosinophilic hyalin mass called "fibrinoid" necrosis. In addition to viruses, the rickettsia and mycoplasmas are also associated with this type of direct vascular injury.

Degeneration and necrosis of the arterial wall may also be caused by inflammation in the vascular supply to the artery, that is, the vasa vasorum. Equine viral arteritis virus produces extensive necrosis of this type in arteries of the intestine, lymphoid tissue, and viscera. Although the virus has been demonstrated in myocytes, it is believed that the mechanisms of injury involve destruction of endothelium in the vasa vasorum. Reinforcing this concept is the first appearance of necrosis at the junction of the two vascular supplies, that is, at the point where the vascular wall is least oxygenated. The myocytes

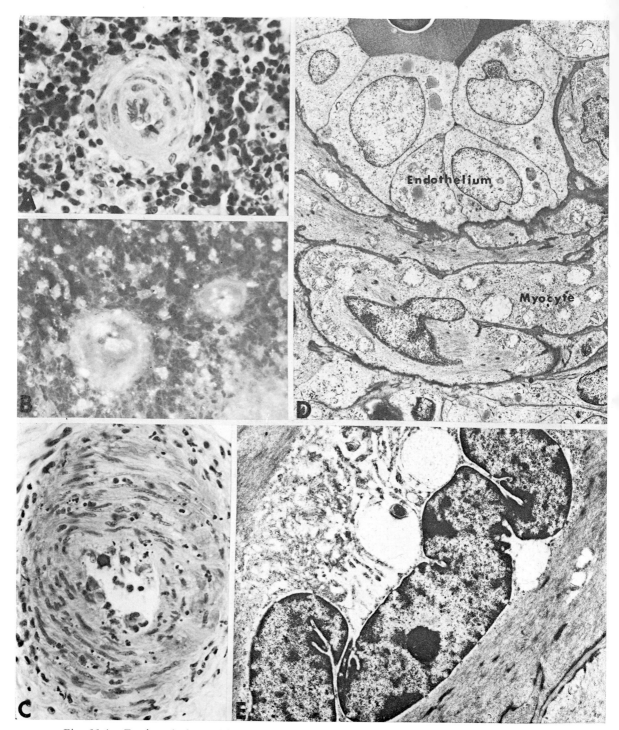

Fig. 11.4. Equine viral arteritis. A. Early swelling of arterial myocytes and necrosis of endothelial cells. B. Distribution of viral antigens
as detected by fluorescent antibody test in central arteries of spleen.
C. Severe necrosis in large muscular artery. D. Ultrastructure of early
change in artery. E. Perinuclear destruction of myofilaments and
pyknosis.

are furthest from their vascular supply and must receive nutrients directly from the lumen of the artery.

Immunologic injury to arterial walls results when immune (antigen-antibody-complement) complexes attach to vascular endothelium. Terminal complement fragments attract neutrophils which liberate proteolytic enzymes and destroy portions of the artery (see the Arthus reaction, Chapter 5). Acute serum sickness has been studied as a model of immunologically induced vasculitis. Naturally occurring lesions are seen in several chronic viral infections where viral antigens and antibodies are known to circulate. Aleutian disease of mink and hepatitis of humans are notable examples. Disseminated arteritis and degeneration are seen very rarely as an idiopathic lesion in dogs (commonly related to renal disease) and may represent an example of immunologic vasculitis.

Healing of the arterial media occurs rapidly after removal of the inciting cause. The fibrinoid material is phagocytized by altered myocytes which allegedly transform into phagocytic cells with expanded secretory mechanisms and altered cell membranes.

Inflammatory lesions which leave scars in the muscular wall of the larger arteries may predispose these structures to the degenerate arteriopathies associated with aging. This point is not settled but it appears that these disturbances, in some cases, act as foci of initiation for arteriosclerotic lesions. Experimental thrombi and hemostatic plugs in injured arteries provoke mitotic activity in smooth myocytes. These cells migrate into the thrombi and foci of hemorrhage in the intima and serve as initiators of fibromuscular plaques.

ARTERIOPATHY

Noninflammatory lesions of the arterial system include a spectrum of confusing and often interrelated degenerative changes. A few are distinct diseases in which the clinical signs may be directly related both to pathologic lesions and to cause. Most, however, are found incidentally during postmortem examination and represent complex lesions to which several mechanisms have contributed. Because their development includes such diverse

entities as hyperplasia, necrosis, thrombosis, and inflammation, we prefer to call these changes arteriopathy. With the exception of acute necrosis of the arterial media, these lesions are distinctly age-related. Whatever the primary cause, they are found with increasing frequency as the animal becomes older.

NECROSIS AND HYALIN DEGENERATION

Hyalin degeneration of arteries is an umbrella term which, like the word hyalin itself, includes lesions of various causes. They have in common the histologic characteristics of smudging and loss of cellular detail in the media. Degenerate smooth muscle cells (myocytes) lose their organized fibrillar character and become dense, amorphous, necrotic masses which stain heavily with eosin and the periodic acid-Schiff technique. These lesions represent dissolution of myocytes with imbibition of plasma proteins into the nonviable muscular wall of the artery.

Hyalin degeneration is most common in aged animals and is most often found in the spleen, heart, kidney, and other viscera. Changes we include as hyalin degeneration are also called "arteriolar hyalinosis," "necrotizing arteritis," and "fibrinoid necrosis" (Biava et al. 1964; Drommer 1972; Dustin 1962; Montali et al. 1970), which indicates the diverse nature of this lesion.

Hyalin degeneration of arteries forms a spectrum of changes. At one extreme are the acute changes characterized by necrosis and plasma infiltration. At the other are chronic lesions which involve recurring episodes of acute damage superimposed upon a healing, sclerosing, and poorly functioning artery. The latter are examples of "hyalinosis" which may be considered a variant of arteriosclerosis.

The staining and appearance depend upon the components that dominate an individual lesion. In the acute lesions, plasma proteins and lipids have exuded into the media. Fibrinogen, albumin, and the different globulins are demonstrable by specific immunologic techniques (Krawczynski 1971). Neutral lipids, phospholipids, and cholesterol may be stainable in these lesions, but mucopeptides are generally not present.

The causes of hyalin degeneration fall into several categories. First, and probably the commonest, are inflammatory conditions: those vasculotropic viral infections (equine viral arteritis, malignant catarrhal fever, Newcastle disease, etc.) that cause necrosis during replication in the vascular wall; and the immunologically mediated diseases (Arthus reaction, Aleutian disease vasculitis). Most of these lesions contain distinct inflammatory components and were properly considered previously under arteritis.

Chronic hyalin changes are found associated with sustained elevations in blood pressure in dogs and humans. In veterinary pathology they are practically limited to dogs with chronic nephritis. Most of these animals have an associated elevation in blood pressure. The mechanism is not established but probably relates to the classic work of Goldblatt, who produced hypertension in dogs by the unilateral clamping of a renal artery. Under the influence of the ischemic kidney, humoral factors were released which caused a sustained elevation in blood pressure. The arteries of the intestine, spleen, and other viscera became progressively hyalinized and in late stages were necrotic. Lesions began subendothelially and progressed until the entire vessels were involved. As models of this type of angiopathy, diets rich in sodium chloride (1% in drinking water) are commonly used. The rat is particularly susceptible to necrotizing angitis under this regimen (Suzuki and Ooneda 1972).

Chemical substances are known to produce acute necrosis and hyalin degeneration of the media of muscular arteries. They do so by a toxic effect upon the endothelial cells. Implicated in this type of injury are endotoxin (Stewart and Anderson 1971), alkaloids (Allen and Carsten 1970), and allylamine (Waters 1948).

It is probable that most agents that cause necrosis and hyalin changes in muscular arteries do so by damaging the endothelial barrier that protects the underlying media. The vascular media is sustained by the constant diffusion of plasma oxygen, nutrients, and proteins that flow from the lumen through the wall to the adventitial zones. When these substances cannot penetrate in sufficient amounts, the myocyte becomes prone to degeneration. When permeability is altered to such an extent that plasma freely flows into the media, severe changes of hyalin degeneration are manifested.

ARTERIOSCLEROSIS

Chronic arterial degenerative changes characterized by induration, loss of elasticity, and narrowing of the lumen are grouped as *arteriosclerosis*. Arteriosclerotic lesions develop as multiple, nodose, or focal sclerotic changes superimposed upon a generalized, age-related increase in connective tissue elements of the arterial wall.

As animals age, subtle but progressive alterations occur in the fibromuscular components of their arterioles. Smooth muscle cells (myocytes) are capable of synthesizing collagen, elastin, basement membrane material, and other mucopeptides. Factors that control the rate and direction of synthesis are not known. In aged animals they appear to be defective and myocyte dysplasia is responsible for irregularities in the vascular wall. In old dogs, for example, this may result in musculoelastic thickenings in the intima and, less often, in the media. Within these lesions are increased numbers of degenerate myocytes and fragmentation of the internal elastic membrane, which blurs the demarcation of the intima and media.

In the aged arterial wall the amounts of mesenchymal matrix material show measurable increases. The presence of random foci of dense, homogeneous, Alcian Blue-staining ground substance is termed *mucodegeneration* (Fig. 11.5). In many species this change precedes the deposition of fibrous materials. Collagen is deposited by myocytes but fibroplasia is extensive only in species such as birds which have significant fibroblast populations in the media (mammals do not). When the cycle of formation-degradation of collagen and elastin is disturbed these substances accumulate. Elastolysis leaves split products of elastin in the intima which are thought to be capable of sustaining an inflammatory reaction.

Arteriosclerosis is found in nearly every vertebrate species and in most is best sought in the abdominal aorta and in the origins of its arterial branches. The hall-

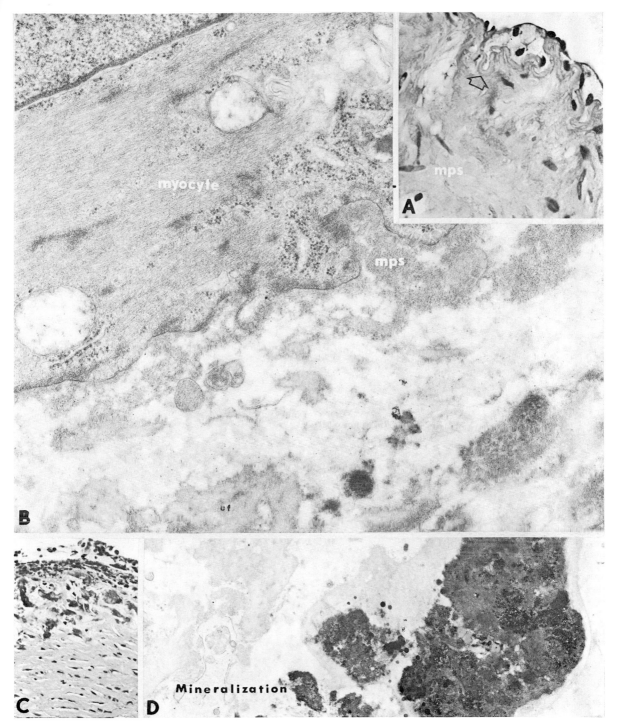

Fig. 11.5. A. Mucodegeneration, aorta, dog. Homogeneous substance
in wall (mps). Disrupted inner elastic membrane (arrow). B. Ultrastructure. Granular material represents mucopolysaccharides (mps).
Broken elastic fibers (ef). C. Extensive calcification (mineralization) of
inner media, dog. D. Mineral is deposited on elastic fibers and is dense,
granular, and irregular.

mark of arteriosclerosis is the fibrous plaque which appears as a white, firm, glistening elevation on the otherwise smooth luminal surface of the artery. It is widely accepted that the early lesion begins as a break in the internal elastic membrane followed by myocyte infiltration through its fenestrae and subsequent proliferation within the intima.

The well-developed *fibrous plaque* (or fibrous streak) consists largely of modified smooth muscle cells surrounded by increased amounts of extracellular matrix. Thickened basement membranes are present and reduplication of and breaks in the internal elastic membrane are common. The hyperplastic smooth muscle cells in the plaque differ from the normal myocytes in the media in being smaller and in lacking tight intercellular junctions. In older plaques, myocytes are degenerate and contain small lipid globules, residual bodies, and disoriented organelles. Lipid deposition, hemorrhage, and calcification are secondary phenomena in most species and the fibrous plaque may develop into a collagenous, calcified, endothelium-covered lesion.

The fibrous plaque and other fibromuscular lesions have been examined in naturally occurring lesions of the dog, pig, cow (Knieriem et al. 1967), monkey (Mc-Combs et al. 1969), rabbit, rat, chicken (Moss and Benditt 1970), turkey (Simpson and Harm 1969), pigeon (Cook and Smith 1968), reptiles, and fish (Manechi et al. 1972). Species differences do occur, but the development of the plaque is remarkably similar in structural pattern (Fankhauser et al. 1965).

How arteriosclerosis is initiated remains vague but it is assumed from established experimental evidence that endothelial injury is of prime importance. It is also assumed that local lesions such as arteritis and systemic changes in blood pressure and flow can be influential. Many arteriosclerotic lesions contain fibrin and platelets (evidence of thrombosis) and the deposition of tiny thrombi has been proposed as initiating some arteriosclerotic lesions. Medial defects follow the experimental induction of hypertension (increased blood pressure) in animals (Boquist and Hassler 1972), although this has never been shown

to be the case in naturally occurring lesions.

Experimental studies have clearly shown that injury to the endothelium can be the principal event leading to the onset of focal arteriosclerotic change. Mechanical injury produces thickening of the arterial wall with narrowing of the lumen. Selective injury to endothelial cells of the artery leads to progressive migration of smooth muscle cells through the internal elastic membrane into the intima. Myocytes can be identified 4 days after injury by their myofilaments, rough endoplasmic reticulum, and associated basement membranes (Bjorkerud 1969; Knieriem et al. 1968; Stehbens and Ludatscher 1973; Stemerman and Ross 1972; Veress et al. 1969).

The myocyte is the cell responsible for the synthesis of the connective tissue components of the media (Ross and Glomset 1973), and it is evident that myocyte hyperplasia in the intimal lesions is followed by deposition of collagen, elastin, and ground substance. It is alleged that the barrier provided by endothelium to the passage of plasma proteins is crucial. Once broken, certain (as yet unidentified) fractions of plasma proteins serve as the stimulus for myocyte migration and transformation. The myocyte is also responsible for the genesis of more serious variants of arteriosclerosis. By accumulating intracellular lipids, it transforms into the large foam cell that characterizes atherosclerosis.

Lesions of arteriosclerosis are reversible if the cause is removed before the vessel wall is fibrotic and calcified. Experimental dietary-induced lesions regress when the diet is readjusted to normal. Degeneration of coronary arteries is common in spawning salmon and trout during and after their migration from sea to fresh water. Salmon die after spawning. In the steelhead trout, which returns again to the sea, the arterial lesions disappear and develop again during the succeeding spawning run (Van Citters and Watson 1968).

The subclassification within the broad category of arteriosclerosis encompasses special types of rare arterial lesions associated with special systemic disease. These include atherosclerosis, amyloidosis, hyaline sclerosis, and systemic medial mineralization. The significance of arterial degeneration and necrosis in animals is overshadowed by the tremendous importance of atherosclerosis as a disease in humans. Although sporadic lesions of atherosclerosis are not uncommon in animals, the diffuse or multifocal distribution which makes this a disease of humans is rarely encountered in animals. Reasons for this relate to genetic differences, diet, and other factors. The life span of most animals is short and, with the exception of pet animals, nutrition is too inadequate in those that survive for long periods for lesions of atherosclerosis to develop. The immense amount of experimental work done in dogs and laboratory rodents relates to human disease and this tends to mask the true incidence and nature of lesions in animals.

ATHEROSCLEROSIS

Atherosclerosis is the accumulation of lipids in larger arteries in the form of elevated, lipid-filled plaques called *atheromas*. Necrosis and fibrosis follow the deposition of lipid and result in a progressively enlarging lesion that expands the arterial wall. Ischemia and infarction may develop in affected organs due to the encroachment of the vascular lumen. Less commonly, aneurysms develop from weakening of the arterial wall.

The atheroma begins as an intimal lesion which progressively extends into and affects the media. The pathogenesis, as reconstructed from serial examination of naturally occurring lesions, involves: (1) endothelial injury, (2) myocyte migration through fenestrae of the inner elastic membrane, (3) proliferation of myoctes in foci within the intima, and (4) the accumulation of lipids within the cytoplasm of the myocyte. Focal clusters of myocytes become ballooned by cytoplasmic lipids, giving these cells the name of *foam cells*. Aggregates of these cells appear grossly as small elevated fatty streaks in the arterial luminal surface. In progressively expanding lesions, foam cells become necrotic and the liberation of free lipid incites fibrosis and calcification which in turn cause more necrosis and so on. Ultrastructurally, lipids vary from small globules to locules which fill the cell. Cholesterol clefts are

represented by empty spaces as they are in histologic preparations. Advanced atheromas are complicated by hemorrhage, thrombosis, ulceration, and the infiltration of the lesion by plasma proteins.

In atherosclerosis in animals the aorta and the small muscular arteries are most commonly affected. When severe systemic atherosclerosis is encountered in dogs, it is associated with advanced age, obesity, and hyperlipoproteinemia. The majority of these dogs have hypothyroidism which leads to the acquired hypercholesterolemia and indirectly to atherosclerosis (Manning et al. 1973). Lesions are prominent in the media as well as intima of large muscular arteries of the heart, kidney, intestine, bladder, and other organs (Fig. 11.6). Lipids are present in the cytoplasm of myocytes and lipid-laden foam cells distort the media (Geer 1965).

Experimental atherosclerosis is classically produced by feeding animals on cholesterol and high-lipid diets. In diet-induced atherosclerosis, the high levels of plasma cholesterol and lipoproteins give rise to large fat-laden foam cells below the intima. Foam cells represent either macrophages or myocytes and these can be differentiated cytologically. Myocytes have distinct myofilaments, elongate nuclei, and surface basement membrane material; their lipid globules tend to be more electron dense (Newman et al. 1971). Their cell surfaces do not have microvilli as do macrophages. In these experimental lesions macrophages dominate the early phases whereas myocytes are the prominent cell in older lesions. Lesions vary from simple intimal lipid deposits to transmural lipogranulomas. The ultrastructural changes in experimental atherosclerosis have been examined in dogs (Suzuki 1972), pigs (Florentin et al. 1965; Imai et al. 1970), monkey (Pucak et al. 1973; Robison et al. 1972), and rats (Marshall and O'Neal 1966).

In general, the morphology of the atheroma is dictated by the type and degree of plasma lipid elevation. The monkey has been valuable as a model for human atherosclerosis because of its close phylogenetic relation to man. The squirrel monkey is particularly useful because of its relatively high incidence of naturally occurring aortic lipid accumulation and

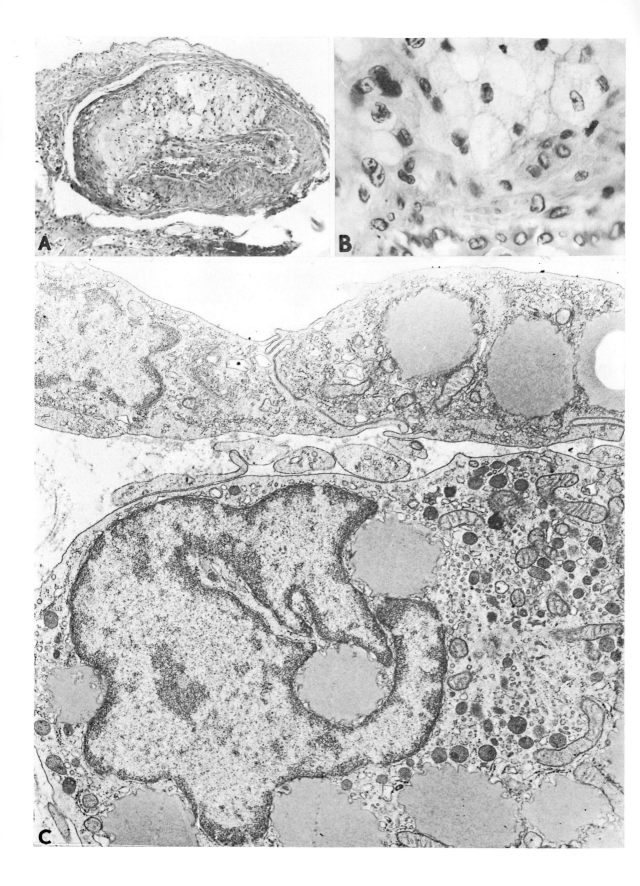

the increase in atherosclerosis which can be induced by changes in diet.

The presence of lipid in the vascular wall does not make these lesions analogous to spontaneous disease and there is doubt that the experimental disease mimics naturally occurring atherosclerosis. Experimental production is too drastic, for it condenses into a few weeks what takes years to develop naturally. The large collection of foam cells in the artery probably represents a generalized storage disease (xanthomatosis) bearing only superficial resemblance to atherosclerosis. On deletion of high-lipid diets, the vascular lesions regress (Tucker et al. 1971).

In aged humans, atherosclerosis is an extremely common lesion and disease. The aorta and iliac, coronary, and cerebral arteries are most often affected. Because atherosclerosis can progressively or abruptly occlude these blood vessels, it often causes serious consequences such as myocardial infarction and stroke. Studies in humans have clearly shown that plasma lipids, elevated blood pressure, and cigarette smoking strongly influence the development of clinical disease but data on the finite pathogenesis of the lesion of atherosclerosis is only suggestive. It may be that elevated plasma lipids, increased blood pressure, and endocrine disturbances convert into atherosclerosis what would, under more normal circumstances, be a reparative response to injury.

In human atherosclerosis the myocyte population of atheromas appears to be monoclonal; that is, it is homogeneous and single cell–derived (Benditt and Benditt 1973). This implicates a specific transformation of the parent myocyte for, if the early atheroma began as an inflammatory lesion, the cell population would be expected to be polyclonal. Sites within the vascular system with a predilection for atherosclerosis are also sites where endothelial and myocyte turnover rates are high. It is therefore reasoned that agents that increase proliferation would also increase the risk of induction of myocyte

transformation. Thus are viruses and mutagenic chemicals implicated in human atherosclerosis.

SKELETAL MYOCYTES

Complete skeletal muscles are composed of groups of muscle fasciculi that extend from the sites of origin and insertion. Each fasciculus contains many individual cells, the muscle fibers (or myocytes). The skeletal muscle fiber is surrounded by a plasma membrane (sarcolemma) and contains groups of myofibrils separated by mitochondria, aggregates of glycogen, and lipid globules. The close association of mitochondria to myofibrils brings the site of energy production close to its point of utilization. Sarcoplasmic reticulum, a modified endoplasmic reticulum, and the tubular (T) systems ramify in the sarcoplasm between the myofibrils.

Myofibrils are constructed of two types of interlocking myofilaments: actin and myosin. Myosin filaments are the principal constituents of the A band and determine its length. The thinner actin filaments of the I band extend both directions from their origin in the Z line. During contraction, actin filaments slide deeply into the A band. The depth to which the ends of the actin filaments penetrate the A band varies with the extent of contraction. The force of contraction is generated by some cyclic process occurring at the cross bridges of overlapping actin and myosin filaments. The breakdown of ATP by ATPase in myosin energizes this process. The connection of the actin filaments at the Z line is of exceptional importance, for it is at this site that many types of muscle degeneration begin. Z lines contain the muscle protein tropomyosin and provide the anchor for the initiation of contraction.

Excitation for muscle contraction is conducted to the myofilaments by the membranes of the sarcoplasmic reticulum and the T system. In some unknown way, the

Fig. 11.6.   Atherosclerosis, dog. A. Histology. Coronary artery. Media is distorted by fat-filled myocytes and macrophages. B. Higher power. Intact foam cells are surrounded by free lipids. C. Ultrastructure (Micrograph, J. Geer). Endothelial cells (top) and subendothelial foam cells (bottom) are filled with lipid globules.

sarcoplasmic reticulum releases Ca++ to the myofibril, triggering contraction. Hypocalcemia is related to reduced contractility. Distortion of the sarcoplasmic reticulum is also the primary site of defect in many of the genetic muscular dystrophies.

The cytologic separation of muscle fibers into type I (red) and type II (white) is based upon differences in oxidative enzyme staining. The smaller red fibers have larger numbers of mitochondria and lipid globules and have wider Z bands. They dominate in metabolically active muscles and are rich in oxidative enzymes but poor in glycogen, glycolytic enzymes, and myofibrillar ATPase. Type I fibers are selectively affected in some myodystrophic diseases. The larger type II white fibers have lower mitochondrial content and predominate in the less active muscles. They are preferentially involved in disuse atrophy, malnutrition, and hyperadrenocorticoidism. Both types of fibers are affected equally in most of the progressive muscular dystrophies, autoimmune muscle diseases, and hypokalemic myopathy.

The dominance of either type I or II fibers determines the nature of a particular muscle. The breast and thigh muscles of the chicken provide a striking difference. Within an individual muscle, such as diaphragm, the fiber content varies. The diaphragm of small animals with fast breathing rates has a high red fiber content; the large animals with slower rates have higher white fiber populations (Gauthier and Padykula 1966). The disease known as malignant hyperthermia of Poland China pigs is associated with a genetically determined increase in number of white, anaerobically metabolizing muscle fibers. Increased ATP depletion in myocytes is triggered by certain anesthetics and leads to skeletal muscle rigidity, hyperthermia, cardiac arrhythmia, and death (Nelson et al. 1972).

Skeletal muscle contains considerable glycogen and glycogen particles may be increased in the sarcoplasm surrounding the myofilaments in some of the dystrophic diseases. Some breeds of pigs have a tendency to produce carcasses with poor quality meat related to a pale, soft, watery quality of the muscle masses. After death, there is utilization of glycogen and rapid fall in muscle pH. Accelerated rates of anaerobic glycolysis lead to extensive coagulation of muscle proteins (Muir 1970).

The motor unit, composed of motoneuron, its axon, and the attached muscle fibers, is the indivisible functional unit in motor activity of muscle tissue. When the motor unit is injured, severe diffuse atrophy characterizes the muscle area that is supplied. Each motor unit goes exclusively to either type I or type II fibers and a selective effect may appear to be operative in some motor end plate diseases. Diffuse or group atrophy is the cardinal myopathic criterion of neural and spinal cord muscle disease. It is in distinct contrast to segmental fiber necrosis that characterizes all primary myolytic disease of muscle where short segments of myofibers, several sarcomeres in length, are destroyed. Some examples of segmental necrosis are the myopathies of intracellular parasitism, viral infection, vitamin E deficiency, and the progressive myodystrophies.

MUSCLE NECROSIS RELATED TO EXTRACELLULAR FACTORS

POTASSIUM DEFICIENCY NECROSIS

Focal rhabdomyolysis and myoglobinuria can occur after severe, prolonged exercise in hot climates. This is well documented in man following extensive training programs in athletes. Normally, K+ is released from contracting skeletal muscle fibers and its rising concentration in interstitial fluid dilates arterioles thereby mediating increased blood flow. When K+ release is subnormal, a relative ischemia may exist and rhabdomyolysis occurs. In normal dogs, muscle blood flow and K+ rise sharply during exercise (Fig. 11.7). In experimental K+-depleted dogs, K+ release and blood flow are markedly diminished despite vigorous exercise. In dogs, at least, ischemia is the final mechanism for K+-deficiency muscle necrosis (Knochel and Schlein 1972).

CLOSTRIDIAL MYOSITIS AND MYONECROSIS

This pattern of muscle necrosis is seen in blackleg of sheep and cattle, in malig-

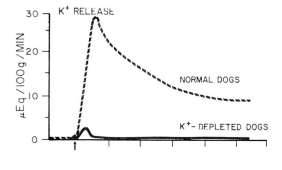

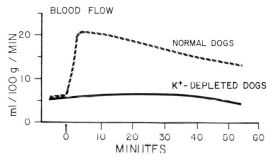

Fig. 11.7. Blood flow and K⁺ efflux in normal and K⁺-deficient dogs.

nant edema of cattle, in gas gangrene of humans, and in muscle infections of many other animals. These diseases follow contamination of wounds with soil and bacteria.

Clostridial exotoxins are elaborated and produce necrosis locally. The chief components of the lesion are: (1) toxin injury to the capillary endothelium which results in altered permeability, edema, and hemorrhage; (2) toxin-induced lysis of myocytes (injury begins in the Z lines of the myofibrils and rapidly spreads causing disintegration of the entire muscle fiber); and (3) gas bubbles which are produced during replication of clostridial organisms utilizing the glycogen within the myocyte. In the initial phases of muscle necrosis, lysis begins in the center of the affected fiber and spreads peripherally. As membranes are disrupted and disintegrate, precipitates of myoglobin accumulate within the dying myocyte (Demello et al. 1974) (Fig. 11.8).

TETANUS AND MYONECROSIS

Tetanus is the syndrome of severe striated muscle spasms that spread pro-gressively from muscle to muscle from a site of wound infection with *Clostridium tetani.* The bacterial toxin suppresses, as does strychnine, all synaptic inhibition. It induces central and peripheral effects that are separable mechanistically. Central effects are characterized by reflex motor convulsions. The peripheral effects, with which we are here concerned, cause an unremitting rigidity of skeletal muscle due to fixation of the toxin to motor end organs. Toxin is activated when bound to membranes of synapses, myocytes, and neurons; the defect produced involves disturbances of ion transport.

In skeletal muscle the toxin, after it binds to membranes, is responsible for sustained contraction of myofilaments. Normal tonicity of the motor end organ is required for tetanic rigidity, and experimental neurotomy results in the absence of a response to tetanus toxin. Toxin-binding sites, when traced by peroxidase-labeled tetanus antitoxin, have been identified in the membranes of the transverse tubular (T) system, at its junction with the sarcoplasmic reticulum, and within the sarcoplasmic reticulum cisternae (Zacks and Scheff 1968). Structural changes develop in myofibrils of affected muscles but are secondary to the extreme contraction and vascular pathology, i.e., they are not due to a direct effect of toxin on myofilaments (Fig. 11.9).

The cause of death in tetanus is usually asphyxia which follows paralysis of the respiratory muscles. *Clostridium tetani* produces a hemolysin that is a cardiotoxin and that induces intravascular hemolysis experimentally (Hardegree et al. 1971). It is probable that some of the cardiovascular and hematologic alterations seen in terminal tetanus are due to this tetanolysin.

MUSCLE NECROSIS AND INTRACELLULAR INFECTION

Diseases discussed under myocarditis generally also affect the skeletal myocyte but the process is overshadowed by the clinical effect upon the heart. Acute purulent myositis is associated with generalized diseases involving several bacteria, notably salmonellosis, tuberculosis, leptospirosis, and infection with *Hemophilus* spp. All

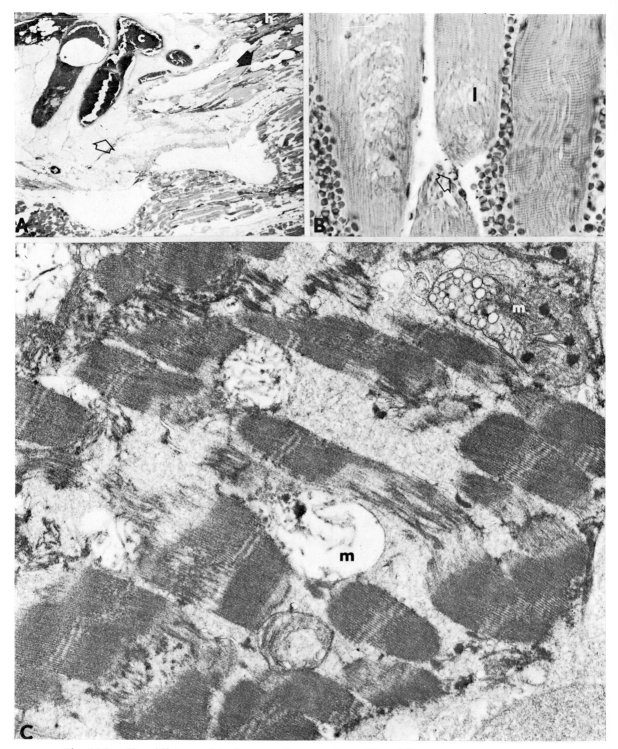

Fig. 11.8. Clostridial myositis, sheep, malignant edema *(Clostridium septicum).* A. Histology. Severe congestion (c), edema, hemorrhage (h), gas bubble formation (arrow), and myonecrosis. B. Lysis of myofibrils (l), extravasated erythrocytes, and bacilli (arrow). C. Ultrastructure. Destruction of myofibril and precipitation of myoglobin. Mitochondria (m).

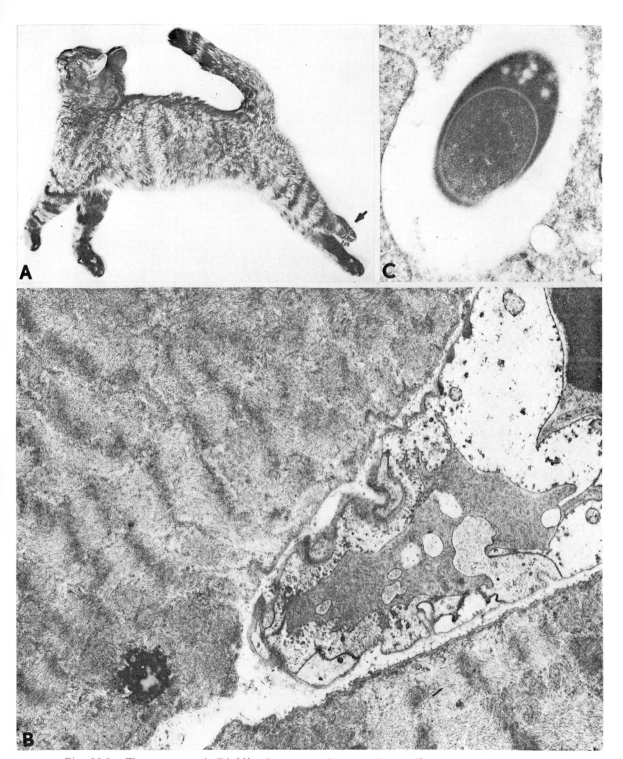

Fig. 11.9. Tetanus, cat. A. Rigidity due to tetanic spasm (note tail and ear). Infection in gangrenous foot (arrow). B. Necrosis of skeletal muscle fibers, cell swelling of capillary endothelium. C. Ultrastructure of sporulated *Clostridium tetani.*

of these infections can be accompanied by muscle necrosis but the processes originate in and are largely confined to the inter-fiber spaces. Organisms that actually enter and destroy the myocyte include some viruses, a few protozoa, and the nematode *Trichinella spiralis*.

VIRAL DISEASE

Although viral infection of skeletal muscles is common, serious disease limited to this tissue is not. Most severe systemic viral infections are capable of producing scattered foci of muscle necrosis. Newcastle disease, hog cholera, canine distemper, feline panleukopenia, foot-and-mouth disease, and bluetongue all produce focal muscle necrosis in which viral antigens can be demonstrated by fluorescent antibody procedures. The pathogenesis of viral replication has only been examined in detail with the picornavirus group which includes avian encephalomyelitis, Coxsack-ieviral infection, and porcine polioen-cephalomyelitis (Bientz et al. 1969; Cheville 1971; Harrison et al. 1971; Rustigian and Pappenheimer 1949).

TRICHINOSIS

Only one nematode, *Trichinella spiralis,* is known to enter cells as part of its life cycle. Larvae encyst in muscle fibers and the host cell thereby provides sustenance and prevents host systems of inflammation and immunity from attacking them. The parasite is protected until the host is killed and its muscle eaten by a new potential carnivore host. Intestinal enzymes of the new host digest the capsule and the liberated larvae burrow into the intestine and begin their life cycle anew.

The adult life of *T. spiralis* is spent in the small intestine of many species of carnivores. The viviparous female burrows into the lamina propria of the intestinal villi and deposits her larvae directly into the intestinal lymphatics. Larvae exit in lymph, pass through the mesenteric lymphatics and thoracic duct, and enter the bloodstream. During circulation through the skeletal muscle fasciculi they enter the myocytes.

Mild transient inflammatory responses may surround migrating larvae in muscle. These usually are limited to edema and a few neutrophilic leukocytes. Larvae are poorly immunogenic (the cutical and enzymic excretions of the oral orifice do not readily induce immune responses in the host) and encystment occurs before these are effective. Adult nematodes may be expelled from the intestine by immunologic means. Both anaphylactic and cellular hypersensitivity develop in response to infection, but it is not known which of these dominates in clinical disease (Catty 1969).

The muscle fiber undergoes striking transformation when invaded by larvae. The fiber becomes swollen and granular for a considerable distance peripheral and distal to the encysted parasite. Within 10 days after infection the larvae are well established. Ultrastructurally, myofibrils within the affected fibers become disoriented and their myofilaments are detached and frayed at the Z lines (Backwinkel and Themann 1972). Most organelles degenerate and disappear; this is especially noticed in mitochondria and lysosomes. By 21 days after infection the cytoplasm of the transformed muscle fiber is filled with large arrays of smooth endoplasmic reticulum.

The larvae exist free in the cytosol of the host cell. They are not associated with lysosomes, intracellular debris, or pathologic membranes. At its periphery, the host myocyte is actively involved in the secretion of acidic mucopolysaccharides which form the hyalin, basement membrane–type material of the capsule (Fig. 11.10). This capsule is formed exclusively by the host muscle fiber and begins about 14 days after encystation (Teppema et al. 1973).

By 2–3 months encapsulation is complete. The cytoplasm of the host cell becomes contracted and dense. The thick hyalin membrane of the capsule shows foci of mineralization which progressively enlarge. In protracted and severe infections antigens may seep into the circulation of the host and antibodies against the larvae and its capsule may arise. Eosinophilic and neutrophilic leukocytes surround the cysts of some larvae and can be seen within their capsules. Lymphocyte aggregates occur around cysts. Plasmacytes that

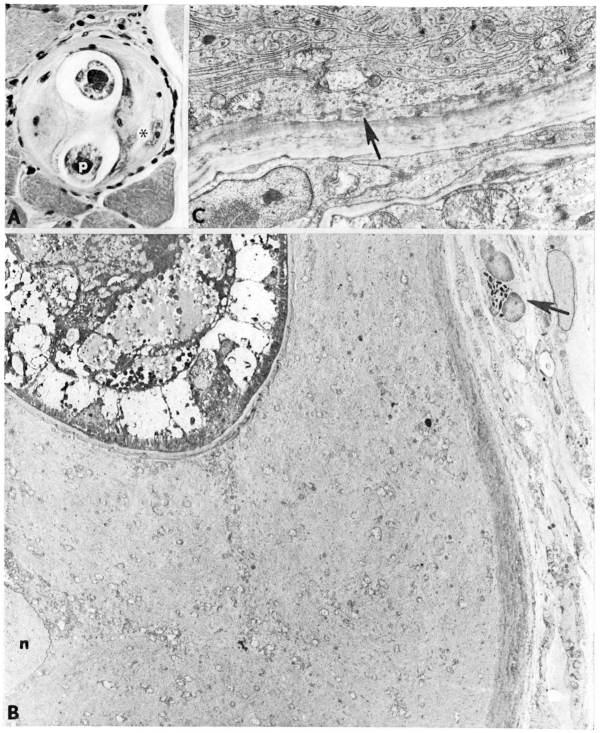

Fig. 11.10. Encystment of *Trichinella spiralis* larvae within skeletal myocyte. A. Cyst includes: parasite (p), modified host myocyte (asterisk), and hyalin capsule. B. Ultrastructure of transformed host cell. Massive reduplication of endoplasmic reticulum, with dense granular material at the basal plasmalemma. Host cell nucleus (n), parasite (upper left). Note eosinophil (arrow) in capsule. C. Deposition of basement membrane material at periphery by altered host cell (arrow).

contain antitrichina antibody are present in these aggregates (Crandall et al. 1967) but their effect on encysted larvae is negligible.

In summary, trichinosis is characterized by two major biologic phases: enteric and visceral. Immunity is acquired in the enteric phase and during circulation of living larvae. These mechanisms may reduce the number of larvae reaching muscle but do not affect migration in muscle, encystment, or larval development (Despommier 1971). The intriguing mechanism whereby larvae induce host muscle cells to transform is unknown. Encysted developing larvae are unique because they are relatively poor antigens and because they are protected by the dense hyalin cyst wall.

TOXOPLASMOSIS

Toxoplasma gondii, a coccidian parasite, has an intestinal epithelial cycle for the production of oocysts only in cats and other Felidae. The organism undergoes schizogony and microgametogony in the feline ileum. Oocysts are shed in the feces and are infectious after sporulation occurs. These asexual forms can propagate in macrophages and myocytes of different mammalian species. Upon entering a secondary host, the endozoites are spread to muscle and other tissues after infecting circulating monocytes. Once inside the muscle cell the organism is confined to a parasitophorous vacuole. Encysted cystozoites appear in muscle in about 2 wks, as immunity becomes detectable. Crescent-shaped daughter organisms develop from the infecting organism (Sheffield and Melton 1968).

Only the encysted parasites are apt to be seen in naturally occurring cases. The thick cyst wall is composed of a dense outer layer of host cell origin and an inner thin membrane of parasite origin (Fig. 11.11). The host reaction consists of necrosis of infected cells and an attendant accumulation of macrophages and neutrophils.

SARCOSPORIDIOSIS

Numerous species of the single genus Sarcocystis parasitize the muscles of mammals, birds, and reptiles. There is virtually no inflammatory reaction around encysted organisms and no known clinical disease is associated with infection. Only the cysts are observed in myocytes. Visible grossly as white dots or streaks, they are intracellular organisms surrounded by a thick cyst wall of both host and parasite origin. The encysted, banana-shaped organisms have a vesicular nucleus and abundant cytoplasmic glycogen; they are motile (Melhorn and Scholtyseck 1973; Simpson 1966).

DYSTROPHY OF SKELETAL MUSCLE

ATROPHY OF CACHEXIA

Wasting syndromes that occur in senility, the nutritional deficiencies, and prolonged chronic infections often result in diffuse atrophy of skeletal muscle. Localized muscular atrophy is also seen in disuse of a particular limb or after the destruction of motor nerves to an individual muscle group. In cachectic atrophy, myofibers vary considerably in size and shrunken atrophic fibers are intermingled with normal fibers. As the myofiber diminishes in size the nuclei become pyknotic and persist in linear arrangement in the destroyed myofiber. The destruction of myoglobin incites lysosomes to develop in perivascular spaces and along the sarcolemmal sheaths. Lipochrome pigments may develop and persist in some myofibers, especially in the cow.

VITAMIN E DEFICIENCY AND MYODYSTROPHY

The dietary deficiency of vitamin E or its excessive destruction in the body is responsible for a wide spectrum of tissue changes. These include muscle necrosis; vascular lesions (see exudative diathesis of chicks); enhanced destruction of erythrocytes; and degenerative lesions in the brain, liver, and heart. Myodystrophy is the commonest manifestation of avitaminosis E and occurs in spontaneous disease in chicks, lambs, calves, and several other species.

Early histologic evidence of muscle degeneration consists of disappearance of

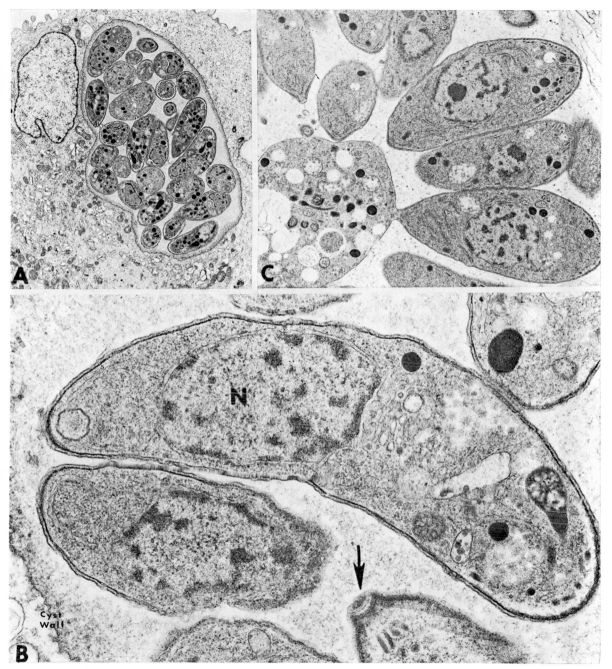

Fig. 11.11. *Toxoplasma gondii.* A. Ultrastructure of cyst in macrophage. B. Individual organisms. Nucleus (N), conoid (arrow). C. Budding of daughter organisms from mother cell (Micrograph, A. Boothe).

striation, central migration of nuclei, and nodose zones of dense eosinophilia (Fig. 11.12). Ruffling of the myofibers and proliferation of interstitial cells along the sarcolemma are typical. In pigs, selective necrosis of type I (red) muscle fiber occurs while the type II (white) fibers remain viable. Macrophages appear late in the lesion in an attempt to remove dead myocytes and myoglobin. The initial ultrastructural injury appears in mitochondria, which are enlarged and distorted. Streaming of the Z lines and disappearance of the I band are followed by total effacement of the myofibrillar structures.

The mechanisms of avitaminosis E–induced injury are intimately related to dietary selenium, for this mineral has much the same action in the cell. Both vitamin E and selenium protect cellular membranes against the destructive action of free radicals that arise from cellular metabolism. Free radicals attack lipid membranes to produce lipid peroxides and these in turn destroy membranes, sulfhydryl-containing enzymes, and other substances.

Selenium participates as a component of the enzyme glutathione peroxidase which acts in the cytoplasmic matrix to destroy lipid peroxides that would otherwise damage cellular membranes (Rotruck et al. 1973). Glutathione peroxidase levels in plasma are directly related to dietary selenium.

Vitamin E is a secondary defense against peroxidative injury. It acts within phospholipid membranes, where it neutralizes free radicals and thereby prevents a chain reaction of auto-oxidation. In other activities, the antioxidant effect of vitamin E appears to act as a brake on mitochondrial metabolism.

HEREDITARY MUSCULAR DYSTROPHIES

These hereditary diseases cause progressive destruction of striated muscle and are of considerable significance in humans. The animal myodystrophies have been reviewed (Hadlow 1962). Most are sporadic isolated cases in which the pathogenesis has not been elucidated. Sex-linked myopathy in five of seven males in a litter of Irish Terriers has been reported (Wentink et al. 1972). The patchy distribution of the muscle lesions, very high serum creatine phosphokinase levels, and ultrastructural alterations of mitochondria and myofibrils were characteristic. The disease was noted at 8 wks of age by difficulty in swallowing. Familial myodystrophy has been documented in chickens (Cardinet et al. 1972), hamsters (Caulfield 1966), and sheep (McGavin and Baynes 1969). Congenital myofibrillar hypoplasia occurs in pigs (Deutsch and Done 1971).

The most significant model of muscular dystrophy exists in a mutant strain of mice (dystrophia muscularis, strain 129) bred at the Jackson laboratory, Bar Harbor, Maine. Progressive atrophy of axial and limb muscles begins at about 3 wks of age and leads to complete paralysis with death in 1–6 months. The initial lesion is located in the sarcoplasmic reticulum (Banker 1967; Platzer and Chase 1964). It becomes increasingly widespread and leads to myocyte necrosis with disorganization of the myofilaments and distortion of the mitochondria. The ability of the altered sarcoplasmic reticulum to take up, store, and release calcium for muscle contraction is impaired early in the disease. Lowered calcium uptake has been demonstrated in affected muscle.

Other models of murine muscle dystrophy include *muscular dysgenesis* (MDG) which is a lethal mutation involving skeletal myogenesis. Death occurs immediately after birth but the lesions resemble those of strain 129 mice and the initial defect is also thought to be in the sarcoplasmic reticulum (Platzer and Gluecksohn-Waelsch 1972). Nuclei in affected myocytes are abnormal and many contain inclusions composed of vacuoles and membranous sacs.

A third model of murine myodystrophy is called, inappropriately, *muscle endplate disease* (MED). The mutant strain of mouse develops primary myopathy that is lethal by 25 days of age (not primary disease of the motor endplate). Lesions are characterized by myofibrillar disorganization with distortion of sarcomere arrangements and extensive lysosomal autophagy (Zacks et al. 1969).

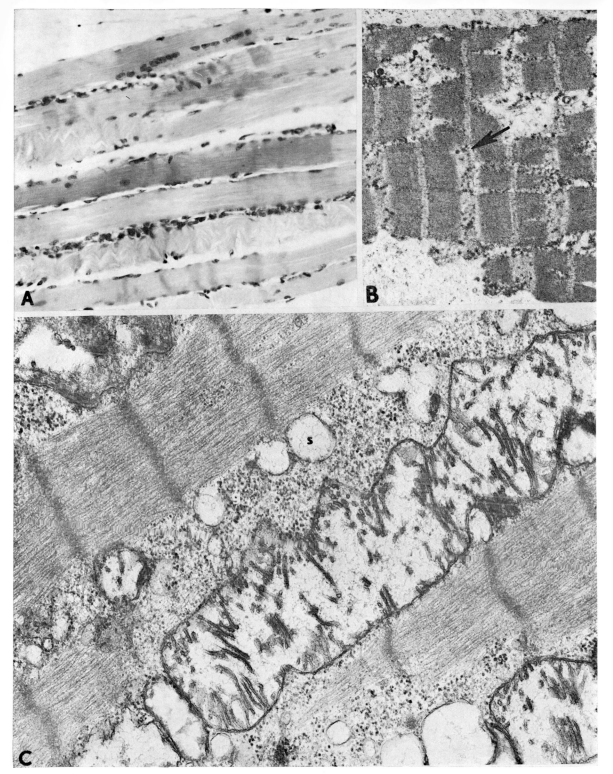

Fig. 11.12. Vitamin E deficiency myopathy, chicken skeletal muscle.
A. Histology. Degeneration and necrosis of muscle fibers. Sarcolemmal
nuclei are increased; myofibrils are contracted and irregular. B. Ultrastructure. Degeneration begins at Z line with precipitation of dense
material (arrow). C. Myofibrils are distorted. Glycogen (g), dilated
sarcoplasmic tubules (s). Mitochondria are markedly enlarged with
reduplication of cristae.

MOTOR ENDPLATE DISEASE

A model for and clinical parallel of human myasthenia gravis occurs in dogs. Affected individuals suffer from severe muscle weakness that responds to anticholinesterase therapy. The defect involves transmission at the neuromuscular junction. Fine structural alterations have been demonstrated in the pre- and post-synaptic elements of the junctional regions of the motor endplate (Zacks et al. 1966).

REFERENCES

Adams, R. D. Thayer lectures: Principles of myopathology. *Johns Hopkins Med. J.* 131: 24, 1972.

Alexander, A. R. et al. Pulmonary hypertension and right ventricular hypertrophy in cattle at high altitude. *Am. J. Vet. Res.* 21:199, 1960.

Allen, J. R. and Carsten, L. A. Pulmonary vascular occlusions initiated by endothelial lysis in monocrotaline-intoxicated rats. *Exp. Mol. Path.* 13:159, 1970.

Backwinkel, K.-P. and Themann, H. Elektronenmikroskopische Untersuchungen über die Pathomorphologie der Trichinellose. *Beitr. Path. Bd.* 146:259, 1972.

Bajusz, E. et al. Hypertrophie des Herzmuskels bei erbbedingter Myopathie. *Naturwissenschaften* 56:568, 1969.

Banker, B. Q. A phase and electron microscopic study of dystrophic muscle. *J. Neuropath. Exp. Neurol.* 26:259, 1967.

Benditt, E. P. and Benditt, J. M. Evidence for a monoclonal origin of human atherosclerotic plaques. *Proc. Nat. Acad. Sci.* 70:1753, 1973.

Biava, C. G. et al. Renal hyaline arteriosclerosis: An electron microscopic study. *Am. J. Path.* 44:349, 1964.

Bientz, K. et al. Identification and arrangement of Coxsackievirus A_1 in muscles of newborn mice. *Brit. J. Exp. Path.* 50:471, 1969.

Bishop, S. P. and Cole, C. R. Ultrastructural changes in the canine myocardium with right ventricular hypertrophy and congestive heart failure. *Lab. Invest.* 20:219, 1969.

Bjorkerud, S. Reaction of the aortic wall of the rabbit after superficial longitudinal mechanical damage. *Virch. Arch. A* 347:197, 1969.

Boquist, L. and Hassler, O. Media defects in arteries. An ultrastructural study of normal and hypertensive rabbits. *Path. Europ.* 7:23, 1972.

Bozner, A. and Meessen, H. Die Feinstruktur des Herzmuskels der Ratte nach einmaligem und nach weiderholtem Schwimmtraining. *Virch. Arch. B* 3:248, 1969.

Brachfeld, N. and Schever, J. Metabolism of glucose by the ischemic dog heart. *Am. J. Physiol.* 212:603, 1967.

Büchner, F. Qualitative morphology of heart failure. *Meth. Achiev. Exp. Path.* 5:60, 1971.

Cardinet, G. H. et al. Morphologic, histochemical and quantitative enzyme study of hereditary avian muscular dystrophy. *Am. J. Vet. Res.* 33:1671, 1972.

Catty, D. The immunology of nematode infections. *Monogr. Allergy* 5:1, 1969.

Caulfield, J. B. Electron microscopic observations on the dystrophic hamster muscle. *Ann. N.Y. Acad. Sci.* 138:151, 1966.

Cheville, N. F. Myopathy associated with avian encephalomyelitis virus. *Am. J. Vet. Res.* 32:979, 1971.

———. The pathology of vitamin E deficiency in the chick. *Vet. Path.* 3:208, 1966.

Cook, P. H. and Smith, S. C. Smooth muscle cells: The source of foam cells in the white carneau pigeon. *Exp. Mol. Path.* 8:171, 1968.

Crandall, R. B., Cebra, J. J. and Crandall, C. A. The relative proportion of IgG, IgA and IgM-containing cells in rabbit tissues during experimental trichinosis. *Immunology* 12:147, 1967.

D'Agostino, A. N. An electron microscopic study of skeletal and cardiac muscle of the rat poisoned by plasmocid. *Lab. Invest.* 12:1060, 1963.

D'Agostino, A. N. and Chiga, M. Morphologic changes in cardiac and skeletal muscle induced by corticosteroid. *Ann. N.Y. Acad. Sci.* 138:73, 1966.

De La Iglesia, F. A. and Lumb, G. Ultrastructural and circulatory alterations of the myocardium in experimental coronary artery narrowing. *Lab. Invest.* 27:17, 1972.

Demello, F. J. et al. Ultrastructural study of clostridial myositis. *Arch. Path.* 97:118, 1974.

Despommier, D. D. Immunogenicity of the newborn larva of *Trichinella spiralis*. *J. Parasit.* 57:531, 1971.

Deutsch, K. and Done, J. T. Congenital myofibrillar hypoplasia of piglets. *Res. Vet. Sci.* 12:176, 1971.

Drommer, W. Permeabilitäts störungen im zentralen Nervensystem des Schweines. Zur. Feinstruktur der cerebrospinalen Angiopathiae. *Acta Neuropath.* 20:299, 1972.

Dustin, P., Jr. Arteriolar hyalinosis. *Int. Rev. Exp. Path.* 1:73, 1962.

Emberson, J. W. and Muir, A. R. Changes in the ultrastructure of rat myocardium induced by hyperkalemia. *J. Anat.* 104:411, 1969.

Fankhauser, R., Luginbühl, H. and McGrath, J. T. Cerebrovascular disease in various animal species. *Ann. N.Y. Acad. Sci.* 127:817, 1965.

Fawcett, D. W. The sporadic occurrence in cardiac muscle of anomalous Z-bands exhibiting a periodic structure suggestive of tropomyosin. *J. Cell Biol.* 36:266–70, 1967.

Florentin, R. A. et al. Dietary-induced atherosclerosis in miniature swine. *Ann. N.Y. Acad. Sci.* 127:780, 1965.

Forbes, M. S. and Sperelakis, N. Ultrastructure of cardiac muscle from dystrophic mice. *Am. J. Anat.* 134:271, 1972.

Garancis, J. C. Type II glycogenosis. Biochemical and electron microscopic studies. *Am. J. Med.* 44:289, 1968.

Gardell, C., Blascheck, J. A. and Kovaks, K. Digitoxin cardiopathy in the rat. *J. Mol. Cell Cardiol.* 1:175, 1970.

Gauthier, G. F. and Padykula, H. A. Cytological studies of fiber types in skeletal muscle. *J. Cell Biol.* 28:333, 1966.

Geer, J. C. Fine structure of canine experimental atherosclerosis. *Am. J. Path.* 47:241, 1965.

Hadlow, W. J. Diseases of skeletal muscle. In *Comparative Neurology.* J. R. M. Innes and L. Z. Saunders, eds., p. 147. Academic Press, New York, 1962.

Hagopian, M., Gershon, M. D. and Nunez, E. A. An ultrastructural study of the effect of reserpine on ventricular cardiac muscle of active and hibernating bats *(Myotis lucifugus).* *Lab. Invest.* 27:99, 1972.

Hardegree, M. C., Palmer, A. E. and Duffin, N. Tetanolysin. *J. Inf. Dis.* 123:51, 1971.

Harrison, A. K., Murphy, F. A. and Gary, G. W. Ultrastructural pathology of Coxsackie A virus infection of mouse striated muscle. *Exp. Mol. Path.* 14:30, 1971.

Heggtveit, H. A. and Nadkarni, B. B. Ultrastructural pathology of the myocardium. *Meth. Achiev. Exp. Path.* 5:474–517, 1971.

Imai, H. et al. Ultrastructural features of aortic cells in mitosis in control and cholesterol-fed swine. *Lab. Invest.* 23:401, 1970.

Jönsson, L. Coronary arterial lesions and myocardial infarcts in the dog. *Acta Vet. Scand. Suppl.* 38:1, 1972.

Kent, S. P. Diffusion of plasma proteins into cells: A manifestation of cell injury in human myocardial ischemia. *Am. J. Path.* 50:623, 1967.

Khan, M. Y. and Ohanian, M. Radiation-induced cardiomyopathy. *Am. J. Path.* 74:125, 1973.

Knieriem, H. J. Electron-microscopic study of bovine arteriosclerotic lesions. *Am. J. Path.* 50:1035, 1967.

Knieriem, H. J., Kao, V. C. Y. and Wissler, R. W. Demonstration of smooth muscle cells in bovine atherosclerosis. *J. Atheroscl. Res.* 8:125, 1968.

Knochel, J. P. and Schlein, E. M. On the mechanism of rhabdomyolysis in potassium depletion. *J. Clin. Invest.* 51:1750, 1972.

Krawczynski, K. Immunohistochemical study of arteriolar (simple) hyalinosis in the spleen. *Am. J. Path.* 62:253, 1971.

Leyton, R. A. and Sonnenblick, E. H. The sarcomere as the basis of Starling's law of the heart in the left and right ventricles. *Meth. Achiev. Exp. Path.* 5:22, 1971.

Lindholm, A., Johansson, H.-E. and Kjaersgaard, P. Acute rhabdomyolysis ("tying-up") in Standardbred horses. *Acta Vet. Scand.* 15:325, 1974.

Mandache, E. et al. The proliferative activity of the heart tissues in various forms of experimental cardiac hypertrophy studied by electron microscope autoradiography. *Virch. Arch. B* 12:112, 1973.

Manechi, H. C. et al. Coronary artery lesions in Atlantic salmon *(Salmo salar).* *Exp. Mol. Path.* 17:274, 1972.

Manning, P. T., Corwin, L. A. and Middleton, C. C. Familial hyperlipoproteinemia and thyroid dysfunction in beagles. *Exp. Mol. Path.* 19:378, 1973.

Marshall, J. R. and O'Neal, R. M. The lipophage in hyperlipemia in rats. An electron microscopic study. *Exp. Mol. Path.* 5:1, 1966.

Martin, A. M. and Hackel, D. B. The myocardium of the dog in hemorrhagic shock. A histochemical study. *Lab. Invest.* 12:77, 1963.

McCallister, B. D. and Brown, A. L., Jr. A quantitative study of myocardial mitochondria in experimental cardiac hypertrophy. *Lab. Invest.* 14:692, 1965.

McCallister, L. P. and Page, E. Effects of thyroxin on ultrastructure of rat myocardial cells. *J. Ult. Res.* 42:136, 1973.

McCombs, H. L., Zook, B. C. and McGandy, R. B. Fine structure of spontaneous atherosclerosis in the squirrel monkey. *Am. J. Path.* 55:235, 1969.

McGavin, M. D. and Baynes, I. D. A congenital progressive ovine muscular dystrophy. *Vet. Path.* 6:513, 1969.

Meerson, F. Z. The myocardium in hyperfunction, hypertrophy and heart failure. *Circ. Res.* 25:(2), 1969.

Melhorn, H. and Scholtyseck, E. Electronenmikroskopische Untersuchungen an Cystenstadien von Sarcocystis tenella aus der Oesophagus-Muskulatur des Schafes. *Zt. Parasit.* 41:291, 1973.

Montali, R. J., Strandberg, J. D. and Squire, R. A. A histochemical and ultrastructural study of intimal bodies of horse arterioles. *Lab. Invest.* 23:362, 1970.

Moss, N. S. and Benditt, E. P. The ultrastructure of spontaneous and experimentally induced arterial lesions. II. The spontaneous plaque in the chicken. *Lab. Invest.* 23:231, 1970.

Mostofa, I. E. A case of glycogenic cardiomegaly in a dog. *Acta Vet. Scand.* 11:197, 1970.

Muir, A. R. Normal and regenerating skeletal muscle fibers in Pietrain pigs. *J. Comp. Path.* 80:137, 1970.

Munnell, J. F. and Getty, R. Canine myocardial Z-disc alteration resembling those of nemaline myopathy. *Lab. Invest.* 19:303, 1968.

Nelson, T. E. et al. Malignant hyperthermia of Poland China swine. *Anesthesiology* 36:52, 1972.

Newman, H. A. I., Muran, T. M. and Geer, J. C. Foam cells of rabbit atheromatous lesions. Identification and cholesterol uptake in isolated cells. *Lab. Invest.* 25:586, 1971.

Onishi, S. et al. Des elektronenmikroskopische Bild der Herzmuskelzelle des Hundes bei experimenteller Herzhypertrophie in der Anpassungsphase. *Beitr. Path. Anat.* 139:94, 1969.

Paplanus, S. H., Zbar, M. J. and Hays, J. W. Cardiac hypertrophy as a manifestation of chronic anemia. *Am. J. Path.* 34:149, 1958.

Paterson, R. A., Layberry, R. A. and Nodkarni, B. B. Cardiac failure in the hamster. *Lab. Invest.* 26:755, 1972.

Pelosi, G. and Agliati, G. The heart muscle in functional overload and hypoxia. *Lab. Invest.* 18:86, 1968.

Platzer, A. C. and Chase, W. H. Histologic alterations in preclinical mouse muscular dystrophy. *Am. J. Path.* 44:931, 1964.

Platzer, A. C. and Gluecksohn-Waelsch, S. Fine structure of mutant (muscular dysgenesis) embryonic mouse muscle. *Develop. Biol.* 28:242, 1972.

Prior, I. A. et al. Calcific heart disease in New Zealand brown trout. *Nature* 220:261, 1968.

Pucak, G. J. et al. Spider monkeys (*Ateles* sp.) as animal models for atherosclerosis research. *Exp. Mol. Path.* 18:32, 1973.

Read, W. K., Pierce, K. R. and O'Hara, P. J. Ultrastructural lesions of an acute toxic cardiomyopathy of cattle. *Lab. Invest.* 18:227, 1968.

Rigdon, R. H. Hereditary myopathy in the white Pekin duck. *Ann. N.Y. Acad. Sci.* 138:28, 1966.

Roberts, J. C., Jr. and Straus, R., eds. *Comparative Atherosclerosis. The Morphology of Spontaneous and Induced Atherosclerotic Lesions in Animals and Its Relation to Human Disease.* Harper and Row, New York, 1965.

Robertson, A. L. and Khairallah, P. A. Angiotensin II. *Science* 172:1138, 1971.

Robertson, O. H., Wexler, B. C. and Miller, B. F. Degenerative changes in the cardio-vascular system of the spawning Pacific salmon (*Oncorhynchus tshawytscha*). *Circ. Res.* 9:826, 1961.

Robison, R. L. et al. Effect of dietary fat and cholesterol on circulating lipids and aortic ultrastructure of squirrel monkeys. *Exp. Mol. Path.* 15:281, 1972.

Ross, R. and Glomset, J. A. Atherosclerosis and arterial smooth muscle cell. *Science* 180:1332, 1973.

Rotruck, J. T. et al. Selenium: Biochemical role as a component of glutathione peroxidase. *Science* 179:588, 1973.

Rustigian, R. and Pappenheimer, A. M. Myositis in mice following intramuscular infection of viruses of the mouse encephalomyelitis group and certain other neurotropic viruses. *J. Exp. Med.* 89:69, 1949.

Sheffield, H. G. and Melton, M. L. The fine structure and reproduction of *Toxoplasma gondii*. *J. Parasit.* 54:209, 1968.

Shen, A. C. and Jennings, R. B. Myocardial calcium and magnesium in acute ischemic injury. *Am. J. Path.* 67:417, 1972.

Simpson, C. F. Electron microscopy of *Sarcocystis fusiformis*. *J. Parasit.* 52:607, 1966.

Simpson, C. R. and Harm, R. H. Aortic dissecting aneurysms. *Adv. Vet. Res.* 13:1, 1969.

Skold, B. H. and Getty, R. Spontaneous atherosclerosis of swine. *J.A.V.M.A.* 139:655, 1961.

Stehbens, W. E. and Ludatscher, R. M. Ultrastructure of the renal arterial bifurcation of rabbits. *Exp. Mol. Path.* 18:50, 1973.

Stemerman, M. B. and Ross, R. Experimental arteriosclerosis. I. Fibrous plaque formation in primates. An electron microscope study. *J. Exp. Med.* 136:769, 1972.

Stewart, G. J and Anderson, M. J. An ultrastructural study of endotoxin induced damage in rabbit mesenteric arteries. *Brit. J. Exp. Path.* 52.75, 1971.

Stoner, C. D., Bishop, S. P. and Sirak, H. D. Normal lysosomal enzyme levels in hypertrophied and failing dog hearts. *J. Mol. Cell Card.* 5:171, 1973.

Suzuki, K. and Ooneda, G. Cerebral arterial lesions in experimental hypertensive rats. Electron microscope study of middle cerebral arteries. *Exp. Mol. Path.* 16:341, 1972.

Suzuki, M. Experimental cerebral atherosclerosis in the dog. *Am J. Path.* 67:387, 1972.

Sybers, H. D. et al. The effect of glucose-insulin-potassium on cardiac ultrastructure following acute experimental coronary occlusion. *Am. J. Path.* 70:401, 1973.

Teppema, J. S. et al. Ultrastructural aspects of capsule formation in *Trichinella spiralis* infection in the rat. *Parasitology* 66:291, 1973.

Tucker, C. F. et al. Regression of early cholesterol-induced aortic lesions in rhesus monkeys. *Am. J. Path.* 65:493, 1971.

Van Citters, R. L. and Watson, N. W. Coronary disease in spawning steelhead trout *Salmo gairdnerii*. *Science* 159:105, 1968.

Veress, B., Kádár, A. and Jellinek, H. Ultrastructural elements in experimental intimal thickening. *Exp. Mol. Path.* 11:200, 1969.

Walker, J. G. and Bishop, S. P. Mitochondrial function and structure in experimental canine congestive heart failure. *Cardiovasc. Res.* 5:444, 1971.

Wallace, C. R. and Hamilton, W. F. Study of spontaneous congestive heart failure in the dog. *Circ. Res.* 11:301, 1962.

Waters, L. L. Changes in the coronary arteries of the dog following injection of allylamine. *Am. Heart J.* 35:212, 1948.

Weaver, D. Q. et al. Structural alterations produced in dogs in sublethal hemorrhagic shock. *Arch. Path.* 93:115, 1972.

Wentink, G. H. et al. Myopathy with a possible recessive x-linked inheritance in a litter of Irish Terriers. *Vet. Path.* 9:328, 1972.

Yarom, M. and Braun, K. Electron microscopic study of the myocardial changes produced by scorpion venom injected in dogs. *Lab. Invest.* 24:21, 1971.

Zacks, S. I. and Scheff, M. F. Tetanus toxin: Fine structure localization of binding sites in striated muscle. *Science* 159:643, 1968.

Zacks, S. I., Shields, D. R. and Steinberg, S. A. A myasthenic syndrome in the dog. *Ann. N.Y. Acad. Sci.* 135:79, 1966.

Zacks, S. I. et al. MED myopathy. *Lab. Invest.* 21:143, 1969.

Pathogenic Intracellular Microorganisms

VIRUSES

To initiate disease, viruses must surmount epithelial barriers. Most do so by attachment to and replication within epithelial cells in the oropharynx, respiratory tract, or intestine. Destruction of overlying epithelium exposes mesenchymal tissues not only to new viral progeny but also to contaminating bacteria which intensify the local inflammatory response. Some viruses are inoculated into tissue through wounds and others by arthropod vectors (by either mechanical or biological transmission). In the latter case, the insect also inserts bacteria and secretions at the site of infection which initiate inflammation.

Systemic disease is provoked when virus-infected cells die. Cellular lysis releases many different host and viral proteins into the lymphatic and blood-vascular systems. These substances act as pyrogens and chemoattractants for inflammatory cells and are responsible for many of the clinical signs of disease. Host reactions to viral infection include fever, leukocytosis, interferon production, and immunoreactivity. Which of these dominates recovery from disease is largely determined by whether infection is localized or systemic. These reactions are an integral part of inflammation, and vascular integrity is required for them to function.

STRUCTURE OF VIRIONS

Viruses are infectious particles that contain only one nucleic acid, either DNA or RNA (Table 12.1). They do not have ribosomes or other structures that synthesize protein, RNA, or metabolic enzymes. *Virions* (the mature, intact, infectious particles) must have the capacity to attach to and enter cells, to shut down host cell synthetic processes, and to subvert the host cell toward replication of new viral nucleic acid and protein.

The *core* of the virion consists of infectious nucleic acid or nucleoprotein. The nucleic acid molecules of the icosahedral viruses (adenoviruses, papovaviruses, reoviruses) are covered by a protein shell, the *capsid,* which is assembled from small protein subunits called *capsomeres*. The number of capsomeres is distinctive for each virus (Fig. 12.1).

The helical viruses (such as influenza), the paramyxoviruses, and other viruses that bud from the plasma membrane during maturation have nucleic acid molecules that are assembled in symmetrical structures called *nucleocapsids*. The nucleocapsid is the helical, ropelike structure composed of a protein shell of structure units that encloses the nucleic acids and can be liberated intact by rupture of the envelope of the virion.

Viral multiplication cycles are artificially divided into phases according to specific events that can be seen or measured. Information is based on work involving one-step growth cycles in cell cultures infected with large doses of virus. This represents a relatively simple experimental system using cloned strains of cells infected with pure strains of virus. In infected animal tissue, replication cycles are going on at different rates and different times. The

Table 12.1. Cytopathology in viral disease

Group	Reference
Poxvirus (Vaccinia subgroup)	
Cowpox	Ichihashi and Dales, *Virology* 51:297, 1973
Smallpox (variola)	Avakyan and Byckovsky, *J. Cell Biol.* 24:337, 1965
Vaccinia	Montasir et al., *Am. J. Path.* 48:877, 1966
Ectromelia (mouse)	Leduc and Bernhard, *J. Ult. Res.* 6:466, 1962
Horsepox	Kaminjolo et al., *Zentr. Vetmed.* B 21:202, 1974
Monkeypox	Wenner et al., *Arch. Ges. Virusforsch.* 27:179, 1969
Rabbitpox	
Buffalopox	
Pseudoswinepox	
Poxvirus (Paravaccinia subgroup)	
Contagious ecthyma (orf)	Kluge et al., *Am. J. Vet. Res.* 33:1191, 1972
Bovine papular stomatitis	Reczko, *Zentr. Bakt.* 169:425, 1957
Pseudocowpox	Cheville and Shey, *J.A.V.M.A.* 150:855, 1967
Poxvirus (avian subgroup)	
Fowlpox	Cheville, *Am. J. Path.* 49:723, 1966
Poxvirus (tumor subgroup)	
Myxomatosis	Purcell and Clarke, *Arch. Ges. Virusforsch.* 39:369, 1972
Rabbit fibromatosis	Pulley and Shively, *Vet. Path.* 10:509, 1974; Prose et al., *Am. J. Path.* 64:467, 1971
Yaba disease	De Harven and Yohn, *Cancer Res.* 26:995, 1966
Squirrel fibroma	Shively et al., *J. Nat. Cancer Inst.* 49:191, 1972
Poxvirus (ungrouped)	
Swinepox	Cheville, *Am. J. Path.* 49:339, 1966
Benign monkeypox	Casey et al., *Am. J. Path.* 51:431, 1967
Sheeppox	Cohen et al., *Ann. Inst. Pasteur* 121:569, 1971
Goatpox	
Camelpox	
Lumpy skin disease	Munz and Owen, *Onderst. J. Vet. Res.* 33:3, 1966
Molluscum contagiosum	Sutton and Burnett, *J. Ult. Res.* 26:177, 1969
Raccoonpox	
Elephantpox	Gehring et al., *Zentr. VetMed.* 19:258, 1972
Marsupialpox	Papadimitriou and Ashman, *J. Gen. Virol.* 16:87, 1972
Scalpox	Wilson et al., *Bull. Wildlife Dis. Ass.* 5:412, 1969
Herpesvirus (human)	
Herpes simplex	Swanson et al., *Lab Invest.* 15:1966, 1966
Herpes zoster	Achong, *J. Gen. Virol.* 3:305, 1968
EB virus	Achong and Epstein, *J. Nat. Cancer Inst.* 36:877, 1966
Cytomegalovirus	Ruebner et al., *Am. J. Path.* 48:971, 1966
Herpesvirus (nonhuman primate)	
Herpesvirus B	Fierer et al., *Ann. Int. Med.* 79:225, 1973
Herpesvirus T	Hunt et al., *Vet. Path.* 3:1, 1966
Herpesvirus saimiri	King and Melendez, *Lab. Invest.* 26:682, 1972
Leukocyte-associated virus (rhesus)	Bissell et al., *J. Inf. Dis.* 128:630, 1973
Herpesvirus (horse)	
Equine rhinopneumonitis	Arhelger et al., *Am. J. Path.* 42:703, 1963
Coital exanthema	
Cytomegalovirus	Kemeny and Pearson, *J. Comp. Path.* 34:59, 1970
Herpesvirus (pig)	
Pseudorabies	Baskerville, *Res. Vet. Sci.* 14:229, 1973; McCraken and Dow, *Acta Neuropath.* 25:207, 1973
Cytomegalovirus	Duncan et al., *Am. J. Vet. Res.* 26:939, 1965
Herpesvirus (cow)	
Infectious bovine rhinotracheitis	Peter et al., *Am. J. Vet. Res.* 27:1583, 1966
Bovine mammillitis	Martin et al., *J. Gen. Microbiol.* 45:325, 1966
Unclassified bovine herpesviruses	Smith et al., *J.A.V.M.A.* 161:1134, 1972; Van Der Maaten and Boothe, Arch. Ges. Virusforsch. 37:85, 1972

Table 12.1 *(Continued)*

Group	Reference
Herpesvirus (sheep and goat)	
Ovine herpesvirus	Malmquist et al., *Lab. Invest.* 26:528, 1972; Smith and MacKay, *J. Comp. Path.* 79:421, 1969
Ovine cytomegalovirus	
Caprine herpesvirus	Saito et al., *Am. J. Vet. Res.* 35:847, 1974
Herpesvirus (bird)	
Infectious laryngotracheitis	Purcell, *Res. Vet. Sci.* 12:455, 1971
Owl herpesvirus	Sileo et al., *J. Wildlife Dis.* 11:92, 1975
Pigeon herpesvirus	Šmíd et al., *Zentr. Vetmed. B* 20:94, 1973
Duck plague	Proctor et al., *Vet. Path.* (in press) 1975
Marek's disease	Cainek et al., *J. Nat. Cancer Inst.* 45:341, 1970
Herpes strigis	Burki et al., *Arch. Ges. Virusforsch.* 43:14, 1973
Falcon herpesvirus	Mare and Graham, *Inf. Immun.* 8:118, 1973
Parrot herpesvirus	Simpson et al., *J. Inf. Dis.* 131:390, 1975
Herpesvirus (other species)	
Canine herpesvirus	Strandberg and Carmichael, *J. Bact.* 90:1790, 1965
Feline herpesvirus	Hoover et al., *Am. J. Path.* 65:173, 1971
Kinkajou herpesvirus	Barahona et al., *Lab. An. Sci.* 23:830, 1973
Guinea pig herpesvirus	Bhatt et al., *J. Inf. Dis.* 123:178, 1971
Frog renal tumor	Zambernard et al., *Cancer Res.* 26:1688, 1966
Carppox	Schubert, *Zt. Naturf.* 196:675, 1964
Channel catfish disease	Wolf and Darlington, *J. Virol.* 8:525, 1971
Adenovirus	
Human respiratory disease	Pinkerton and Carroll, *Am. J. Path.* 65:543, 1971
Infectious canine hepatitis	Given and Jezequel, *Lab. Invest.* 20:36, 1971
Canine laryngotracheitis	Yamamoto, *J. Gen. Virol.* 4:397, 1969
Piglet diarrhea	Koestner et al., *Am. J. Path.* 53:651, 1968
Bovine respiratory infection	Cutlip and McClurkin, *Am. J. Vet. Res.* (in press) 1975
Equine adenovirus	Ardans et al., *Am. J. Vet. Res.* 35:431, 1974
Murine adenovirus	Hareley and Rowe, *Virology* 11:645, 1960
Simian adenovirus	Slifkin et al., *Exp. Mol. Path.* 11:285, 1969
Avian adenovirus	Lim et al., *Avian Dis.* 17:690, 1973
Papovavirus	
Rabbit papilloma	Stone et al., *J. Exp. Med.* 110:543, 1959
Bovine papilloma	Brobst and Hinsman, *Vet. Path.* 3:196, 1966
Canine oral papilloma	Cheville and Olson, *Am. J. Path.* 45:849, 1964
Human papilloma	Chapman et al., *Am. J. Path.* 42:619, 1963
Equine papilloma	Fulton et al., *J. Ult. Res.* 30:328, 1970
Polyoma (mouse)	Mattern et al., *Virology* 30:242, 1966
Murine pneumonitis	Compans et al., *J. Exp. Med.* 126:267, 1967
Simian leukodystrophy	Gribble et al., *Nature* 254:602, 1975
Parvovirus	
Feline panleukopenia	
Mink enteritis	
Rat parvovirus	Baringer and Nathanson, *Lab. Invest.* 27:514, 1972
Adeno-assoc. virus	Henry et al., *Virology* 49:618, 1972
Bovine parvovirus	Bates et al., *Exp. Mol. Path.* 20:208, 1974
Porcine parvovirus	
Iridovirus	
African swine fever	Breese et al., *Virology* 31:508, 1967
Lymphocystis virus	Howse and Christmas, *Virology* 44:211, 1971
Tadpole edema virus	Wolf et al., *J. Inf. Dis.* 118:253, 1968
Frog iridovirus	Maes et al., *Virology* 33:137, 1967
Myxovirus	
Influenza	Blaskovic et al., *Arch. Ges. Virusforsch.* 38:250, 1972; Dourmashkin and Tyrrell, *J. Gen. Virol.* 9:77, 1970
Paramyxovirus	
Newcastle disease	Cheville and Beard, *Lab. Invest.* 27:129, 1972
Mumps	Duc-Nguyen, *J. Virol.* 2:494, 1968

Table 12.1 *(Continued)*

Group	Reference
Parainfluenza	Ane, *J. Microsc.* 6:31, 1967, Howe et al., *J. Virol.* 1:215, 1967; Prose et al., *J. Exp. Med.* 122:1151, 1965
Measles	Baringer and Griffith, *Lab. Invest.* 23:335, 1970; Nakai et al., *Virology* 38:50, 1969
Canine distemper	Koestner and Long, *Lab. Invest.* 23:196, 1970; Richter and Moize, *Vet. Path.* 7:346, 1970; Tajima et al., *Am. J. Vet. Res.* 32:913, 1971; Watson and Wright, *Res. Vet. Sci.* 17:188, 1974
Respiratory syncytial virus	Bachi and Howe, *J. Virol.* 12:1173, 1973; Ito et al., *Arch. Ges. Virusforsch.* 40:198, 1973
Mouse pneumonitis	Compans et al., *J. Exp. Med.* 126:267, 1967
Rhabdovirus	
Rabies	Dierks et al., *Am. J. Path.* 54:251, 1969; Miyamoto and Matsumoto, *J. Exp. Med.* 125:447, 1967
Vesicular stomatitis	Bergold and Munz, *J. Ult. Res.* 17:233, 1967; David-West and Labzoffsky, *Arch. Ges. Virusforsch.* 23:105, 1968
Green monkey disease	Murphy et al., *Lab. Invest.* 24:279, 1971
Bovine ephemeral fever	Murphy et al., *Arch. Ges. Virusforsch.* 38:234, 1972
Aerocystitis (carp)	Bachman and Ahne, *Nature* 244:235, 1973
Hemorrhagic septicemia (trout)	Zwillenberg et al., *Arch. Ges. Virusforsch.* 17:1, 1965
Infectious hematopoietic necrosis (fish)	McAllister et al., *Arch. Ges. Virusforsch.* 44:270, 1974
Reovirus	
Human reovirus	Silverstein and Dales, *J. Cell Biol.* 36:197, 1968
Murine reovirus	Jenson et al., *Am. J. Path.* 47:223, 1965
Avian reovirus	Simmons et al., *Avian Dis.* 16:1094, 1972; Walker et al., *J. Ult. Res.* 41:67, 1972
Reo-like Viruses	
African horse sickness	Breese et al., *J.A.V.M.A.* 155:391, 1969
Epidemic hemorrhagic disease (deer)	Tsai and Karstad, *Am. J. Path.* 70:379, 1973
Infectious pancreatic necrosis (fish)	Moss and Gravell, *J. Virol.* 3:52, 1969
Infectious bursal disease	Cheville, *Am. J. Path.* 51:527, 1967
Orbivirus	
Bluetongue	Bowne and Jochim, *Am. J. Vet. Res.* 28:1091, 1967
Colorado tick fever	Murphy et al., *Virology* 35:28, 1968
Rotavirus	
Enteritis of calves	Stair et al., *Vet. Path.* 10:155, 1973
Enteritis of man	Kapikian et al., *Science* 185:1049, 1974
Epizootic diarrhea of mice	Adams and Kraft, *Am. J. Path.* 51:39, 1967, Banfield et al., *Virology* 36:411, 1968
Coronavirus	
Infectious bronchitis of chickens	Becker, *J. Virol.* 1:1019, 1967
HEV encephalitis of pigs	Mengeling, *Am. J. Vet. Res.* 33:297, 1972
Transmissible gastroenteritis of pigs	Thake, *Am. J. Path.* 53:149, 1968
Calf enteritis	Stair et al., *Am. J. Vet. Res.* 33:1147, 1972
Murine hepatitis	Ruebner et al., *Am. J. Path.* 51:163, 1967
Arenavirus	
Lymphocytic choriomeningitis	Abelson et al., *J. Nat. Cancer Inst.* 42:497, 1969
Togavirus	
Western encephalitis	Morgan et al., *J. Exp. Med.* 113:219, 1961
Eastern encephalitis	Murphy et al., *Exp. Mol. Path.* 13:131, 1970
Semliki forest virus	Grimely and Friedman, *Exp. Mol. Path.* 12:1, 1970
Venezuelan encephalitis	Jelinkova et al., *Acta Virol.* 18:154, 1974
Japanese B encephalitis	Oyangi et al., *Acta Neuropath.* 13:169, 1969
Louping ill	Doherty and Vantsis, *J. Comp. Path.* 83:481, 1973
Yellow fever	Bearcroft, *J. Path.* 83:59, 1962; McGavran and White, *Am. J. Path.* 45:501, 1964
Rift Valley fever	McGavran and Easterday, *Am. J. Path.* 42:587, 1963
Toga-like Virus	
Equine arteritis virus	Estes and Cheville, *Am. J. Path.* 58:235, 1970

Table 12.1 *(Continued)*

Group	Reference
Hog cholera	Cheville and Mengeling, *Lab. Invest.* 20:261, 1969
Bovine viral diarrhea	Peter et al., *Am. J. Vet. Res.* 29:939, 1968
Rubella	Murphy et al., *J. Virol.* 2:1223, 1968
Picornavirus	
Avian encephalomyelitis	Cheville, *Am. J. Path.* 58:105, 1970
Mouse poliomyelitis	Nelson et al., *Am. J. Path.* 44:29, 1964
Porcine enterovirus	Koestner et al., *Am. J. Path.* 49:325, 1966
Poliomyelitis (man)	Anzai and Ozaki, *Exp. Mol. Path.* 10:176, 1969; Dales et al., *Virology* 26:379, 1965
Coxsackievirus	Haas and Yunis, *Lab. Invest.* 23:442, 1970
Echovirus	Skinner et al., *Virology* 36:241, 1968
Vesicular exanthema (pig)	Zee et al., *Am. J. Vet. Res.* 29:1025, 1968
Swine vesicular disease	
Foot-and-mouth disease	Breese, *J. Gen. Virol.* 4:343, 1969
Encephalomyocarditis	Adachi et al., *Acta Neuropath.* 25:169, 1973
Rhinovirus	Gauntt et al., *Arch. Ges. Virusforsch.* 41:382, 1973; Kawana and Matsumoto, *Jap. J. Microbiol.* 15:207, 1971
Feline picornavirus	
Duck hepatitis	Richter et al., *Virology* 24:114, 1964
Oncornavirus	
Lymphoid leukosis (chicken)	Di Stefano and Dougherty, *J. Nat. Cancer Inst.* 37:869, 1966; Heine et al., *J. Nat. Cancer Inst.* 29:211, 1962; Mladenov et al., *J. Nat. Cancer Inst.* 38:251, 1967
Feline lymphoma	Herz et al., *J. Nat. Cancer Inst.* 44:339, 1970; Laird et al., *J. Nat. Cancer Inst.* 41:867, 1968
Murine lymphoma	Aoki et al., *Proc. Nat. Acad. Sci.* 65:569, 1970; De Harven, *J. Exp. Med.* 120:857, 1964; Feldman and Gross, *Cancer Res.* 27:1513, 1967
Mouse mammary gland tumor	Feldman, *J. Nat. Cancer Inst.* 30:477, 1963; Moore et al., *J. Nat. Cancer Inst.* 44:965, 1970
Unclassified Viruses	
Visna	Coward et al., *Virology* 40:1030, 1970
Bovine visna-like virus	Boothe and Van Der Maaten, *J. Virol.* 13:197, 1972
Reticuloendotheliosis	Zeigel et al., *J. Nat. Cancer Inst.* 37:709, 1966
Equine infectious anemia	Ito et al., *Arch. Ges. Virusforsch.* 28:411, 1969; Tajima et al., *J. Virol.* 4:521, 1969
Aleutian disease (mink)	Yoon et al., *Nature* 245:205, 1973
Lactic dehydrogenase virus	du Buy and Johnson, *J. Exp. Med.* 123:985, 1966
Bovine syncytial virus	Boothe et al., *Arch. Ges. Virusforsch.* 31:373, 1970
Rabbit syncytial virus	Brown et al., *Proc. Soc. Exp. Biol. Med.* 133:587, 1970

cells involved are not simple homogeneous cell systems, for even the simplest tissues include cells of differing function and structure (Cheville 1975).

The early events of replication are associated with entry of virions into the cell and disappearance of infectivity until new virions are assembled (Fig. 12.2). One of the few defined mechanisms of adsorption is that of influenza in which the hemagglutinin is contained in projections from the surface of the virion. Attachment of the virion to the host plasma membrane occurs by the complexing of hemagglutinin projections on the virion's envelope with mucoprotein components of the host cell plasma membrane.

Penetration is the entry into the cytoplasm of the intact virion or that part containing the nucleic acid. In general it occurs by fusion with the plasma membrane. Ultrastructural evidence of degradation of influenza virions following attachment is characterized by smudging and continuity of virion and plasma membrane. After release of the viral genome into the cytoplasmic matrix, synthesis of new viral proteins and nucleic acids begins.

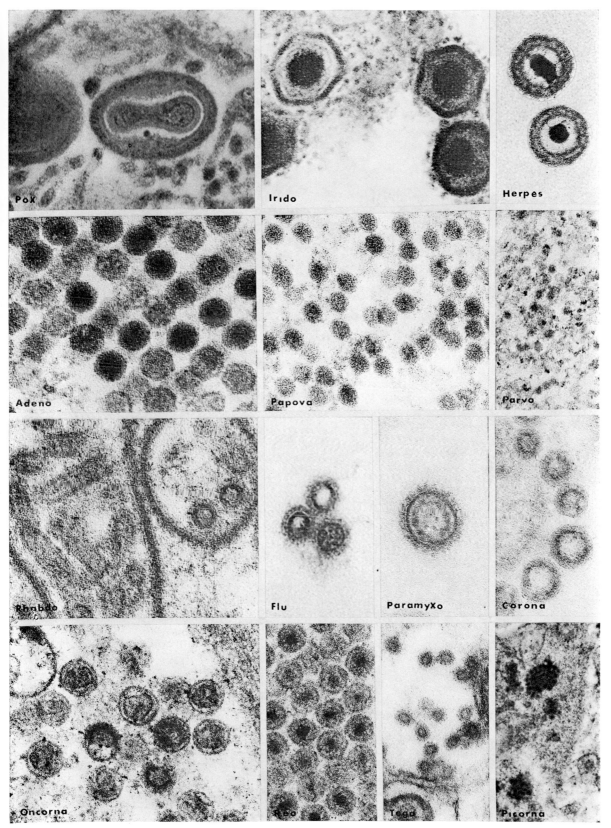

Fig. 12.1. Ultrastructure of virions in thin sections of tissue.

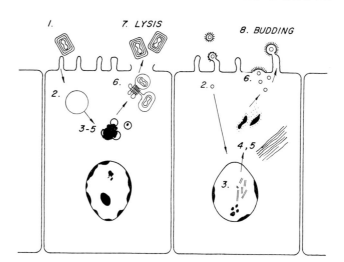

Fig. 12.2. Diagram of stages of infection of poxviruses and influenza virus.

ANTIVIRAL HOST MECHANISMS

FEVER IN VIRAL DISEASE

Fever usually precedes other clinical signs of viral disease and its disappearance heralds recovery. Experimental studies have shown decreased fatality and tissue virus levels in animals in which elevation of body temperature has been artificially produced (Carmichael et al. 1969). Similar depression of viral replication has been demonstrated in vitro. The artificial elevation of body temperature is associated with decreased growth and release of virus in target cells (Bennett and Nicastri 1960; Cole and Wisseman 1969).

The way in which fever acts is not known; it is assumed that there is some thermal inactivation of circulating virus. Animals with fever, however, have secondary increases in metabolism, hormone secretion, immune response, and phagocytosis and the true beneficial role of elevated body temperature is difficult to assess.

PHAGOCYTOSIS

Following invasion of virulent viruses into mesenchymal tissue of a susceptible host, replication occurs at the point of entry and, because of the flow of lymph, in the draining lymph node. This may be accompanied by a primary viremia, but usually blood levels of virus are low and are cleared by phagocytosis by granulocytes

and by sinusoidal macrophages in the liver and spleen. Clearance of larger virions generally occurs more quickly than that of smaller virions.

Macrophages are of primary importance in the clearance of viruses from tissue. They may destroy virions following phagocytic uptake. If the virus is able to replicate within the macrophage, dissemination occurs. Several experiments have demonstrated that different strains of the same virus may differ in virulence because of their differing capacities to replicate in macrophages. This in turn determines their capacity to produce systemic infection and replication in critical target organs. Blockade of the reticuloendothelial system with carbon or thorotrast or inhibition of macrophage lysosomes with cortisone will result in increased susceptibility to many viral infections.

Immaturity of the reticuloendothelial system is responsible for the increased susceptibility of young animals to some viruses. Newborn mice are killed by encephalitis after intraperitoneal injection of herpes simplex virus. Adult mice are not. Furthermore, newborn mice that have been injected with syngeneic macrophages from normal adult mice show increased resistance to encephalitis and death (Hirsch et al. 1970). In vitro, "neonatal" and "adult" macrophages show no difference in resistance to infection but there are clearcut differences in transmission of virus to neighboring cells; suckling mouse macrophages will and adult macrophages will not transmit the virus.

The regional lymph node provides the first great barrier to viral infection. Virions enter the node through the cortical afferent lymph and are phagocytized by macrophages in the cortical or peripheral sinuses. The effectiveness with which the virion is degraded for immunogenic activity is determined by the susceptibility of the macrophage to infection. The balance between the early production of antibody and the effect of virus on the adjacent lymphoid tissue often determines the course of the disease. Numerous studies in vitro have shown that the susceptibility of the macrophage and its lysosome to a particular virus may determine the extent of infection. Some viruses have an affinity for macrophages and may exist in massive numbers in lysosomes following replication.

INTERFERON

The *interferons* are proteins of cell origin that are induced and released following stimulation by foreign substances. They were discovered as virus-inhibiting soluble substances released by cells inoculated with inactivated influenza virus; the myxoviruses are potent inducers of interferon. Interferon is not itself antiviral; that is, it does not inactivate virus. It blocks intracellular viral synthesis by inducing an antiviral protein in the cell that acts upon ribosomal synthesis. Interferon is produced locally in all cell types within hours after viral infection.

The spleen may be an important source of interferon since splenectomized animals produce much less interferon than intact animals. Although species specific, interferon is nonspecific in activity; it will inhibit many viruses. This is in contrast to antibody, which is specific, extracellular in action, and produced by specific lymphoid cells distant from primary infection at a delayed time following infection.

Interferon is one of the first host defense mechanisms to appear in viral infection. When stimulated by initial viral infection it appears about the same time as progeny virus. It diffuses to surrounding cells and spreading virus thus meets an intracellular barrier to its continued replication. Considerable amounts of interferon also occur in the blood but interferonemia rapidly disappears due to loss via the renal glomerulus (Fig. 12.3). Interferonuria develops rapidly and levels of interferon are often higher in urine than in blood. Salivary secretion also occurs and may be significant in infections such as mumps (Baron 1970).

The interferon system, like antibody production, is influenced by other mechanisms such as corticosteroid injections, immunosuppressive therapy, stress, temperature elevation, and changes in oxygen tension. An immature interferon system is present at early age and the lack of interferon in fetuses may play a role in the production of viral-induced congenital malformations.

ANTIBODY

The importance of antibody in recovery from viral infection was established long

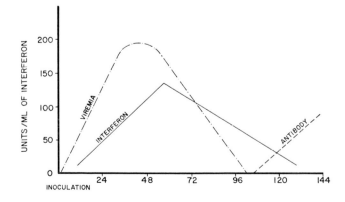

Fig. 12.3. Rise and fall of interferon in circulating blood relative to viremia and antibodies in an acute infection with an interferon-inducing virus.

ago by the observation that viruses disappeared from the host as antibody appeared. Conversely, suppression of antibody synthesis led to disastrous and fatal disease in viral infections which resolved without sequelae in normal animals. The end result of infection came to be viewed as a race between viral replication and the host's antibody response (Nathanson and Cole 1971). Acceleration of the antibody response by active immunization or by passive administration of antisera clearly demonstrated the value of antibodies.

Infected animals may produce many types of antiviral antibodies. Large complex viruses such as the poxviruses induce more than ten different antibodies. Most are directed against internal components of the virion and are of little consequence in viral neutralization. The important antibodies are those that react with the surface of the virion to neutralize infectivity. For example, the antibodies that neutralize influenza are those that are formed against the hemagglutinin within the envelope of the virion (Svehag 1968).

Serum antibody of the IgG class is the prime mediator of immunity for viruses that undergo a systemic phase of dissemination. IgA, which is produced by local plasmacytes, is present in nasal or gut secretions and is the functional immunoglobulin for viruses that localize in these organs. In these situations serum antibody may be relatively ineffective. Circulating antibodies are particularly effective during viremia in preventing the spread of virions to distant target organs.

CELL-MEDIATED MECHANISMS

It is recognized that cell-mediated immunity, in contrast to immunity induced by plasmacytes and antibody, plays a role in recovery from viral infection and in suppression of "latent" viruses. The cells involved are "immune" lymphocytes, that is, thymic-dependent, nonantibody forming cells. Their action involves (1) the specific attachment to virus-infected cells with liberation of lymphotoxins that destroy the target cells and/or (2) the secretion of lymphokines which nonspecifically attract monocytes and macrophages to sites of infection that then function to destroy the infected cells (Blanden 1971; Hapel and Gardner 1974).

The functions of cell-mediated immune reactions of lymphocytes are best illustrated by animals and children with hereditary absence of antibody-forming cells (agammaglobulinemia). These patients are highly susceptible to bacteria yet develop delayed hypersensitivity reactions and progress through most viral diseases normally.

BACTERIA

Pathogenic bacteria elaborate inflammatory agents and substances that modify the host's inflammatory response (Table 12.2). Edema-producing factors are especially important for they not only allow organisms to multiply in a liquid environment but also permit spread throughout the tissues. Cellular degeneration and death may be caused by exotoxins, toxic bacterial components, or direct intracellular replication. The pathogenicity or virulence of an organism is largely determined by how effectively that organism produces toxic factors.

Although true virulence of bacteria is detectable only in the living animal, microbiologists use structural components that develop in cultures (capsules, pili, cell walls) and secretions (exotoxins, coagulase, hyaluronidase, etc.) as markers of virulence. When produced by the bacterium in sufficient concentrations these substances cause the organism to resist the opsonic and lytic effects of antibody and complement.

STRUCTURE OF THE BACTERIAL CELL

Bacterial cells are delimited by a plasma membrane and most are surrounded by a dense, rigid cell wall that defines the shape of the cell (Fig. 12.4). Gram stain–retaining (gram-positive) bacteria have thick walls composed of mucocomplexes containing muramic acid (Fig. 12.5). Those whose cell walls are solely of mucocomplexes are susceptible to lysozyme which solubilizes this substance. The cell walls of many gram-positive bacteria also contain simpler polysaccharides and teichoic acid. Electron micrographs have shown that teichoic acid chains penetrate into the polysaccharide

Table 12.2. Ultrastructure of pathogenic bacteria

Family	Genera	Reference
MYCOPLASMALES		
Mycoplasmataceae	Mycoplasma	Jones and Hirsch, *J. Exp. Med.* 133:231, 1971
RICKETTSIALES		
Rickettsiaceae	Rickettsia	Brinton and Burgdorfer, *J. Bact.* 105:1749, 1971
	Neorickettsia	Frank et al., *J. Inf. Dis.* 129:257, 1974
	Cowdria	Pienaar, *Onderst. J. Vet. Res.* 37:67, 1970
	Coxsiella	Krauss and Leyk, *Zentr. Vetmed. B* 21:271, 1974
	Ehrlichia	Hildebrandt et al., *Inf. Immun.* 7:265, 1973
		Simpson, *Am. J. Vet. Res.* 33:2451, 1972
	Rickettsiella	
	Unclassified	Tuomi and von Bonsdorff, *J. Bact.* 92:1478, 1966
Chlamydiaceae		Swanson et al., *J. Inf. Dis.* 131:678, 1975
	Chlamydia	Doughri, *Vet. Path.* 10:114, 1973
Bartonellaceae	Bartonella	Cuadra and Takano, *Blood* 33:708, 1969
	Eperythrozoon	McKee et al., *Am. J. Vet. Res.* 34:1196, 1973
	Hemobartonella	Demarce and Nessmith, *Am. J. Vet. Res.* 33:1303, 1972 (cat)
		Simpson and Love, *Am. J. Vet. Res.* 31:225, 1970
		Venable and Ewing, *J. Parasit.* 54:259, 1968
	Grahamella	
Anaplasmataceae	Anaplasma	Simpson, *J. Cell Biol.* 27:227, 1965
EUBACTERALES		
Lactobactereaceae	Streptococcus	Swanson and Gotschlich, *J. Exp. Med.* 138:245, 1973
		Huls in'T Veld and Linssen, *J. Gen. Microbiol.* 74:315, 1973
	Diplococcus	
Micrococcaceae	Staphylococcus	Conti et al., *J. Bact.* 96:554, 1968
		Horn et al., *Lab. Invest.* 21:406, 1969
	Neisseria	Froholm et al., *Acta Path. Microbiol. Scand. B* 81:525, 1973
		Garcia-Kutzback et al., *J. Inf. Dis.* 130:183, 1974
Corynebacteriaceae	Corynebacterium	Hard, *J. Med. Microbiol.* 5:483, 1972
	Listeria	North and Mackaness, *Brit. J. Exp. Path.* 44-601, 1963
		Racz et al., *Lab. Invest.* 26:694, 1972
		Tenner et al., *Virch. Arch. B* 14:35, 1973
	Erysipelothrix	Drommer et al., *Vet. Path.* 7:455, 1970
Bacillaceae	Bacillus	Hachisuka et al., *J. Bact.* 91:2382, 1966
		van Iterson et al., *J. Bact.* 121:1189, 1975
	Clostridium	Ellison et al., *J. Bact.* 108:526, 1971
		Schallehn and Wecke, *Zentr. Bakt. A* 228:63, 1971
Brucellaceae	Brucella	Hatten et al., *J. Bact.* 108:535, 1971
		Obertini et al., *Path. Biol.* 22:471, 1974
	Pasteurella	
	Bordatella	Richter and Kress, *Lab. Invest.* 16:187, 1967
	Malleomyces	
	Actinobacillus	Kurashima and Fujiwara, *Jap. J. Exp. Med.* 42:139, 1972
	Bacterioides	Bladen and Waters, *J. Bact.* 86:1339, 1963
	Spherophus	
	Hemophilus	
	Moraxella	Froholm, *J. Ult. Res.* 42:411, 1973
Enterobacteriaceae	Escherichia	Bertschinger et al., *Inf. Immun.* 5:505, 1972
		Staley et al., *Am. J. Path.* 56:371, 1969
		Burdett and Murray, *J. Bact.* 119:1039, 1974
	Aerobacter	Kennell and Kotoulas, *J. Bact.* 93:367, 1967
	Klebsiella	Thornley and Horne, *J. Gen. Microbiol.* 28:51, 1962
	Proteus	Seibert et al., *Zentr. Bakt. A* 228:210, 1974
		Leene and van Iterson, *J. Cell Biol.* 27:25, 1965
	Salmonella	Takeuchi and Sprinz, *Am. J. Path.* 51:137, 1967
	Shigella	Takeuchi, *Curr. Topics Path.* 54:1, 1971
Pseudomonadaceae	Pseudomonas	Diedrick and Cota-Robles, *J. Bact.* 119:1006, 1969
		Cheng et al., *J. Bact.* 107:325, 1971
	Vibrio	Moon et al., *Am. J. Vet. Res.* (in press), 1975
		Ritchie et al., *J. Gen. Microbiol.* 43:427, 1966
	Aeromonas	

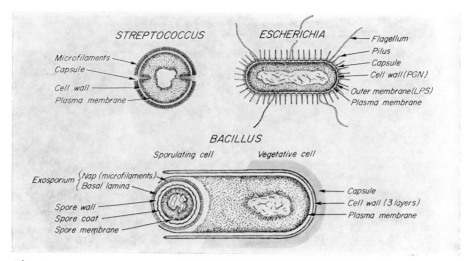

Fig. 12.5. Diagram of ultrastructure of Streptococcus, Escherichia and Bacillus.

taining lysosomes. The phagolysosomes are the sites of destruction for nearly all organisms of low virulence. Many highly pathogenic bacteria contain powerful exotoxins that destroy the membrane of the phagosome, allowing the organisms to be liberated into the cytoplasmic matrix where they more readily cause cell death.

The fusion of bacteria-containing phagosomes with lysosomes is prevented by some microbial substances. Tubercle bacilli in some unknown way prevent this fusion and they can persist within the phagosome to kill the cell. The heavy lipid-containing cell wall of the tubercle bacillus enables this microbe to resist enzymic degradation within phagolysosomes if fusion does occur.

INTRACELLULAR REPLICATION

The simplest bacterial cells may require an intracellular environment to replicate. Rickettsiae and Chlamydiae have evolved transport mechanisms that enable them to exploit host-generated ATP and other intermediates for their own use. The way in which they exist within the cell is not known. The facultative intracellular bacteria such as *Listeria monocytogenes*, *Brucella* spp., and some others have the capacity to activate macrophages inducing an enhanced state of reactivity.

MECHANISMS OF BACTERIAL DESTRUCTION

ANTIBODY AND THE BACTERIAL CELL

Selective immunological destruction of bacteria is mediated by immunoglobulin molecules in two ways: (1) by opsonization, that is, attaching to bacterial surfaces and enhancing their phagocytosis by macrophages and circulating granulocytes and (2) by affecting the complement system on the surface of the bacterial cell and inducing plasmolysis.

The simplest way to demonstrate opsonization is to mix two dilute suspensions of bacteria with leukocytes obtained from the buffy coat of centrifuged blood. To one sample saline is added; to the other, specific antiserum. When smears are made after several minutes of incubation, it can be seen that neutrophils have engulfed large numbers of bacteria in the preparation containing antibodies. In the control, the neutrophils contain few if any bacteria. The *phagocytic index* is the number of bacteria ingested by 100 neutrophils. When this is determined on immune and normal (control) sera, an *opsonic index* can be calculated as a ratio between the phagocytic indices of the two sera. It is the measure of the sensitizing power of the serum of an infected animal for phagocytes.

Antibody functions in the initial phase of plasmolysis. The antibody molecule must recognize antigens on the invading bacterium, activate complement, and fix it to the bacterial cell surface. Complement completes the actual work of lysis. When antibodies are added to bacteria containing their respective antigens in cell-free media, complement is needed before structural damage to the bacterial cell can be demonstrated. When antibodies are added to *E. coli* labeled with radioactive phosphorus, structural changes occur in the cell surface and P^{32} leaks into the medium. Ultrastructurally, the bacterial cell swells and there is smoothing of the normally undulant cell walls (Wilson 1968). Bacterial plasma membranes contain tiny holes which are sites of complement activity in the process of lysis (Bladen et al. 1966). Breaks occur with fibrillar fragmentation in the mucopeptide layers. In some instances, lysozyme is allegedly required for complete plasmolysis. After its addition, the cells break up. Cell wall "ghosts" are common, remnants of cells remaining after release of internal components.

COMPLEMENT

Complement is an intricately linked set of enzymes which cooperates with antibody in the destruction of bacteria. Invading organisms are identified by antibody and are then attached by the components of the complement system. The antibody molecule, when it combines with antigens in the bacterium, serves to activate complement which actually does the work of destroying the organism. Complement must recognize the antibody molecule, respond to it, and fix to the bacterial cell surface.

During lysis of the bacterial cell, the complement components C5, C6, C7, C8, and C9 become enmeshed in the bilayer of lipid molecules which constitute the plasma membrane of the bacterium. They aggregate to form a doughnut-shaped arrangement with the central hole penetrating through the membrane. This allows leakage of water and ions. Bacterial cells swell until the plasma membrane ruptures and the cytosol spills out.

INTRACELLULAR DESTRUCTION OF BACTERIA

The most effective mechanisms of animals for the destruction of bacteria involve phagocytosis and intracellular digestion. This occurs on first contact during initial infection or later, and more efficiently, by specific immunologic mechanisms. Even in immune reactions, the effector process involves phagocytic action of monocytes and fixed macrophages.

When bacteria enter an animal through breaks in epithelial surfaces they are phagocytized and digested by macrophages located within the connective tissues (Suter and Ramseier 1964). The efficiency of the two phases (uptake and digestion) is determined largely by the characteristics of the bacterium which are markers of virulence. For example, Streptococci, Pasteurellae, and Klebsiella resist phagocytosis because of components of their capsules which block the action of macrophages. These obligate extracellular bacteria produce acute infections with a tendency to septicemia. Infection is characterized by neutrophilic leukocytosis and accumulation of neutrophils at sites of infection.

In contrast, facultative intracellular bacteria such as Brucella, Listeria, Salmonella, and the Mycobacteria are readily phagocytized but resist intracellular digestion and have the capacity to replicate within macrophages. These bacteria tend to produce subacute and chronic infections.

When bacteria are shed into the bloodstream, fixed macrophages in the liver and spleen are responsible for removing organisms. Efficiency of clearance depends upon the type of bacteria, the species of animal, and several factors in individual animals that relate to previous "experience" of the reticuloendothelial systems; that is, whether complement levels are high, antibodies are present, and macrophages are activated (Landy et al. 1965; Wood 1960).

An accurate method of measuring clearance of bacteria experimentally is to radioactively label bacterial cells, inject them intravenously, and follow the rate of disappearance of radioactivity in blood samples

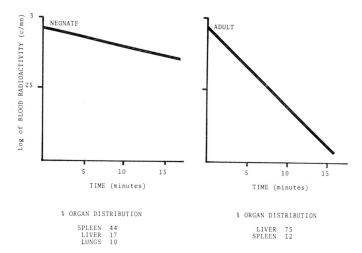

Fig. 12.6. Comparison of the removal of bacteria from bloodstream of newborn and adult pigs and importance of spleen, liver, and lungs (after Mouton 1963).

taken periodically. When newborn piglets (which lack antibodies and other opsonins) are injected intravenously with labeled Salmonellae, clearance is slow (Mouton 1963). The bacteria are taken up chiefly in the spleen; small numbers of organisms are removed in the liver and lung (Fig. 12.6). In adult pigs, which have activated macrophages, opsonins, and higher levels of complement, bacteria are more rapidly removed by the liver. Small numbers are also removed by the spleen, but only traces are found in other organs.

Although avirulent bacteria are rapidly removed, clearance varies according to the species of bacteria; Salmonellae are removed much faster than *E. coli*. Clearance also depends upon the host animal: given proportionately equal numbers of bacteria

according to weight, the rabbit clears *E. coli* in 5 min, the guinea pig in 25 min, while the mouse requires over 50 min (Benacerraf et al. 1966). Virulent bacteria generally are not totally removed from the blood but numbers remain low until a secondary bacteremia occurs, which may then lead to death or to activation of immune response and recovery of the host animal (Fig. 12.7).

MACROPHAGE ACTIVATION AND ACQUIRED CELL RESISTANCE

Metchnikoff believed that macrophages underwent intrinsic changes in their functional ability and that this was responsible for increased antimicrobial capacity following bacterial infection. When studies

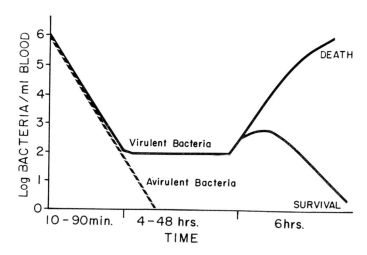

Fig. 12.7. Persistence of bacteremia in infection with bacteria of varying virulence.

on opsonization joined this cellular theory with the humoral theory (which had previously been predominant), the concept of macrophage activation in the absence of antibody was dismissed. It is now again believed that, in fact, macrophages do acquire an "innate" resistance to reinfection to some types of bacteria (Mackaness 1964; McGregor et al. 1971).

Virulent facultative intracellular bacteria such as Listeria, Brucellae, and the Mycobacteria replicate successfully within macrophages. During the initial infection, an acquired cellular resistance develops which lasts for several weeks following infection and is unrelated to specific antibacterial antibody. Subsequent infection with the same or similar organisms is followed by a more rapid and efficient destruction of bacteria. For example, in cells from normal mice, inactivation of the Salmonellae does not begin for about 10 min and hardly more than 50% of the bacteria are killed. The killing of *Salm. typhimurium* in cells of previously infected mice begins immediately after phagocytosis and proceeds rapidly until every intracellular organism has been killed.

Antibacterial antibody does not exert an effect on this type of reactivity. Animals infected with Salmonellae are equally microbicidal for Listeria (Blanden et al. 1966). The augmented cells, once activated, are not specifically directed against the infectious agent that induces their activation.

DESTRUCTION OF BACTERIAL CELLS BY ANTIBIOTICS

The specific bacteriostatic, and in some cases bacteriolytic, effect upon the bacterial cell varies with individual antibiotics; the structure affected may be the cell wall, plasma membrane, or sites of protein synthesis in the cytoplasm. Although there is generally a primary site of action, many antibiotics interfere in several metabolic processes.

Penicillin interferes with synthesis of peptides of the cell wall by virtue of being an analog for the D-alanyl-D-alanine end of the pentapeptide. In effect, it blocks the transpeptidase that initiates final cross-linking of peptides. This occurs at the outer surface of the cell membrane and penicillin need not enter the bacterial cell to exert its effect (Lorian 1971). The three successive events in the penicillin-injured cell are swelling with thinning of the cell wall, breakup of the cell wall, and plasmolysis.

During normal bacterial cell division, controlled lysis at sites of separation of daughter cells is produced by autolytic enzymes in the cell wall such as acetylmuramidase. When penicillin is added to cultures of gram-positive cocci, cell wall synthesis stops abruptly but autolysis continues to lyse and erode the wall. The cell continues to increase in volume, for general protein synthesis is not significantly depressed and osmotic pressure within the cell leads to plasmolysis. The failure of penicillin to affect gram-negative bacteria is due chiefly to its inability to penetrate the lipopolysaccharide layer of the cell wall. Although mucopeptides and cross-linking may be inhibited, other cell wall structures tend to preserve the wall.

The polymyxins act on the cytoplasmic membranes of gram-negative bacterial cells. Molecules of polymyxin are inserted between lipid and protein layers of the membrane and produce a chemically disruptive cleavage which leads to rupture of the membrane. Membrane function is destroyed and substances can pass freely in and out of the cell. Polymyxin acts as a disinfectant, that is, by quick and simple surface contact. Its effect is bactericidal and occurs whether the bacterial cell is metabolically active or inactive. Polymyxins are not active on gram-positive bacteria for they are unable to cross the cell wall.

Several antibiotics act by inhibiting protein synthesis. Tetracycline blocks the binding of tRNA–amino acid complex in the ribosomes and amino acids are not available to mRNA to sustain the construction of polypeptides. Chloramphenicol blocks the amino acid transfer on the growing polypeptide chain. Streptomycin interferes with the translation function of mRNA. Amino acids are aligned improperly in the peptide sequence and unusable proteins are formed. The antibiotics of the above types are bacteriostatic. They inhibit protein synthesis in the bacterial cell but the damage is reversible when the drug is removed.

FUNGI

Fungi are single-celled, nucleated plant organisms that include not only a wide variety of pathogenic species but also the yeasts, molds, mushrooms, mildews, and other similar organisms. The simplest structural form is the single-celled budding yeast. In culture, most fungi consist of networks of hyphae called mycelia. Individual hyphae form by the elongation of the fungal cell without separation into new cells. Fungi grow by producing new hyphae at the edge of the mycelium (vegetative growth).

Many fungi form specialized reproductive bodies or *spores* (sporulation) and the spore structure and its mode of development are the characteristics by which different fungi are classified and identified. Two kinds of spores are distinguished: asexual and sexual. Sexual spores are produced by fusion of two cells; asexual arise by differentiation of cells of spore-bearing hyphae without fusion. Three classes of fungi (Phycomycetes, Ascomycetes, and Basidiomycetes) are "perfect fungi" (with both sexual and asexual spore forms) which are differentiated on the basis of differences in fruiting bodies. A fourth group, the Deuteromycetes or Fungi Imperfecti, have no sexual state. With few exceptions, fungi pathogenic for vertebrate cells are classified as Fungi Imperfecti. The important groups within the Fungi Imperfecti are the pathogenic yeasts and the dermatophytes.

Most of the important pathogens are dimorphic; that is, their typical growth forms in tissue and in saprophytic stages in culture are different. For example, in histoplasmosis the causal organism *(Histoplasma capsulatum)* is found as small budding yeast cells within macrophages. In culture, this organism grows as septate mycelia with microconidia and tuberculate chlamydospores.

ULTRASTRUCTURE OF FUNGI

Fungal cells are identified in tissue according to their size, cytoplasmic structure, type of reproductive bodies, and distinctive cell wall (Table 12.3). The thick cell walls are usually layered and may contain homogeneous, fibrillar, and granular components of varying electron density (Fig. 12.8).

The eukaryotic fungal cell is composed of cytoplasmic matrix filled with ribosomes, lipid (or lipoid) globules, vacuoles,

Table 12.3. Ultrastructure of pathogenic fungi

Organism	Reference
Aspergillus flavus	Merkow et al., *Am. J. Path.* 62:57, 1971
A. fumigatus	Campbell, *Sabouraudia* 8:133, 1970
A. niger	Tsukahara, *Sabouraudia* 8:93, 1970
Blastomyces dermatitidis	Garrison and Lane, *Mycopath. Mycol. Appl.* 52:93, 1974
	Collins and Edwards, *Sabouraudia* 7:237, 1970
Candida albicans	Belcher et al., *Lab. Invest.* 29:620, 1973
	Miller et al., *J. Bact.* 119:992, 1974
Chlorella sp.	
Cladosporium trichoides	
Coccidioides immitis	
Cryptococcus neoformans	Al-Doory, *Sabouraudia* 9:113, 1971
	Lurie et al., *Sabouraudia* 9:15, 1971
Dactylaria sp.	
Emmonsia crescens *E. parva*	
Geotrichum candidum	
Histoplasma capsulatum	Dumont and Robert, *Lab. Invest.* 23:278 1970
H. farciminosum	San-Blas and Carbonell, *J. Bact.* 119:602, 1974
H. duboisii	
Loboa loboi	Woodward et al., *Lab. Invest.* 27:606, 1972
Oidiodendron kalrai	Swenberg et al., *Lab. Invest.* 21:365, 1969
Paracoccidioides braziliensis	Carbonell and Rodriguez, *J. Bact.* 96:538, 1968
Penicillium sp.	
Prototheca sp. (algae)	
Rhinosporidium seeberi	Kannan-kuty and Teh, *Pathologica* 6:63, 1974
Rhodotorula sp.	
Sporothrix schenkii	Lurie and Still, *Sabouraudia* 7:64, 1969
Torulopsis glabrata	

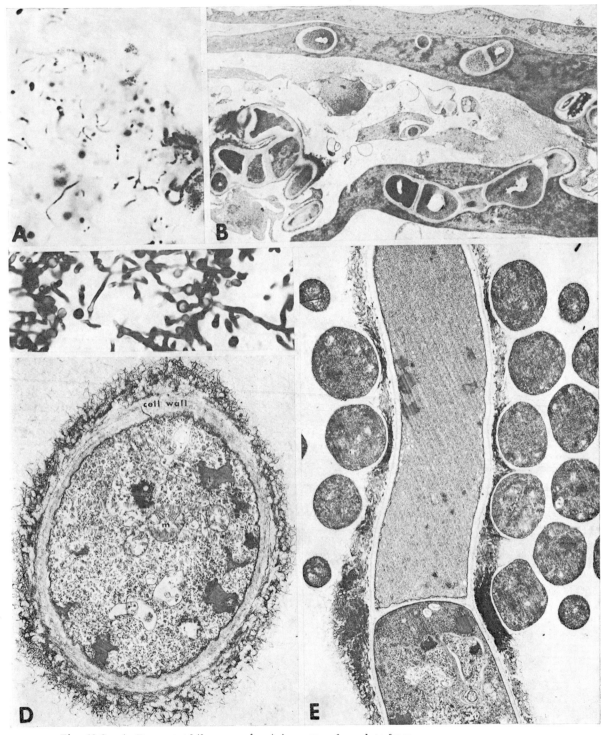

Fig. 12.8. A. *Dermatophilus congolensis* in smear of exudate from skin lesion, cow (Giemsa stain). B. Cross section of invading hyphae of *D. congolensis* in cornified keratinocytes of epidermis, horse. C. *Aspergillus fumigatus* in lung granuloma (methenamine silver stain). D. Spore of *A. fumigatus*. Note many ribosomes, lipid (1), mitochondria (m), and loose fibrillar structures peripheral to cell wall. E. Longitudinal and cross sections of hyphae in various stages of differentiation.

and mitochondria. A defined nucleus and nuclear membrane are present in all true fungi as distinct from bacterial cells (Fig. 12.9).

Histologically, the special stains used to identify cell walls include the periodic acid-Schiff stain and the silver methenamine reaction. These procedures can also be used in electron microscopy in cases where the cell walls are electron-lucent.

PATHOGENESIS OF FUNGAL INFECTION

Most fungi are omnipresent in the environment. Host resistance is therefore a dominant factor in disease. Opportunistic fungal infections result when animals are immunosuppressed, when their mechanisms of inflammation are inhibited, and when stress is placed upon their systems over long periods. Newborn and very old animals are most often affected by these factors.

Inhalation is the most significant factor in enabling fungal infections to become established. The size of the fungal cell inhaled is important. In the mammalian lung, nothing over $10\,\mu$m that penetrates the nose reaches the lungs while almost everything under $2\,\mu$m reaches the alveoli

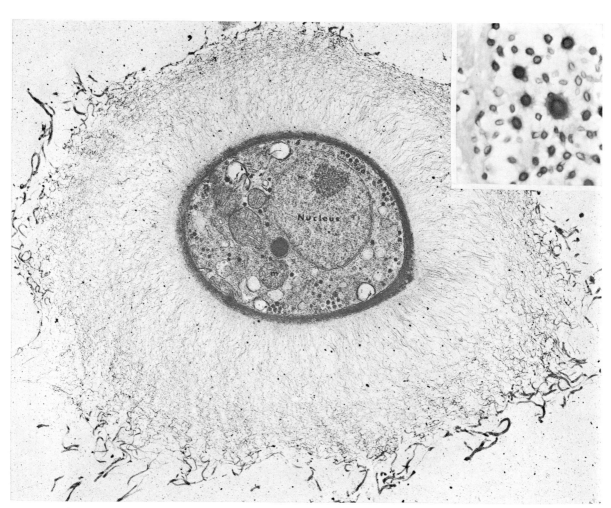

Fig. 12.9. Cryptococcus neoformans. Note nucleus, mitochondria (m), glycogen granules, dense granules. Cell wall is thin lamellar structure. Capsule contains thin dense lamina and very thick fibrillar layer. *Inset:* Histology of C. *neoformans* in brain tissue.

and is retained. The gastrointestinal tract, despite the ingestion of large numbers of spores, is seldom the site of primary fungal infection. One notable exception involves fungi associated with bovine mycotic placentitis and abortion in which the disease appears to follow ingestion of spores. The urogenital tract is rarely affected for fungi are swept away by mucous secretions. The bovine teat is an important orifice for infection and mycotic mastitis results from several species of fungi.

One distinctive pathogenetic feature of hyphal growth in tissue is the tendency to enter and grow within the lumens of blood vessels, usually inciting thrombosis. Dissemination may occur as with *Mortierella wolfii* as a cause of bovine mycotic placentitis. Hyphal fragments from the placenta enter the bloodstream at parturition and are carried to the lungs of the mother where they lodge and grow. The calf acquires infection from the umbilical vessels and may die of generalized infection.

Fungi cause three types of disease in animals: (1) *mycosis,* the direct invasion of tissue by fungal cells; (2) *allergic disease,* the development of hypersensitivity to fungal antigens; and (3) *mycotoxicosis,* the ingestion of toxic fungal metabolites. It is not unusual for mycosis and allergic disease to occur together, especially when infection of the lung is involved.

Hyphal pneumonia results from direct damage to lung parenchyma. When inhaled into the adult lung, spores are killed by phagocytosis and digestion in alveolar macrophages. Factors that suppress these processes allow germination in a percent of phagocytized spores sufficient to cause disease. During germination and growth, fungal metabolites are elaborated that act upon cell membranes and suppress the activity of alveolar macrophages. Experimentally, normal adult mice exposed to aerosols of *Aspergillus flavus* are resistant to lethal infection. In contrast, mice pretreated with corticosteroids and then exposed to spores develop over 90% fatal hyphal bronchopneumonia. Phagocytosis occurs normally in treated mice but the contact of lysosomes with spore-containing phagosomes is inhibited by the corticosteroid.

PROTOZOA

The phylum Protozoa is composed of one-celled animals. Some species exist in clusters, but, although colonized in organization, individual cells have no dependency on each other. Only a few of the thousands of protozoal species are pathogenic for animals. Most of these are associated with disease of the blood, reticuloendothelial system, or intestinal tract.

Four classes are considered under the phylum Protozoa: (1) Mastogophora, the flagellates; (2) Sarcodina, the amebas; (3) Sporozoa, which have complex sporelike stages (and are all parasitic); and (4) Ciliophora, the ciliates (Table 12.4).

Long, whiplike flagellae, which are used for locomotion, characterize the flagellates. All pathogenic forms require a bloodsucking insect vector as an intermediate host. During their life cycle, these protozoa display a variety of structural manifestations which are typical for the growth phase in a particular host and tissue. Four forms, based upon the type and position of the flagellum, are known: trypanosomal, crithidial, leptomonad, and leishmanial (Fig. 12.10). In general, the flagellated stages inhabit body fluids in vertebrates and the alimentary canal in insects. In the vertebrate hosts the leishmanial stages are found intracellularly.

Trypanosomiasis includes a group of animal diseases that are important in the tropical regions of the world. Most of these parasites occur in the blood as mature, elongate trypanosomes. The basic life cycle involves a vertebrate host (which at some stage manifests a parasitemia) and a bloodsucking invertebrate. When taken into the gut of the latter, the parasite undergoes transformation through one or more stages such as leishmanial, leptomonad, or crithidial forms which are not infective to the vertebrate host. The final, infective stage is the trypanosome stage.

Trypanosomes have a single nucleus and several distinctive organelles. The kinetoplast is a DNA-containing, self-duplicating cytoplasmic organelle located at the base of the flagellum adjacent to the tiny blepharoplast from which the flagellum arises. The kinetoplast divides by binary fission prior to nuclear division of the organism.

TABLE 12.4. Ultrastructure of Protozoa pathogenic for vertebrates

Class	Genus and Species	Reference
MASTIGOPHORA (flagellates)		
	Trypanosoma avium	Baker and Bird, *J. Prot.* 15:298, 1968 (canary blood)
	bouffardi	Molyneux and Robertson, *Ann. Trop. Med. Parasit.* 68:369, 1974
	brucei	Goodwin et al., *Parasitology* 67:115, 1973 (rabbit)
	congolense	Vickerman, *J. Prot.* 16:54, 1969 (mouse blood)
	conorhini	Milder and Deane, *J. Prot.* 15:65, 1967 (in vitro)
	cruzi	Deane and Milder, *J. Prot.* 20:586, 1973 (in vitro)
		Meyer and De Sousa, *J. Prot.* 20:590, 1973 (in vitro)
		Voigt et al., *Zt. Parasit.* 41:255, 1973 (mouse blood)
	lewisi	Anderson and Ellis, *J. Prot.* 12:483, 1965 (in vitro)
		Lee and Barnabas, *Zt. Parasit.* 44:93, 1974 (rat liver)
	raiae	Preston, *J. Prot.* 16:320, 1969 (in vitro)
	theileria	Moulton and Kraus, *Cornell Vet.* 62:124, 1972
	vivax	Vickerman, *J. Prot.* 20:394, 1973 (fly eye)
	Leishmania donovani	Dwyer et al., *Zt. Parasit.* 43:227, 1974 (hamster spleen)
		Rudzinska et al., *J. Prot.* 11:166, 1964 (hamster spleen)
	Histomonas meleagridis	Lee, *Parasitology* 59:877, 1969 (*Heterakis* sp. gut)
		Lee et al., *Parasitology* 59:171, 1969 (turkey liver)
	Trichomonas vaginalis	Brugerolle and Metenier, *J. Prot.* 20:320, 1973 (in vitro)
		Nielsen et al., *J. Microsc.* 5:229, 1973
	gallinae	Mattern et al., *J. Prot.* 14:320, 1967 (in vitro)
	gallinarum	Lee, *Parasitology* 65:71, 1972 (chicken cecum)
	Tritrichomonas foetus	Honigberg et al., *J. Prot.* 18:183, 1971 (in vitro)
		Muller, *J. Cell Biol.* 57:453, 1973 (in vitro)
	muris	Daniel et al., *J. Prot.* 18:575, 1971 (hamster feces)
	Hypotrichomonas acosta	Mattern et al., *J. Prot.* 16:668, 1969 (in vitro)
	Pentatrichomonas sp.	Honigberg et al., *J. Prot.* 15:419, 1968 (in vitro)
	Giardia muris	Bockman and Winborn, *J. Prot.* 15:26, 1968 (hamster gut)
	Hexamita	
	Lamblia duodenalsis	Cheissin, *J. Prot.* 11:91, 1964 (in vitro)
SARCODINA (*Amoebae*)		
	Entamoeba histolytica	Feria-Velasco and Trevino, *J. Prot.* 19:200, 1972 (hamster liver)
		Eaton et al., *Ann. Trop. Med. Parasit.* 64:299, 1970
		Lushbaugh and Miller, *J. Parasit.* 60:421, 1974 (guinea pig feces)
	Acanthamoeba sp.	Martinez et al., *J. Inf. Dis.* 131:692, 1975
	Hartmannella sp.	Ito et al., *J. Prot.* 16:638, 1969 (in vitro)
	Naegleria sp.	Schuster, *J. Prot.* 10:313, 1963 (in vitro)

Table 12.4. *(Continued)*

Class	Genus and Species	Reference
SPOROZOA COCCIDIA		
	Eimeria acervulina	Fernando, *Zt. Parasit.* 43:33, 1973 (chicken)
	aubumense	Hammond et al., *J. Prot.* 14:678, 1967 (cow)
	necatrix	Fernando, *Zt. Parasit.* 45:105, 1974 (chicken)
	maxima	Melhorn, *Zt. Parasit.* 40:243, 1972 (chicken)
		Sheffield and Hammond, *J. Parasit.* 53:831, 1967 (calf)
	magna	Speer et al., *J. Prot.* 20:274, 1973 (rabbit intestine)
		Danforth and Hammond, *J. Prot.* 19:454, 1972 (rabbit)
		Colley, *J. Prot.* 15:374, 1968 (rat)
	nieschulzi	Scholtyseck, *J. Prot.* 9:107, 1962 (rabbit)
	perforans	Scholtyseck and Melhorn, *Zt. Parasit.* 40:281, 1972 (mouse colon)
	falciformis	
	steziae	Scholtyseck and Piekarski, *Zt. Parasit.* 26:91, 1965 (mouse liver)
	Isospora felis	Pelster, *Zt. Parasit.* 41:29, 1973 (cat)
	canis	Roberts et al., *Zt. Parasit.* 40:183, 1972 (Sporozoites, dog feces)
		Schmidt et al., *J. Prot.* 14:602, 1967 (gecko)
	Klossiella helicina	Schulte, *Zt. Parasit.* 56:193, 1971 (snail kidney)
	Cryptosporidia agni	Barker and Carbonell, *Zt. Parasit.* 44:289, 1974 (lamb intestine)
	bovis	Meuten et al., *J.A.V.M.A.* 165:914, 1974 (calf)
	sp.	Kovatch & White, *Vet. Path.* 9:426, 1972 (monkey)
		Proctor and Kemp, *J. Prot.* 21:664, 1974 (goose)
	wrairi	Vetterling et al., *J. Prot.* 18:248, 1971 (guinea pig)
	Lankesterella sp.	Heller, *Acta Vet. Acad. Sci. Hung.* 24:151, 1974 (fish)
	cuicis	Sanders and Poinar, *J. Prot.* 20:594, 1973 (mosquito larvae)
	hylae	Sheffield et al., *J. Prot.* 18:98, 1971 (mosquito)
	garnicami	Steihens, *J. Prot.* 13:63, 1966 (frog)
		Garnham et al., *J. Prot.* 9:107, 1962 (sparrow spleen cells)
	Toxoplasma gondii	Ferguson et al., *Acta Path. Microbiol. Scand.* B 82:167, 1974
		Sheffield and Melton, *J. Parasit.* 54:209, 1968 (in vitro)
		Zaman and Colley, *Trans. Roy. Soc. Trop. Med.* 66:781, 1972
		Gavin et al., *J. Prot.* 9:222, 1962 (mouse peritoneal exudate)
		Pelster and Piekarski, *Zt. Parasit.* 37:267, 1971 (cat intestine)
		Van Der Zypan, *Zt. Parasit.* 28:31, 1966 (mouse brain cyst)
	Sarcocystis fusiformis	Melhorn et al., *Zentr. Bakt. Hyg. A* 231:301, 1975
	sp.	Vetterling et al., *J. Prot.* 20:613, 1973 (grackle muscle)
	tenella	Melhorn and Scholtyseck, *Zt. Parasit.* 45:227, 1975 (sheep esophagus)
		Melhorn and Scholtyseck, *Zt. Parasit.* 43:251, 1974 (cat intestinal wall)
	Frenkelia sp.	Scholtyseck et al., *Zt. Parasit.* 42:185, 1973 (mouse brain)
	Hepatozoon muris	
	Haemogregarina sp.	Desser and Weller, *J. Prot.* 20:65, 1973 (frog)

Table 12.4. (Continued)

Class	Genus and Species	Reference
HAEMOSPORIDIA	Plasmodium berghei	Seed et al., J. Prot. 20:603, 1973 (intraerythrocytic rat)
		Ladda et al., J. Parasit. 55:633, 1969 (mouse blood)
	chabaudi	Kelly and Silverman, J. Prot. 16:354, 1969 (mouse erythrocyte)
		Scalzi and Bahr, J. Ult. Res. 24:116, 1968 (mouse blood)
	coatneyi	Rudzinska and Trager, J. Prot. 15:73, 1968 (monkey erythrocyte)
	cynomolgi	Terzkis, J. Prot. 18:62, 1971 (mosquito)
	gallinarum	Ristic and Krier, J. Trop. Med. Hyg. 67:509, 1964
	falciparum	Miller, Trans. Roy. Soc. Trop. Med. 66:459, 1972
	lophurae	Beaudoin and Stone, Exp. Parasit. 34:313, 1973 (in vitro)
		Bodammer and Bahr, Lab. Invest. 28:708, 1973 (mouse blood)
	tropiduri	Scorza, Parasitology 63:1, 1971 (lizard blood)
		Sterling and Aikawa, J. Prot. 20:81, 1973 (bird blood, gametocyte)
	sp.	Langreth and Trager, J. Prot. 20:606, 1973 (in vitro)
	sp.	Aikawa, Exp. Parasit. 30:284, 1971 (review)
	Leucocytozoon	Aikawa et al., J. Ult. Res. 32:43, 1970
		Trefiak and Desser, J. Prot. 20:73, 1973 (bird blood)
	Hemoproteus columbae	Bradbury and Trager, J. Prot. 15:700, 1968 (microgam.)
		Bradbury and Gallucci, J. Prot. 19:43, 1972 (schizonts, pigeon blood)
		Bradbury and Gallucci, J. Prot. 18:679, 1971 (merozoites)
		Klei, J. Prot. 19:281, 1972 (sporozoites) (insect salivary gland)
	metchnikovi	Sterling, J. Prot. 19:69, 1972 (turtle)
		Sterling and Degiusti, J. Parasit. 58:641, 1972 (turtle spleen)
PIROPLASMIDA	Babesia ovis	Friedhoff et al., Zt. Parasit. 38:132, 1972 (tick salivary gland)
		Friedhoff and Scholtyseck, Zt. Parasit. 30:347, 1968 (sheep tick)
		Simpson, Am. J. Vet. Res. 31:1763, 1971; 35:701, 1974
	rodhaini	Rudzinska and Trager, J. Prot. 9:279, 1962 (mouse rbc)
	Theileria parva	Jarrett and Brocklesby, J. Prot. 13:301, 1966 (cow lymph node)
		Moulton et al., Lab. Invest. 24:187, 1971
	Nuttallia	MacMillan and Brocklesby, Res. Vet. Sci. 12:185, 1971
CILIOPHORA	Paramecium sp.	McKanna, J. Prot. 20:631, 1973 (in vitro)
	Balantidium sp.	
Unclassified	Pneumocystis carini	Barton and Campbell, Arch. Path. 83:527, 1967 (human lung)
		Shively et al., Cornell Vet. 64:72, 1974 (horse lung)
		Vavra and Kucera, J. Prot. 17:463, 1970 (rat lung)
	Encephalitizoon	Sprague and Vernick, J. Prot. 18:560, 1971 (mouse ascitic fluid)
		Brown et al., J. Med. Primatol. 2:114, 1973 (monkey)
	Besnoitia sp.	Sheffield, J. Parasit. 52:583, 1966 (mouse ascitic fluid)
	jellisoni	Sénaud et al., Parasitology 40:165, 1972 (mouse viscera)
	Myxosporidium sp.	Spall, J. Parasit. 60:169, 1974 (fish gill)

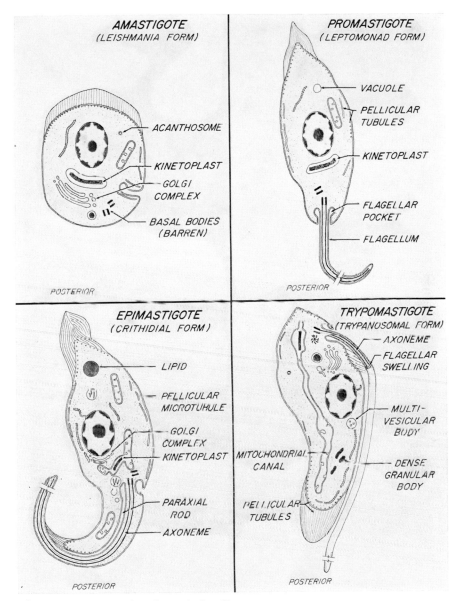

Fig. 12.10. Forms of pathogenic flagellates.

Trypanosomes localize in the brain, myocardium, subcutis, lymphoid organs, and mesenchymal tissues of other organs. At these sites, they replicate extracellularly. The basic tissue reaction involves reticuloendothelial hyperplasia and the perivascular infiltration of monocytes, lymphocytes, and granulocytes. Plasmacytes are prominent in chronic trypanosomiasis. Interstitial myocarditis and meningitis are the most striking lesions. In addition to parenchymal cell necrosis, these lesions contain large numbers of organisms, necrotizing vasculitis, and thrombosis. The release of toxins is the basis of tissue injury.

Amebae commonly infect the intestine of animals but are rarely implicated (and less often responsible) in disease processes. Parasites replicate in the intestinal lumen and live on digested food, erythrocytes, and other microorganisms. They are amorphous, large (15–50μ) cells which move by the sudden extension of pseudopodia.

Ultrastructural studies have been limited to pathogenic amebae cultivated in vitro. Trophozoites from these cultures are large, amorphous bodies. The cytoplasm is bound by a plasma membrane and contains ribosomes, food vacuoles, lysosomes, lipids, and tubular bodies of unknown origin. Neither mitochondria nor Golgi complexes have been reported. Amebae appear to kill cells in culture by a lysosomal mechanism. Cell death can occur within a few minutes of contact and dead cells can be partially phagocytized by the ameba. Ultrastructurally, a group of lysosomes has been described at the surface of *E. histolytica,* each with a vermiform protrusion which is alleged to be a triggering mechanism. It is proposed that in pathogenic amebae these organelles have become adapted to function at the surface of intestinal epithelial cells enhancing attachment and penetration.

All members of the class Sporozoa are parasitic. They produce spores, as indicated by the name, that contain one to several sporozoites. In species whose life cycle is completed in one host, the spore membrane is thick and resistant and protects the sporozoites while they are outside the host. The spore membrane is always thin and fragile in species that require two hosts. The organism is protected in an invertebrate host where replication is required for it to infect the primary vertebrate host.

In general, the three stages in the sporozoan life cycle are: (1) *schizogony* of sporozoites to produce many merozoites; (2) *gametogony,* or sexual reproduction; and (3) *sporogony,* in which the zygote divides to form multiple sporozoites. Sporogony may take place within delicate oocysts in the body of invertebrates or take place outside the body of the host in protective oocysts. In either case, the sporozoites are infective when swallowed by or injected into the appropriate host.

REFERENCES

Aikawa, M. The fine structure of malarial parasites. *Exp. Parasit.* 30:284, 1971.

Baron, S. The defensive role of the interferon system. *J. Gen. Physiol.* 56:193, 1970.

Benacerraf, B., Sabestyen, M. M. and Schlossman, S. S. A quantitative study of the kinetics of blood clearance of P^{32}-labeled *E. coli* and *Staphylococci* by the reticuloendothelial system. *J. Exp. Med.* 124:585, 1966.

Bennett, I. L. and Nicastri, A. Fever as a mechanism of resistance. *Bact. Rev.* 24:16, 1960.

Bladen, H. A., Evans, R. T. and Mergenhagen, S. E. Lesions in *Escherichia coli* membranes after action of antibody and complement. *J. Bact.* 91:2377, 1966.

Blanden, R. V. Mechanisms of recovery from a generalized viral infection: Mousepox. III. Regression of infectious foci. *J. Exp. Med.* 133:1090, 1971.

Blanden, R. V., Mackaness, G. B. and Collins, F. M. Mechanisms of acquired resistance in mouse typhoid. *J. Exp. Med.* 124:585, 1966.

Carmichael, L. E., Barnes, F. D. and Percy, D. H. Temperature as a factor in resistance of young puppies to canine herpesvirus. *J. Inf. Dis.* 120:669, 1969.

Cheville, N. F. Cytopathology in viral disease. *Monogr. Virol.* 10:1–224, 1975.

Cole, G. A. and Wisseman, C. L., Jr. The effect of hyperthermia on dengue virus infection of mice. *Proc. Soc. Exp. Biol. Med.* 130:359, 1969.

Darekar, M. R. and Eyer, H. The role of fimbriae in the process of infection. *Zt. Bakt.* 225:130, 1973.

Hapel, A. and Gardner, I. Appearance of cytotoxic T cells in cerebrospinal fluid of mice with ectromelia virus-induced meningitis. *Scand. J. Immun.* 3:311, 1974.

Hirsch, M. S., Zisman, B. and Allison, A. C. Macrophages and age-dependent resistance to herpes simplex virus in mice. *J. Immun.* 104:1160, 1970.

Landy, M., Sanderson, R. P. and Jackson, A. L. Humoral and cellular aspects of the immune response to the somatic antigen of *Salmonella enteritidis. J. Exp. Med.* 122: 483, 1965.

Lorian, V. The mode of action of antibiotics on gram-negative bacilli. *Arch. Int. Med.* 128:623, 1971.

Mackaness, G. B. The immunological basis of acquired cellular resistance. *J. Exp. Med.* 120:105, 1964.

McGregor, D. D., Koster, F. T. and Mackaness, G. B. The mediator of cellular immunity. *J. Exp. Med.* 133:389, 1971.

Mouton, D. et al. Phagocytosis of Salmonellae by reticuloendothelial cells of new-born piglets lacking natural antibody. *Nature* 197:706, 1963.

Nathanson, N. and Cole, G. A. Immunosuppression: A means to assess the role of the immune response in acute viral infection. *Fed. Proc.* 30:1822, 1971.

Suter, E. and Ramseier, H. Cellular reactions in infection. *Adv. Immun.* 4:117, 1964.

Svehag, S.-E. Formation and dissociation of virus-antibody complexes with special reference to the neutralization process. *Progr. Med. Virol.* 10:1, 1968.

van Iterson, W. Symposium of the fine structure and replication of bacteria and their parts. *Bact. Rev.* 29:299, 1965.

Wood, W. B. Phagocytosis with particular reference to encapsulated bacteria. *Bact. Rev.* 24:41, 1960.

APPENDIX ONE

Glossary of Cytologic Terms in Ultrastructure

Acanthosome. Small membrane-bound vesicle containing characteristic surface projections. Allegedly transports soluble protein. Originates in Golgi complex; moves to and fuses with plasma membrane.

Ameboid movement. Movement by pseudopod formation with streaming of the cytoplasm into the pseudopod.

Apoptosis. Condensation of nucleus and cytoplasm with budding of small membrane-bound cell fragments which are phagocytized and digested by adjacent cells.

Autectomy. Shedding of portions of damaged cytoplasm by blebing with pinching off of bleb from cell surface (see ecdysis).

Autolysosome. Autophagosome.

Autophagic vacuole. Autophagosome.

Autophagosome. A secondary lysosome containing cellular organelles and other debris.

Autophagy. Accumulation of degenerate organelles, inclusions, and other cell substances in lysosomes for the purpose of enzymic degradation. *Syn:* autophagocytosis.

Basal body. Centriolelike structure bearing a flagellum or cilium. *Syn:* kinetosome, blepharoplast.

Basal lamina. Limiting lamina of collagenlike protein and carbohydrate that lies below certain epithelial and endothelial cells. *Syn:* external lamina, basement membrane.

Basement membrane. 1. The granular substance of collagenlike protein and carbohydrate that makes up the basal lamina. *Syn:* basement membrane material. 2. *Syn:* Basal lamina (ultrastructure). 3. *Histol:* The membrane at the basal aspect of epithelium which is composed of the basal lamina and thicker, electron-lucent, periodic acid-Schiff staining substance.

Caveoli. Pinocytotic vesicles that are fused with the plasma membrane and open to the extracellular space. *Syn:* Plasmalemmal vesicles.

Chondriospheres. Giant mitochondria. *Syn:* megamitochondria.

Cytopempsis. Exocytosis.

Cytoplasmic matrix. Soluble, nonparticulate milieu that fills the cytoplasmic areas of cells. Transparent and structureless on microscopic examination.

Cytosegresome. Autophagosome.

Cytosol. Cytoplasmic matrix.

Cytosome. The body of the cell excluding the nucleus.

Dictysome. Stacks of Golgi lamellae containing open cisternae. Dictysomes are polar—one side associated with the nuclear membrane; the other with endoplasmic reticulum.

Diplosome. Pair of centrioles.

Ecdysis. Blebing of portions of cytoplasm from the cell surface within membrane-bound vesicles.

Emiocytosis. Exocytosis.

Empiripolesis. Entrance and residence of one cell within another, e.g., the presence of small lymphocytes within larger target cells during immunologic reactions.

Endocytic vacuole. Phagosome.

Endocytosis. Entrance of material into the cell by invagination of the plasma membrane, fusion of indentation margins, and separation of the membrane-bound material to form a phagosome or pinocytotic vesicle free within the cytoplasmic matrix (see phagocytosis, pinocytosis).

Esotrophy. Invagination of a membrane into the cytoplasmic matrix (turning in of a membrane).

Exocytosis. Mechanism of exit of vesicles and secretory granules from the cytoplasm. Includes movement to the plasma membrane, fusion of membrane of the vesicle with the plasma membrane, and exit of contents of the vacuole from the cell. *Syn:* emiocytosis, reverse pinocytosis.

Exotropy. Protrusion of a membrane into a space (turning out of a membrane).

Filopodium. Slender filamentous pseudopodium (L. filum = thread + foot).

Glycocalyx. Broad designation for all polysaccharide-containing structures on the external surface of cells. Includes glycolipids and glycoproteins.

Hyaloplasm. Cytoplasmic matrix.

Internalization. Cell uptake of external material by invagination of a portion of the plasma membrane or by fusion of vacuoles with emptying into the cell cytoplasm.

Kinetosome. Basal body.

Langerhans' cell granules. Cytoplasmic rod-shaped granules with dense outer limiting membrane and dense central linear structure with periodicity.

Lectins. Plant proteins that bind to specific carbohydrate residues on the cell surface.

Ligand. Substance that binds specifically to the outer aspect of the plasma membrane.

Ligand capping. Movement of surface ligands into a single large aggregate.

Liposome. Small lipid globule within the endoplasmic reticulum of lipid metabolizing cells composed of triglycerides and various amounts of lipoproteins.

Lysosome. Single membrane-bound granule containing hydrolytic enzymes produced by th Golgi complex and fusing with phagosomes to initiate the process of intracellular digestion. Primary lysosomes are small dense granules that have not interacted with other organelles; enzymes are inactive.

Microbody. Old term for peroxisome, especially as it occurs in liver. Acid phosphatase negative. Homogeneous granular matrix surrounded by 6–7 nm membrane. Generally 0.2–1μ in diameter.

Microfilaments. Slender, threadlike filaments which function in cell movement.

Microtubules. Cylindrical tubules (18–30 nm diameter) associated with cell movement. Present in dividing cells as the spindle apparatus. Also part of normal cilia, spermatozoa, and nerve cells.

Multivesicular body. Large $(0.2–1\mu)$ membrane-bound cytoplasmic body containing several small (about 10 nm diameter) vesicles.

Myelin figure. Myeloid body.

Myeloid body. Abnormal dense laminar lipoprotein membranes which form as a response to cell injury; usually occur in residual bodies. Development into whorls allegedly resembles the process of myelin formation.

Nucleoplasm. Soluble matrix material of the nucleus. *Syn:* karyoplasm.

Peroxisome. Small $(0.2–1\mu)$, dense, membrane- bound granules containing peroxidase and other enzymes. Acid phosphatase negative. Occur in liver and other organs and are associated with intracellular digestion. *Syn:* microbody.

Phagocytosis. 1. Uptake of material by endocytosis. *Syn:* endocytosis. 2. *Restrictive:* uptake of solid material by endocytosis.

Phagolysosome. Digestive vacuole formed by fusion of a primary lysosome with a phagosome in which enzymatic degradation of ingested material takes place. A secondary lysosome.

Phagosome. A vacuole formed during the process of endocytosis in which material resides following its entrance into the cell. Acid phosphatase negative.

Pinocytosis. Uptake of soluble material by the cell by endocytosis.

Pinocytotic vesicle. Vesicle formed during pinocytosis which functions to transport soluble material within the cell.

Plasmalemma. Plasma membrane.

Plasmalemmal vesicles. Regularly spaced invaginations that form vesicles on the plasmalemma of certain endothelial and other cells. Also called pinocytotic vesicles.

Plasma membrane. Membrane surrounding the cells which maintains cell shape. *Syn:* cell membrane, plasmalemma.

Polyribosome. Chain of single ribosomes connected by a strand of mRNA.

Polysome. Polyribosome.

Potocytosis. Cortical edema of the cell. *Syn:* blistering.

Protolysosome. Golgi vesicles.

Residual body. Large secondary lysosome containing dense granular debris.

Secondary lysosome. Broad category including all lysosomes formed by the interaction of primary lysosomes and other vesicles; includes autophagosomes, cytolysosomes, phagolysosomes, and residual bodies.

Sphaeroplast. Acanthosome.

Telolysosome. Dense body or primary lysosome.

Uropod. A large blunt pseudopod.

Zeiosis. Projection of knobby protuberances on the cell surface due to herniation of cytoplasm through defects in the cortical microtubular net. *Syn:* blebing.

Anatomical Terminology of Inflammation

Bile duct	cholangiitis
Bladder	cystitis
Blood vessel	vasculitis
Bone	osteitis
Bone marrow	osteomyelitis
Brain	encephalitis
Bursa	bursitis
Cecum	typhilitis
Connective tissue	cellulitis
Cornea	keratitis
Dura mater	pachymeningitis
Ear	otitis
Eye	ophthalmitis
Eyelid	blepharitis
Fascia	fasciitis
Fat	steatitis
Gall bladder	cholecystitis
Gill (branchia)	branchiitis
Glans penis	balanitis
Heart	carditis
Intestine	enteritis
Iris	iritis
Kidney	nephritis
Knee	gonitis
Ligament	desmitis
Lip	cheilitis
Liver	hepatitis
Lung	pneumonitis
Lymph vessel	lymphangiitis

Meninges	meningitis
Mouth	stomatitis
Muscle (skeletal)	myositis
Myocardium	myocarditis
Nerve	neuritis
Ovary	oophoritis
Oviduct	salpingitis
Pancreas	pancreatitis
Pericardium	pericarditis
Peritoneum	peritonitis
Pleura	pleuritis
Prepuce	posthitis
Renal glomerulus	glomerulitis
Renal pelvis	pyelitis
Sinus	sinusitis
Skin	dermatitis
Spinal nerve root	radiculitis
Spleen	splenitis
Stomach	gastritis
Testicle	orchitis
Tongue	glossitis
Trachea	tracheitis
Tympanum	tympanitis
Uterus	metritis
Vagina	vaginitis
Vas deferens	vasitis
Vein	phlebitis
Vertebra	spondylitis
Vessel	vasculitis

Ultrastructural Pathology in Models of Hepatotoxicity

TOXIN	ANIMAL	REFERENCE
Acetylsalicylic acid	Rat	Hruban et al. *Lab. Invest.* 30:64, 1974
Aflatoxin	Rat	Bernhard et al. *Compt. Rend.* 261:1785, 1965
	Duck	Theron, *Lab. Invest.* 14:1586, 1966
	Monkey	Lin et al. *Lab. Invest.* 30:267, 1974
Alcohol (ethanol)	Rat	Iseri et al. *Am. J. Path.* 48:535, 1966
		Rubin et al. *Lab. Invest.* 23:620, 1970
Amantin (mushroom)	Mouse	Derenzini et al. *Lab. Invest.* 29:150, 1973
Aminoacetonitrile	Rat	Hadjiolov et al. *J. Nat. Cancer Inst.* 50:979, 1973
Beryllium	Rat	Goldblatt et al. *Arch. Env. Hlth.* 26:48, 1973
Bis-1-10-decase	Rat	Feldman, *Path. Biol.* 22:179, 1974
Carbon tetrachloride	Mouse	Leduc, *Lab. Invest.* 29:186, 1973
Chlorobiphenyl	Monkey	Nishizumi, *Arch. Env. Hlth.* 21:620, 1970
	Comp.	Vos, *Env. Hlth. Persp.* 1:105, 1972
Clindamycin	Comp.	Gray et al. *Toxic. Appl. Pharm.* 21:516, 1972
Copper	Rat	Barka et al. *Arch. Path.* 78:331, 1974
Corticosteroid	Mouse	Kodama and Rodama, *Cancer Res.* 32:208, 1972
Diazofluoranthen	Rat	Thys et al. *Lab. Invest.* 28:70, 1973
Dieldrin	Rat	Hutterer et al. *Lab. Invest.* 20:455, 1969
Diethylnitrosamine	Rat	Bruni, *J. Nat. Cancer Inst.* 50:1513, 1973
Dimethylnitrosamine	Rat	Emmelot and Benedetti, *J. Cell Biol.* 7:393, 1960
Endotoxin	Dog	Boler and Bibighaus, *Lab. Invest.* 17:537, 1967
Ethionine	Rat	Goldblatt et al. *Lab. Invest.* 28:206, 1973
		Steiner et al. *Am. J. Path.* 44:169, 1964
Ferrous sulfate	Rat	Ganote and Nahara, *Lab. Invest.* 28:426, 1973
Galactosamine	Rat	Koff, *Exp. Mol. Path.* 19:168, 1973
Halothane	Rat	Ross and Cardell, *Am. J. Anat.* 135:5, 1972

TOXIN	ANIMAL	REFERENCE
Hydrazine	Rat	Amenta and Johnston, *Lab. Invest.* 11:956, 1962
Iodoform	Rat	Sell and Reynolds, *J. Cell Biol.* 41:736, 1969
Kepone	Quail	Atwal, *J. Comp. Path.* 83:115, 1973
Lantana	Sheep	Seawright, *Vet. Path.* 2:175, 1965
Lead	Rat	Hoffman et al. *Exp. Mol. Path.* 17:159, 1972
	Pig	Watrach, *J. Ult. Res.* 10:177, 1964
Mercury	Rat	Oudea, *Lab. Invest.* 12:386, 1963
Mirex (insecticide)	Rat	Gaines and Kimbrough, *Arch. Env. Hlth.* 21:7, 1970
Ngaione (plant)	Mouse	Seawright and O'Donahoo, *J. Path.* 106:251, 1972
Nickel carbonyl	Rat	Hackett and Sunderman, *Arch. Env. Hlth.* 19: 337, 1969
Penicillin	Man	Goldstein and Ishak, *Arch. Path.* 98:114, 1974
Phalloidin	Rat	Weiss et al. *Beitr. Path.* 150:82, 1973
Phenobarbitol	Rat	Herdson et al. *Lab. Invest.* 13:1032, 1963
Phosphorus	Rat	Barker et al. *Lab. Invest.* 12:955, 1963
Pregnenolone-carbonitrile	Rat	Tuchweber et al. *J. Ult. Res.* 39:456, 1972
		Garg et al. *Acta Anat.* 85:190, 1973
Pyrrolizidine alkaloid	Monkey	Van der Watt et al. *J. Path.* 107:279, 1972
	Rat	Afzelius and Schoental, *J. Ult. Res.* 20:328, 1966
		Svoboda and Soga, *Am. J. Path.* 48:347, 1966
Orotic acid	Rat	Jatlow et al. *Am. J. Path.* 47:125, 1965
Tannic acid	Rabbit	Arhelger et al. *Am. J. Path.* 46:409, 1965
	Rat	Reddy et al. *Cancer Res.* 30:58, 1970
	Chicken	Konstantinov and Ivanov, *Ab. Vetmed. A* 20: 426, 1973
Thioacetamine	Rat	Barker and Smuckler, *Am. J. Path.* 74:575, 1974
		Thoenes and Bannasch, *Virch. Arch.* 335:556, 1962
Thiohydantoin	Rat	Herdson and Kaltenbach, *J. Cell Biol.* 25:485, 1963
		Elfont et al. *Proc. Soc. Exp. Biol. Med.* 141:184, 1972
Trichlorethane	Rat	Ortega, *Lab. Invest.* 15:657, 1966
Viridicatin (mycotoxin)	Rat	Rafiquzzamen, *Acta Vet. Scand. Suppl.* 47:1, 1974
Vitamin A	Man	Hruben et al. *Am. J. Path.* 76:451, 1974

INDEX

Abscess, 155
  in brain, 157
  in lung, 339
Acanthoma, 303
Acanthosome, 501
Acid-base balance, 11
  in uremia, 375
Acidosis, 11
  in cardiac ischemia, 446
  in diarrhea, 403–4
  metabolic, 362, 375
  in nephron, 362
  in uremia, 375–76
ACTH, 408–12
Actinobacillus, 483, 485
Actinomycin
  nucleolar damage and, 35
Actomyosin, 175
Adenocarcinoma, 261
  of mammary gland, 305–7
  of nasal cavity, 312
  of thyroid, 311
Adenovirus, 476
  in nucleolus, 36
  in nucleus, 33–35
Adenyl cyclase, 29–30
Adipocyte, 55
ADP, 128
  in platelet aggregation, 107
Adrenal cortex, 408–13
  and electrolytes, 412
  and infection, 412–13
  in pyometra, 364
  and stress, 412
Adrenal medulla, 413–15
Adrenocorticosteroids, 409–13
  and adrenal structure, 411, 415
  and eosinophils, 167
  and erythrocytes, 114
  in fungal infection, 493
  in glomerulonephritis, 364
  in immunosuppression, 228
  in inflammation, 161
  in milk fever, 428
  in neoplasia, 281
  in septicemia, 413
Aerocystitis, 346
Aflatoxin, 60–62, 504
  and liver carcinoma, 285
  site of action, 62
  types, 62
Aging, 12–13
  in alveolar wall, 340
  in cell culture, 13

in erythrocytes, 118
in fish, 13
and wound healing, 177–80
Air sac, 350
Albinism, 69
Albumin, 90
  dye-complexes, 148
  in inflammation, 150
  in kidney, 375
  in plasma, 90
  in urine, 359
Alcohol toxicity, 61, 504
Aldosterone, 409
  and angiotensin, 361, 412
  and nephron, 362
Aleutian disease, 478
  and glomerulopathy, 366
Alkalosis, 11
Allergy, 229
  atopic, 232
  and pneumonitis, 234
Alpha-fetoprotein, 310
Alveolar wall, 325–30
  aging, 340
  in chronic injury, 340
  fibrosis, 133
Alveoli, 332
  and fungi, 493
Alveolitis, 331
  allergic, 298, 333
Ammonia, 375
Amoeba, 494
Amphotericin
  toxicity, 360, 371
Amyloid, 247–52
  in diabetes mellitus, 248
  in renal glomerulus, 250
Amyloidosis, 247–52
  and kidney, 247–48, 250, 366
Anaphylaxis, 230–32
  adrenal cortex in, 410
  in fibrin, 86
  in shock, 231
Anaplasia, 266, 269
Anaplasmosis, 124
Anasarca, 92
Anemia, 120–30
  autoimmune, 233
    in anaplasmosis, 124
    erythrocytes in, 115
  in heart disease, 450
  hemolytic, 121
  hereditary, 127
  immunologic, 233

iron-deficiency, 129–30
and liver, 18
in sickle cells, 128
in uremia, 376
Angiogenesis factor, 273
Angiotensin, 87
  in artery, 451
Anisocytosis, 111
Annulate lamellae, 41
  in cell, 43, 272
Anoxia, 10
  and heart, 444
  and nephrosis, 373
Anthrax bacilli, 176, 486
Antibiotics
  and bacterial lysis, 489
Antibodies, 201–6
  and bacteria, 486–87
  classes, 201–3
  in colostrum, 202, 212
  cytophilic, 203
  in eye, 203
  in fetus, 211
  in immunity, 200
  in inflammation, 150
  in intestine, 212–13
  in neoplasms, 280
  in newborn, 212
  precipitating, 203
  and viral infection, 481–82
Antidiuretic hormone, 134
  action on nephron, 361–62
  in pituitary, 134–35
  in shock, 96
Antigen, 199–200
  of bacteria, 484
  in neoplasms, 280
Antimycin, 27
Aortic body, 87
Aplasia, 9
  of thymus, 216, 227
Apoptosis, 9, 500
Argentaffin cell. See Enterochromaffin
Arteriopathy, 453
Arteriosclerosis, 454–57
Arteritis, 451–53
Artery, 450–59
  immune injury, 233, 451–53
  neurologic control, 83
Arthus reaction, 233–34
Ascites, 92
Asparagine, 271